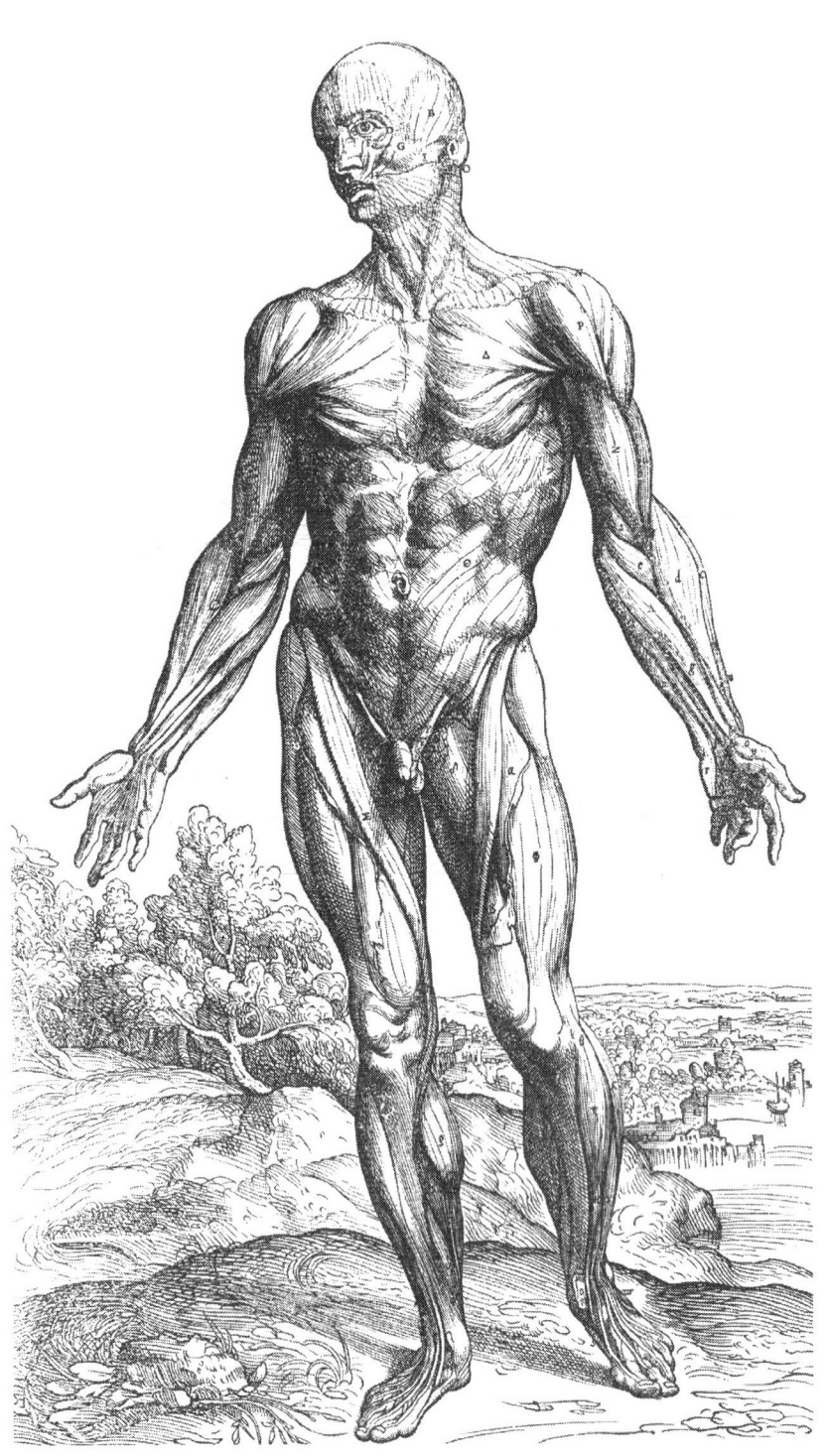

Zen of Dumbbell Training

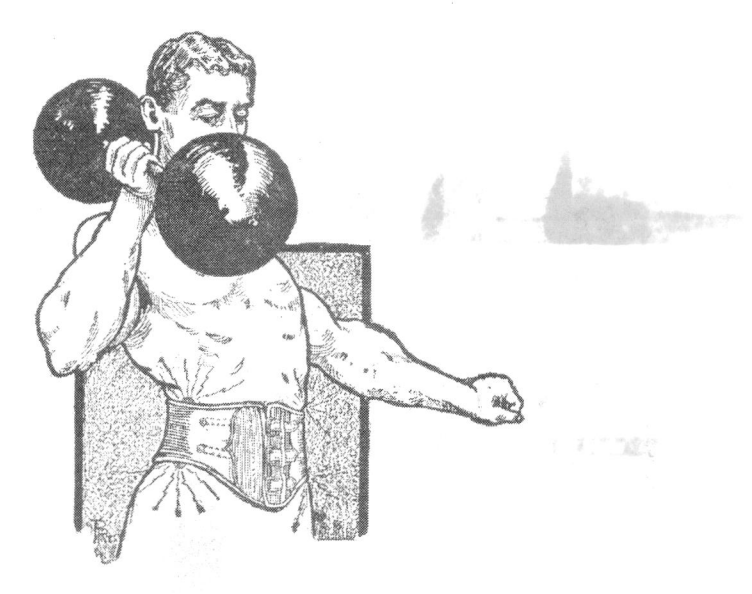

How to

use a Dumbbell for

Health, Strength, Figure and Therapy

ALAN STUART RADLEY Ph.D.

Dedicated

to

Philip, Ellen, Nigel and Caroline Radley

Copyright (©) Alan Stuart Radley 2013
Published and distributed by Alan Radley
Printed and bound by Radley Press, Blackpool, UK.
www.alanradley.com

All rights are reserved. No part of this publication may be reproduced or utilised in any form or by any means, electronic or mechanical, including photocopying, recording, or by any internal storage and retrieval system, without the express permission of the author(s).

Zen of Dumbbell Training
ISBN 978-0-9539945-9-5 (paper - Black and White)
First Edition [Version 1.8.0]
Third Printing, November 2013.
~ 1200 illustrations

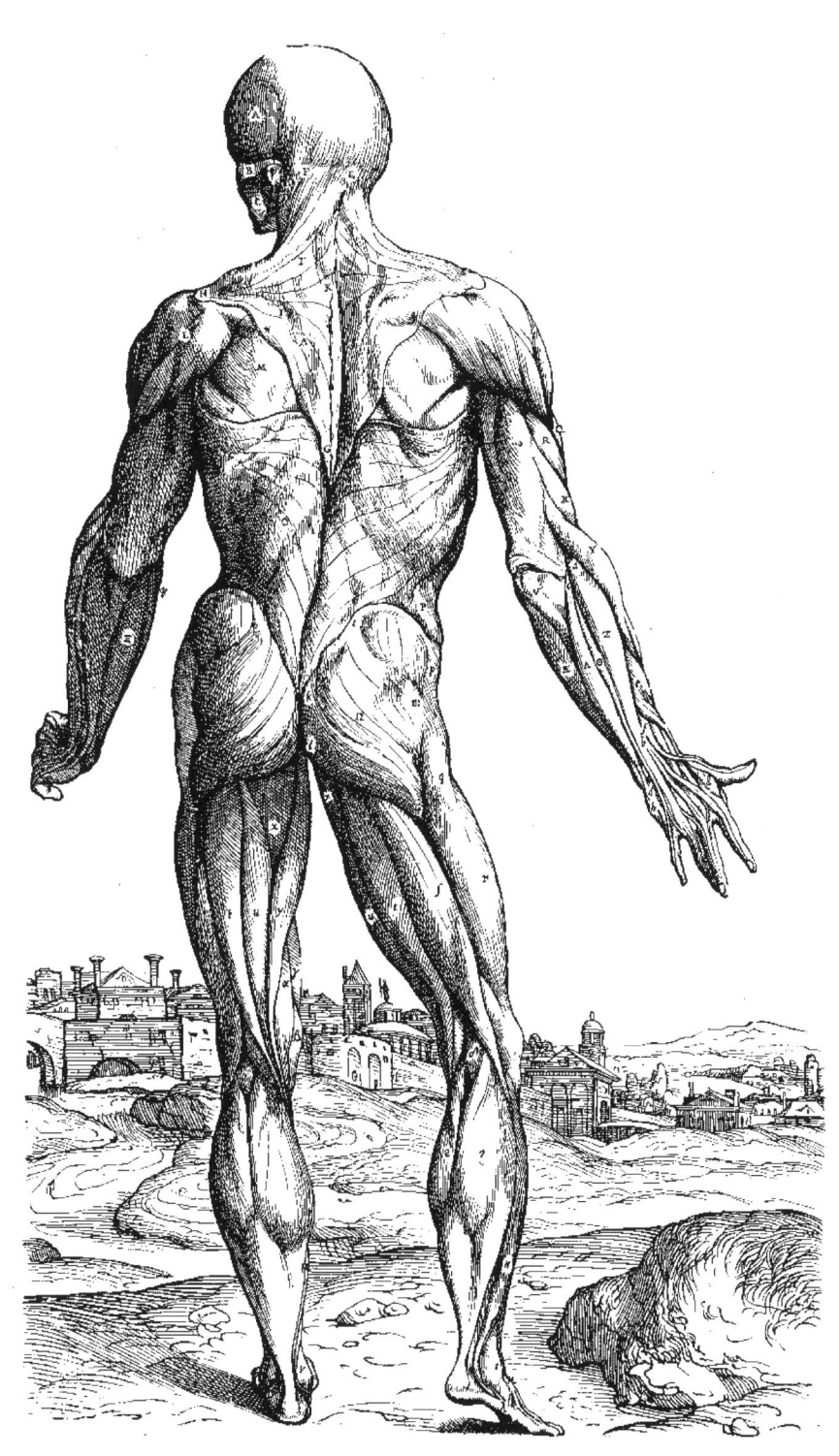

Contents

Synopsis
Acknowledgements
Preface

1. Introduction
2. Theories
3. Fitness
4. Training Systems
5. Zen Training
6. Movement Anatomy
7. The Trunk
8. The Shoulder
9. The Elbow
10. The Wrist and Hand
11. The Hip and Knee
12. The Ankle and Foot
13. Gravity
14. Techniques
15. Training for Health
16. Training for Strength
17. Training for Figure
18. Training for Therapy
19. Conclusions
20. Bibliography
21. Anatomy Charts
22. Glossary
23. Dangers of Machines
24. Exercises to Avoid
25. Exercise Charts
26. Natural Movement Patterns
27. Mechanics of Dumbbell Training

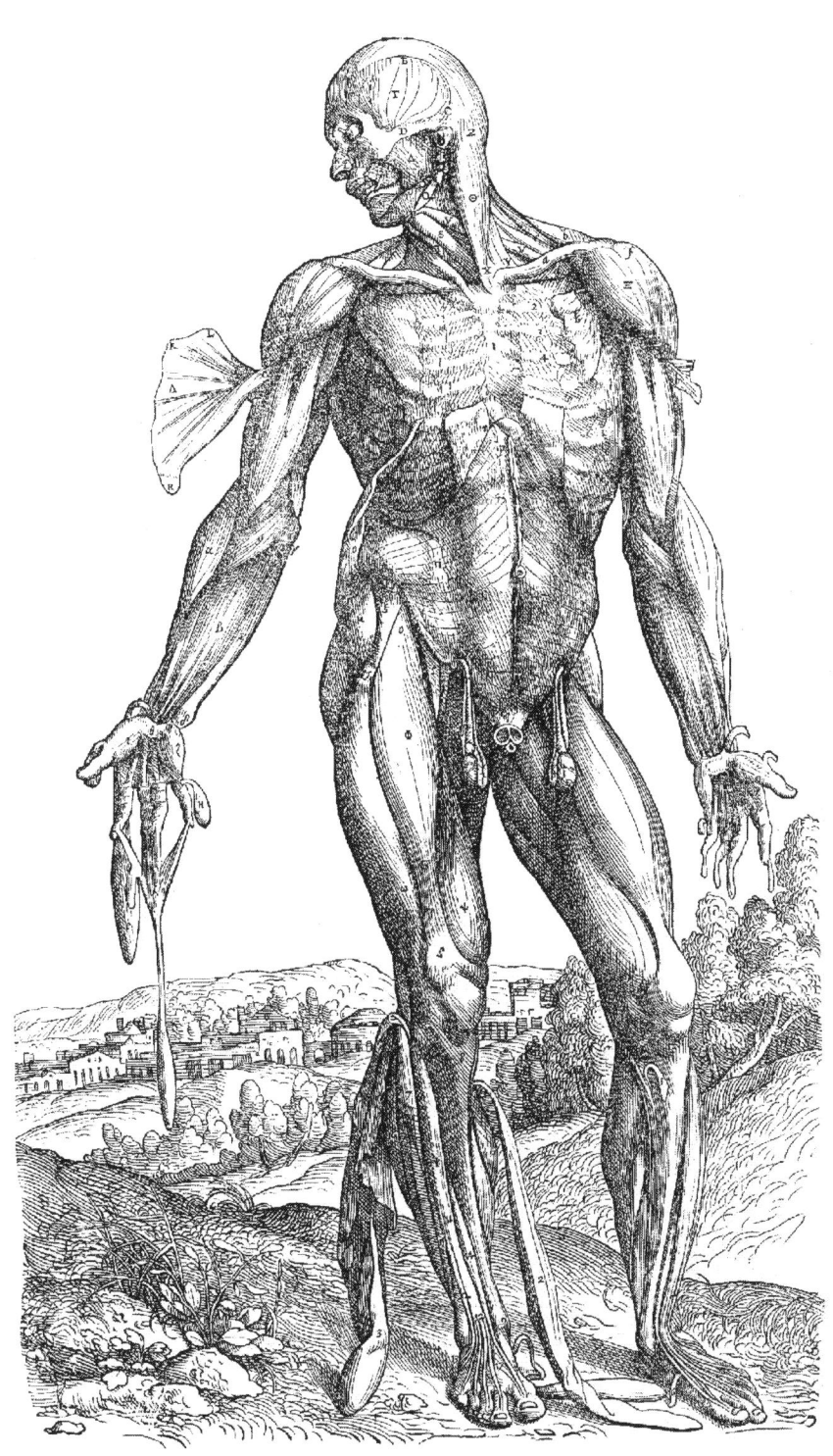

Synopsis

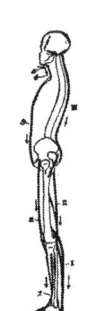

ALAN RADLEY has written a comprehensive book on the zen of dumbbell training. Developed is a thoughtful approach to dumbbell practice, with emphasis on natural movement patterns, deep concentration and technically informed practice.

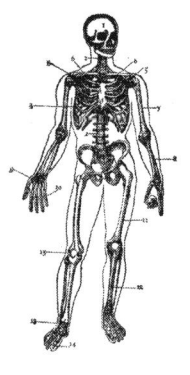

Alan aims to inspire and enlighten us as to the health, strength, and spiritual benefits of mindful training with the "ultimate fitness tool". The "zen" trainee performs exercises according to the law of harmony in order to free himself from incorrect technique, dogma and mind/body illusions.

This book highlights the close relationship between form and function in the human body. It is beautifully illustrated throughout with classic physique art and anatomical drawings. You will learn how to spice-up your routine with ~50 "lost" exercises; including arm, shoulder, body and triceps circles and various twisting, stretching and bending moves.

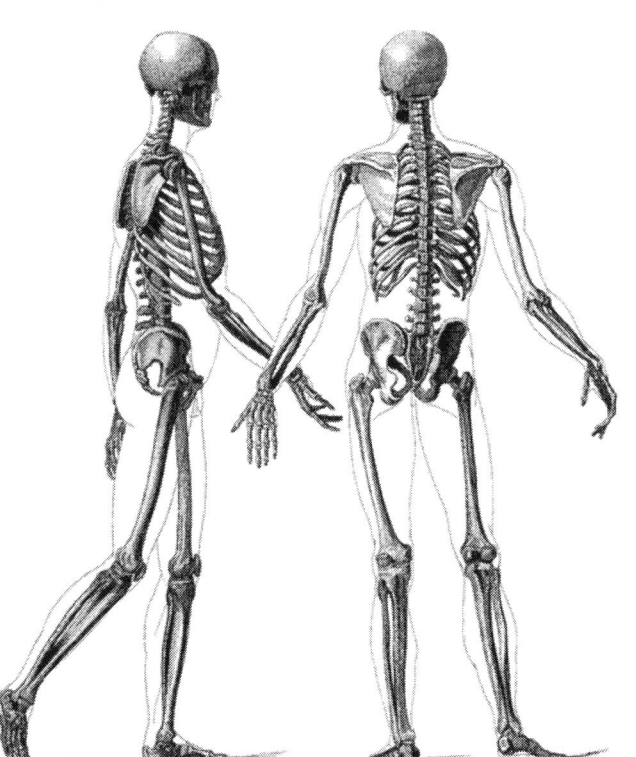

Both men and women can use the *Zen of Dumbbell Training* to attain their fitness goals. The how and why of dumbbell training is explained in greater detail than ever before, and laid-out is a well-defined path to physical perfection.

Enjoy!

Acknowledgements

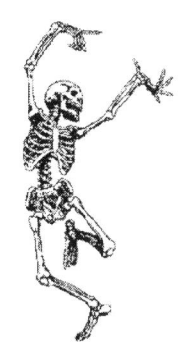

FIRSTLY I acknowledge all of the magazines, books, websites, friends, mentors, training partners, writers, teachers, and others who took the time to time to impart various nuggets of wisdom. Full copyright is acknowledged (where known) for all works and quoted in the captions or else the original publication is given or else the publication date is provided wherever possible.

Thanks to Roy Adams (featured artist), Burne Hogarth (featured artist), Dave and Rose Gentle, David Chapman, David Webster O.B.E., Restie and Rowena Wight, Roy Edwards, Dave Prowse M.B.E., Bill Cook, Philip, Ellen, Nigel, Arlene, Joshua, Emma, Ben, and Caroline Radley, Dr Kim Veltman, Nigel Pugh, Chris Green and others.

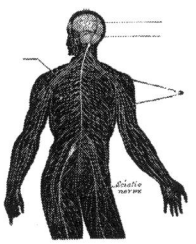

Warning

THIS BOOK is presented only as a means of preserving some ideas on exercising with weights. We make no representation, warranty or guarantee that the techniques described or illustrated in this book will be safe or effective. You may be injured if you apply or train according to the techniques herein described, and the author and publisher(s) are not responsible for any injury that may result.

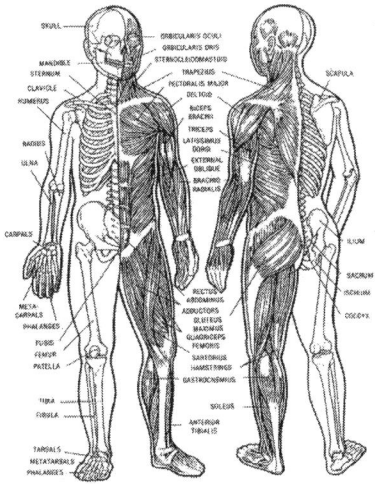

Consult a Physician and/or Medical Doctor regarding whether or not to attempt any exercise and/or technique described in this book.

10 ZEN OF DUMBBELL TRAINING

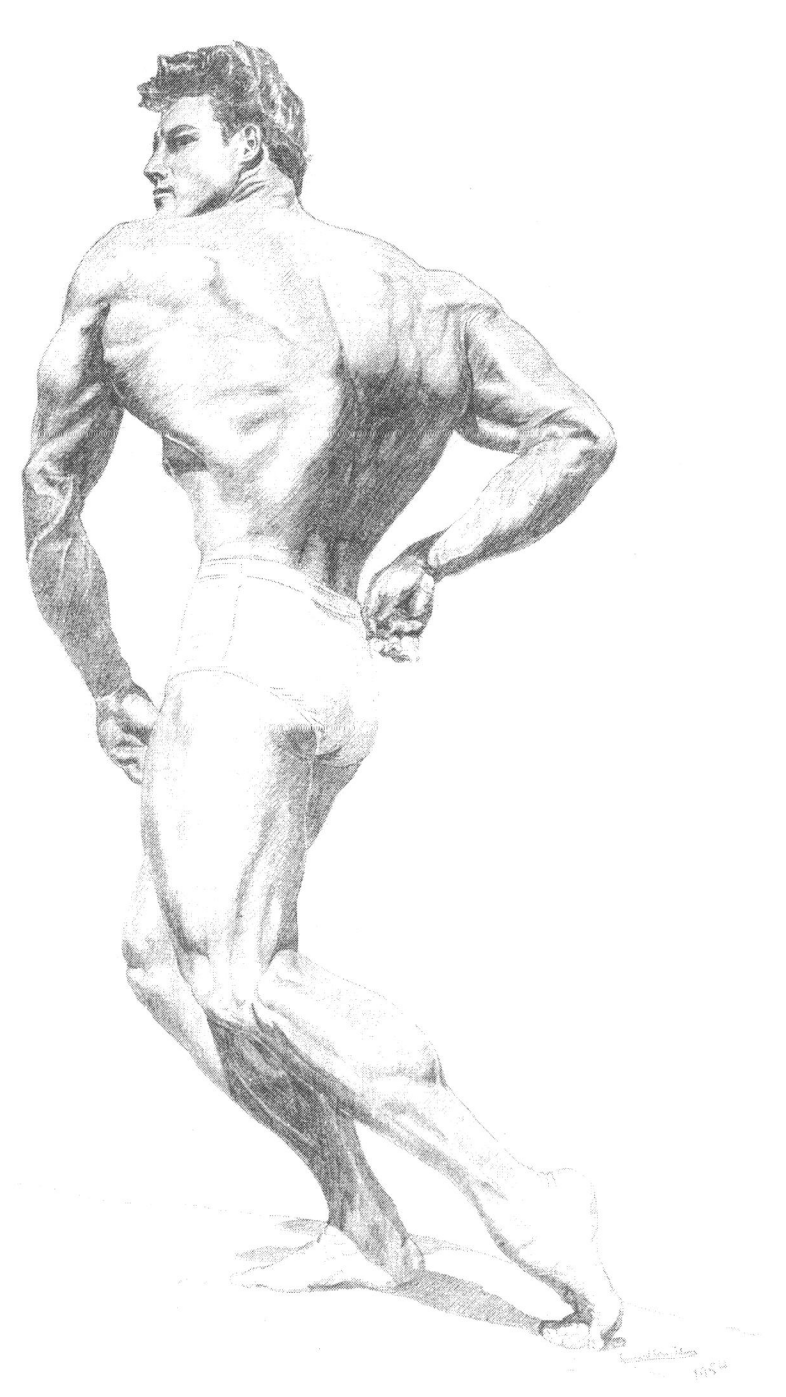

Preface

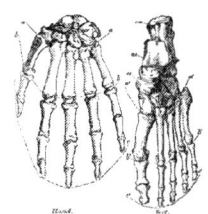

I HAVE spent my life studying the great writers, scientists and thinkers. And I was lucky enough to meet a few.

What have I learned?

To trust one's heart, mind, and body in all that you do. To love what you do, and to be a free-thinker. Do not live with the results of other peoples thinking. Be an *individualist*. Strike out on your own. Self-actualise. Listen to your inner-voice.

Question everything. Start with: who am I, what can I offer, and how shall I be remembered?

In writing this book, my goal is to impart useful ideas, unfettered by self-importance, conventional thinking, dogma, false beliefs, incorrect assumptions, and over-simplification.

How did I come to write this book? To start with, I own a **Physical Culture** (PC) library consisting of a large magazine and book collection. And I am a life-long weight-trainer.

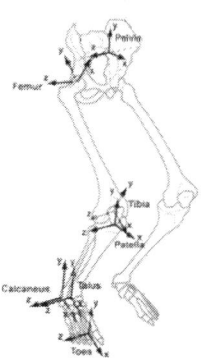

I am the author of The Illustrated History of Physical Culture, and I have written articles in Milo and Health and Strength magazine. In 2011 with David Gentle I wrote: Classic Muscle Art: Muscular Ideals and Inspirations, and then: 1001 Dumbbell Exercises, volumes 1, 2 and 3.

As stated in the sub-title of this book, I will teach you how to use a dumbbell for health, strength, figure and therapy. But all knowledge is ultimately self-knowledge. And because we are all so different, each needs a specific, flexible and continually evolving life-philosophy.

So take what is useful and disregard the rest.

Alan

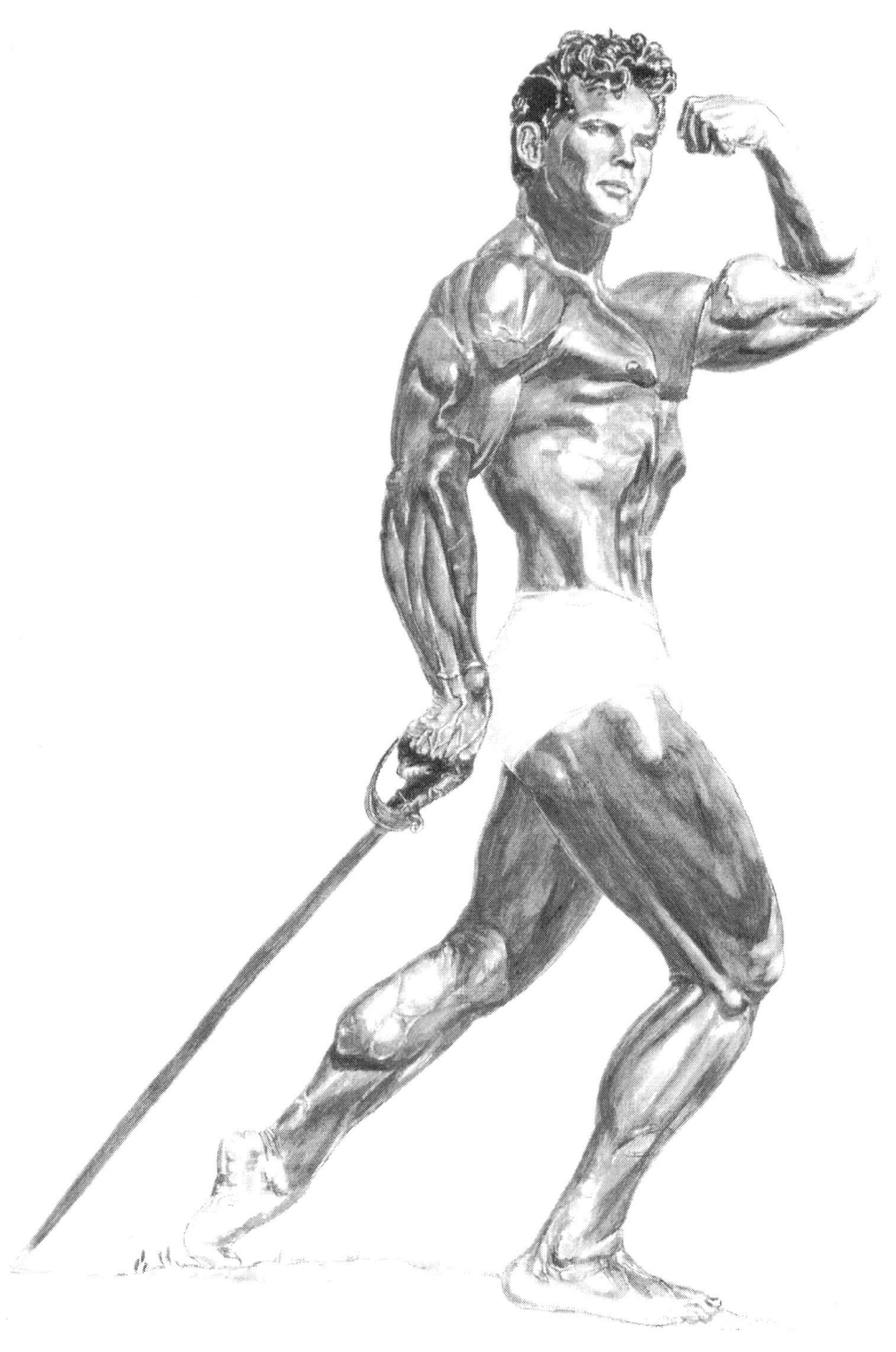

CHAPTER ONE

Introduction

Yoga is 99% practice and 1% knowledge

Krishna Pattabhi Jois

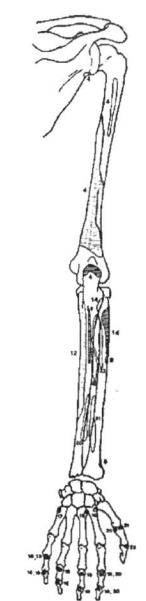

WHY WRITE another manual on fitness, because it seems that every possible type of book on physical training has already been written. In part, my aim has been to discover effective workouts and exercises. This goal is a response to the widespread confusion about which are the most useful training methods.

And it is no wonder that people are confused, because the fitness industry is flooded with a tremendous amount of misleading and often contradictory information. Also many people exhibit poor exercise technique, and possess low levels of knowledge as to what an effective fitness program might actually be. Paradoxically, in the information age, the process of getting fit is more of a puzzle than it ever was.

This book will help you to develop a truly effective personal fitness program. And along the way you will learn how to use a dumbbell! Now you might think that everybody already knows how to use a dumbbell, but, as we shall see, it's not so easy, and most do not.

A second motivation came about as a result of David Gentle's and my own: *1001 Dumbbell Exercises*; which surveyed weight-training exercises. In that book we highlighted the fact that old-time athletes had employed

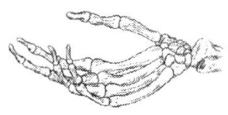

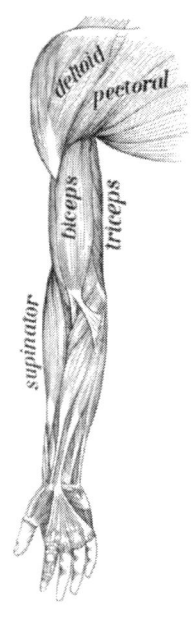

a large number of unusual and little-known dumbbell movements. Furthermore these athletes did possess excellent physical development, plus superior skills and technical knowledge in relation to resistance training.

What is the nature of this lost training knowledge, why is it important, and how and when should we apply it? In the following chapters we embark on a journey of discovery, and in order to address each of these questions.

And there is much to learn. It is an interesting fact that fantastic, but little-known, dumbbell exercises were commonly used 50-100 years ago. And these lost exercises include various dumbbell stretching movements, shoulder circles, arm circles, hand circles, triceps circles, body circles, leg swings, lean backs, forearm extensions, the bent-press, torso twisting/bending exercises, static holds, unusual squats and arm peak-contraction curling techniques etc. I have counted over 100 exercises that are completely unknown to the general public of today, and many are explained here.

These exercises gave men and women of the past tremendously muscular, flexible, and trim bodies; plus real-world strength. And all of this from natural methods, and from what (to us) are very unusual, but obviously effective, training techniques. I thought it would be useful to re-introduce these methods, using detailed performance descriptions and movement pattern diagrams.

Another motivation for the present book relates to my personal observation that many people, and especially the majority of so-called experienced trainees, follow ill-conceived, ineffective and poorly-suited fitness programs.

Perhaps they lack the necessary information.

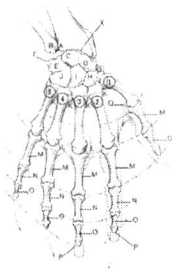

Most books on weight-training focus on muscles. They attempt to explain which muscles are involved in specific exercises. However this knowledge is next to useless in practical terms. There are 650 muscles in the human body, and remembering the functions of each is impossible - and pointless. Muscles normally work in combination, with perhaps a dozen or more involved in even simple movements. Of-course it is interesting to know that the squat exercise works the thighs, hips, and buttocks. But nobody needs to know the names of all of the different muscles involved, including: erector spinae, quadriceps femoris, gluteus maximus, rectus femoris, biceps femoris, vastus lateralis medialis, vastus internus, and intermedius etc. Knowing the functions and locations of all of these different muscles is quite frankly, complex and entirely redundant information.

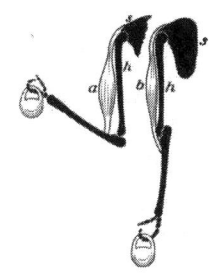

In this book we take a simpler and more practical route to training knowledge. Firstly we identify the joints and fundamental movement patterns that are possible in the human body. Next we analyse how to move in a natural and beneficial manner whilst exercising.

We consider the body as a type of "machine". In contrast to other "muscle" based books, we emphasise the skeleton. We start by learning how the various joints move - prior to studying natural movement patterns. Deeper and practical understanding is the result.

The modern obsession with muscles, as opposed to joints, has other consequences. Modern trainees seem to think that the only benefit to be derived from from weight-training is muscular enlargement. For example, bulky bodybuilder types often use (and over-use) the wrong exercises, being ones that mitigate against the creation of joint flexibility,

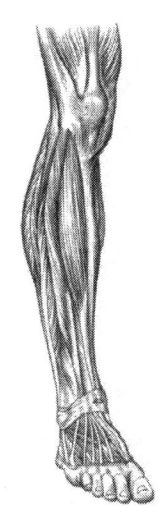

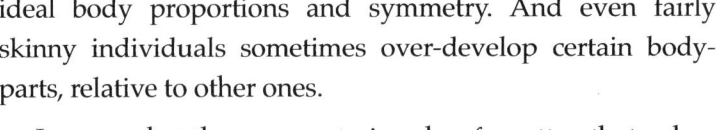

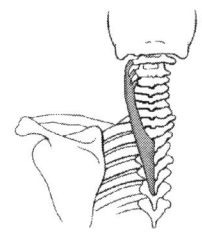

ideal body proportions and symmetry. And even fairly skinny individuals sometimes over-develop certain body-parts, relative to other ones.

It seems that the average trainee has forgotten that, when properly conceived and executed, resistance training is especially beneficial for other physical attributes. For example, dumbbell training can transform a person's ability to perform everyday movements easily and with a good range of motion or ROM. But most people do not obtain such benefits, and largely because they do almost everything wrong when it comes to weight-training. My conclusion here is based on the evidence: the abysmal exercise choices, dangerous techniques and outright sloppy form displayed by modern trainees.

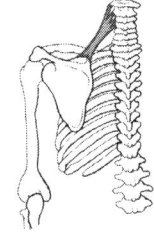

People also commonly use too much weight, and exhibit sloppy movements. But technique is everything in weight-training. You waste your own time when you move with less than precision, and loose all of the benefits that would have otherwise accrued.

Correct exercise choices, combined with effective techniques, can result in tremendous physical improvements for anyone. Lifting is especially beneficial in terms of functional capabilities and also the flexibility of the various body-parts. To say nothing of the improved energy levels, plus the attendant systematic benefits, provided to the heart and cardiovascular system.

Today the Doctors and health specialists recommend that we should all spend time at the gym. But sadly they also assume that the formulation of a beneficial fitness program is easy to achieve and/or that the correct methods are already well known and easily obtainable. Perhaps they

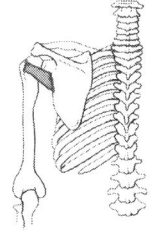

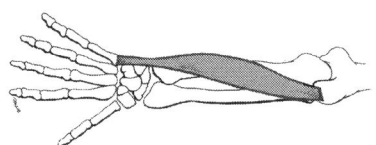

assume that knowledgeable personal trainers will be available to help. But they are often wrong in this respect, because the typical gym instructor has only a limited of knowledge of the field of resistance training.

Instructors exhibit little understanding of even basic factors such as how a person should go about choosing beneficial exercises. And they give no advice on exercise / weight selection or how to develop (that is to evolve) good movement forms (patterns). Rather they usher people towards machines, and demonstrate a few repetitions without much, if-any, explanation at-all.

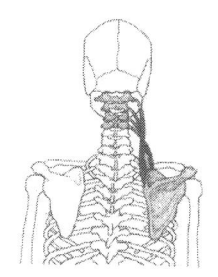

And it also seems as if everyone is on the same routine, consisting of multiple sets of barbell bench presses, bicep curls and a few machine based exercises; being exercises largely done for the chest, upper back and arms.

Ignored are the more important areas (in functional terms) such as the abdominals, shoulders, legs, hips, lower back, feet and calves, hands and forearms. And completely lacking are exercises for the twisting muscles of the torso, and range-of-motion (ROM) exercises are non-existent.

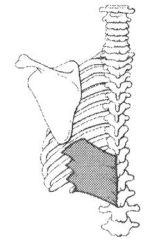

Yet bodybuilding used to be such a very different sport. Some 50 years ago it was all about development of the body-beautiful and healthful Physical Culture (PC).

The old-time PC enthusiast (pre 1960), focussed on his health as much as his figure. That is, he attempted to create overall strength and fitness, plus an excellent symmetry of body-part development. Ideal here were well-developed calves and thighs, wide shoulders, narrow waist and flowing lines everywhere.

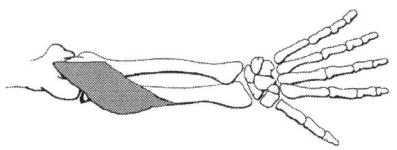

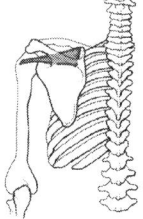

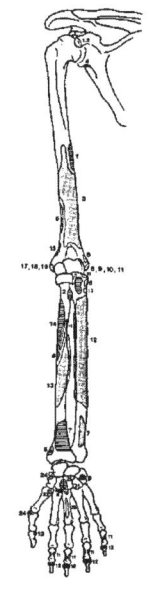

The overall look of Steve Reeves was considered an ideal for men. In other words, the "classic" physique was very much in-vogue, as in the Ancient Greek ideal.

The poor flexibility, constant rigid body position and stiff movements of a modern bench press "addict" are a dead giveaway of a poorly planned and executed fitness program. Perhaps some people like this look, but I much prefer the overall capability of a gymnast, martial artist, athlete or swimmer, being someone with an obvious looseness and freedom of physical movement.

In a nutshell, I want to have a functional body. And it is not widely-known that dumbbell training can develop this type of body. Being one produced with the free-space dumbbell movements that bring athletic grace and symmetry to one's physical form.

We also live in an age of fancy machines, cross training and kettle-bell routines. But the "ultimate fitness tool" - the dumbbell - has become somewhat neglected of late. My aim in writing this book has been to bring attention back to the dumbbell. It is without doubt the most versatile, effective and widely available tool for improving the human body. Dumbbell training brings unrivalled benefits including superior strength, flexibility, balance and coordination. More on my thinking later on.

Another motivation for the present book relates to my own personal journey, over many years, to find the ideal fitness routines; and then apply them to myself. Ever since I first began training at 13 years of age, I have attempted to select the most effective program, choose beneficial exercises, and then experiment to discover how far each method could take me.

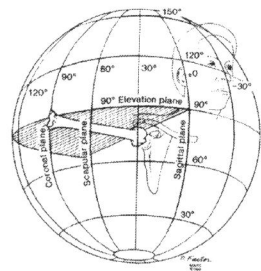
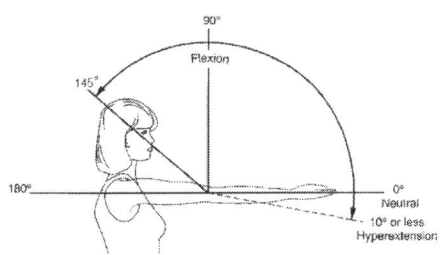

Before beginning to write this book, I performed a detailed literature survey in order to study past training systems. The "Zen" system of dumbbell training that follows is based on what I learned as a result of this large literature survey. And at the same time, it is routed in basic human anatomy, and on scientific range-of-motion (ROM) studies.

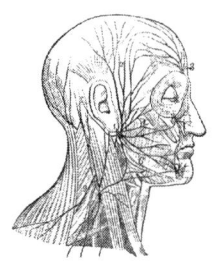

A key idea is to learn how your own body works - or moves - at the most basic level. Each of us moves about in unique ways, and the focus here is on listening to your body whilst you exercise. Use of natural movement patterns is essential, allowing the trainee to discover for himself the most effective ways in which he - and he alone - moves. And it is vital that you do so without any interference from a "bossy" know-it-all personal trainer. Plus the switch to a simplified (daily) dumbbell routine that can be performed at home produces fast results, and saves money and also time travelling to a gym.

In conclusion to this introduction, and overall, it seems that trainees of today do not tailor their routines according to their own specific needs. People follow convention and dogma (other peoples thinking) when it comes to the design of a personal fitness program. As a result they choose standard exercises, poor form and limited-range-of-motion movements. And if it all seems like it's not for them, then they simply don't bother. Most trainees use a very narrow range of exercises, and rarely (if ever) try any new ones. Perhaps they simply don't know any.

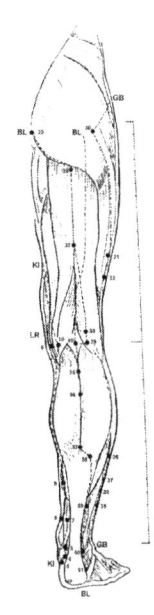

However a vast range of exercises are at their disposal using only the simplest of tools - the common dumbbell. And I have also noticed that people often select positively dangerous exercises, or else choose a movement variation that

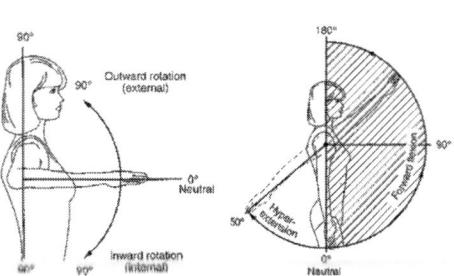

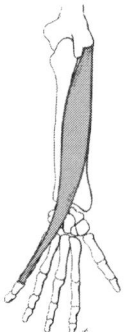

has a far more productive alternative. It is almost as if when they come to the gym, people just wonder about copying, and trying out, anything they happen to see. Poor technique, bad exercise choices and random progress are the result.

In a word, people fail to *tailor* their personal routines to their own specific needs, to say nothing of the fact that they use the same routine constantly. And the results speak for themselves, being a fat or skinny body, or else an unbalanced (and often tight) physique with low levels of functional fitness. Tragically, trainees of today seem to be stuck with the accepted wisdom of the drug taking bodybuilders and other specialist strength athletes who have a "get big at all costs" mentality, and survive on a very limited range of exercises. Many of these same "experts" eat massive amounts of protein and take drugs to build overly large, ugly, unbalanced and/or unhealthy physiques.

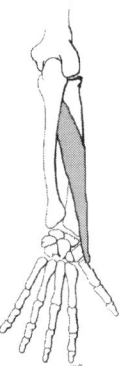

Paradoxically such "body-bulking" training principles have become widely adopted by men. The accepted "macho" mantra is to get a bulky chest, and large shoulder and arm muscles fast, and to forget about function, proportion and symmetry. And not bothering to train the legs, abdominals or lower back is normal. Not really the body beautiful then. Trainees in general have accepted the dogma that every routine should be based on machine movements, the barbell bench press and some curls. These exercises can indeed be useful, but a far wider range of superior exercises exist.

As a result of such "brainwashing" of the general public, people show little imagination in putting together a balanced program of exercise. Therefore it is no wonder that the typical trainee's progress stagnates and development fixes. Likewise the mind becomes bored, and excitement plus motivation are lost.

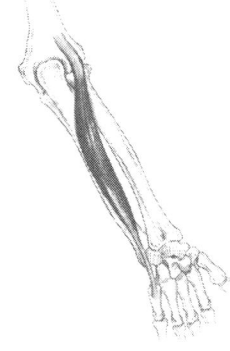

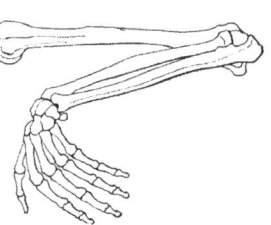

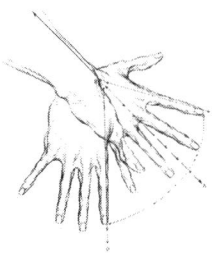

Another problem relates to the use (and over-use) of machine movements. Many choose to go down this route because of the supposed "danger" of free-weights. Or else they use a machine because it (conveniently?) sets the movement "arc" for you, thus reducing effort - mental and physical. However reduction of effort should be a warning signal, because improving one's strength and fitness is supposed to be reasonably hard work!

With this book we aim to break down many of the misconceptions that surround weight-training, and to introduce a new dumbbell-based training system which contains within itself sufficient variety to feed both mind and body. We supply detailed performance descriptions for around 80 excellent exercises. We think that these are the very best exercises, in general, that you could do. Feel free also to seek out other exercises and performance techniques, and as required.

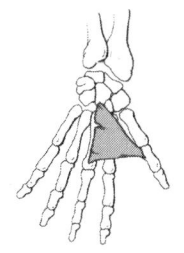

Hopefully you will not be put off by the detailed anatomical drawings presented here, which serve to instruct.

Someone once said that: *a dumbbell/barbell looks dumb but you have to be intelligent to use it, whilst a machine looks intelligent but you have to be dumb to use it.* This statement lies at the core of the training philosophy that follows.

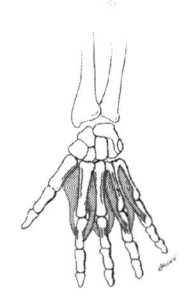

It is my hope that the present book can give you, dear reader, renewed knowledge and inspiration so that you can formulate your own "Zen" of dumbbell training. I would urge you to avoid all dogma, conventional wisdom and other people's thinking in relation to fitness training. Follow your own path and make up your own mind.

Only be certain to arm yourself with appropriate knowledge, and in order to make informed decisions.

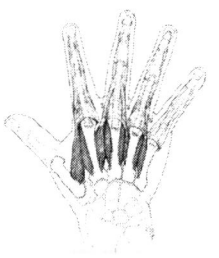
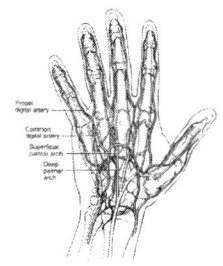

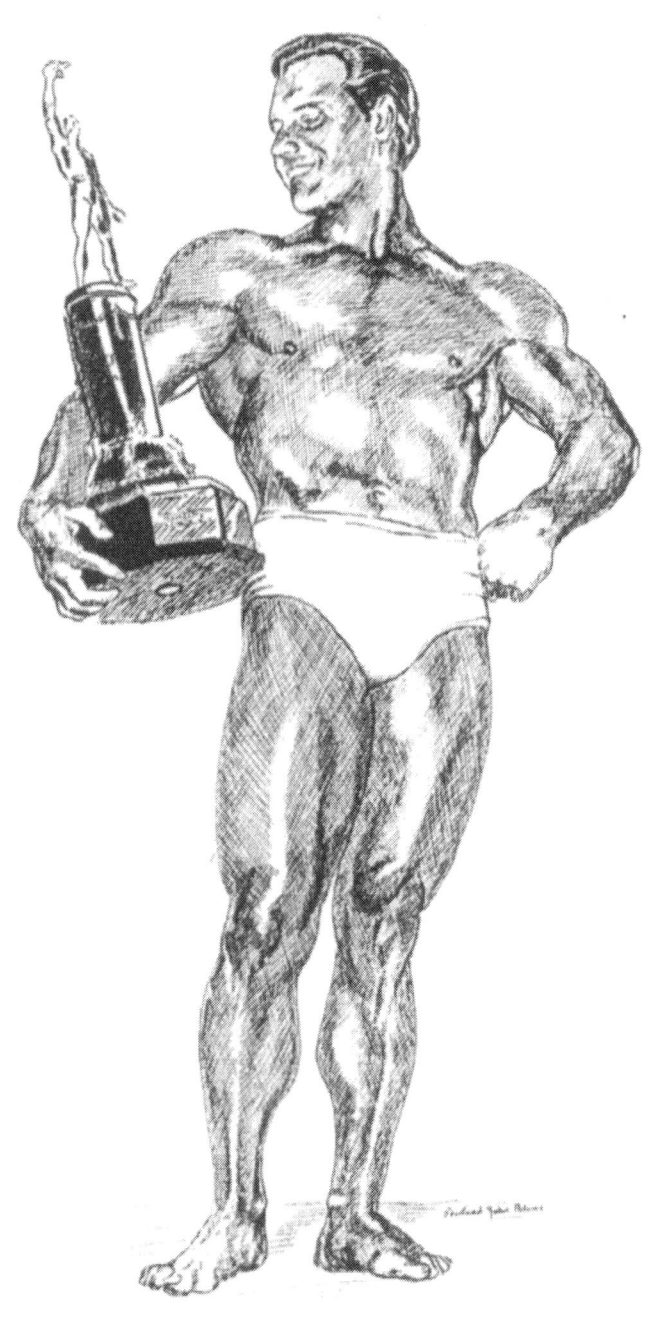

Method

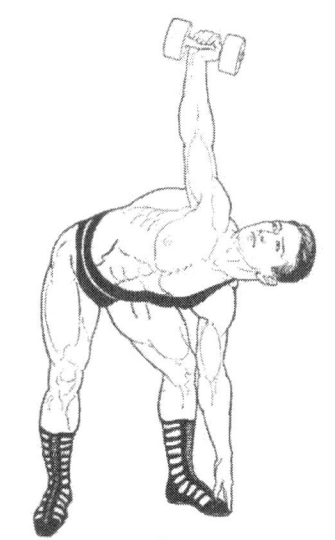

As a scientist (by profession) I feel compelled to relate the research methods that were used to create the "Zen" dumbbell training theory described herein. Firstly I performed an in-depth literature survey. This consisted of time looking back over the weight-training books, courses and papers produced in the past 150 years. [1]

My survey revealed that weight-training has developed a relatively large literature base. Also clear is that no one system or study has managed to capture an ultimate guide to weight-training. And nobody has developed a complete system of dumbbell training.

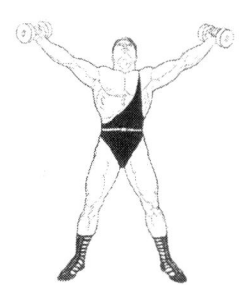

It is my belief that the dumbbell is the most versatile training tool imaginable; and although it looks "dumb" it takes intelligence to use properly. Many of the useful dumbbell techniques are inaccessible, and scattered about amongst a huge variety of publications. Thus I set about collating dumbbell related training knowledge from all of the systems and courses published in the last 100 years.

A key aim of the present book is to bring together in one place a complete and scientifically organised system of dumbbell training. Movements are explained to the fullest degree, core principles are developed, and the minutiae of dumbbell practice are discussed in greater detail than ever before.

---

[1] See: *1001 Dumbbell Exercises* - by A. Radley & D. Gentle

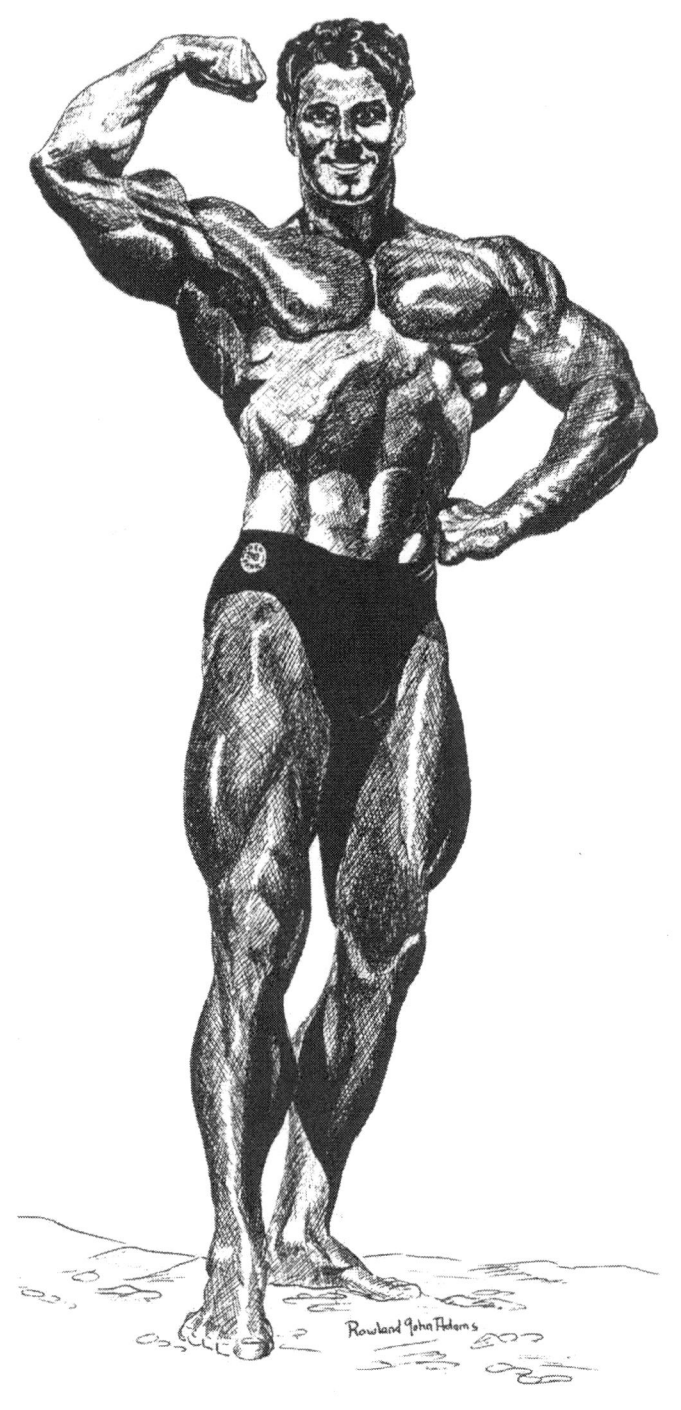

CHAPTER TWO

Theories

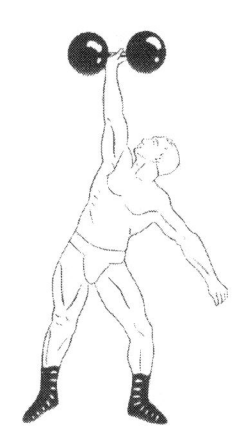

A QUICK google search for the keywords barbell, dumbbell, resistance training, and/or weight-training reveals literally hundreds of different systems, techniques and exercises.

My own library includes over one hundred books and thousands of magazines on these same topics, ranging from the earliest written in 1860 to one published in 2013.

A cursory glance through many of these references reveals some interesting facts in relation to the so-called "science" of exercise. Firstly, it is not really a science, but a field that has been developed by the practitioners themselves, as opposed to scientists. Of particular note is how great is the variety of opinions on fitness training. Training principles and points of view often contradict one another.

I think part of the reason for this diversity, is that the human body is capable of adapting to many different types of physical environments and also to diverse stress conditions. Therefore, and to a degree, any training system that does not kill you, will often result in some kind of physical improvement - at least for a while.

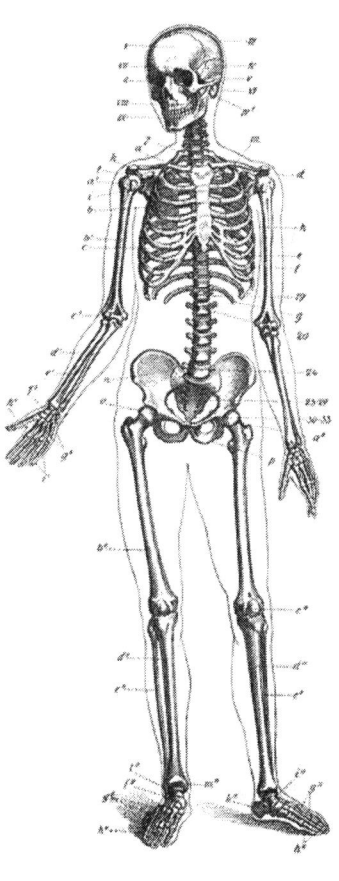

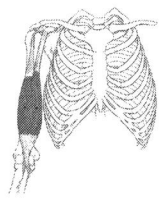
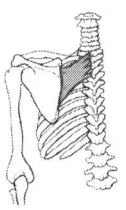

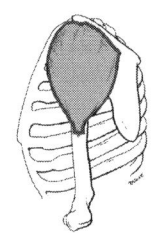

But the athlete is looking for optimal results, that is fast improvements in health, strength and functional capabilities. The question arises as to which kind of training system is the most effective; or gives the best results.

Results are often desired in the least time, and perhaps also for the minimum work input. This latter point has been the golden offering by the muscle hucksters through the ages. And it's the one that the experts have argued about over the last 100 years, and continue to debate today. And it has not helped that many have lied about the effectiveness of methods, products, foods etc; and in order to make money.

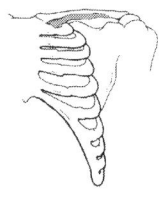

In a way, the debate has been simplified to one dimension alone, being muscle-growth production.

Whereas any generally useful exercise system would result in a wide range of benefits that relate to other aspects of physical fitness, including body structure and posture, flexibility, joint stability, aerobic capacity, muscular endurance and coordination etc, as discussed below.

Hopefully the present book can clear up some of the confusion, and identify a truly effective way to get fit using dumbbells alone.

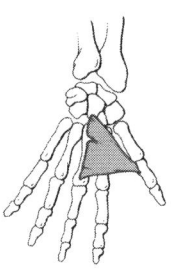

But don't expect to find all of the answers in any one book, or even to get most of your knowledge from any one teacher. You may (or will) also want to incorporate non-dumbbell routines, such as barbells, machine training (limited) and/or other forms of training into your program (e.g running).

Here we shall focus on dumbbell training (largely), and in order to illuminate that topic fully, plus to give the humble dumbbell its proper place as the pre-eminent training tool.

However the answers to your own individual physical development must be discovered by you, and you alone.

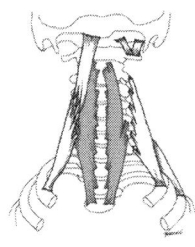

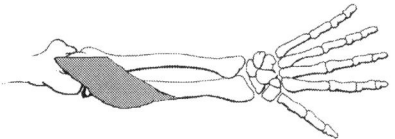

We all have different needs, capabilities, and genetics; plus our tolerance to physical exercise varies. Thus the process of getting fit, in each person's case will require specific methods. I do however, make the claim that you can get incredibly fit using dumbbells alone, and this fact is not widely known.

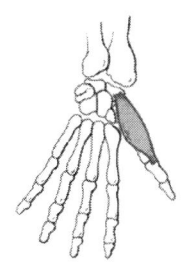

Another point being addressed here is that a far wider range of weight-training training systems had once been in common use, and especially prior to the second world war. But later on, from around 1960 onwards, one type of training system and a rather small set of "favourite" exercises began to dominate. Today there is a great deal of perceived wisdom (most of it wrong) that a few basic barbell and/or machine exercises are best for physical improvement, including the barbell bench press, curls and pulldowns etc.

Undoubtably there are elements of truth here, for such exercises do (sometimes) result in fast development of the larger muscles, in terms of the most bulky. But these movements by no means result in the best physiques or the most flexible joints. Machine training (the current king) tends to work larger muscles over smaller ones, and often does not work all of the many important coordinating and supporting muscles that are present. Plus barbells often only work the muscle over a limited range of motion, and there are only a small number of barbell moves that are practical or even possible (perhaps 10-15).

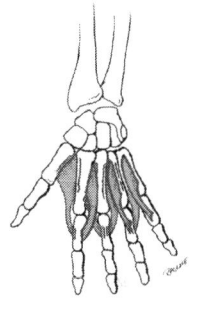

The joints and levers of the human body, by contrast, are designed to work over a great variety of limb positions. And literally hundreds of unique movement paths are possible using nothing more than a dumbbell.

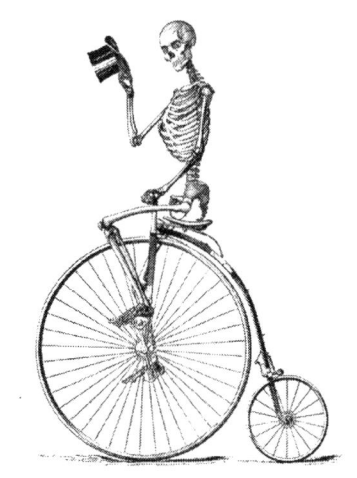

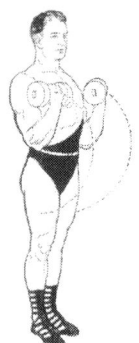

Dumbbells offer true *three-dimensional or "3D" training* because they offer natural, and "spatially free" movement paths or patterns. Dumbbells allow constantly changing movement paths, as opposed to the more fixed movement paths of a machine or even a barbell.

It is interesting to look briefly at the views of a veritable titan of fitness. Arthur Jones, of Nautilus fame, was an intelligent individual. His *Nautilus Bulletins,* produced in the 1970s, contain many unquestionable truths about the nature of weight-training. But like us-all he was sometimes wrong. For example, I think he missed the mark when he spoke about the need for super-intense weight-training, largely because it is unnecessary and also dangerous, and it can result in frequent injuries.

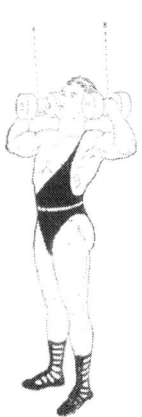

Arthur also said that his Nautilus machines were an improved form of barbell, being a tool that adapted to the human, as opposed to the need for a human to adapt to the tool (as in a barbell). In a sense I can see what he is talking about here. Jones attempted, with his Nautilus off-centre "cam" to provide a resistance profile that closely matched that of the human being; thus making the exercise constantly difficult throughout the full movement path. However I think that Arthur's analogy doesn't work; because the trainee must adapt himself more to a machine, than he ever would to a free-weight such as a dumbbell.

A major drawback of Nautilus (and Hammer etc) machines is that they fail to provide exercise for the various supporting and balancing muscles; plus each machine provides only one fixed movement pattern (the same one) for everyone. Thus they really only provide exercise over a very limited range of motion(s).

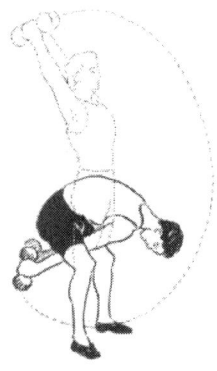

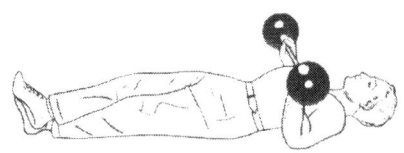

For example, a dumbbell pullover potentially allows movement, and produces resistance, along quite literally hundreds of different 3D movement paths as opposed to the single path offered by a pullover machine. Thus with a dumbbell, the trainee can alter the path on different occasions, and/or choose a path that suits him/her best.

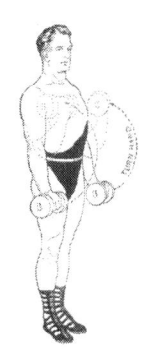

Nevertheless, we live in a machine age. When they were first introduced in the 1950s, cable machines offered a tremendous advance. They allowed the trainee to exercise his/her muscles from new and unusual angles, and to create resistance (for example) at the peak of the bicep curl where resistance normally drops off. Cable machines remain useful today as a result, largely because unlike most other machines, they allow a range of different movement paths.

But now a whole plethora of new machines have appeared. And whilst many machines apparently seem to have further evolved and become more "advanced", in future chapters I shall explain the inherent drawbacks that most of these new machines posses.

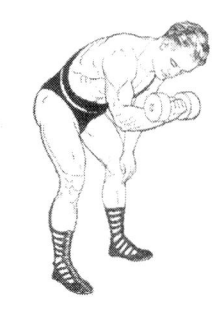

Back to the long-running dumbbells versus barbells debate. The great natural bodybuilder/weightlifter John Grimek once told David Gentle that in the old days (1930s-1960s), that they (the York champion lifters), never really used barbells much, but preferred a great variety of dumbbell movements. John was Mr Universe and the USA weightlifting champion long before tissue growth drugs came on the scene. Grimek is also worth studying because he was so unusual. He was a strongman who could perform back-flips, the splits and tumbled about like a cat.

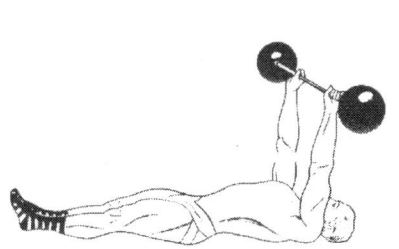
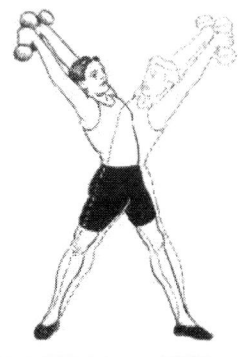

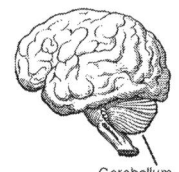

By the way, the movements that John alludes to were often not performed in a fixed pattern of sets and reps, but were completed as movements and partial movements in a variety of set combinations and repetition ranges, and even changing movement paths. For example, John sometimes stopped the weight in one position for a few seconds (or even minutes), before twisting the dumbbell in the hand into a different direction, and going forwards/backwards along a different movement path. Sometimes he would even turn one exercise into another within a movement arc.

So none of the boring and repetitive movements performed as in a military marching style, but rather going by feeling and doing what (your body tells you) seems the right thing to do on a moment-by-moment basis. Very free and "Zen" like - I think you will agree.

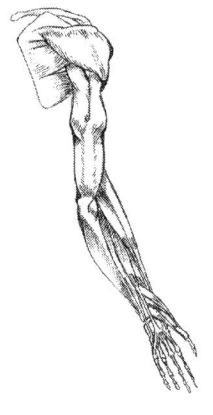

John also much preferred standing movements as opposed to seated or lying down ones. Perhaps his ideas relate to the fact that a human being's most natural and also strongest position is a standing one. Or maybe he believed (correctly) that standing exercises worked the most muscles at once, and also worked the many supporting and inner structures, including those around the hips, spine and the balancing muscles and ligaments in the legs and feet etc.

John also said; that he used to come into the gym and do whatever he felt like in terms of exercises - and so he did not even have a routine ! How un-scientific I can here many piping up. Yet Grimek had 19 inch biceps long before steroids and could easily bench press for reps, or standing push press, 400 lbs. It seems that John used the muscle-confusion principle, realising that one's system quickly becomes accustomed to an exercise stress and stops adapting. So routine

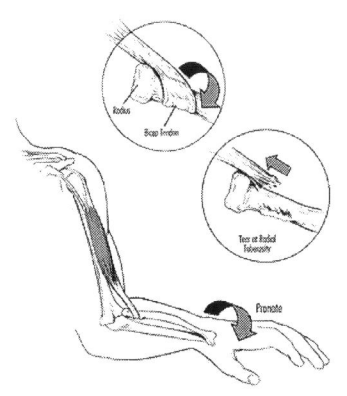
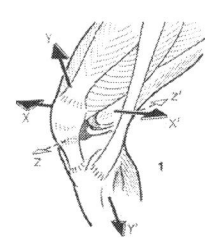

variance is key. John also recommended playing about with dumbbells almost as a child would do. Here the notion of having a "routine" or following a schedule has been abandoned. Perhaps it seems more scientific to lift weights for sets and reps and on a fixed "routine" which never varies. This can work for a while, but you soon become stale, and progress falters and your mind becomes bored.

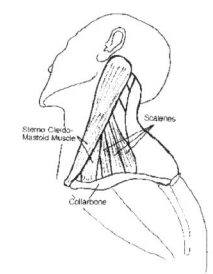

In fact, training knowledge is never complete, and you should constantly experiment with new techniques and theories. Try to be in a constant state of learning in relation to your body. In terms of its capabilities, responses and adaptions to training, rest and food etc. And challenge yourself.

The great martial artist Bruce Lee is today remembered for his amazing physical conditioning, low body-fat and superior musculature. Bruce was an accomplished weight-trainer and had weights scattered all over his house including barbells, dumbbells and machines of all kinds. Bruce took every opportunity to train, and he was constantly moving about exercising (according to his wife and a friend of mine who knew Bruce at school). Bruce was also very intelligent, and had a large book collection on fitness training, which indicates that training is not for dummies and requires careful and constant study in order to achieve superior performance. Knowledge is power, so-to-speak.

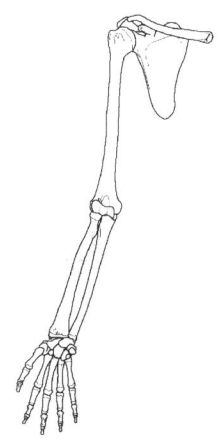

In the chapters that follow, we identify a set of core principles and methods which underpin the "Zen" system of dumbbell training. Our quest is to find the ultimate training routine, and to then have the knowledge and means to adapt it to our own specific requirements.

A tall-order, but one that I think we can meet.

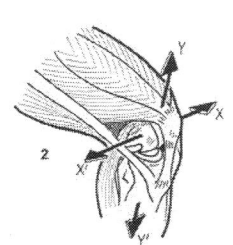
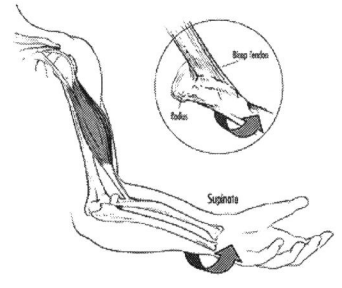

32 ZEN OF DUMBBELL TRAINING

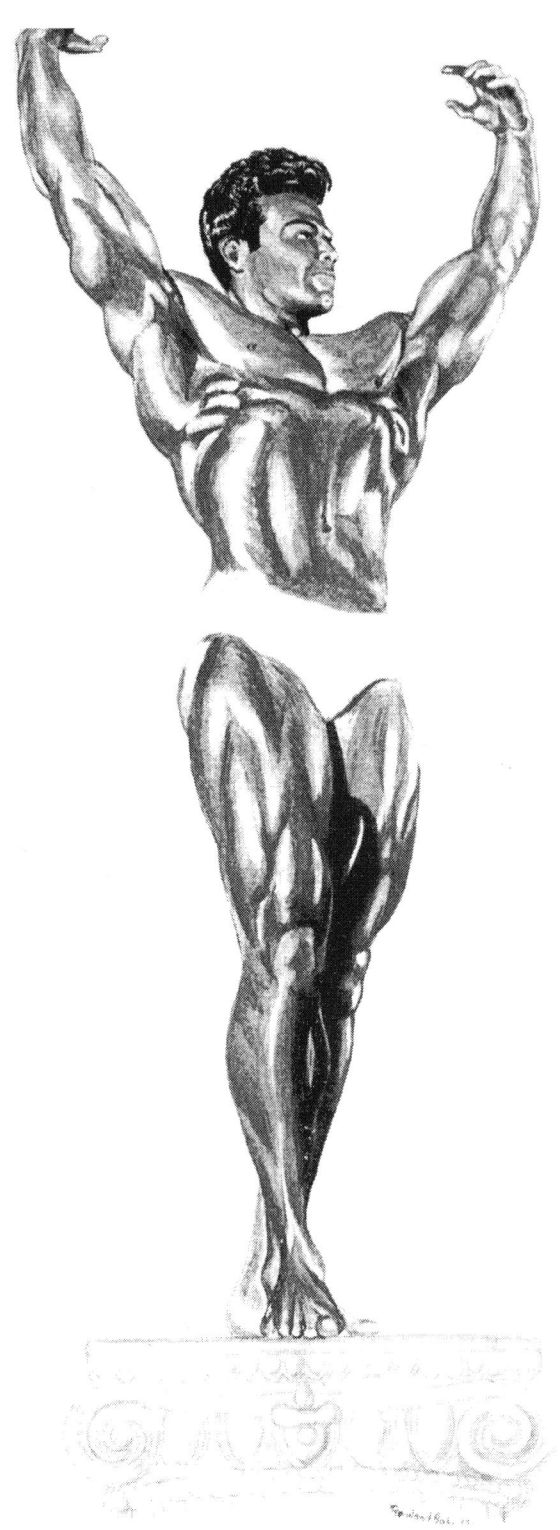

CHAPTER THREE

Fitness

PHYSICAL FITNESS can be split into two basic types. General fitness (a state of health and well-being), can be separated from specific fitness, which is a task-oriented definition and based on the ability to perform specific aspects of sports or occupational requirements. Physical fitness has also been defined as a set of attributes or characteristics that people have and/or achieve, and that relate to the ability to perform physical activity.

Fitness is generally achieved through correct nutrition, exercise, hygiene and rest. The american president's council on Physical Fitness and Sports developed the following chart to help define physical fitness (hereafter just fitness).

Physiological	Health Related	Skill Related	Sports
Metabolic	Body Composition	Agility	Team
Morphological	Cardiovascular Fitness	Balance	Individual
Bone Integrity	Flexibility	Coordination	Lifetime
Other	Muscular Endurance	Power	Other
	Muscle Strength	Speed	
		Reaction Time	
		Other	

Table 1: Elements of Physical Fitness

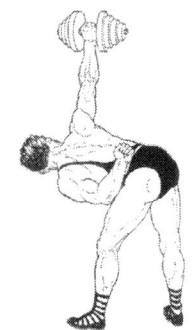
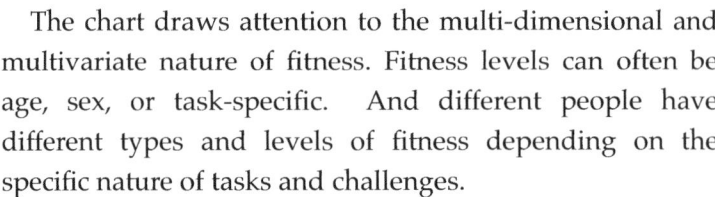

The chart draws attention to the multi-dimensional and multivariate nature of fitness. Fitness levels can often be age, sex, or task-specific. And different people have different types and levels of fitness depending on the specific nature of tasks and challenges.

Without a doubt genetics, lifestyle and training impinge on one's physical capacity. And it has also become well understood that one can develop or improve fitness in both specific and general ways through engaging in a physical fitness program.

Experts often talk about the physical, mental and emotional facets of fitness and how they interrelate and so impact on the healthy lifestyle. The present book is a practitioners guide, and so we do not have the space to examine the different aspects of fitness from a theoretical perspective. Rather in this book we shall refer to some exercises and methods that affect specific aspects as listed in Table 1.

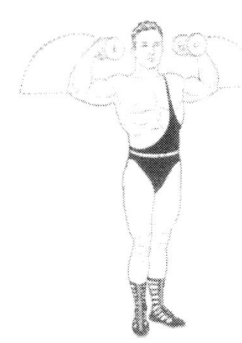

And we shall not attempt to prove or else validate our claims and any predicated results, but rather we leave it to the reader to assess the truth or otherwise of the system here described.

A brief caveat on the "scientific" basis of what follows is important at this point. *I make no claims that the principles and methods that I shall describe have any basis in science whatsoever*. And nobody could.

Let me qualify that statement. I have examined the findings of the so-called "exercise scientists", and I am in agreement with Nautilus inventor Arthur Jones on this topic. He said (in effect) that many claims and findings of exercise scientists and coaches are completely worthless,

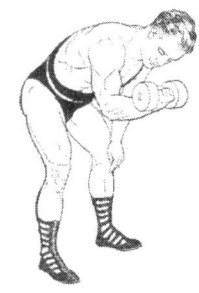
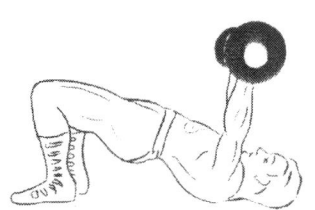

baseless and "not worth a damn". It is not that we haven't learned much; but only that people and individual circumstances are so different so as to require highly specific advice - or one-to-one coaching - and in order to tailor recommendations to the individual.

Many "experts" also talk a good talk, spouting lots of "scientific" principles etc, but most have never walked-the-walk, so-to-speak. In other words some are arm-chair practitioners who never tested what they preach and who look like they are very unfit individuals indeed.

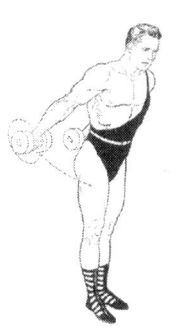

Conversely, there are today several truly capable kinesiologists, exercise scientists and physiotherapists such as Gray Cook and Stuart McGill etc. What these men have to say is really worth listening to. But they are not the norm.

Sadly passed are other excellent weight-training examples and teachers such as Steve Reeves, Arthur Jones, Bruce Lee, and Mike Mentzer. Although they left writings in order to study their beliefs in detail.

Additionally today we have other knowledgeable coaches and teachers such as Pavel Tsatsouline, Frank Zane, and Bill Pearl. And the systems of older men like Alan Calvert, Joe Weider, Eugene Sandow, Charles Atlas, and many others are worth a look as well.

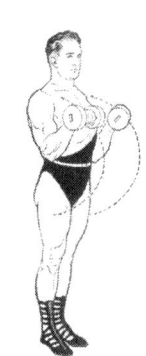

But unfortunately at the same time, sometimes your average fitness instructor, coach or physiotherapist has limited knowledge of how the body works in an integrated way. And they often make baseless claims of the benefits/drawbacks of specific movements, spout blatant falsehoods, and even make incorrect claims about which movements affect which specific body-parts.

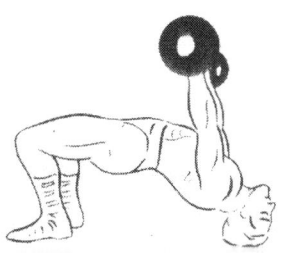

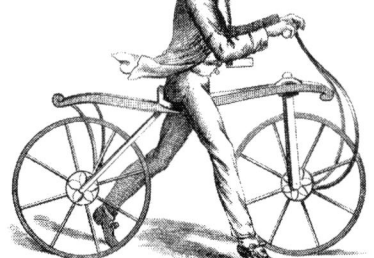

The "Dandy Horse"

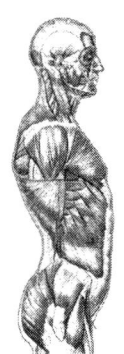

Unfortunately, some of today's "experts" have little knowledge of the fact that the human body can move in hundreds of different ways, and likewise they fail to recognise the vast array of exercise forms that are possible. It's not that they aren't intelligent or don't have the best intentions; but only that they lack the breadth of knowledge to give good advice.

Largely here I am talking about the knowledge of those instructors and medical professionals who make themselves available to the general public. By contrast, the coaches and medical professionals who are available to the professional athlete, who can pay for the best, must be far superior (we can but hope).

Recently I visited a physiotherapist, and after one hour spent talking to me, she stated "You know more about how the body works and remedial exercise than I do!" I was flabbergasted.

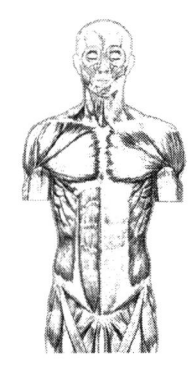

Let us take a step backwards. By all means listen to the scientific experts - but take what's said with a pinch of salt. You must make up your own mind when it comes to your own body, and in terms of its unique capabilities and responses to lifestyle. Remember that we are all far more diverse physically than we may think. And I am not only talking about genetic differences, but rather I want you to remember that the way we have lived our lives strongly affects our physical capabilities as they are today. Plus the food we eat and our personal schedules mean that we should not compare ourselves to others, but rather proceed as individuals in all things physical.

I do not think (personally) that exercise science has evolved sufficiently to even claim to be a science. Not yet. I say this because in relation to most other fields which have

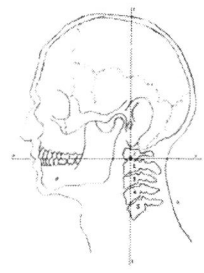
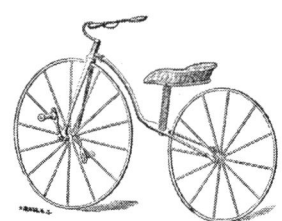

been developing for hundreds of years, exercise science has only been seriously studied for (at best) the last 30 years or so. It's core principles are still evolving and developing, and perhaps some key features have yet to be discovered.

I do not want to dwell on the failings of the scientists, because it may not actually be their fault that the field has not advanced very far.

Exercise science crosses the boundaries of several scientific disciplines, and it is very complex indeed. It is difficult to test principles here because many aspects of fitness are highly specific to the individual and also to the type of fitness being measured.

Finding widely applicable training principles for the general public becomes very difficult and/or impossible. This is because of the requirement to extrapolate results, simplify findings and convey the information to ordinary people who may have highly specific needs; and in fact being needs that they may not be aware of.

But at the same time the science of health, exercise and fitness training is today rapidly developing. However it is with the coaches and athletes themselves that the real advances are being made. Fitness is a practical, experimental field, but it is also one that relies on theory.

Let us get back to you and the reason that you are reading this book. Hopefully, in the Chapters that follow, I can impart sufficient knowledge to you, and so that you are able to formulate an effective personal fitness program.

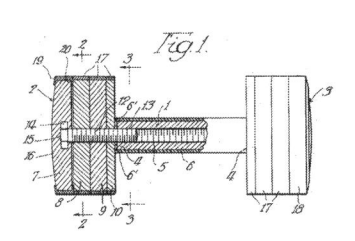

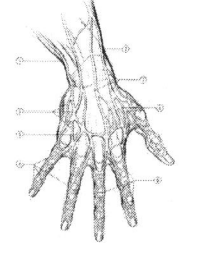

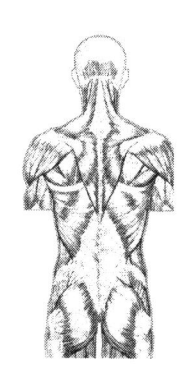

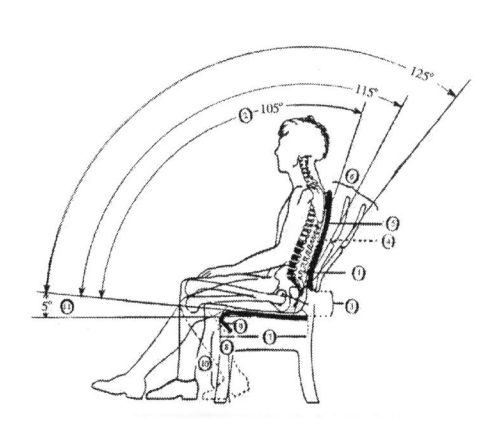

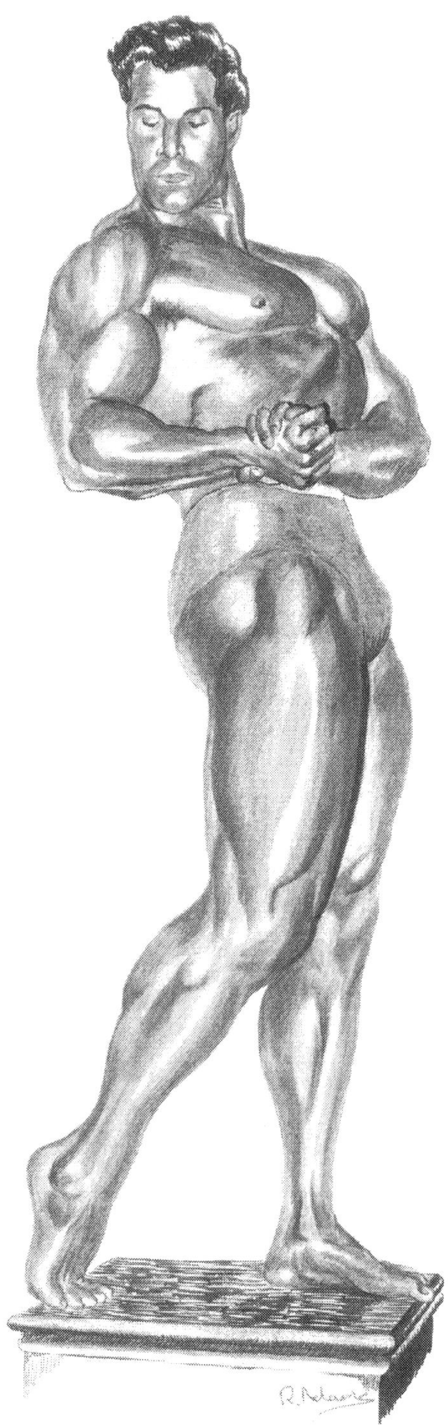

Personal Fitness

A S INDICATED, the concept of fitness has two aspects, general and specific. Now it goes without saying that you want the general aspects, being the health, strength and even spiritual benefits that just go along with being a fit individual.

Yet the specific aspects of fitness are just that - specific to the individual and to particular task(s). If an athlete wants to improve his/her specific fitness, several actions must be taken. To begin with one has to look at the person's goals, their current physical condition and capabilities, and at their strength, flexibility, endurance, skill etc. Next we see if a training program can be devised to close the gap between capabilities and requirements.

Often one's fitness goals come from the requirements of the sport(s) that one is engaged in, for example sprinting or gymnastics etc. Sometimes performance of the discipline itself develops sufficient fitness to achieve one's goals. However as athletics (and sport in general) has developed and become professionalised, so athletes have sought means to improve their basic physical capabilities, whilst leaving skill training to the discipline itself.

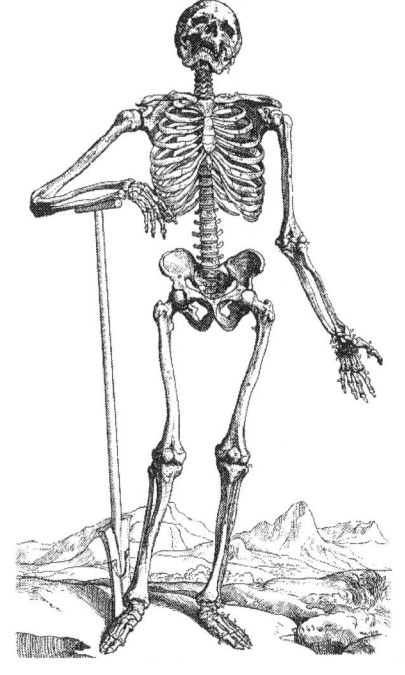

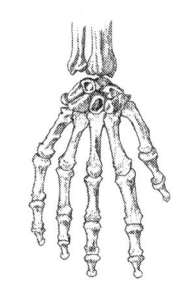

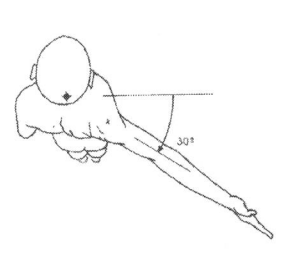

Weight-raining has become the de-facto method for athletes in all disciplines to improve muscular strength and endurance. In fact, during the last 30 years or so, it has been realised that weight-training improves aspects such as speed, flexibility and balance, and it can also improve the the overall structural stability plus resilience of the body in general. To say nothing here of the improvements in strength that can be the result of a properly applied resistance training program.

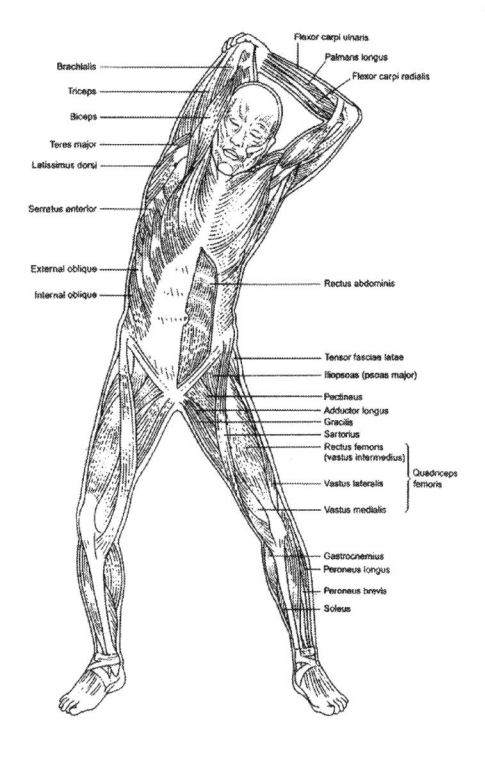

I cannot know what your personal goals are in terms of the application of the fitness program(s) here given. Therefore in what follows I shall present a general program of exercises, listing the likely outcomes of the same. It is then up to you to pick and chose methods/exercises, and as your needs dictate. In addition, I shall also give you some effective training principles to follow, in order that you may progress from a sound foundation.

The goal of this book is to provide a system of fitness training that you may adapt to your own particular needs.

Height	Weight
5 feet 9 inches	180 lbs
5 feet 10 inches	185 lbs
5 feet 11 inches	190 lbs
6 feet 0 inches	200 lbs
6 feet 1 inches	210 lbs
6 feet 3 inches	230 lbs

Table 2: Ideal Body Weight (Men)

Fitness Assessment

AS INDICATED, fitness is specific to the individual. You will have to decide for yourself what amounts to sufficient fitness in your own case.

It may be useful to define a few simple fitness measures that you can use to assess your own fitness levels. We shall focus here on the most basic attributes of a human being; body appearance and measurements.

Let us begin with bodyweight and percentage body-fat. Now it is true that some sports require a high body-fat percentage, but in general it is healthier, and the athlete performs better, when they possesses a fairly low to medium body-fat percentage.

Many people feel much healthier with a low body-fat percentage, for example moving about more freely and experiencing less stress and strain on the joints and digestive organs etc.

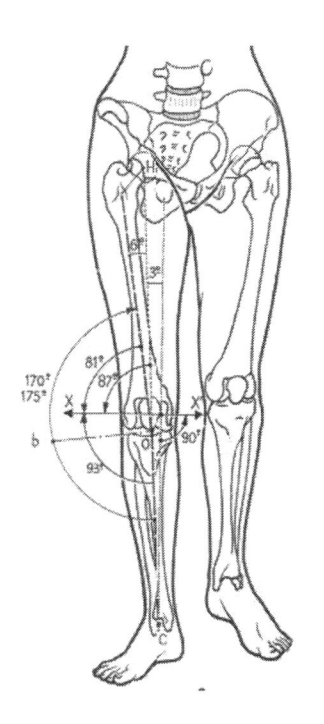

Description	Women	Men
Essential Fat	10-13 %	2-5 %
Athletes	14-20 %	6-13 %
Fitness	21-24 %	14-17 %
Average	25-31 %	18-24 %
Obese	32 % +	25 % +

Table 3: Ideal Body Fat Percentage

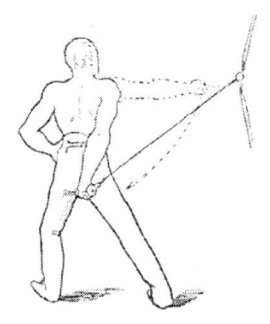

The above table gives standard values of body fat for different cases. Ideal for a male trainee would be 10-15 percent body-fat. But people can vary quite a bit and some athletes (i.e. Clarence Bass) have managed to get down into single figures.

Calculating your body-fat percentage is not easy, although the new electric scales can do a pretty good job by measuring body electrical impedance.

Remember everyone is different, and I would not use a table to completely determine my own goals for this reason. Also a better evaluator is often the bathroom mirror or simply your athletic capabilities as measured against requirements. Use the table as one of several fitness indicators appropriate to yourself.

Another possible method from which to judge your current physical condition is the taking of body measurements. Let us begin with bodyweight. In his book, the natural bodybuilder Steve Reeves gave the previously listed Table 2 for an ideal bodyweight.

I am not sure what type of athlete Steve is talking about here; (he was a bodybuilder) and so perhaps we can assume he was talking about someone with a significant amount of muscle. The table seems to work well for me, I am 6 feet 3 inches tall (with heavy musculature), and I have noticed that my best bodyweight is around 230 lbs.

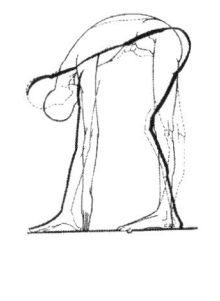

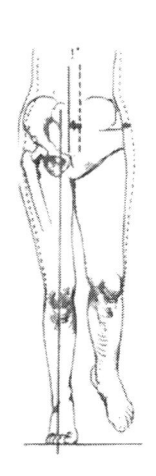

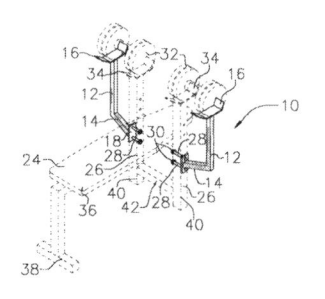

Rather than use this table however, I would be inclined to use one of the on-line "Grecian Ideal" calculators that takes a wrist measurement, and as output gives ideal body-part measurements. Often these take into account variations in bone structure, but be aware that resultant ideal body-weights can still vary by around 10 - 15 lbs. Any one of these assessment methods can be useful to a person who wants to create the ideal proportionate and symmetrical physique.

But ideals are simply not attainable for everyone due to genetic limitations and other factors.

We are all aware of the different types of physique; for example of the long distance runner, weightlifter and swimmer etc. Perhaps it is a better approach to emulate an athlete who is involved in a sport that you are also participating in. Or rather choose an athlete who seems to have a build similar to your own, or one that you think is achievable for you, and then find out his/her measurements, and go for that look.

The reason we have focussed on appearance, bodyweight and measurements in this section is that these relate to some of the most basic elements of fitness. It would seem sensible to be aware of what one's body should be like in the most general way, before focussing in on weak points and on which particular elements of fitness you would like to improve.

As discussed, fitness has many elements, and your own capabilities and goals will be somewhat unique. You will also have to formulate a top-level plan in order to achieve any desired changes. And there are many routes and methods to achieving those same goals.

The present book is obviously about improving those elements of fitness that dumbbell training can be used to improve. And dumbbells are, in fact, a very efficient way to improve many of the elements of fitness, including muscular strength, flexibility and coordination etc.

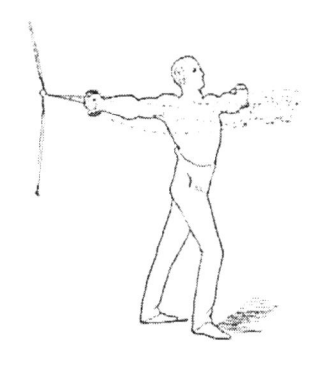

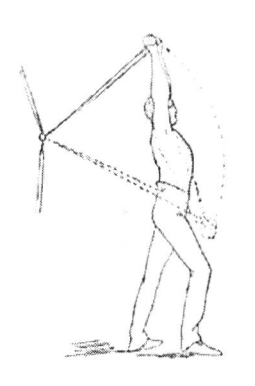

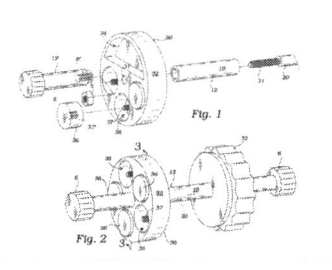

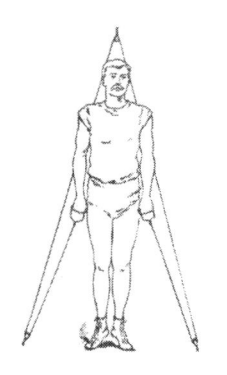

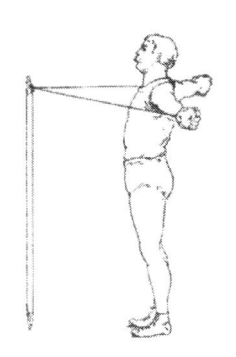

But I advise getting yourself close to your ideal bodyweight before beginning a serious weight-training program. Look at the above table, and make a visual assessment of your naked body, and decide if you are within 15-20 pounds of your ideal bodyweight. Here I am talking about over-weight individuals.

If you are over-weight then I advise embarking on a program of daily cardiovascular exercise (walking/running/swimming for 60 minutes (combined) per day). Join this approach with a natural-foods and low-fat diet, low in sugar, and in order to bring your bodyweight close to the ideal.

Over-weight individuals should do no weight-training until they are within about 20-30 pounds of their ideal weight. Remember also that it is not really possible - or safe - to loose more than 2 lbs per week.

Consider that the table of ideal bodyweight does not account for differences in bone-structure. So if you are thin-boned subtract 10 pounds from the calculated figure, and if you are heavy-boned add 10 pounds. A long distance runner or another type of endurance athlete, would perhaps want to subtract as much as 10 - 40 lbs from the figures given in table 2.

It is you and nobody else who must decide what is your ideal body form, from the perspective of health and fitness, and in order to meet daily physical challenges and requirements. Remember that if you have any doubts about your capability to exercise safely, then get a doctor's checkup before embarking on an exercise program (in fact do so anyway).

Later in this book we shall recommend various dumbbell exercises, and show standard movement

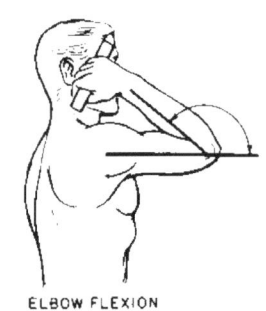

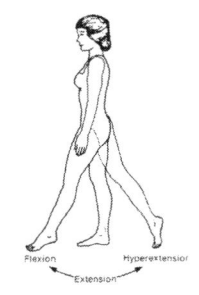

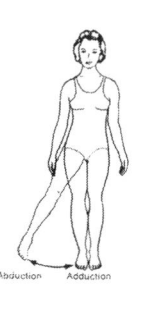

ELBOW FLEXION

patterns for the same. You will notice that we have gone to great lengths to explain exercise form and so movement performance in sufficient detail. We have done so in part because we think that knowledge of dumbbell usage is today very poor, on average.

And many people are simply not aware of the great diversity of training exercises and methods that are possible using only a dumbbell and perhaps an incline bench. But do not be fooled into thinking that everyone would be able to do each and every one of these exercises, or that everyone can even attempt to do them. We are all unique, with differing physical structures, including individual strengths and limitations. As a result, every individual's program of exercise will be singular. This uniqueness extends to choice of exercises, movement patterns, frequency of exercise and especially the weights lifted.

Myself I am a big believer in working all of the different elements of fitness, thus performing exercises for strength, flexibility (ROM) and also cardiovascular capability. I believe that everyone who can, should run or walk each day, because moving from A to B is the fundamental human activity.

Listen to your heart before taking advice from others; and always test out ideas before accepting them into your own body of knowledge. [2] Remember also, that exercise and fitness systems are supposed to be personalised and fun, but not torture! If it really hurts - then something is wrong.

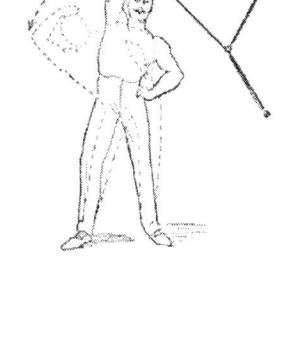

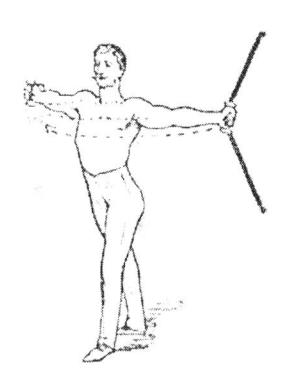

---

[2] N.B. It is prudent to get a Doctor's approval before embarking on any exercise regime.

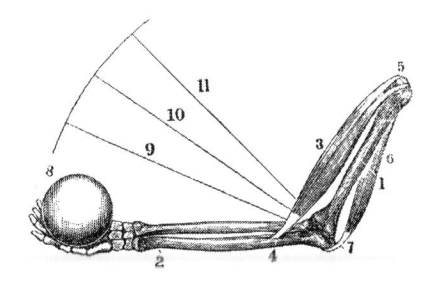

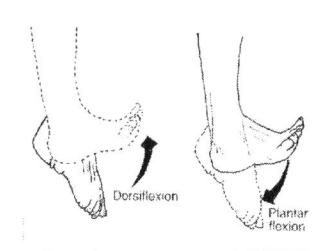

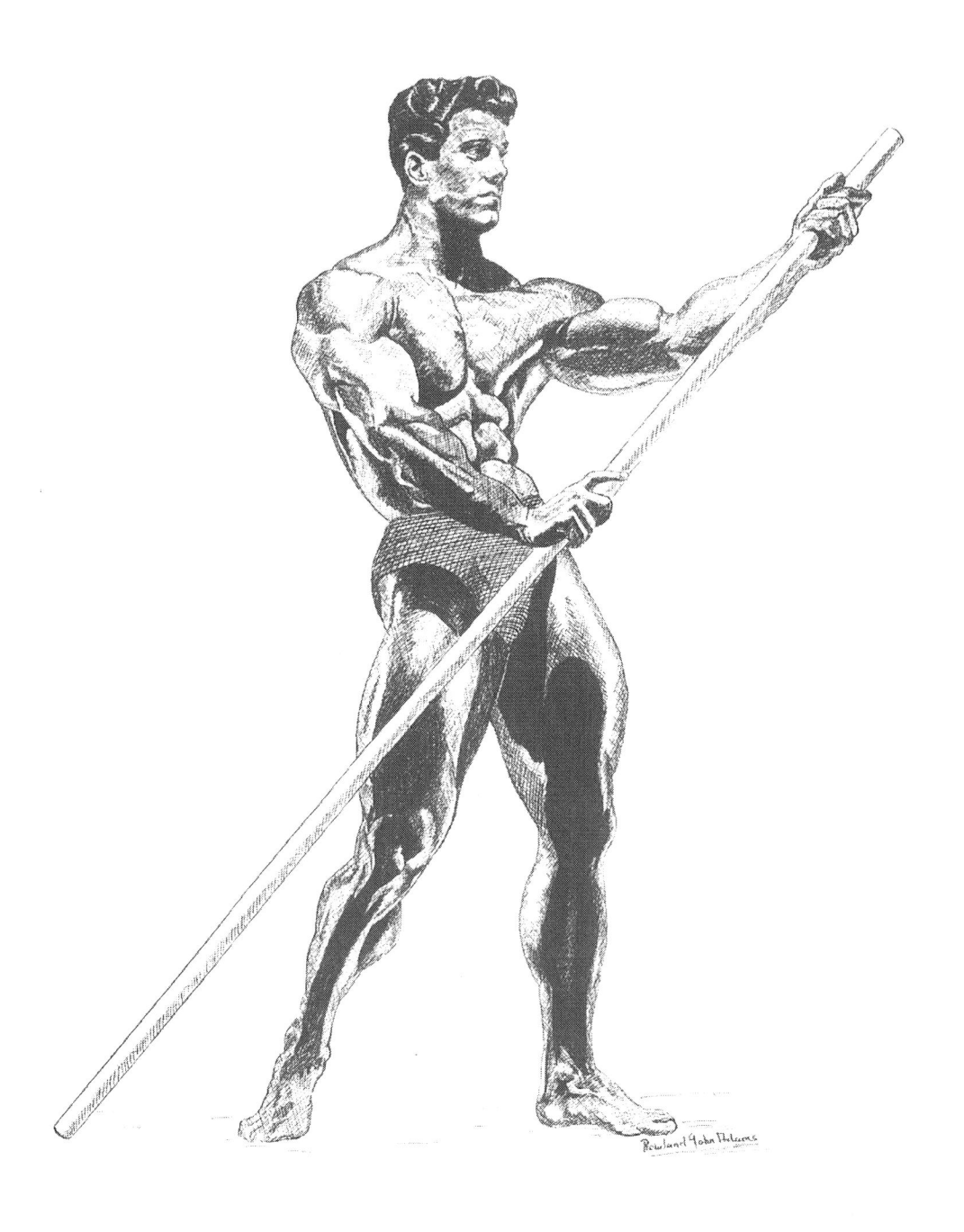

Diet

BODYWEIGHT AND body-fat percentage are the first items to work on in most people. And it's not rocket-science to get to the correct weight (N.B for some people it may take some time - even up to 1 year to approach an ideal body-weight, and especially if you are overweight).

How do you get to an ideal bodyweight? Simply calculate how many pounds over or under-weight you are and work to adjust your weight accordingly. Since most people who are past the teenage years want to loose weight, a few simple calculations can point the way ahead.

For every 1 lb that you want to loose you will need to take in approximately 3500 calories less than your body burns. This is called being in a calorific or energy deficit. An example is the best way to explain this.

Let's say you are 10 lbs overweight and wish to loose that in 5 weeks. That's a loss of 2 lbs a week or 2 * 3500 / 6 = 1167 calories per day deficit. An energy deficit of 1167 calories per day is quite allot to attain, but it is not impossible. It is best to split this up into taking in 600 calories less each day (dieting), and exercising to burn up the other 500 or so calories.

Now it turns out that if you weigh 200 lbs and do 30 minutes of vigorous weight-training, then that will burn up 275 calories. And 30 minutes of running will burn up 370 calories - totalling around 640 calories burned. So you can easily loose the weight if you follow this program 6 days per week. After 5 weeks you should end up around 10 pounds lighter. Nice and simple, I think you will agree.

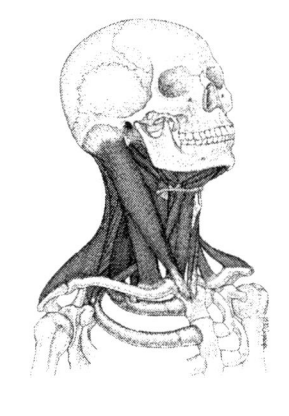

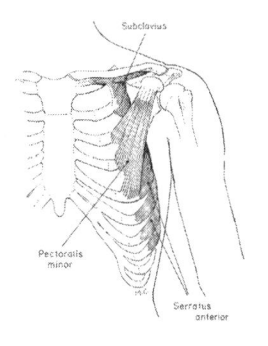

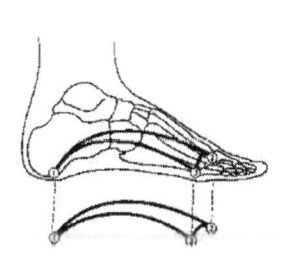

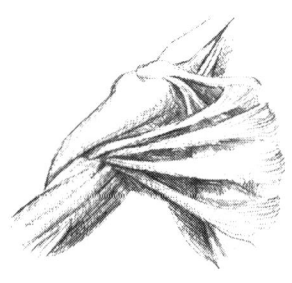

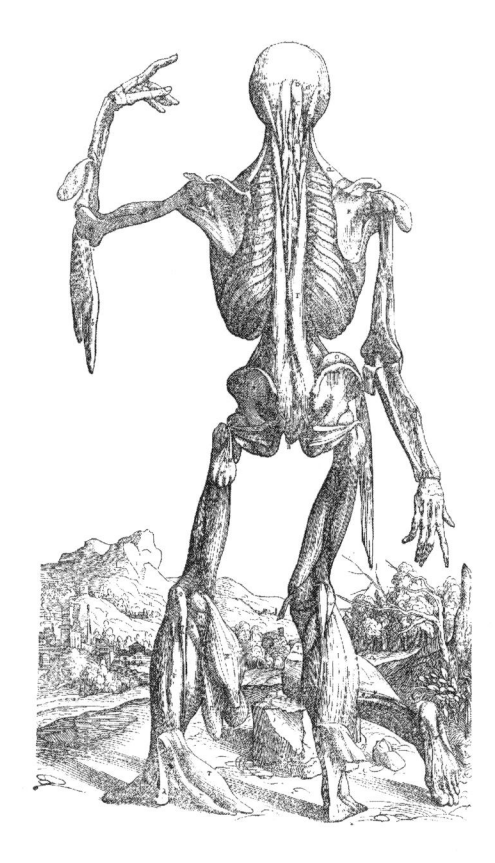

Although such a "simplistic" approach can work, others have spoken about the need for certain individuals to address their unusual metabolic condition, and specifically in order to loose fat.

Writer Gary Taubes speaks about carbohydrate as a driver (that is a cause) of excessive body-fat, and in his view we should restrict carbohydrates (refined and simple sugars) to obtain an ideal body-weight. I think that Gary has a point, and it is a good idea to avoid excessive refined carbohydrates (mostly sugar) to attain an optimal body-weight. However remember that athletes often require larger amounts of carbohydrates for energy.

Gaining weight (that is lean muscle) is more difficult than losing fat, and there are many factors that determine a person's success rate in meeting any goal in this respect. Normally it is a youth (12-18 years old) who needs, and wants to, gain muscular bodyweight.

There are obviously different ways of gaining muscle - both healthy and the unhealthy (drug) methods. We recommend natural methods, and taking your time. Try to gain no more than 5-10 lbs of muscle each year, and by use of a wide range of exercises, a high protein diet and lots of rest and relaxation when you are not training.

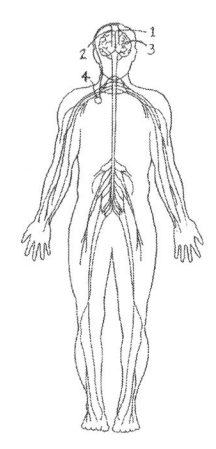

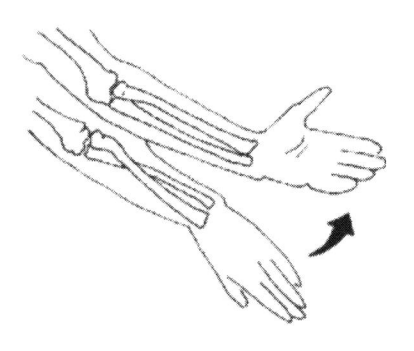

Weight-gainers should also avoid excessive restriction of exercise variety. Employ a wide variety of movements to develop flexibility (ROM), coordination and to develop a balanced and proportionate physique. More on that later on.

Now we are not going to get into the details of dieting or nutritional calculations here, because there are many excellent books on those topics. However it is important to note that if you do go on a specialised diet, be sure that you get the correct amounts of macronutrients and also micronutrients. Often supplements can help here. Perhaps the best bodybuilding and fitness supplement to come along in recent years is whey protein.

Mother's milk is around 60-80 percent whey proteins, and so whey is the most natural and easily digestible protein that is available for humans. I strongly urge you to use whey. If you do, then you will find yourself looking and feeling better when taking 2-3 scoops of whey each day. Another diet tip is to drink lots of water, and to eat plenty of fruits and vegetables. Shun all sweet products, and anything that contains white flour - and especially sugar.

In my experience, making and drinking raw vegetable juices can help the trainee with progress. The juices are health promoting and can really help you to attain super fitness. Finally, I urge you to read everything you can about diet and its relation to health and fitness, and especially books by Clarence Bass, Bruce Lee, Bill Pearl, Frank Zane etc.

Once again remember to take what the nutritional scientists say with a pinch of salt, because they have recently completely changed their minds on what constitutes a healthy diet. Previously they had been down on fats of all kinds, but now it seems that simple sugars and trans-fats are the ones to be avoided at all costs.

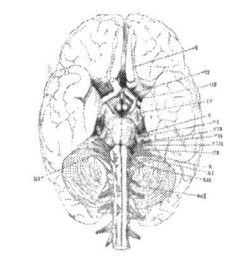

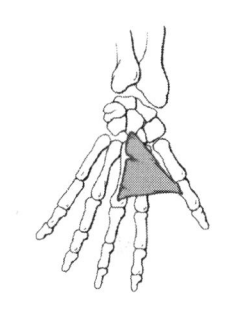

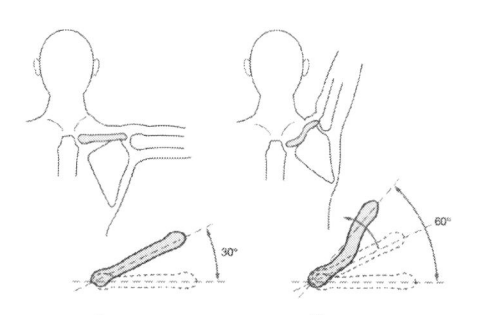

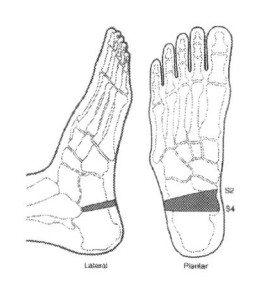

50 ZEN OF DUMBBELL TRAINING

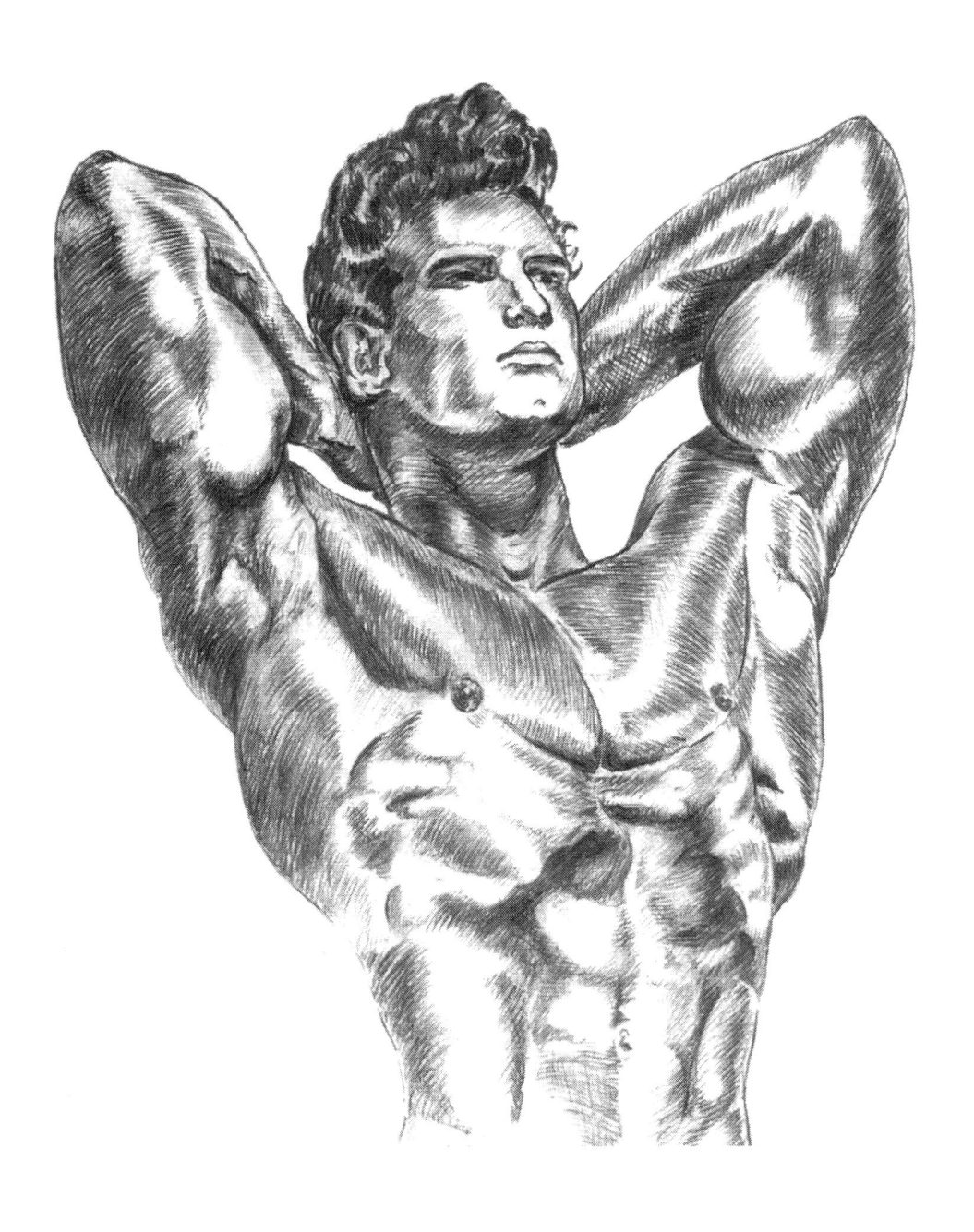

Yoga

SOME TIME ago, and right in the middle of a workout, a friend said to me "You know that weight-training is a form of Yoga". At once these words struck me as true; yet full of mystery and contradictions.

If you look into the history of exercise, then you will find that Yoga is the oldest system known, being perhaps 5000 - 10,000 years old. It is also one of the most developed of the disciplines, in philosophical terms, also being a direct ancestor to every known Physical Culture method, including weight-training.

The most well-known form of Yoga in the Western culture relates to the practice of Asana postures, and it is a discipline of the body. Here one adopts rules and postures to keep the body disease-free and to preserve the vital energy. You can think of Yoga as being the means and tools to realign and rebalance the body.

Yoga is a well-developed system of exercise (postures), that can lead you to a sense of peace and well-being, and it also develops a feeling of "being at one" with the environment. The ultimate aim is self-development and self-realisation. And because your body is finely tuned you will perhaps find that your chances for injuries and illnesses will drop; as you are in a much more attuned state.

As you continue with yoga practice, you may notice other changes in your body.

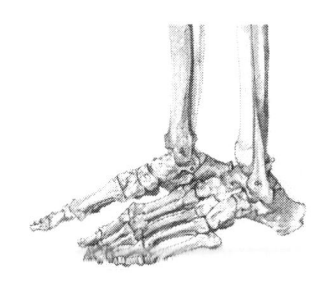

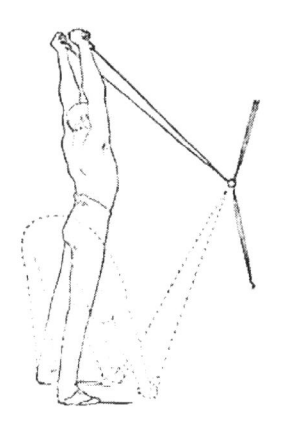

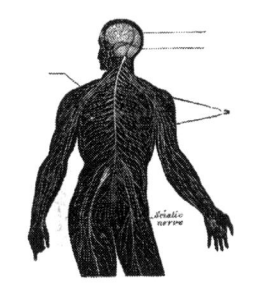

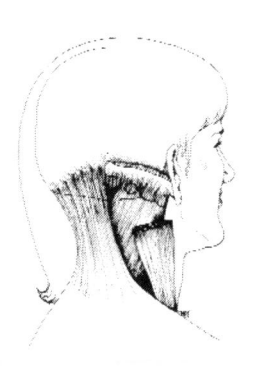

Maybe your legs are more flexible, or your shoulders less tense. Your posture may be better or your breathing more relaxed. When this starts to happen, you have begun to *integrate* what you've learned into your body. Plus as you become more aware of how you are functioning physically, you may become more conscious of your emotions and how they affect your body.

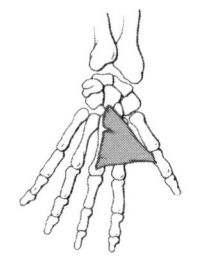

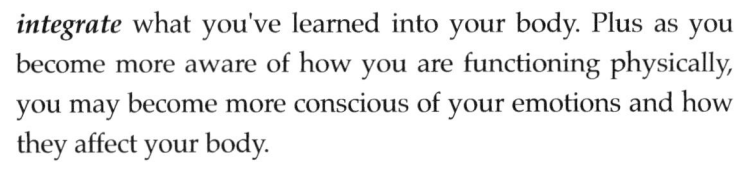

Without this type of integration, we tend to live with underlying fear, anger, or sadness. With this integration, we create more beauty, more awareness, more elevated consciousness, more love. Part of the aim of "Zen" dumbbell training is to likewise benefit from this type of integration of training "knowledge" or capability into your daily life - and hence obtain useful benefits in terms of a new sense of physical and mental well-being.

Over the years I have taken quite a few Yoga classes. And even though my large frame and heavy musculature prevented me from attaining anything more than average levels of flexibility (in terms of Yoga postures), I did notice benefits from this form of physical culture. In particular I found that the Yoga exercises gave me a strong sense of the position of my spine, limbs and torso in everyday life, and especially when moving about. It was as if I had a wider number of body positions to choose from when moving. The same leads to a great relaxation of effort when walking, changing body-positions and/or articulating limbs.

Similarly, properly performed "Zen" dumbbell training increases the number - and choice of - movement paths that you can perform; leading to relaxed and effortless life postures.

More on the links between dumbbell training and Yoga later. But remember that weight-training = Yoga!

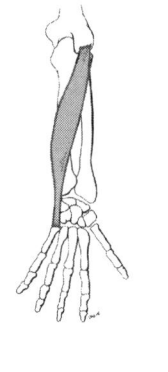

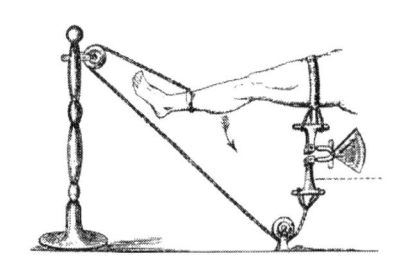

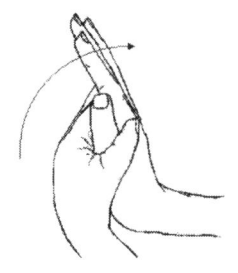

Law of Harmony

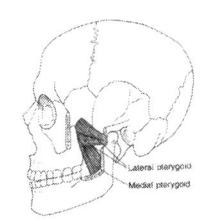

ZEN IS the process of meditation and its results in consciousness or, in some way, super-consciousness. It also relates to the process of going beyond thought and "self" and becoming enlightened by satori, that is, seeing right into something to penetrate its true nature.

Zen refers to finding something quite new which is known with great clarity, and which illuminates the whole of life. In view of all the problems experienced by trainees, and as related in the introduction, it is clear that exercise enlightenment is badly needed by today's trainees. But how can the principles of zen have any practical bearing on something as "physically real" as dumbbell training?

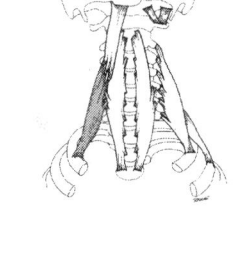

My answer relates to the principle of Yin and Yang. These are the well-known Chinese principles that are said to underly reality, being positive and negative, male and female etc. They are said to unite the world, in processes of life and death, and action and thought.

The principle is expressed in the Law of Harmony.

It states that there should be harmony with, and not rebellion against, the strength and force of opposing forces. This means that one should not do anything that is not natural or spontaneous. And the important thing is not to strain in any way when facing any challenge in life.

When lifting a heavy weight for example, one should not over-strain in any way - but find a path of movement which seems most natural and which takes the least effort to achieve.

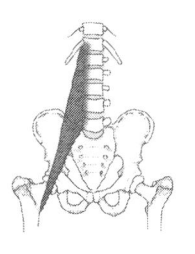

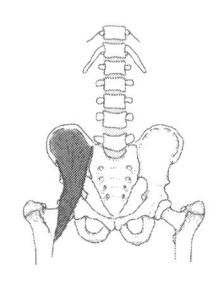

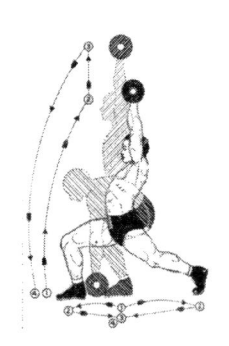

With harmonious training, one listens to the body, in real time and especially during the exercise movement itself. You are mindful of what all of the different parts of the body are up to. Watching, feeling and listening to the body is essential, whilst all-the-time paying close attention to the limbs, spine, muscles, and joints.

It's all about feelings as opposed to thinking.

In fact the listening goes far beyond the ordinary sensation, and relates even to the choice and frequency of exercises, plus factors like weight selection, location of body, gym choice, footwear, mood, training partner, clothing, etc. We shall come back to these details as and when we deal with training techniques in later chapters.

The Law of Harmony gives rise to a closely related law, the law of non-interference with nature, which teaches a trainee to forget about himself, and to follow the weight being lifted instead of his own body (solely). He/she does so to ensure that he/she does not move ahead, but responds to the fitting influence.

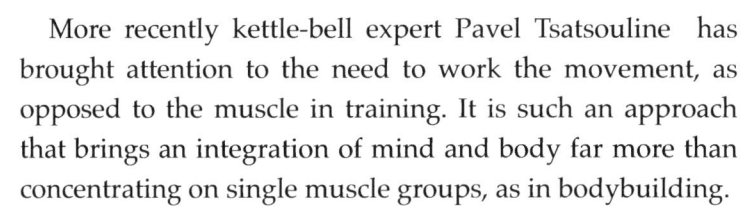

More recently kettle-bell expert Pavel Tsatsouline has brought attention to the need to work the movement, as opposed to the muscle in training. It is such an approach that brings an integration of mind and body far more than concentrating on single muscle groups, as in bodybuilding.

The basic idea is to lift the weight by yielding to the path of least resistance, when it comes to the force of gravity, and so (in real-time) to find one's own movement pattern, being the one that seems most natural.

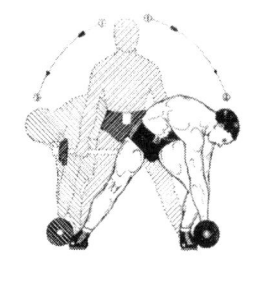

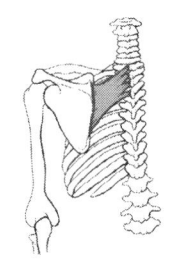

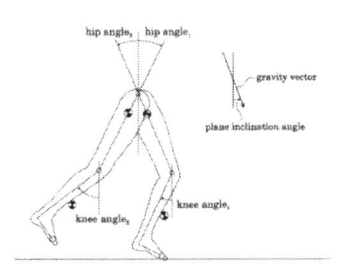

The concept here is in direct opposition to that dictated by most of today's western trainers, who instruct us in the one ideal way to move, being a movement pattern which is the same for everyone (more or less).

In zen dumbbell training there is no such thing as an ideal movement path that is known and can be told from one person to another. Because if there was it would be too complex to convey in any case. Rather one has to discover the movement path himself, through mindful training and constant practice.

In zen training, despite the fact that you are lifting a weight with positive force (yang), you must at the same time, and on a moment by moment basis, yield to and find, the yin path through softness of movement and pliability. And so the body is not held in too rigid a stance, but is held in a kind of loose-tension or tense-looseness. The movement of weights in zen dumbbell training is closely related to the movement of the mind. The mind is trained to direct the body, but not in an unnatural way. Constant feedback from the body is listened to as the movement progresses. A certain degree of physical and mental loosening is required to make it work - and to allow the mind to be not only agile but free. When lifting dumbbells, do not concentrate on merely the position of the dumbbell in space, and do not simply focus on the primary muscle(s) involved. Rather be aware of all aspects at once, being the position/tension of every body-part - and which muscles are held firm, semi-firm and/or soft at each moment.

The zen devotee employs his mind as a mirror, it grasps nothing, and it refuses nothing, it receives but does not keep. You want to act in a like manner as you exercise. There is nothing special to try to do, just let the movement happen, for whatever comes up moment by moment is accepted. Try to employ the whole mind, just as we use the

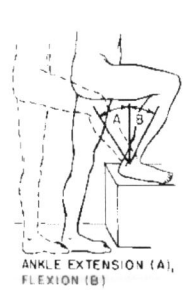

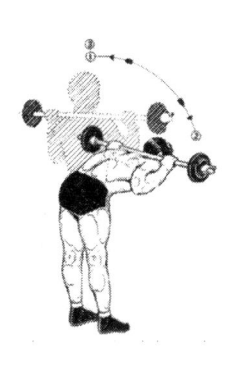

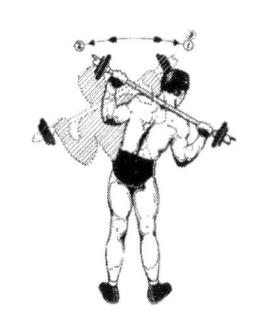

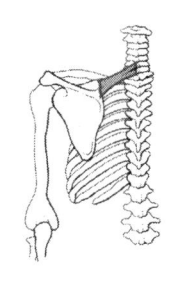

ANKLE EXTENSION (A), FLEXION (B)

eyes when we look at various objects all-at-once but do not fix on any one in particular.

The trainee forgets about himself and follows the movement of the weight, leaving the mind to make its own movements without any interfering deliberation. As soon as he stops to think, the flow of movement will be disturbed and he is immediately in danger of being dominated by the weight and loosing "the groove" or path of least resistance.

Do not worry if my description of Zen Training seems a bit esoteric or else is difficult to achieve right away. It is a training philosophy that you need to practice to understand. Plus you don't necessarily have to become a believer in each and every aspect of the method. You can pick and choose those aspects that interest you and apply them individually. You will still see important physical and mental benefits even by applying just a few of these techniques - of that I am confident. In conclusion, Zen Dumbbell Training takes the middle path when it comes to weight-training; whereby the trainee selects a not-too-heavy weight; and proceeds to lift without excessive speed or strain. You must open up to the feelings of the movement in all of its different aspects. It's a matter of listening to the body to the fullest degree possible, and opening oneself up to constant feedback from muscles, joints, ligaments, and the bones etc.

And above all; training should be both fun and refreshing to partake in; and after the workout is over you should feel like you could do it all over again if required (an old Steve Reeve's comment). Zen Dumbbell Training leaves you energised, glowing, massaged and reborn anew.

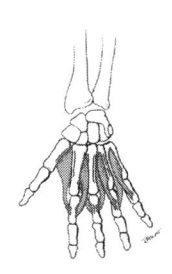

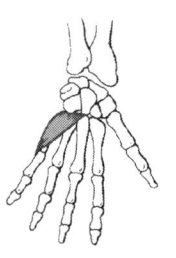

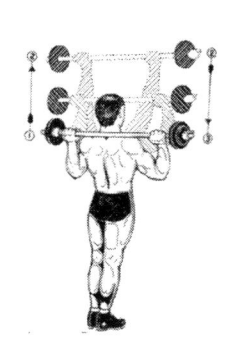

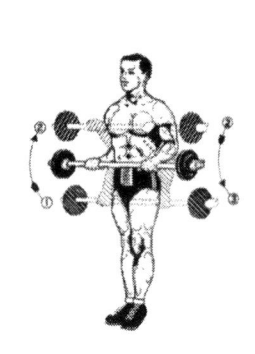

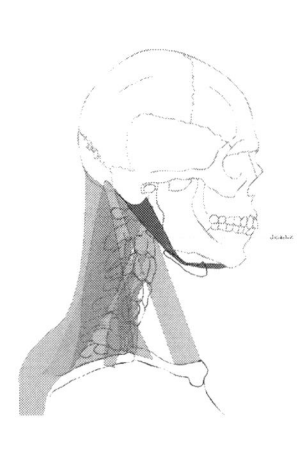

CHAPTER FOUR
Training Systems

A STATED aim of this book is to identify the most efficient training system. And what could that be apart from an amalgamation of the best parts of the many other systems that are already known.

I am not talking about simply throwing together various unconnected features from these different systems.

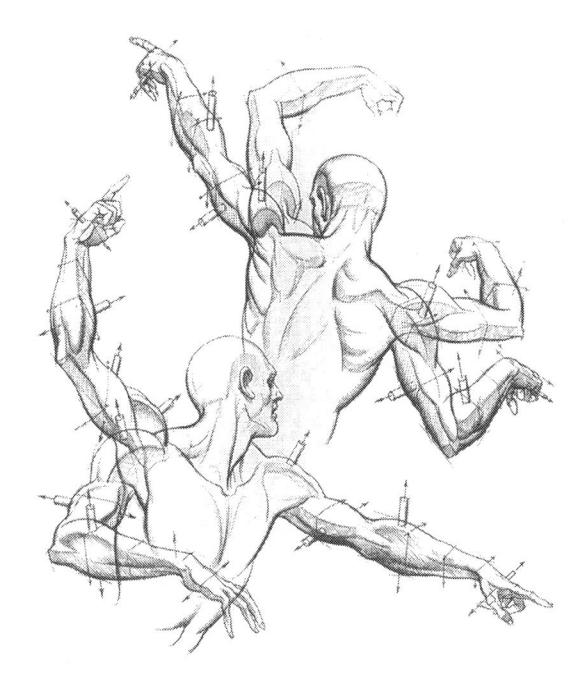

Rather we aim to develop a new system which takes the best elements of the old, and then looks at these anew and systemises them in light of the present dumbbell training method. In this respect if a principle fits, then we take it and absorb it into our practice, and if not, we leave it alone. In what follows much of the information comes from the original literature, but some has come down by means of personal meetings with coaches and trainees from a variety of disciplines.

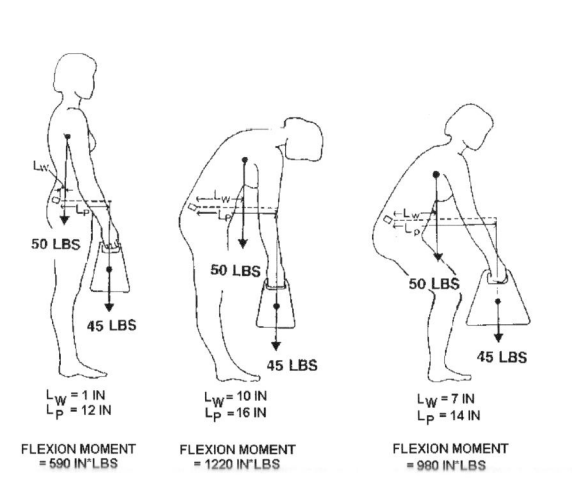

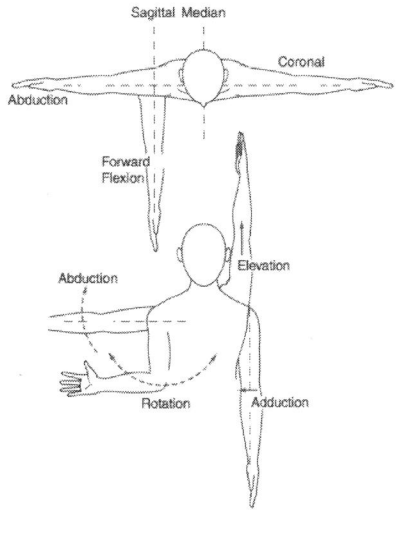

50 LBS
45 LBS
$L_W = 1$ IN
$L_P = 12$ IN
FLEXION MOMENT = 590 IN*LBS

50 LBS
45 LBS
$L_W = 10$ IN
$L_P = 16$ IN
FLEXION MOMENT = 1220 IN*LBS

50 LBS
45 LBS
$L_W = 7$ IN
$L_P = 14$ IN
FLEXION MOMENT = 980 IN*LBS

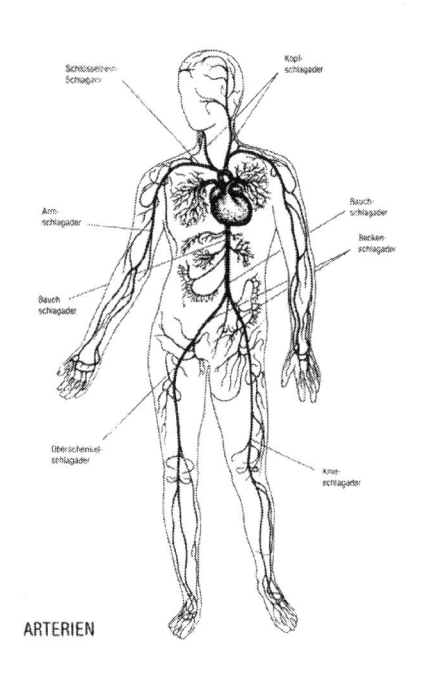

Unfortunately, and due to space limitations, not all of the various systems and/or techniques are represented. The following should thus be taken more as an introduction, rather than a comprehensive guide to all of the different kinds of training systems that are possible.

Historical discussion gives insight into the development of dumbbell training and healthful exercise in general. An interesting aside relates to the human body as a mechanical machine. It was Arthur Jones who (I think) first called the body a rotary machine, pointing out that in order to press a barbell overhead (for example), the body uses 3 circular motions to achieve such a lift. In a shoulder press, required rotation is about the joints of the shoulder, elbow and wrist. Here a linear motion is achieved by three rotary motions.

Arthur said that all human movements were similarly combinations of circular motions, and on this point he was quite correct and also being somewhat profound. I don't think many people (even today) would be aware of - or be able to visualise - such combined circular-motions. And neither do many people take any interest in how human anatomy works. I think this ambivalence is a mistake, because a major tenant of the present book is that you must become your own personal trainer. Because nobody else knows, or feels, what is going on in your body, its responses, and limitations, like you do. It is my belief that ultimate athletic excellence requires good (functional) knowledge of human physiology by the athlete himself; hence all of the anatomical and movement information provided in this book.

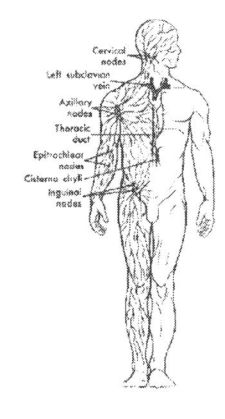

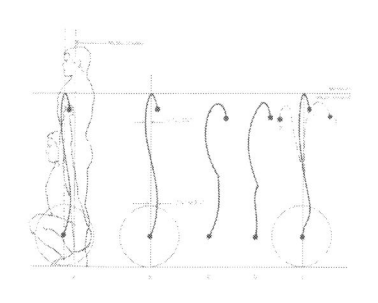

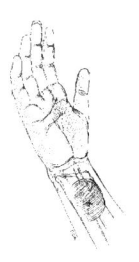

Ancient Systems

MEN HAVE long been interested in finding ways to improve the health and strength of the human body. David Webster in *Bodybuilding: An Illustrated History*, and also myself in *The Illustrated History of Physical Culture*, have examined this topic in depth.

Early peoples noticed that those who lifted heavy objects became stronger and developed an improved musculature. In Greece we see the first examples of dumbbells - also called Halteres - which were often used by swinging them to allow the athletes to jump further.

Ancient athletes tended to specialise, just as they do today, into strength and endurance based events. It is worth noting that the Ancient Greeks believed that it was a young man's scared duty to develop his mind and body to the highest possible degree. And such a balanced development of qualities was named "Arete".

Arete refers to a man's total worth as a human being, to his physical and mental capabilities, his level of vital force, his degree of training, and readiness for war. But it relates also to intelligence, kindness, morality and even to his capability as a teacher and musician etc.

The Ancient Greeks believed in the saying: *a sound mind in a sound body*, and so in a holistic concept of health.

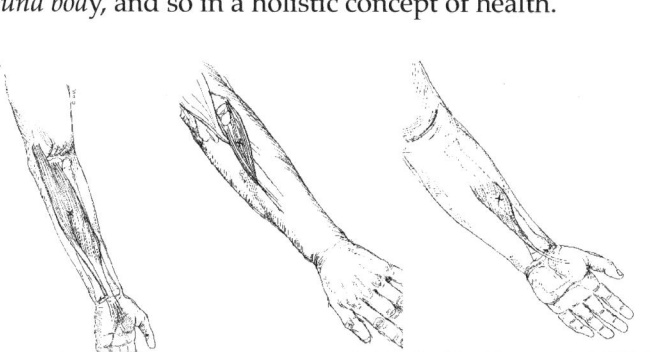

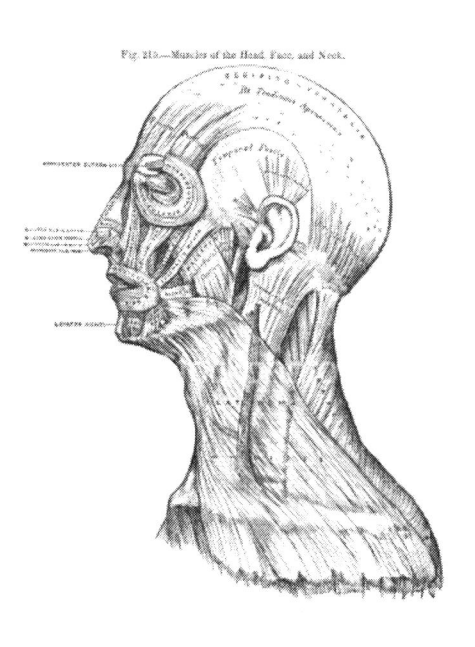

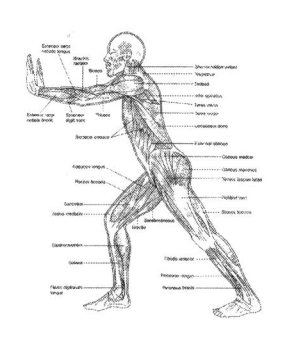

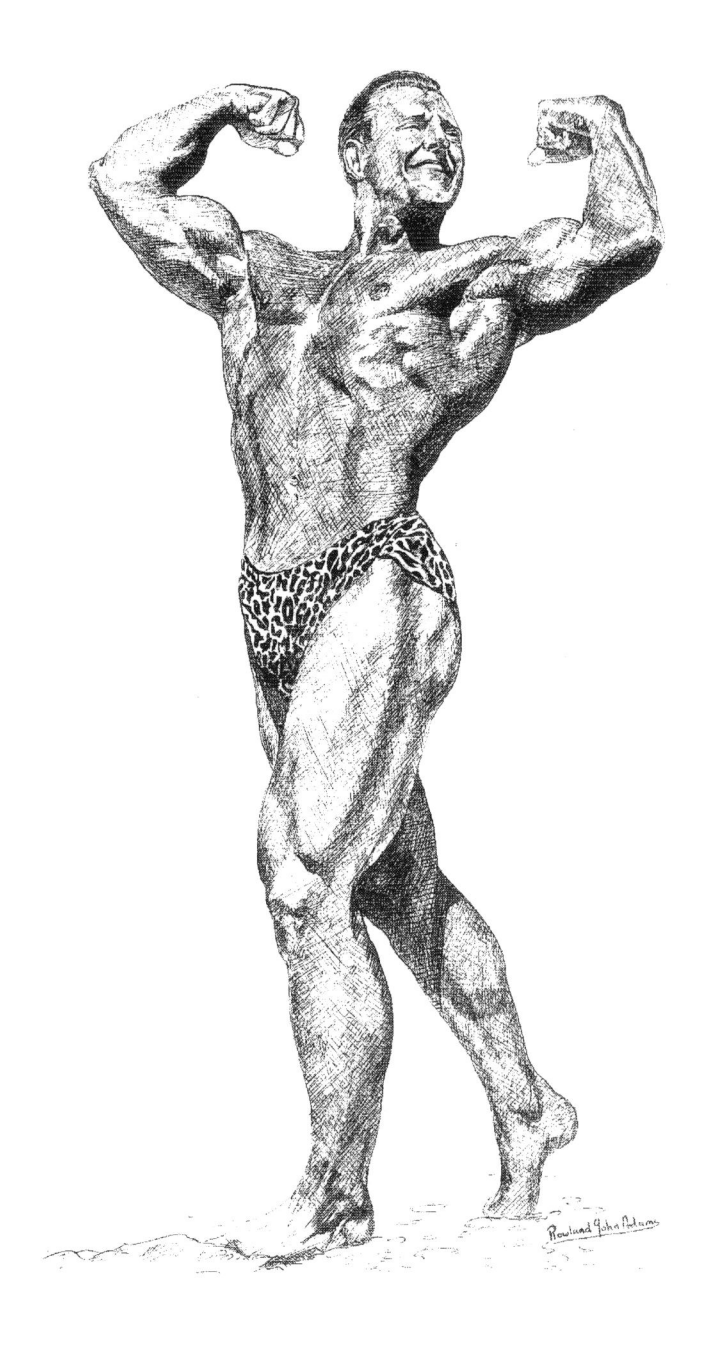

Early European Systems

DURING THE middle ages knights developed strong bodies for war by wielding swords, axes and other heavy implements. Later in 1587 the Italian Physician Mercurialis published his *De Arte Gymnastica*, which contained illustrations and descriptions of physical exercises and also bodybuilding exercises.

In the 16th and 17th centuries others began to popularise the athletic lifestyle including gymnastics, wrestling and running. Sometimes systems were taught at schools and universities, and at other times in private institutes and home gymnasia. In particular Pehr Ling taught his pupils how to perfect the body using gymnastics and apparatus which he then used to create a unique and effective system. Around 1850, victorian Englishmen began a *Physical Culture* craze in which all kinds athletic sports and healthful fitness activities became popular. In 1859 the Oxford University Gymnasium was opened for the first time, and Triat's gym in France was also active in this period. Both gyms had all kinds of trapeze, and pommel horses, plus dumbbell training was very much in evidence.

As the 20th century dawned a whole range of different types of Physical Culture became common, including athletics, football, running swimming, cycle-riding and weight-training or bodybuilding. As today, each sport had its own famous athletes, well-known adherents, marketers and stars.

Perhaps the most famous turn of the century Physical Culturist was Eugene Sandow.

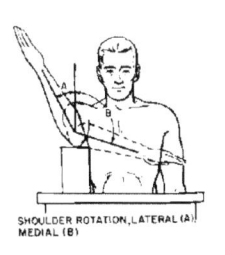

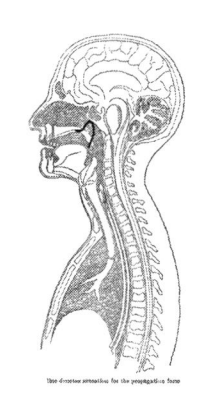

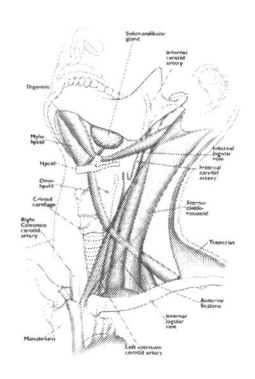

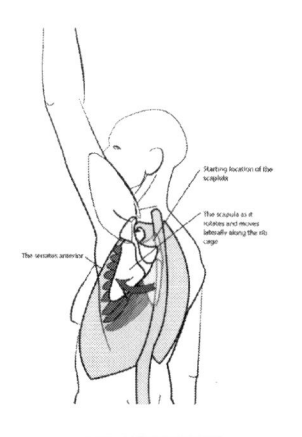

FINGER STRENGTH

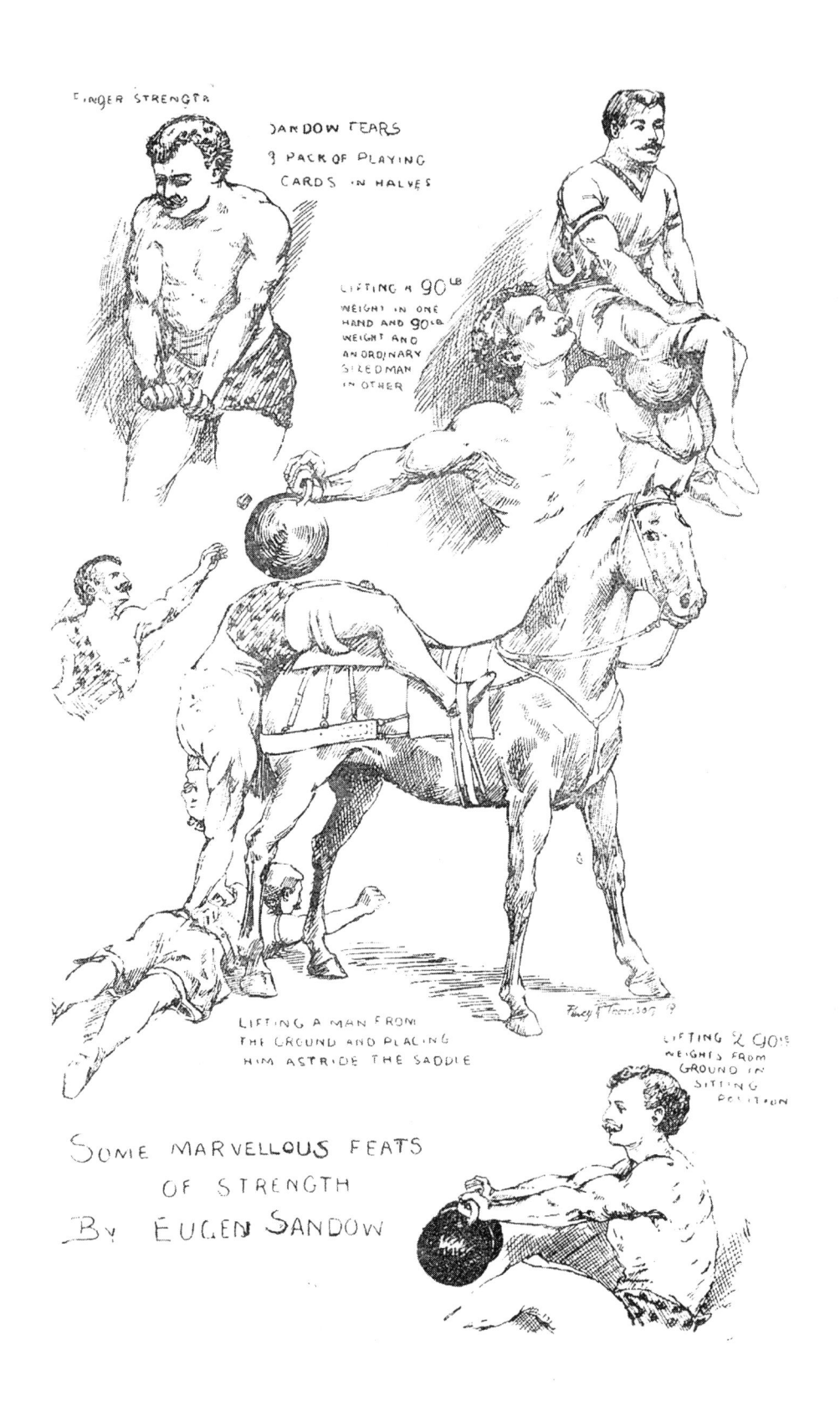

SANDOW TEARS
A PACK OF PLAYING
CARDS IN HALVES

LIFTING A 90 LB
WEIGHT IN ONE
HAND AND 90 LB
WEIGHT AND
AN ORDINARY
SIZED MAN
IN OTHER

LIFTING A MAN FROM
THE GROUND AND PLACING
HIM ASTRIDE THE SADDLE

LIFTING 2 90 LB
WEIGHTS FROM
GROUND IN
SITTING
POSITION

SOME MARVELLOUS FEATS
OF STRENGTH
BY EUGEN SANDOW

Eugene Sandow

EUGENE SANDOW [1867-1925] is today remembered as the first bodybuilder. Sandow was a vaudeville star, a health-club/gymnasium chain owner, and he wrote and sold books and special "grip" dumbbells, plus expander sets.

He was also the first moving picture star when he posed for Thomas Edison's movie camera. Famous right across the world, Sandow was a multi-millionaire known to stand at the centre of the Physical Culture mania and he was its chief proponent and evangelist on a world-wide basis.

What made him world famous was his incredibly defined and muscular physique, combined with the wherewithal to be able to market it to the general public in both England and the USA. And he was a forerunner of the future, in this respect.

How Sandow obtained his muscles is shaded in mystery. But we do know that he was a practiced gymnast in his youth, and that background might very well have been responsible for much of his natural muscular development. Nevertheless we also know that he practised heavy weightlifting moves later on, which would have developed his muscles to full maturity.

The reason we say that his muscles are shaded in mystery is because the so-called *Sandow System* of exercise, which was much advertised, consisted mostly of exercising with very light dumbbells (2-5 lbs). He also sometimes railed against the use of heavy weights. The exercise drawings shown on these pages form part of the famous *Sandow System*. Note the details depicted; including supination and pronation of wrist, plus hand and foot positions etc.

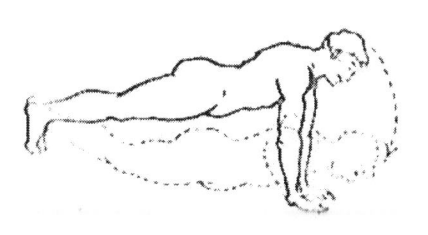

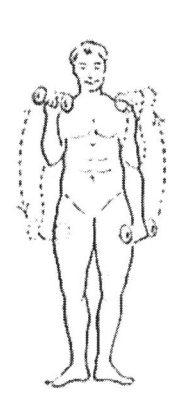

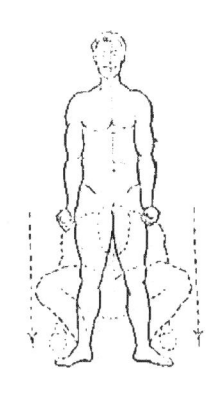

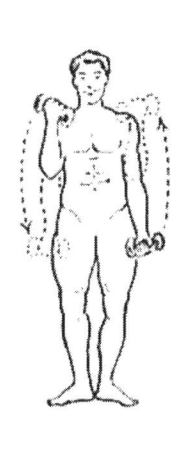

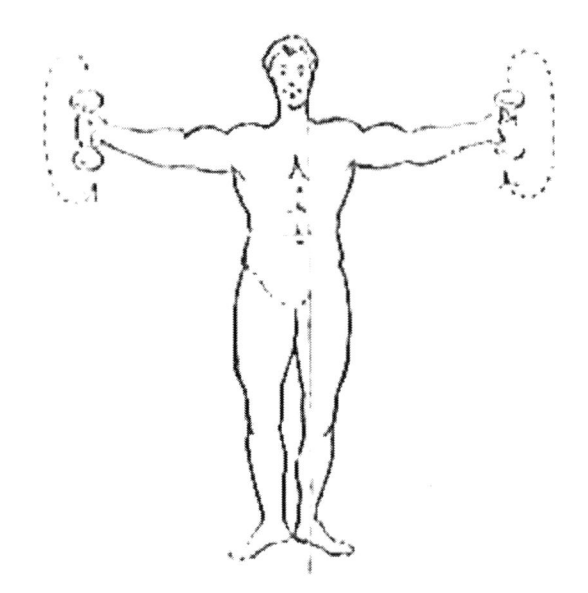

Nevertheless perhaps he let his true feelings out in *Sandow's System of Physical Training* published in 1894:

The system I specially commend, is dumbbell and barbell exercise, **and for beginners especially***, of very light weights ... Nothing, in my opinion, however, is better than the use of the dumbbell, for developing the* **whole** *system, particularly if it is used intelligently, and with a knowledge of the location and function of the muscles ... it will surprise how much can be done and what a vast complexity of muscles can be brought into play ..*

Sandow continues:

It has been said that the muscular system of a man is not made up alone of chest and bicep; yet to expand one and enlarge the other is almost all that is thought of by the untrained learner. It is also foolishly supposed that this is the limit of work to be done by the dumbbell .. but there is hardly a muscle that cannot be effectively reached by the system of dumbbell exercise which I use .. and .. all exercises should be performed on the ground, as nature intended .. man to stand erect ..

This quote is quite a telling one, especially when he calls novices "foolish" who stick to exercising chest and bicep muscles alone. It seems that the trainees of today are making the very same mistake, in particular when they stick to a few sets of curls or bench presses, and leave it at that.

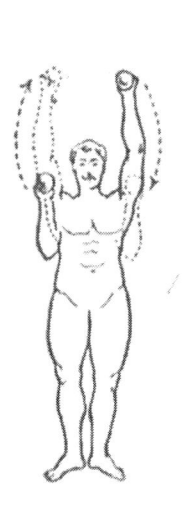

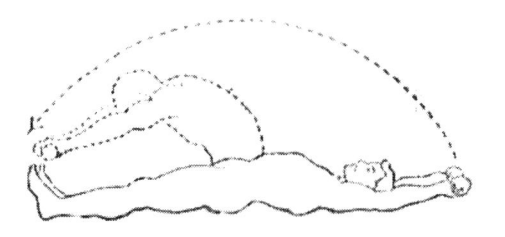

Sandow believed in developing *"grace and symmetry of form"* and in obtaining *"uniform and harmonious development"*. He also talked about *"intelligent methods of physical training"*. Sandow recommended that a wide-range of dumbbell exercises be performed, and he believed that only the simplest of equipment (the dumbbell) could produce the highest possible degree of physical development.

Sandow would undoubtably have disapproved of today's bench press fetish, because he believed that only the ill-informed trainee would focus on the accomplishment of one or two feats.

Rather than simply advertise his own abilities, Sandow was the first of the muscle pedlars, beginning the long-standing tradition of musclemen who sold their own methods, secrets and muscle-building courses and systems, and with which anyone might (supposedly) attain superior muscular development.

He is quoted as saying *"my system will enable even the weakest to attain a perfect physical development"*. As you can imagine this was of immense interest to all, and especially appealed to young men who wanted to attain the muscles of manhood sooner rather than later. In fact, most of the muscle-hucksters of the next 100 years or so, would claim that they had started out as relative weaklings, before embarking on a system of training which had in a short space of time transformed them into veritable supermen.

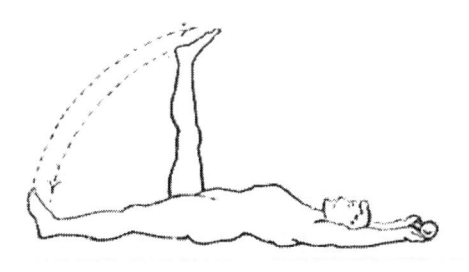

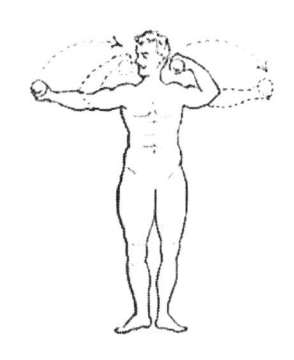

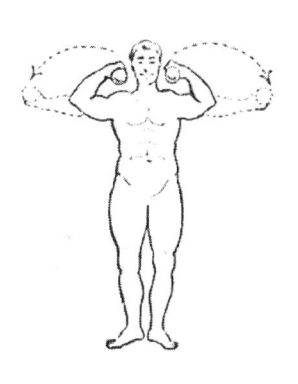

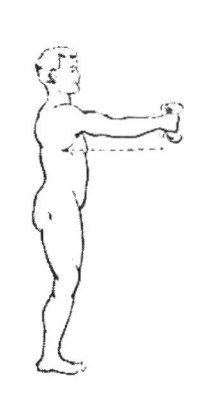

And there was often some truth in their claims. Because a skinny youth could, through **several years** of hard weight-lifting and put on 10-30 lbs or so of pure muscle and sinew. The latter progress would probably be made only by youths who were pre-pubescent when beginning a training regime, and so that much of the structural changes could be attributed to attainment of manhood. Nevertheless it was to a large extent true that muscles could be "grown" or developed with the help of adequate training.

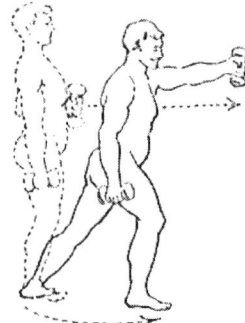

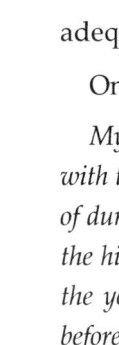

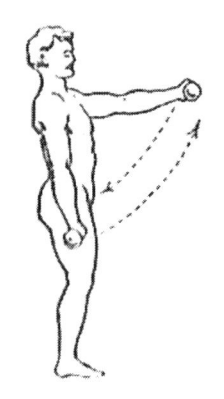

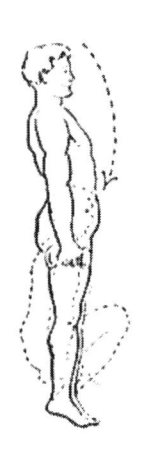

On training Sandow said:

My faith is pinned to dumbbells, and I do all of my training with their aid, supplemented by weightlifting .. by the constant use of dumbbells any man of average strength can bring his muscles to the highest possible development .. exercise, I would impress upon the young reader, ought to be taken in a well-ventilated place .. before proceeding to the movements proper, the pupil-in-training would do well to devote some little time to a number of exercises with dumbbells, so as to give suppleness to the limbs, and accustom himself to easy and well-balanced postures of the body .. and if thirty minutes cannot be given continuously to the exercises, perhaps fifteen can be snatched twice a day ..

the preliminary exercises with the dumbbells may now be entered upon. Those of immediate benefit are the movements tending to give free play to the muscles and joints which, in the later exercises, will be drawn more heavily into service; to relaxing and rendering them supple ..

On exercises (2-3 lbs dumbbells for ladies; men use 3-5 lbs):

A: The flexing, or bending, the hands inwards and outward upon the wrist; and rotating or turning it round, long enough until the muscles ache. B: Keeping the shoulders perfectly square, the body erect, the arms pendant and close to the sides, move the head slowly backwards and forwards, from side to side, and then roll it around the right and left, as far as possible. Now raise and

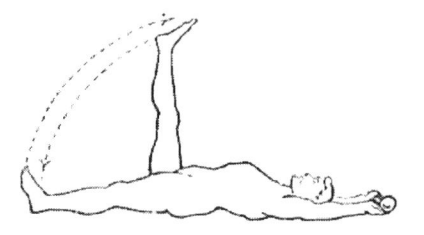

depress the shoulders, after which, elevate the arms at full length and in-line with the body, and rotate them in both directions until the muscles are tired. C: Resuming the attitude of attention, the dumbbells still in hand, rotate or twist the body on its hip-axis alternately to the left and right, keeping the back and legs straight during the movement, then sway the trunk on the hips from side to side, bending sideways as far as may be comfortable; after which, bend the body backwards and forwards, care to keep the legs straight, the chest out and the head un-drooped. D: Keeping the body straight and the head erect, knee-bending and stretching may now be exercised, in which the body is allowed to drop until the buttocks are in contact with the heals ..

The above example is a Sandow recommended 5-minute warm-up and daily stretching and calisthenic routine with very light weights. He intends this to be performed by all trainees (as a warm-up), and on a daily basis; but he also expects them to engage in heavier and more systematic training to fully develop the bodies capacities.

The second set of exercises that Sandow recommends he names "*Light-Weight Exercises*". You can see these moves in the margins of the present pages. Also recommended are heavier weight-lifting moves, but this time only for athletes. Here he says that dumbbells from 12-56 pounds can be used at first as a way to improve one's physical strength. See **Sandow's System of Physical Training**.

We do not have space to examine the detailed history and development of the different training principles and all of the interesting personalities who followed. We have mentioned Sandow merely because he was the first, and also the instigator of much that was to come.

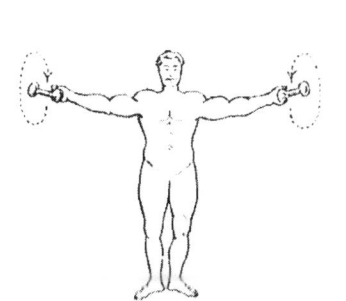

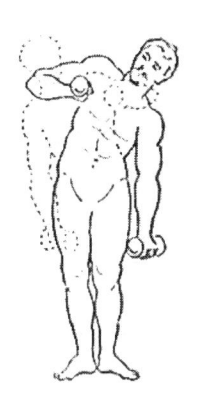

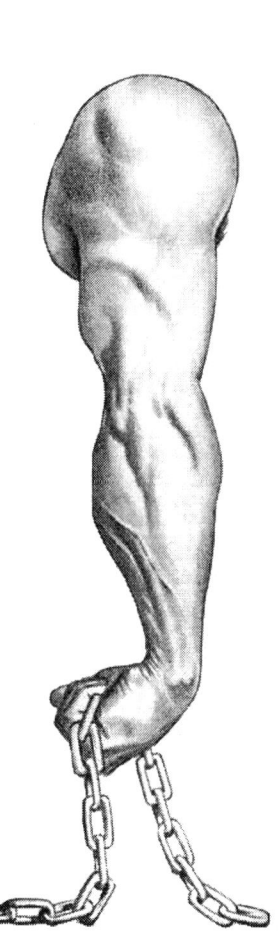

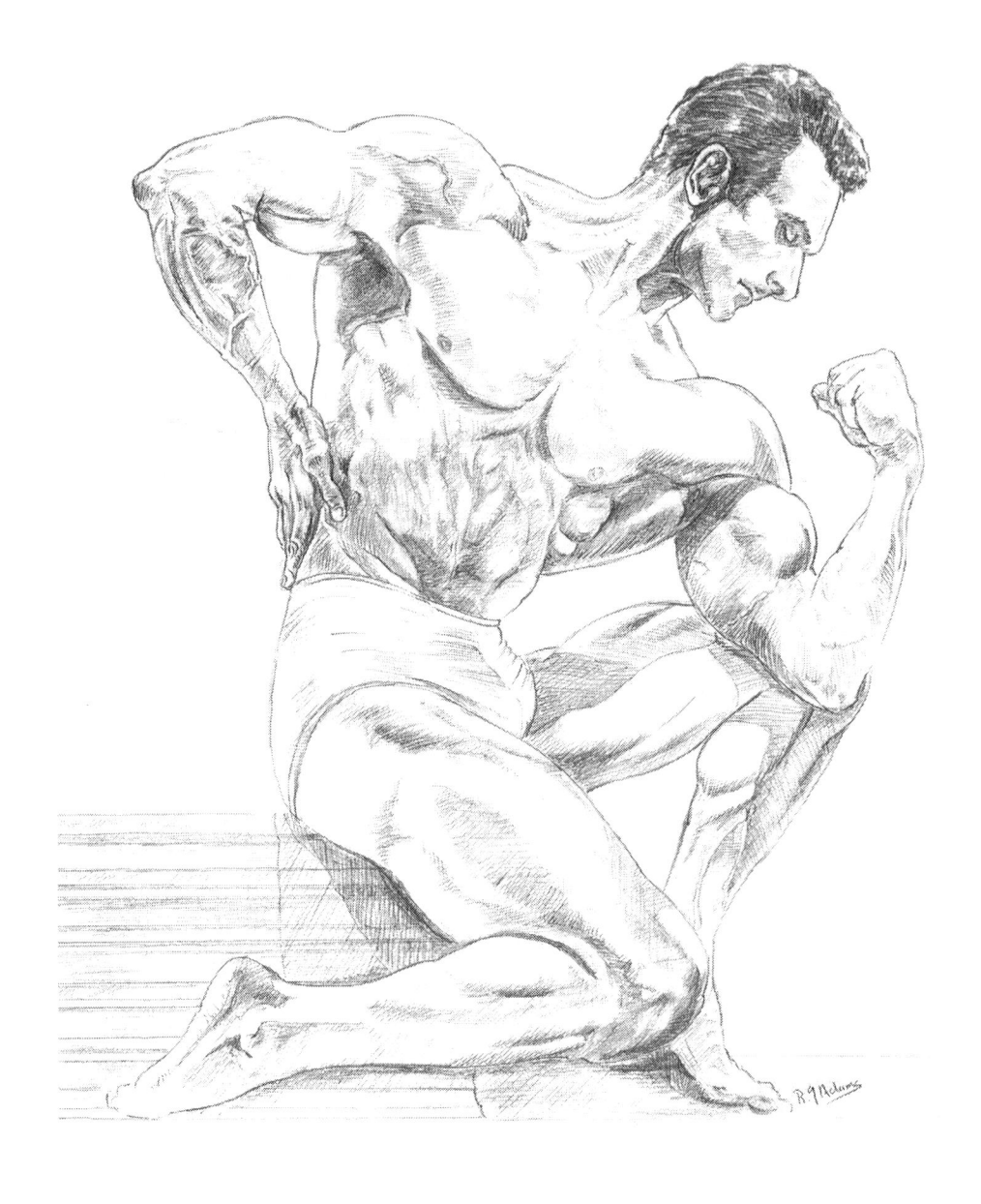

General Principles

WEIGHT-TRAINING HAS been around in a semi-scientific form for more than 100 years. As we saw in our discussion of Sandow, early partitioners understood that there was a right, and also a wrong way, to lift heavy objects such as barbells and dumbbells. Sandow was the first of many who developed so-called "scientific" principles of training, which continued with men such as Thomas Inch and Georges Hackenschmidt.

Although weight-training did not develop into a cut-and-dried science, for example as in farming principles, we can see that the sport and activity of resistance training did steadily develop through the adoption of special routines, principles and methods.

Perhaps the first principal of weight-training is that it should be progressive; that is, in order to improve the size and strength of one's muscles (and structure), the intensity and/or weights being lifted must slowly increase over time. Muscles will then adapt and grow, and in in order to cope with an increasing workload; and so the weights used must be gradually increased in order to give the body a chance to adapt to the increasing stress over an extended period of time (at least for beginners).

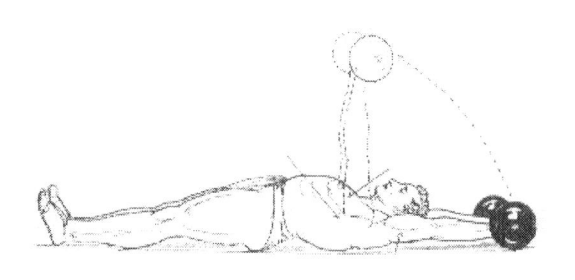

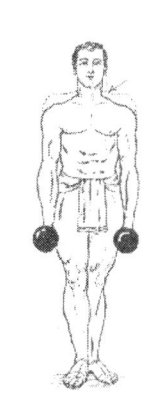

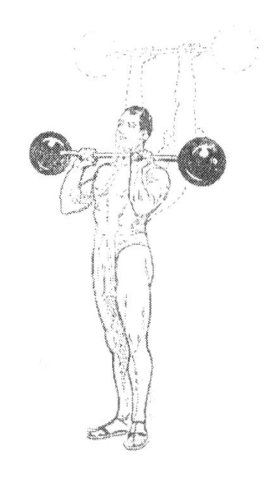

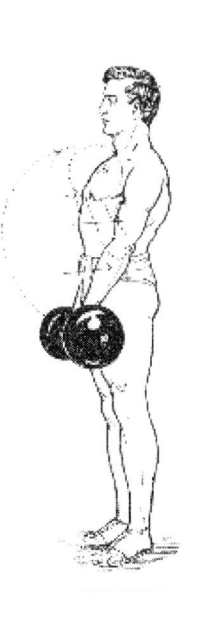

But muscles don't continue to grow and develop forever, and progress will soon stall and stop, and at such times new movements and/or resistance angles and/or other techniques to increase the intensity of muscular exercise, and so to spur the muscles into new growth, must be adopted.

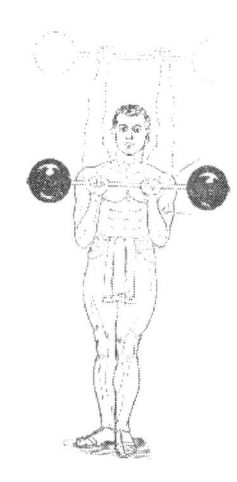

This is all a bit strange. What on earth is going on here?

Perhaps the main message is that muscles don't magically grow larger and become stronger by themselves. When you exercise by stressing the muscles beyond the degree of resistance that they are used to, you actually cause the muscle fibres to become torn and damaged.

In response (and over a period of a few days) they repair themselves and grow extra fibres in order to be prepared to face that very same stress again. And so it is damage to the fibres that causes the muscles to develop. Alternatively, if you only ever use the same resistance, the muscles will never become damaged and so they will stay at the same size and strength forever. [3]

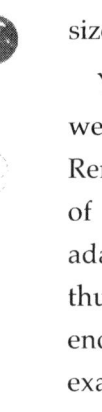

You should be aware however that the benefits of weight-training are not restricted to muscles alone. Remember that the body is composed of a large number of systems and structures, and many of these will also adapt to stress, becoming stronger and more efficient; thus one's entire physical structure can benefit enormously from the effects of muscular exercise. For example, bones became stronger, joints improve in strength and stability as well as in terms of flexibility or an extended range of motion. And thats not all; the circulatory and cardiopulmonary systems, including veins, heart and lungs can become vastly improved in

---

[3] N.B. As we age (or if we are optimally developed); then maintaining strength is progress, and in any case physical abilities have limits.

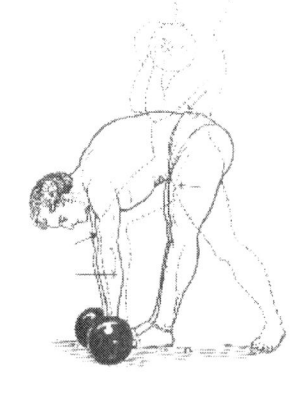

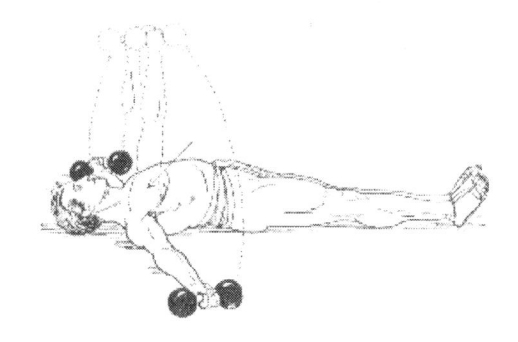

efficiency and capacity when you exercise with weights over a period of time.

What many forget is that weight-training has additional benefits to provide the body as a whole; and being ones that are potentially far more important than muscular development alone. Especially vital here are the potential improvements to the systems and structures involved in joint articulation; and in terms of (for example) arm, leg and back strength, plus capabilities related to lifting and moving about from one place to another.

I hardly feel it necessary to even mention the benefits to the human body in a systematic sense of a well-planned exercise regime. Many experts have done studies that basically prove that you can keep your body in top condition by combining weight-training sessions with some form of aerobic training for the cardiovascular system. And although weights have long been used for physiotherapy; it is my belief that we have just merely scratched the surface in terms of the potential of weight-training to treat a whole range of illnesses and movement based disfunction(s).

I take myself as a good example here. Over the years I have engaged in heavy powerlifting with barbells (perhaps too much). However, over the last 10 years or so, I noticed increasing back-pain, and after an MRI scan my Doctor informed me that I had developed degraded or damaged discs in my spine that causes pressure on the nerves - hence some pain and difficulty moving about. So I began a program of very light stiff-legged dumbbell dead-lifts and twisting dumbbell bend-overs, and the pain improved and almost disappeared (but not completely - perhaps due to age).

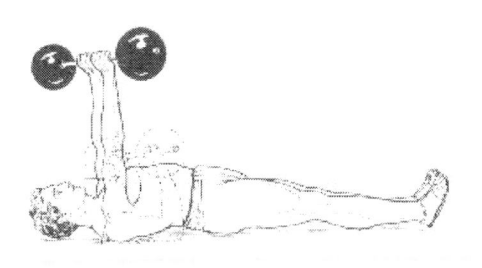

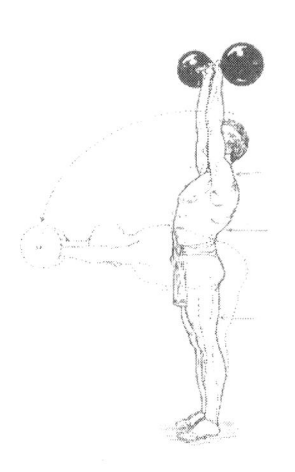

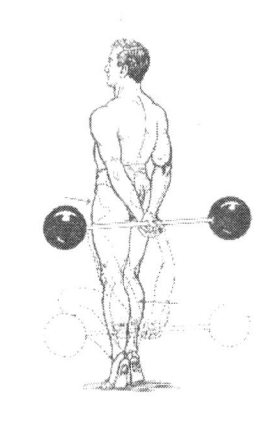

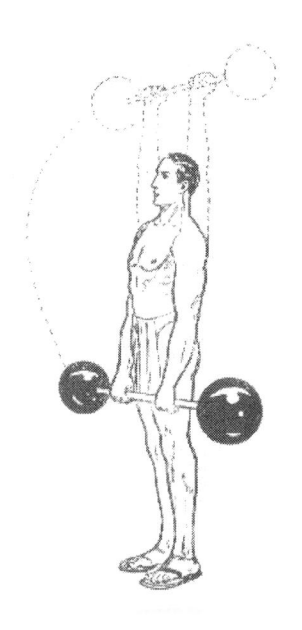

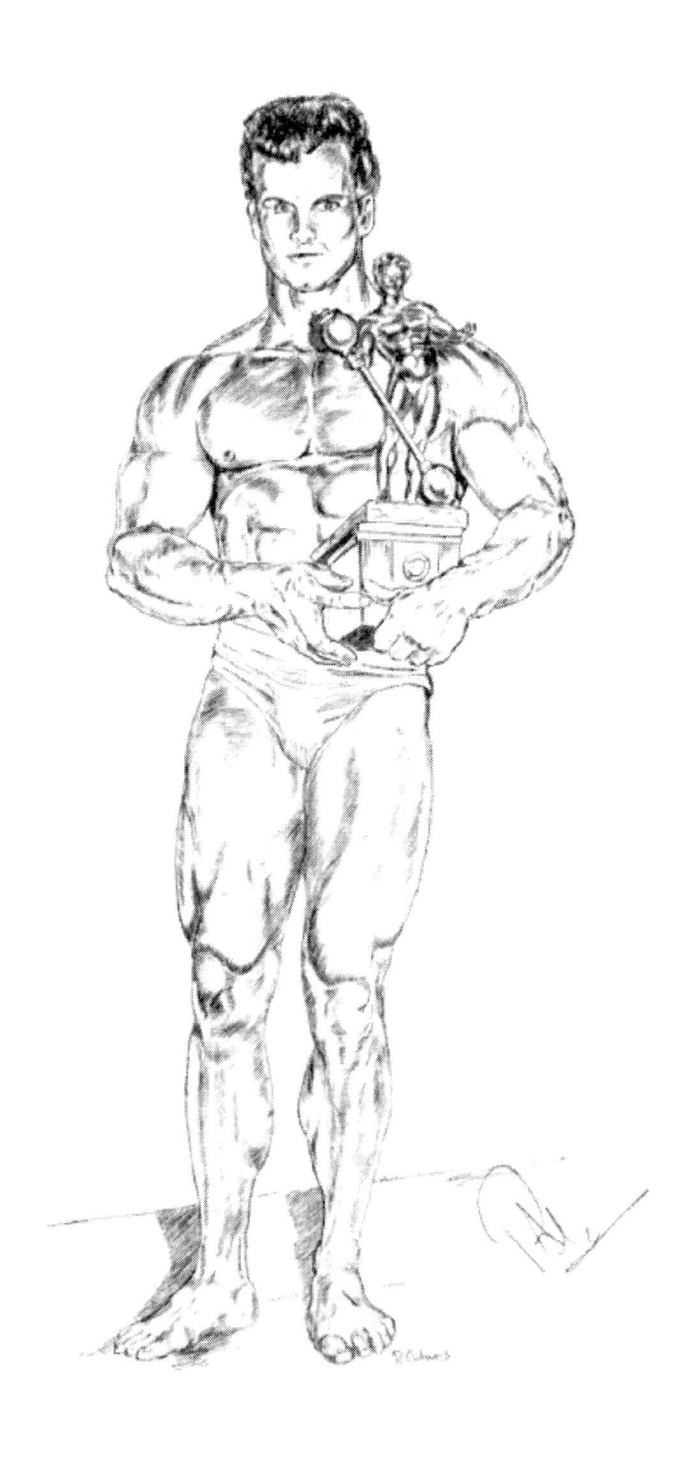

Key Principle

AS WITH most ventures, there are in fact many different paths to the same fitness end; and possible are a number of alternative ways to train the body in order to get it into top condition. The benefits of running, cycling and swimming are well-documented. And activities like martial arts, yoga, athletics and gymnastics are complete systems of Physical Culture that may provide all that is necessary for perfect health.

However I do think that a properly performed weight-training routine with dumbbells can rival any of these activities for efficiency and effectiveness, so far as providing a fast, simple, and progressive way to condition the body (including also perhaps a few selected barbell moves).

Obviously weights develop the visible muscles. But it is not so-well known that weight-training is just as beneficial for the hidden (deep inner) muscles and structures, including the bones, tendons, ligaments, joints and also the circulatory system, heart and lungs.

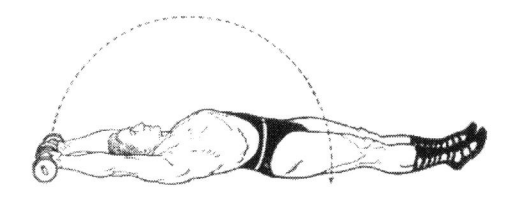

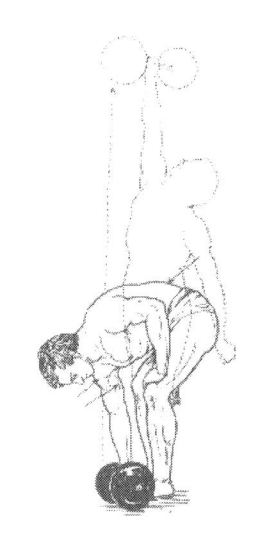

I should not have to defend the barbell and dumbbell sports today; because by now multiple scientific studies have proven their effectiveness on the systems mentioned. But as with any physical activity, the key is to tailor the method to the individual, and in terms of needs, limitations and in order to achieve specific results. Not everyone can perform every exercise, and movements should be carefully chosen, and neither can each of use the same resistance or even make it to the gym.

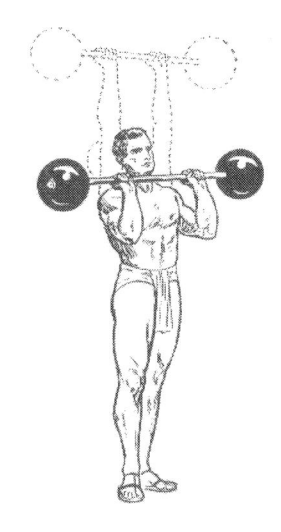

As with so many things in life, a little knowledge can be a bad thing. Before embarking on a program of exercise one should do quite a bit of research. And get some expert advice if possible. This book is a good place to start, but remember that I do not know anything about you and your specific physical capabilities and any limitations. Take my advice with a pinch of salt therefore, and likewise in terms of information obtained from others. Because at the end of the day it is you who must do the exercises, and only you can judge their effects (beneficial or otherwise) on your body.

It may surprise you that certain exercises can be bad for you, and especially so for you as opposed to even your own brother/sister. You will need different exercises at different times, and you should choose different ones as you age/develop and in order to produce specific results.

But this fact has escaped many. Have you noticed how everyone in the gym is giving everybody else advice on exercise selection. It's almost as if people think that some exercises are universally superior to other ones.

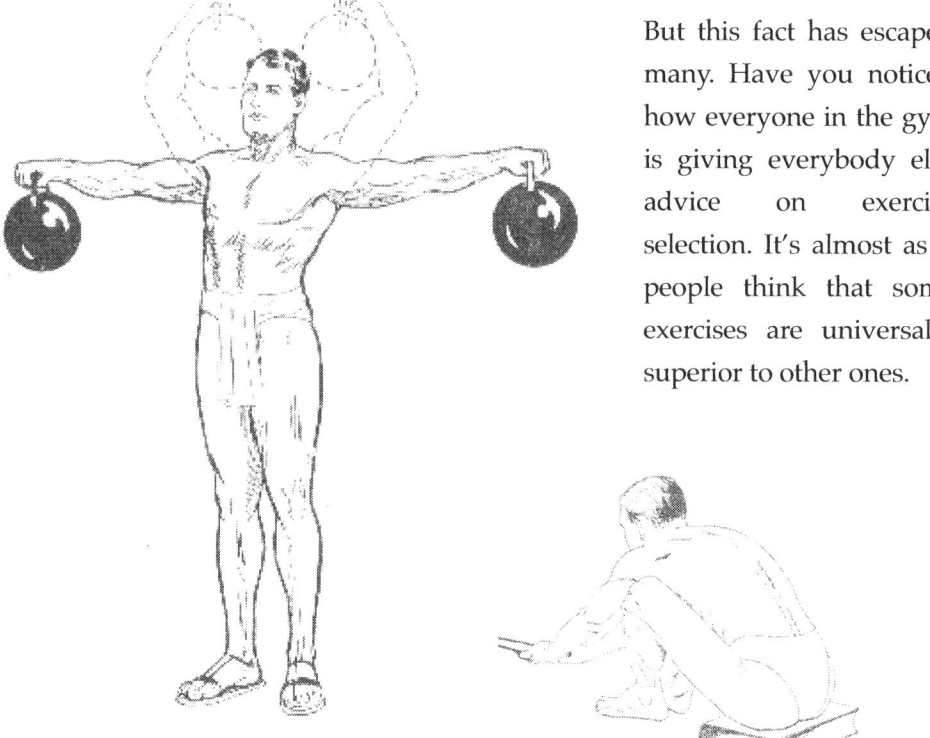

People should probably not give advice here, unless they know you very well, because it is important to realise that choosing appropriate exercises is something only you can do for yourself (unless you have a truly knowledgable coach).

And everyone should be doing different exercises according to their needs. My own brother needs completely different exercise choices and fitness training methods; and in part because he has lived a different life from me. We all will also, at any particular time, have specific levels of conditioning, strength, and flexibility etc.

Remember also that you should probably switch your exercises around every so often because the body quickly becomes adapted to a particular routine and stops improving.

Also as the saying goes, too much of anything will make you sick. If you do an exercise too often, and with too much weight, then something has to give and you will either become injured or else stop making progress (you may even regress in development/capability when you over-exercise). Frequency of exercise, weight, and number of sets and repetitions, must all be carefully chosen to meet the needs of the individual.

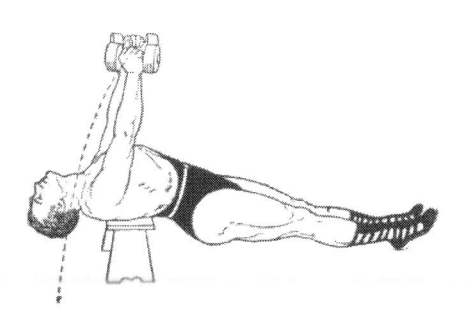

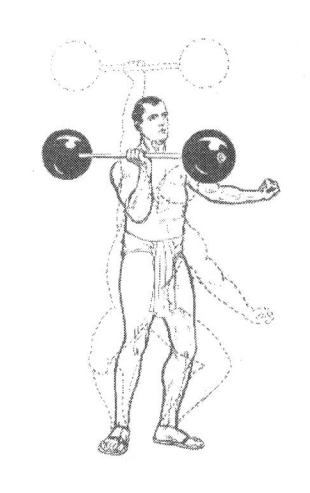

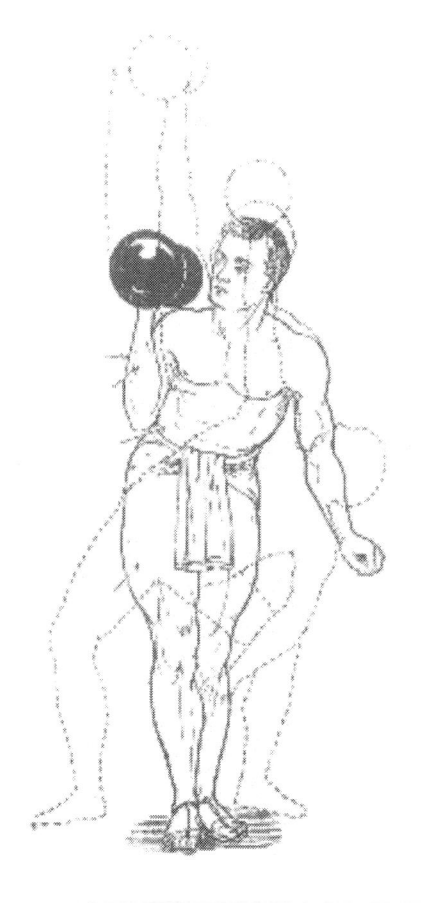

Even though I do not believe that there are universally ideal exercises for everyone, I do think that (in general) some exercises are better than others. Certain exercises are just safer to perform, whilst others are quite bad for the joints and human system generally. In fact this point goes to the heart of the reasons why I have written this book.

I believe that dumbbells are superior to barbells, and that free-weights are superior to machines.

Why are dumbbells better than barbells - isn't a barbell just a long handled dumbbell? Yes and no. It comes down to the fact that you hold a barbell with two hands. This duel attachment to the bar, to some extent, and in some exercises, limits the range of motion and also the freedom of movement of the limbs (normally this effect is worse for pressing, rowing and curling moves).

Think about it this way; your arms and legs naturally move about independently one from one another. When one arm moves in this direction - the other can (and often does) move in an entirely different direction. Even slight changes in elbow, shoulder, and joint positions matter significantly in terms of the resulting hand position in space. And so the ligaments, joints and bones move in slightly different ways (3D paths in space) as we move about normally. Nothing could be more natural than independent and free movement of the joints. Thus many of our natural movement patterns depend on the independence of our limbs, and hence multiple joint-hinged movements without any restrictions.

Of-coarse whilst performing some multi-lever movements such as walking, running, jumping; or even when lifting weights overhead etc; then multiple joints move and work in unison. Only in each cases the joints are free (in terms of natural paths) to move independently one-from-another.

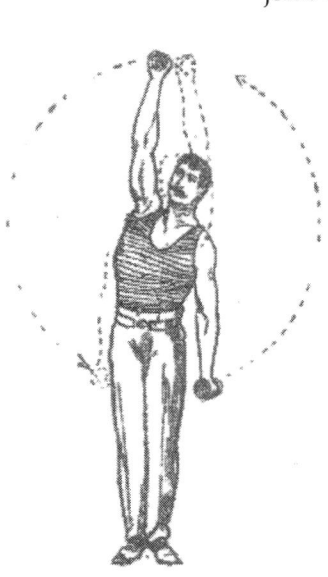

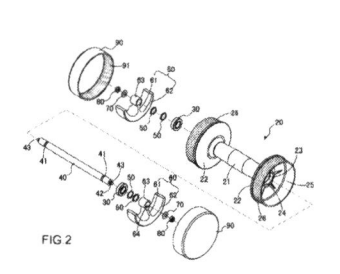

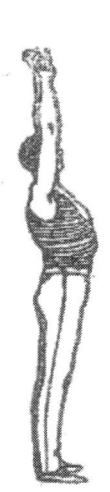

FIG 2

Movement in one joint, does not (usually) and by definition, result in tension or required movement in another joint. Overall body movement(s) may (and often do) cause movement in multiple joints simultaneously, but this is by choice - and is not forced upon the body in an "external" sense.

Put simply, human joints are supposed to move freely and independently (with respect to each other). Thus limbs are to a large extent normally free to move separately, one from another. Combining the possible movements of the different joints gives rise to many different types of potential movements; and as a result of the large (almost infinite) number of combinations. Thus the human body is free to move about in countless ways. The number of ways in which you can move your limbs and body is equivalent to thousands of different movement patterns. In every case an individual movement emanates from a joint or multiple joints, which in each instance moves in a circular motion.

But when you hold a barbell with 2 hands, then the number of movement patterns is severely reduced, and each of these new movement paths happens over a limited range of motion. Your movements are greatly restricted here, in both the number of ways you can move and also in terms of the range of motions (ROMs) possible. When performing the barbell bench press for example, you are "tying" together the shoulder and elbow joints (with the barbell). You then are asking, no forcing, the joints to do their job(s) as normal - but within a severely restricted range of motion. Crunching and grating of joints is the inevitable result.

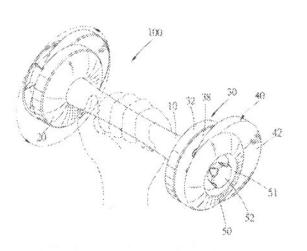

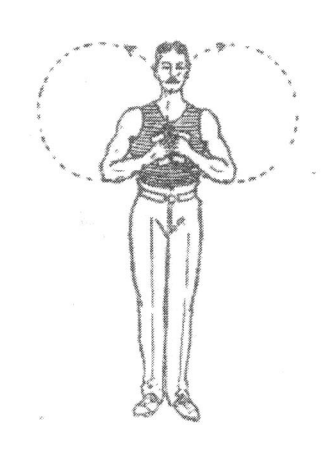

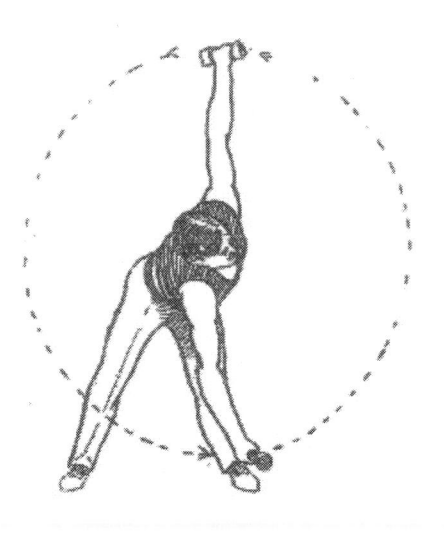

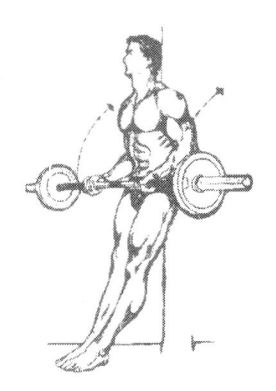

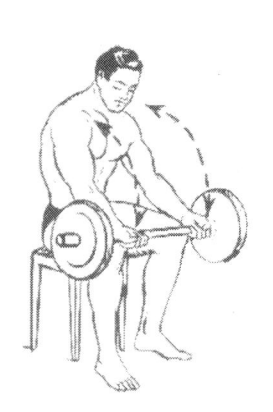

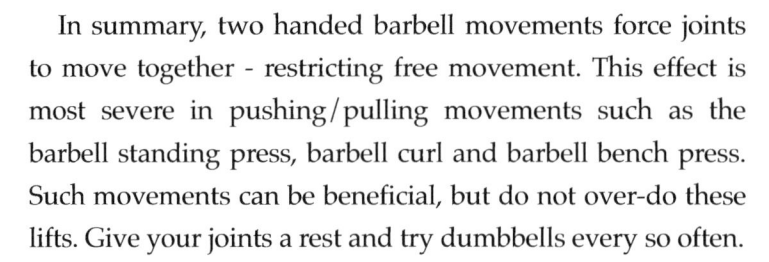

In summary, two handed barbell movements force joints to move together - restricting free movement. This effect is most severe in pushing/pulling movements such as the barbell standing press, barbell curl and barbell bench press. Such movements can be beneficial, but do not over-do these lifts. Give your joints a rest and try dumbbells every so often.

Movements such as the barbell squat, dead-lift and barbell clean (the best and most productive of the barbell exercises), do not suffer from this reduced (and restricted) range of motion because your arms are operating more as "hooks" than as levers. Here the shoulder and elbow joints are not prime-movers, and so the joint restriction(s) and joint "crushing" effects do not occur.

It stands to reason that you cannot exercise muscles and joints from as many different angles with barbells, as opposed to dumbbells, because of the restricted movements. You get less training results - in terms of ROM flexibility - as a result, and inevitably less development and strength capability. With barbells, exercises are optimised over a far smaller range of movement than is the case if the same motions are performed with dumbbells.

Barbells are worse for you, in terms of joint health, than are dumbbells. As Arthur Jones once said, the human body moves in circular motions, because the limbs move basically in circular paths and around circular and rounded joints.

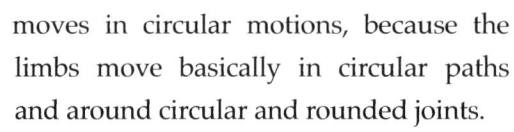

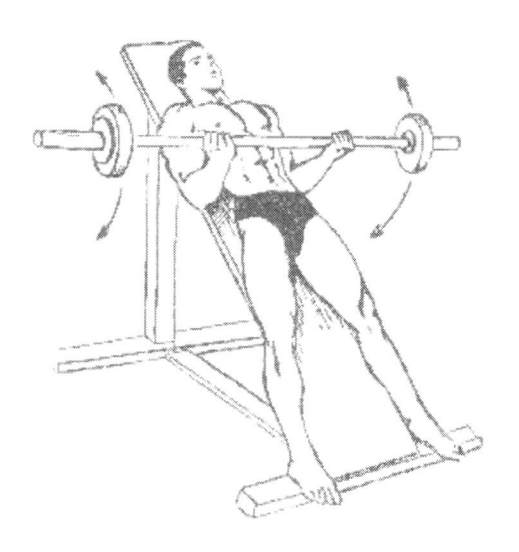

Dumbbells often let you work "around" the joint in natural and circular movement arcs, whilst barbells tend to push "against" the joint. This is because movement is restricted due to the lever being held in 2 different locations where your hands meet the bar, and possibly two more positions (for example) at the joints where the body meets the bench pads. With a barbell, the weight bears down on the joint, actually pushing into, or against it.

One might say that the dumbbell is far superior because it allows you to perform a wider range of motion (ROM) on any exercise, working muscles over their full ROM. Plus you can perform a great many more exercises (lots of different 3D movement patterns); and each pattern is being performed in a natural movement arc. Let me qualify what I have said, because I like barbell training very much, but just not as much as training with dumbbells. I know that certain barbell exercises can be very beneficial because they allow you to use lots of weight efficiently in exercises like the squat, dead-lift and clean and press. If you want to get really strong; barbells can help, but it is a mistake to focus solely on barbells at the expense of dumbbells (note that the fun curling variations depicted on these pages can also be performed with dumbbells).

Incidentally even though I have enjoyed performing many barbell bench presses in my life, this is a potentially dangerous exercise (if performed constantly), and from a theoretical perspective. The movement arc is further restricted because the body is held in a firm position on the bench at the shoulders, and when combined with restriction at each hand position due to holding the bar, the "pushing' affect on the shoulder joint is most severe.

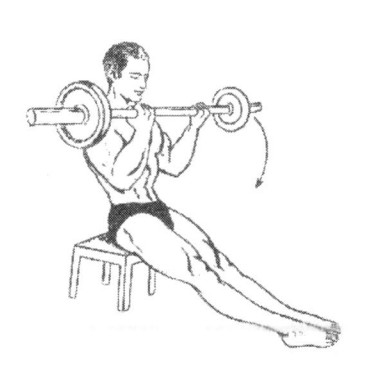

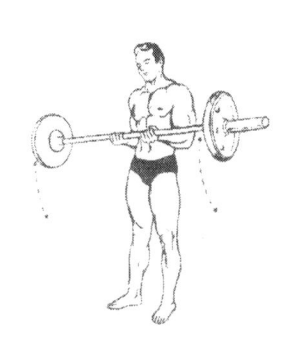

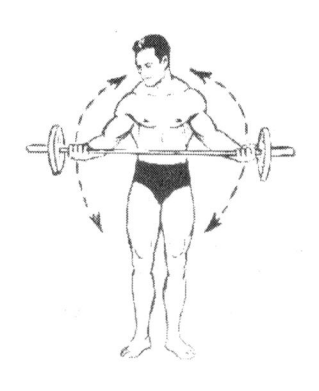

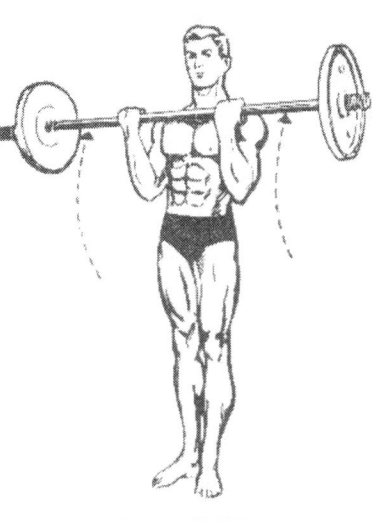

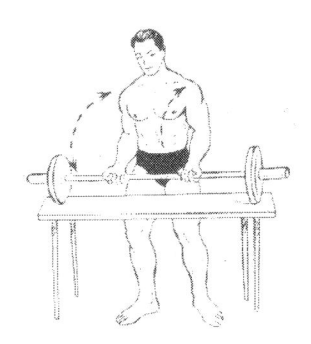

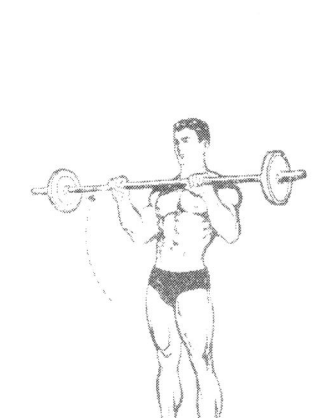

Part of our new "Zen" training system has now been identified; which can be stated in a principle as follows:

in general, the torso, limbs, and levers of the human body; and hence the joints of the human body; should move freely and (sometimes) independently of one another along unrestricted paths; in this way preserving the range of motion and natural movement patterns of the various articulated components.

- Zen Training Principle no. 1

The above principle is more of a guide than a fixed rule. It indicates that dumbbells are perhaps the most natural form of training; although we do happily recommend certain barbell exercises. Largely we do so where the first principle is not broken. As mentioned barbell squats, cleans and dead-lifts use the arms more as hooks than as prime levers, and so they are basically OK in terms of natural upper body articulations. Note that these exercises do tie the legs to the floor in a sense because both feet are both planted to the ground, and thus the legs do often move together, but the legs naturally move together in this way anyway.

In later chapters I shall give my recommended exercises, and discuss the merits of each in turn. I shall miss out all exercises that I consider to be useless, dangerous or just a plain waste of time. I shall include useful machine, free-body and barbell exercises where I think that no better exercise can be performed with dumbbells. I do recommend movements like chin-ups, dips and press-ups, even though they apparently (partially) break the first rule. I do so because these movements are performed with only one's body-weight as resistance, and so they do seem to be quite natural as a result.

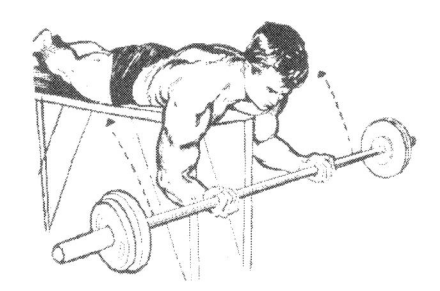

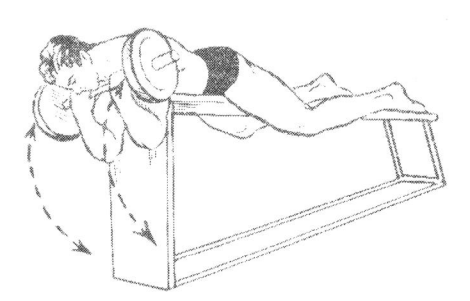

Now I would like us to consider machine exercises. Let us start with cable machines and expander exercises. Cable/expander movements do allow free-and unrestricted movement paths and so facilitate natural (free) movement patterns. I find these methods excellent, and I rarely suffer the joint "crushing" or pushing problems - and especially if I stick to using a moderate resistance and slow performance speed.

We now consider other types of machines, and in particular those machines that force the trainee to use a pre-determined movement path such as Universal, Nautilus and Hammer machines etc. Now these machines may look very scientific, but in fact they are not. Whilst dumbbells seem very un-scientific, but in fact they are highly scientific.

Let me explain. I think we have established that the most natural form of training allows the limbs and various body parts to move freely and along unrestricted movement paths. This is without doubt how we move in real-life. If that is so, then why would we do anything so unnatural as to fix a movement path, especially when we are all so different, and each and every one of us has unique movement path(s).

If you think that barbells force you into a fixed movement pattern, and so push against the joints; then the effect is only ten times worse with machines. At least with a barbell you are often free to move your body in space - whereas with many machine exercises your body is pinned to a seat. And your limbs (and torso etc) have to try and move in a pre-determined way even though they are not free to adjust themselves, and in order to find an ideal body position from which to push/pull with full efficiency.

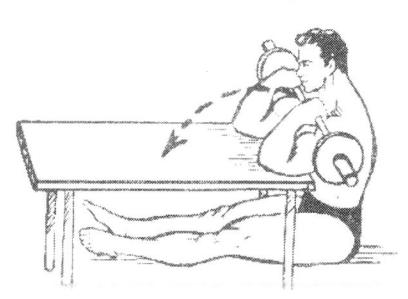

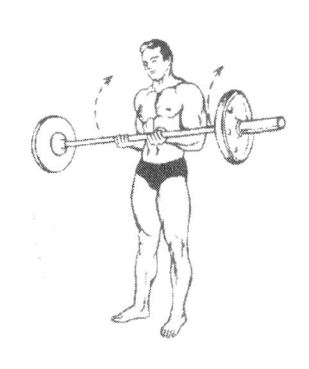

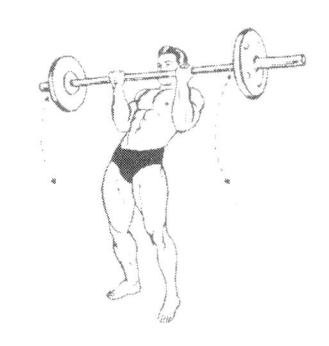

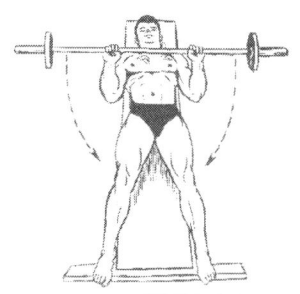

With most machines this is just not possible; and you feel more like you are being tortured than exercising.

Machines (in general) are really bad for your joints, tendons, bones and other moving parts. When using a machine, I often feel like the bones are being pushed and pulled in wholly unnatural ways, and in fact it sometimes feels as if the machine is trying to break my bones and/or grind my joints into dust ! (perhaps they are so doing).

It's not that the concept of a machine is a bad idea. Only that it is very, very difficult to manufacture a machine that provides natural movement paths; and especially considering the need to adjust movement paths for each individual (I have never seen/used such a machine).

I have one small caveat here; machines can be useful for physical therapy and in cases where the person is for some reason unable to use free-weights. But never forget that they severely limit the choice of movement patterns. Machines often force your body to lift from unnatural and disadvantageous mechanical position(s), and also they take balance right out of the equation. Machines can never come close to mimicking real-world physical tasks.

Progress and development will be lower (with machine training) as a result, and there will be an upper limit on how far you can go by use of such methods alone. Note that some machines (particularly the cable type) are very good; and I shall refer to these again later on. And thats about it for my discussion of the key principle behind Zen Dumbbell Training. I have laid my beliefs, and experience, on the table (35 years of training has been my teacher).

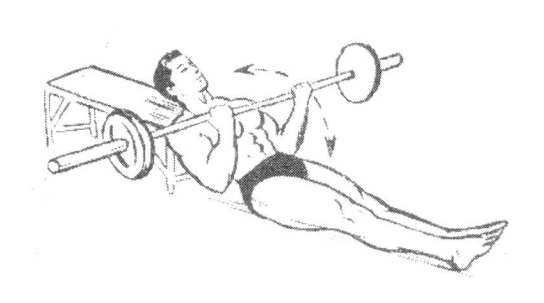

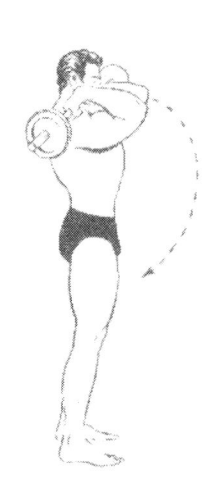

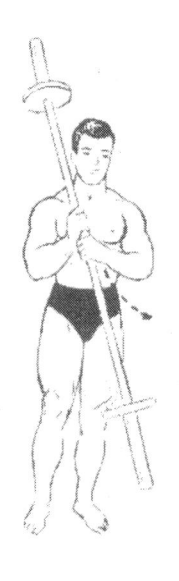

Good / Bad Exercises

IN a way I hesitate to provide information on good and bad exercises, and largely for all of the reasons mentioned relating to the individuality of need and capability. However, we are all human, and it is my belief that some exercises are so dreadfully bad - and also dangerous - that nobody should perform them under any circumstances. Likewise certain exercises are so good that everyone should use them, that is unless they cannot do so due to injury or other physical imitation and/or should not do so for medical reasons.

I have decided to identify those exercises that are average, poor, and dangerous below. Note that not every single type of exercise is listed, and you may have to extrapolate the recommendations to the actual movements that you are considering.

Dumbbell Exercises: These are almost universally good, as long as you choose the correct weight, do not use excessive momentum/bouncing and do not try to move in unnatural ways (i.e. don't make up new [crazy] exercises).

Barbell Exercises: These are mostly average or good; with a few bad examples that you should never do. Especially good are barbell squats, dead-lifts and the clean (with good form). I would say that the barbell bench press can range from a good exercise for beginners when they want to bulk up the chest muscles, to average for the developed trainee, to bad where the trainee has a shoulder injury or is prone to over-development of the pectoral muscles.

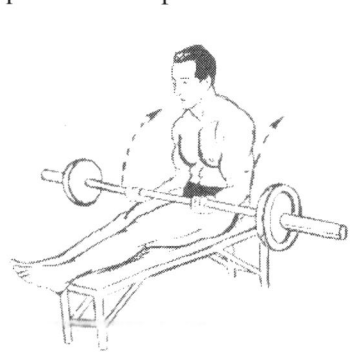

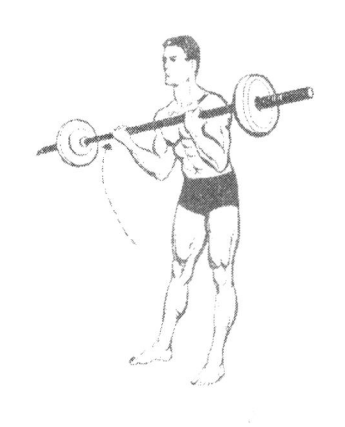

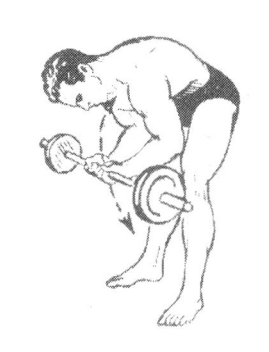

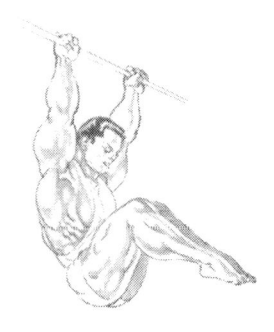

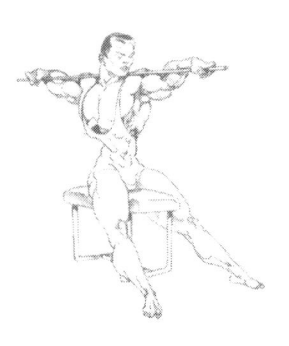

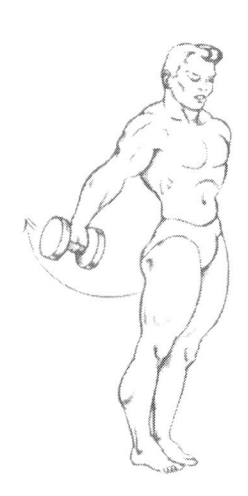

I would rate the barbell pullover (straight-armed) as an excellent exercise. Examples of universally bad barbell moves are the lunge and the seated behind the neck press. Good to average are barbell curls, barbell bent-over rows, lying triceps extensions and the barbell standing press.

Please do not think that I am down on barbell exercises; because I have experienced really tremendous improvements in size and strength myself using many of the above exercises (I have dead-lifted 500 lbs for 20 non-stop reps, and bench pressed 400 lbs). It is only that as I have become older I have re-evaluated my thinking; and I now believe that the barbell is best (exclusively) used in your early teens up until your mid-20s, and for gaining initial strength and size. Barbells can be bad for your joints as you age and when flexibility and joint health becomes more important, which happens as you move out of the initial youth phase. That said, I do recommend barbell squats and dead-lifts to almost everyone.

Cable Exercises: These are almost universally good, as long as you do not use too much resistance, and also do not try to move in unnatural ways by making up strange and unwieldy exercises that the human body was never meant to perform.

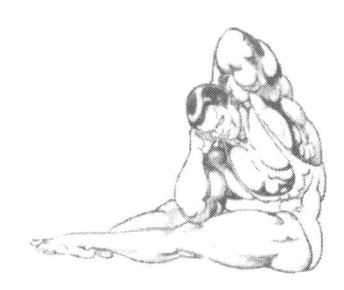

Machine Exercises: [fixed movement path type - e.g. Hammer, Nautilus, Universal] These are universally bad, with a few major exceptions (in particular Nautilus curl machines). The reasons why I do not recommend use of machines is due to the logic stated elsewhere in this book; that they are very bad for your joints and also (in general) they limit the range of movement(s) that the trainee can perform. Basically they are not very natural in terms of the restricted movement paths offered. Good machine exercises include standing and seated calf machines raises, cable rowing machine, and a few others. Some of the new hammer machines can be average/OK to use when you are injured or for use when you are unable to exercise with free weights. On the whole however, myself I would not go anywhere near most machines under normal circumstances, and especially when the alternative barbells and dumbbells are available. One caveat here is that if I were injured, then I would consider using such machines, but only until such time as the injury healed.

Bodyweight Exercises: These are almost universally good. In fact, always in your routine should be chin-ups, press-ups and dips. Plus a wide variety of leg-raises, crunches, sit-ups, twisting and forward/sideways bending exercises should be performed as well.

Running: This is the supreme exercise (along with walking) and is almost universally good. No matter what else you do, please find time for at least 30-60 minutes of daily walking or running. Your heart and cardiovascular system will thank you before very long, and your chances of developing some kind of systematic illness will be significantly reduced. Remember the well-known saying: "when the legs go - you go too" !

Bicycling and swimming: These are excellent exercises and are almost universally good. In conclusion, there are many different and marvellous ways to train for improved fitness, but all superior methods have one key factor; being that they involve healthy and natural movement patterns.

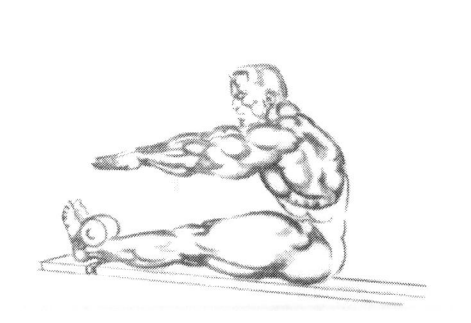

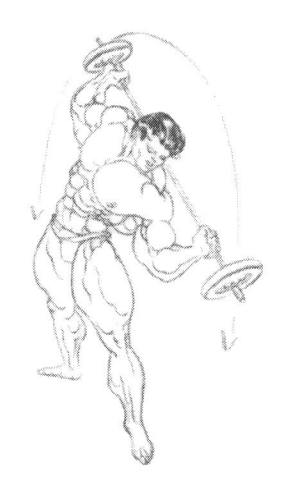

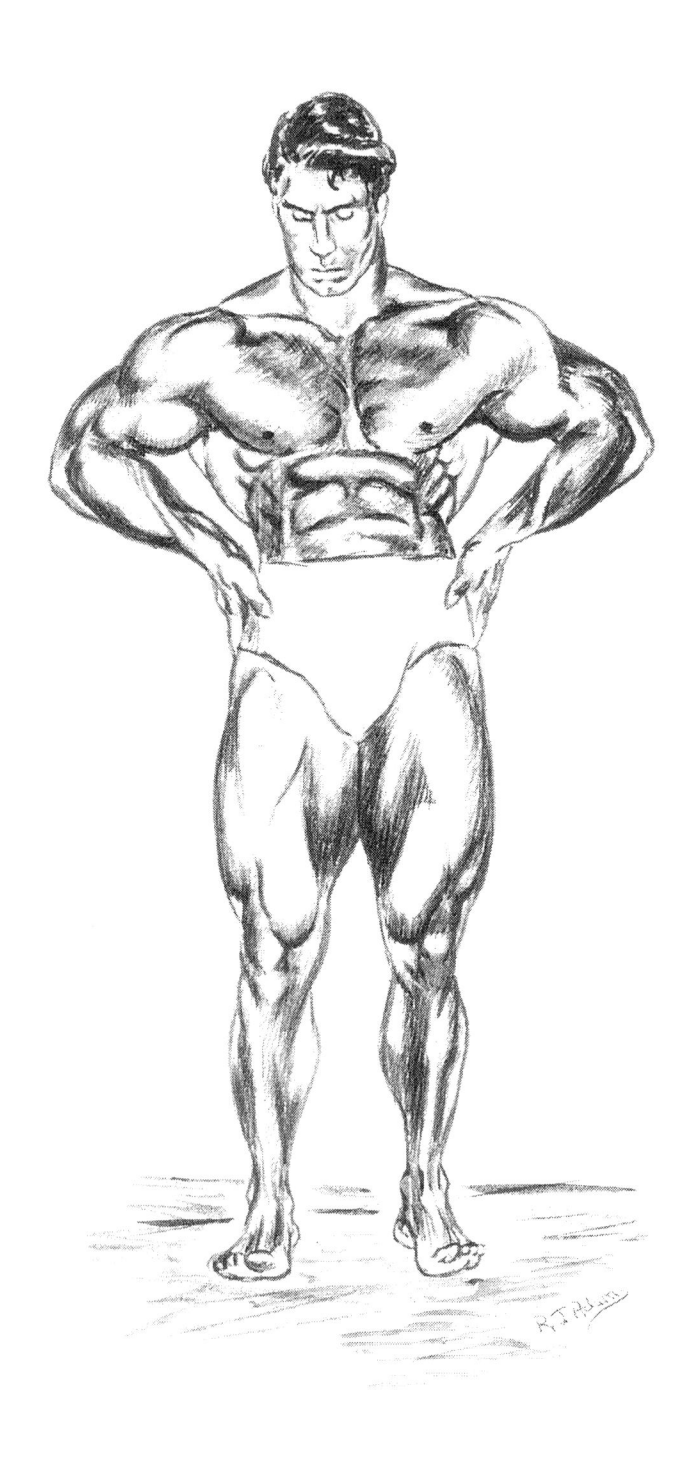

CHAPTER FIVE
Zen Training

MY AIM in writing this book is not to repeat lots of information that you will find elsewhere; but rather I intend to succinctly present the system of Zen Dumbbell Training. I shall focus on how this method differs from all other training systems, and in so doing hopefully provide new information to the trainee.

As with most books, almost everything I have got to say has been said before (somewhere). And leaving out information is the most difficult task faced by the writer. To produce this book I had to sift through hundreds of books and also thousands of magazines in my personal library. In so doing, one finds a great many useful pieces of information. To save space, I present (largely) only those ideas that differ from the normal fitness training principles familiar to all. Remember that my observations are not *entirely* correct for everyone, or even for one individual at any particular time.

I only say that you may find benefit if you try mindful training with dumbbells according to the principles herein described. Before we begin, I thought it would be useful to define some terms, being those that are particularly useful, or that have special meaning as defined here.

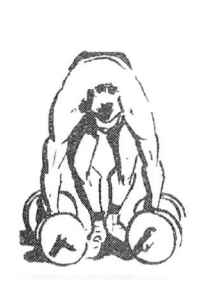

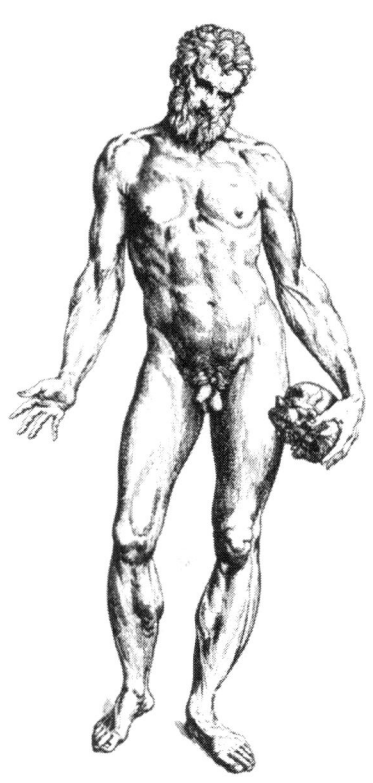

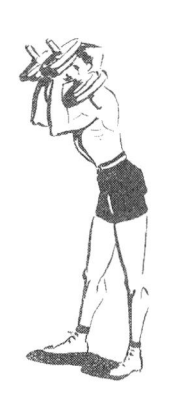

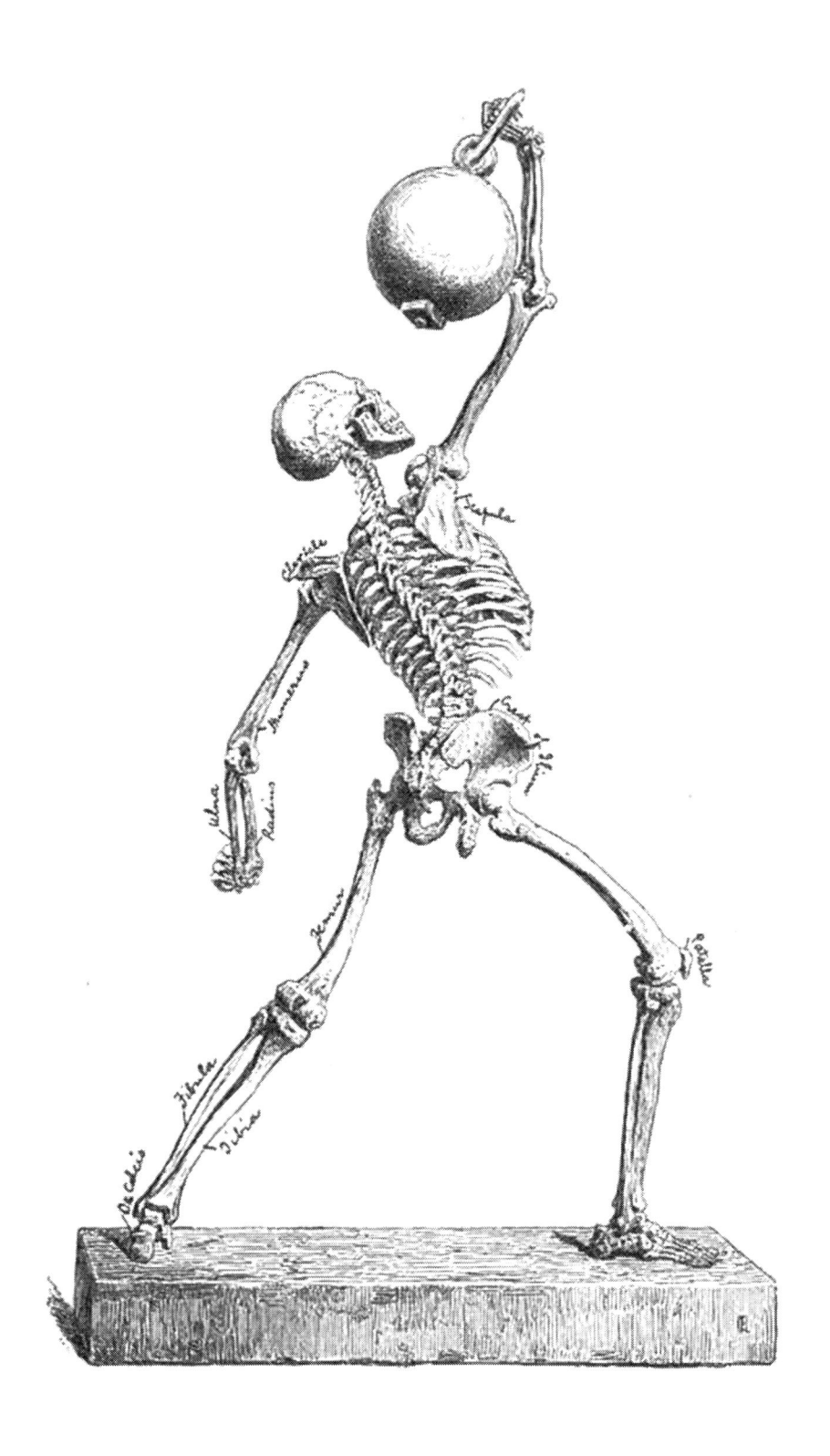
Scapula
Clavicula
Humerus
Ulna
Radius
Femur
Patella
Fibula
Tibia
Os Calcis

Beginners Mind

THE STUDENT of Zen seeks truth and knowledge of the world. Zen also teaches the pupil to distrust written knowledge and thought - but rather attempt to see things as they really are. The focus is on perception as opposed to dogma.

Many people have written books on fitness training, and much has been said that is useful. But the zen approach teaches us another way of attaining knowledge, whereby we realise and accept that we are in a state of constant relationship to the environment, and so in a state of constant change. If we think too much - then we loose this connection to reality - and life. The zen approach relates to the innocence of the beginners mind in any activity. In a sense one should always approach training as a beginner, and be open to listening to the body and what it has to teach. Here the focus is on learning about the self.

Flexibility

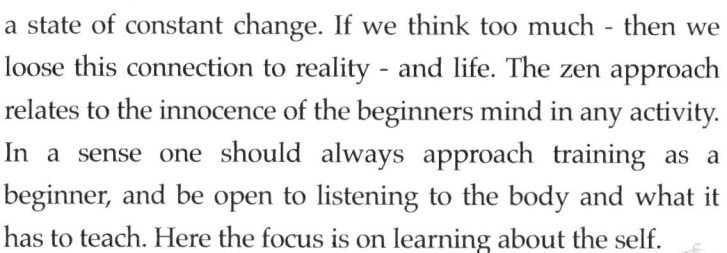

Flexibility has been defined as mobilisation, freedom to move, or technically as range of motion (ROM). The amount or degree of range of motion is specific for each joint. There are two types of flexibility, static and dynamic.

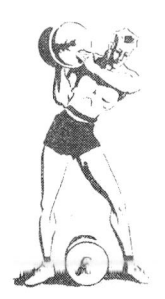

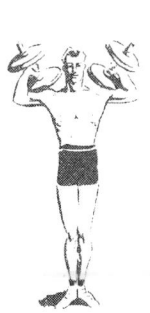

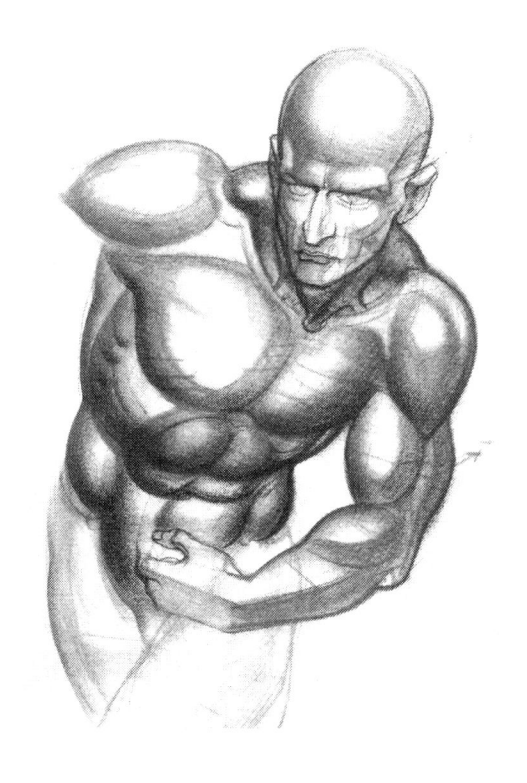

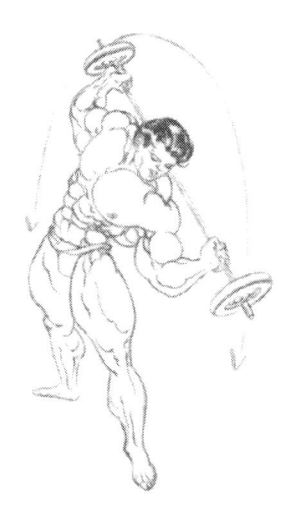

Static refers to ROM about a joint with no emphasis on speed, whilst dynamic considers speed ROM. This is not a book about stretching or flexibility training however; since all weight training is basically stretching and contracting muscles against resistance; and it stands to reason that a properly performed dumbbell training program will improve both types of flexibility, and increase joint ROMs.

Choices

The outcome of any training program can be made more predictable and less haphazard if certain biological and biomechanical principles are understood and applied. Part of the reason for writing this book has been to explain that dumbbells are the most natural, advanced and also versatile training tools available to us. When choosing dumbbells as the prime training method; the trainee has taken a major step forward in terms of the formulation of a scientific and systematic training methodology. But he/she must know which exercises to choose and how to perform them correctly. This is the *raison d'être* for the present book.

In evaluating one's fitness and formulating a dumbbell training program, one must consider not only the benefits of increased strength, flexibility, and better functional movement. Also consider the potential for injury and impairment of function, and how to maximise performance and progress without imposing injury / suboptimal conditions.

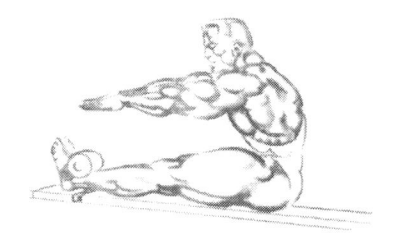

You should take every opportunity to manipulate the various factors that affect physical improvement. All I can do is to point the way. Unfortunately I will not be with you to guide you. But remember that even if I was present when you workout, the Zen approach states that it is still up to you to listen to your own body and make the right choices; specifically in terms of choosing beneficial exercises, weights, and movement paths, etc.

Benefits of Dumbbells

To obtain maximum benefit from a dumbbell training program, you must know and understand what can and cannot be achieved by so doing. We define 2 basic types of dumbbell training program. Firstly a dumbbell training program that is a planned, deliberate, and regular program of exercises that it is hoped will progressively and permanently increase one or more of the elements of strength for an individual (named *strength training*). Whereas a dumbbell calisthenics / warm up/ cool down program is defined as a regular program of lighter exercises that are done immediately before or after an activity (or as a wake-me-up after slumber/inactivity) and to improve ROM performance or else to reduce the risk of injury in any activity (*ROM training*).

When one begins a dumbbell training program, the potential benefits are (in a sense) virtually unlimited. The quality and quantity of improvements are determined firstly by the ends, being an individual's goals. Secondly the benefits are dependant upon the means, which determine whether and to what extent the ends are achieved. The means are the methods and techniques used to attain one's goals - and are largely what this book is about. Ends can include emotional, psychological as well as biological or physiological factors.

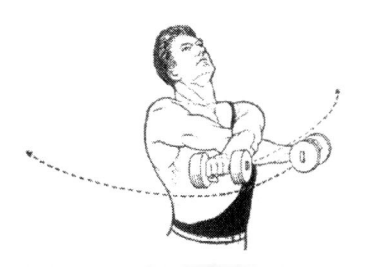

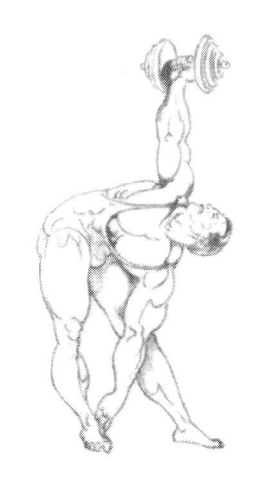

Union of Mind, Body & Spirit

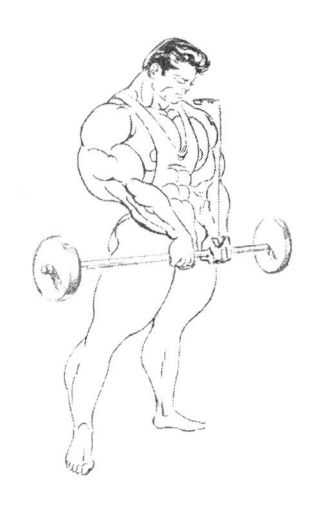

A dumbbell training program can serve to unify one's mind, body and spirit. A friend of mine once told me that weight-training was in fact a form of yoga. That thought immediately struck a note of truth with me - and I have remembered it ever since.

Yoga is probably the most widely known of many disciplines that seek to achieve a perfect harmony between mind, body and spirit. The word yoga is derived from the Sanskrit root yui, meaning *to bind, attach and yoke; to direct and concentrate one's attention; to use and apply*. It also means union or communion. The many books on yoga emphasise certain basic principles that are mystical; and transcendental, yet highly logical and rational.

Yoga is based on the following principles:

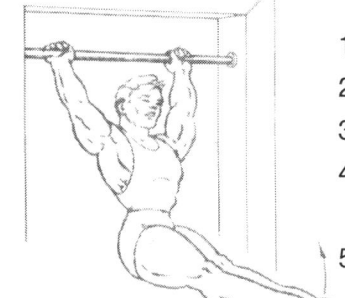

1) The body is a temple that houses the **Divine Spark**
2) The body is an instrument of attainment
3) The Yogi masters the body by the practice of asanas (postures)
4) The Yogi performs asanas to develop the complete equilibrium of body, mind and spirit
5) The body, mind and spirit are inseparable

To the Yogi then, the body is the prime instrument of attainment. If the vehicle breaks down, the traveller cannot go far, and he can achieve little. Therefore physical health is important for mental development, as normally the mind functions through the nervous system.

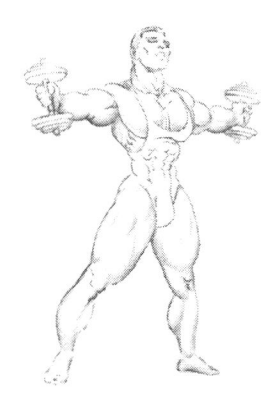

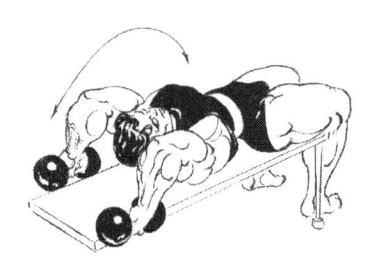

It may seem a bit esoteric, and your training buddies/partners might think that you have gone a little mad if you mention these motivations; but I would suggest that each and every one of these same principles can become the real reason why you train with weights.

At least these should be important motivations - since nobody else (not even your girlfriend or boyfriend) really cares how big your biceps are, or what you can bench press.

Another important reason to train is to reduce one's overall stress levels. Stress can be described as the "wear and tear of life". Stress occurs in varying degrees and in different forms - mental , emotional and physical. Normal levels of stress are healthy and desirable, but intense and persistent stress such as continuos fear, anger, and frustration can become bottled up inside and threaten health. It is the buildup of stress that leads to problems.

Without a doubt Zen dumbbell training is an excellent way to reduce stress, in part because of what we previously said about the integration of body movements and feelings into very day life. By improving ROM, strength, coordination and general fitness; you will feel much fitter, happier and healthier. Wait and see!

The knowledge that illness must be considered and treated in relation to the whole person forms the basis of many holistic medicine practices. When you are upset, angry, or frustrated you can perhaps reduce these negative feelings through exercise. Try to find a few minutes each day to use dumbbells; and I feel certain that the chances of illness will be reduced, and further that how you cope with illness will be more positively managed.

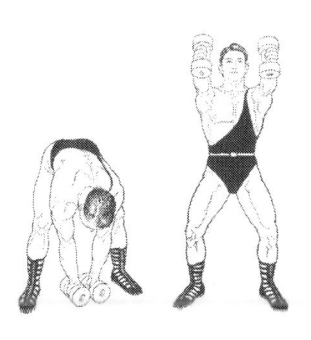

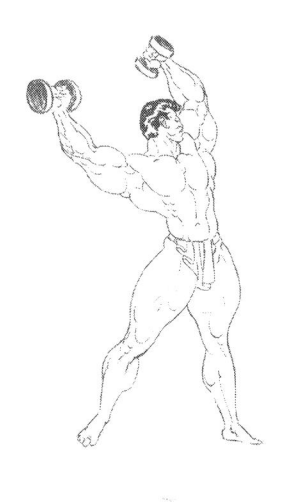

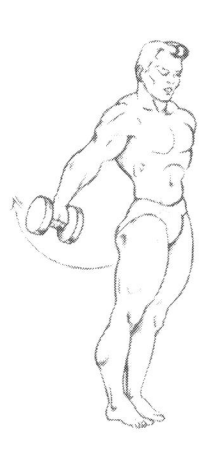

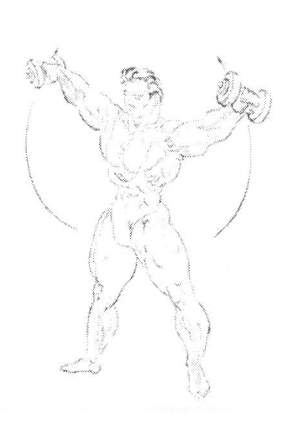

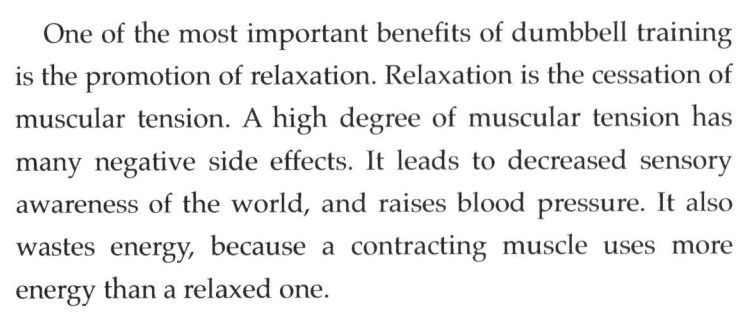

One of the most important benefits of dumbbell training is the promotion of relaxation. Relaxation is the cessation of muscular tension. A high degree of muscular tension has many negative side effects. It leads to decreased sensory awareness of the world, and raises blood pressure. It also wastes energy, because a contracting muscle uses more energy than a relaxed one.

A habitually tensed muscle tends to cut off circulation over time, and toxic and waist products build up in the muscle. This situation in turn causes fatigue, aches and even pain. This discussion of relaxation goes to the heart of what is wrong with many weight training programs. Macho types spend all of their time training chest, shoulders and biceps. And they do often end up with huge pectorals, deltoids and biceps - but also they have relatively week legs, back and abdominals as a result of in-balanced training. Thus their body kind of sags or slumps forward (as they walk about) in a hunched and round-shouldered look. Many times, the muscles of the back and stomach are simply too weak to support the bulk of the over-developed muscles in the top/front of such bodies. Often "benchers" have a belly sticking out front, and very skinny legs, and the whole physique package looks ridiculous.

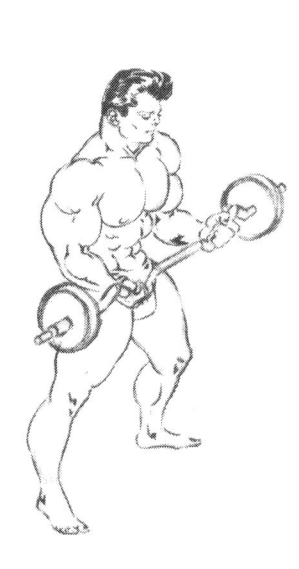

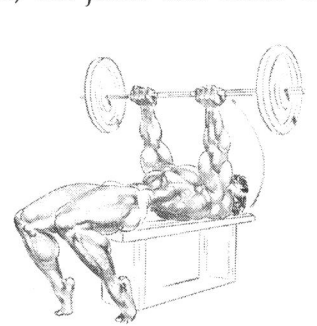

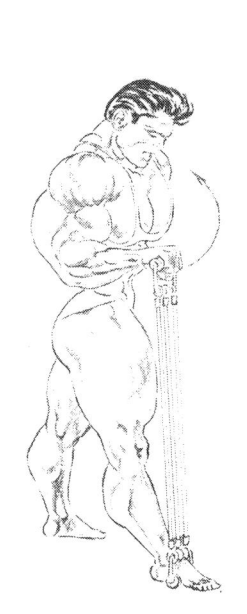

Can you develop muscles that are too large? In an era of steroids and advanced proteins - I would say definitely yes. My point is that if you do develop such an unbalanced physique, are you not placing yourself into a state of constant tension, as opposed to relaxation. You must tense certain muscles to support others, and because you have over-used certain exercises, the joints and limbs settle into the most unnatural of positions. Unfortunately, you may not even be able to get limbs back into their normal location(s), one-relative to another, because of poor flexibility and ROM.

Using weights that are too heavy also tends to throw the body into a state of permanent imbalance. Joints, tendons, and muscles became fixed into unnatural positions. But you don't *need* to lift hundreds of pounds in the bench press, squat or dead-lift - because it simply is not natural to do so in any case. Any person training like this will eventually be forced to change the way that he/she trains in any case because they will became injured (eventually). Focussing on a narrow range of exercises will further limit your flexibility, coordination and joint ROMs.

Is it not better to exercise with moderate weights, using dumbbells, and with a wide-range of exercises. You will be constantly mentally and physically challenged by such training, and it is also more fun.

The desire to be healthy and attractive is almost universal. The way to achieve your best physically in terms of body symmetry (right and left sides of the body identical) and proportion (body parts well-sized one relative to another), is through appropriate diet and exercise. Physical fitness and health can be greatly enhanced by daily physical activity. And daily training is the most natural way to train, but on a varying program of light to medium resistance exercises; just as we do in nature.

We now go onto describe the recommended dumbbell training program(s); including exercises and movement patterns.

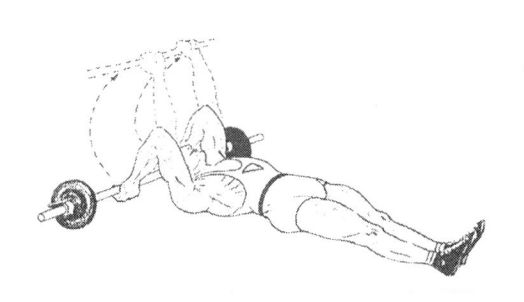

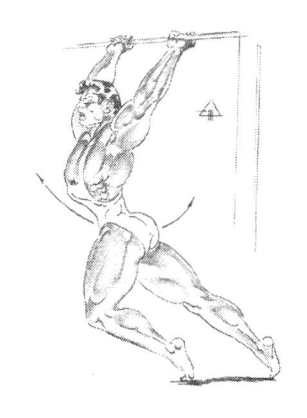

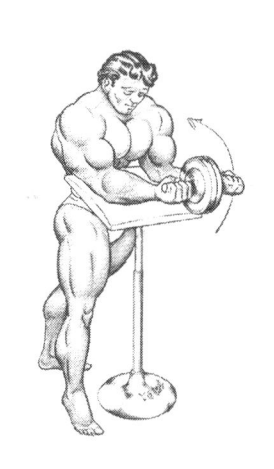

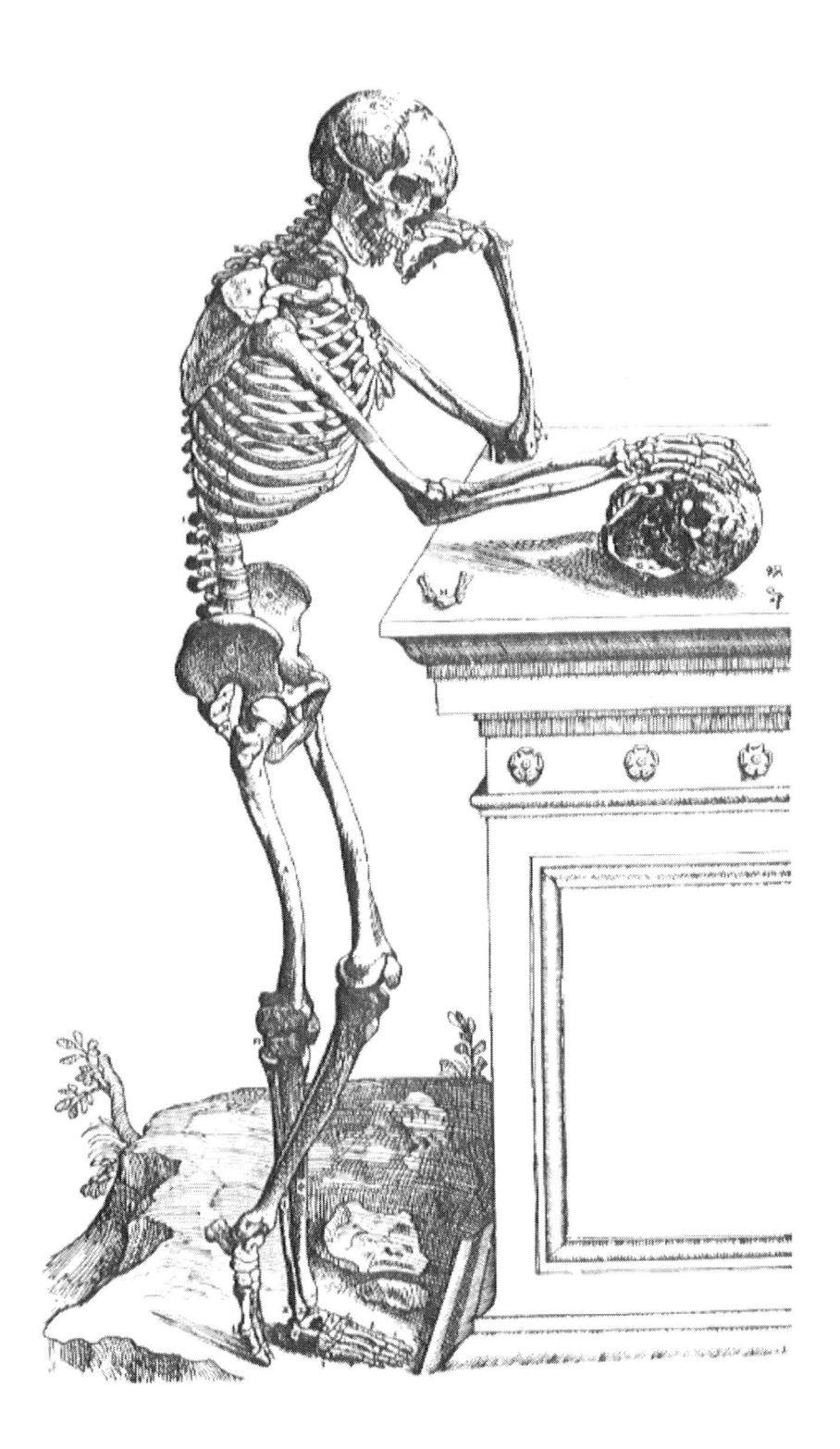

Light Dumbbell Training

EXPERTS ON physical training universally recognise that any exercise period should be preceded by a series of calisthenics and loosening exercises to warm up individual muscles. The benefits obtained from warm-up exercises are believed to be derived from the increased body temperature generally and also locally in specific body-parts.

The use of light dumbbell exercises to increase flexibility is also commonly based on the idea that it may decrease the incidence, intensity or duration of muscular pulls and joint injuries. Advantages of light dumbbell training include:

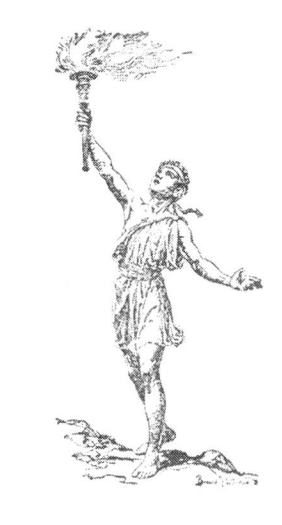

1. Union of mind, body and spirit
2. Relaxation of stress
3. Muscular relaxation
4. Improved health and strength
5. Improved cardiovascular system
6. Spiritual growth and learning about oneself
7. Improvement in posture, symmetry and proportion
8. Reduction in lower back pain - and joint pain generally
9. Increased range of motion (ROM)
10. Improved coordination, balance of body when lifting
11. Improved movement pattens - specific and generally
12. Enhanced performance skills
13. Reduced risk of injury
14. Personal enjoyment and gratification

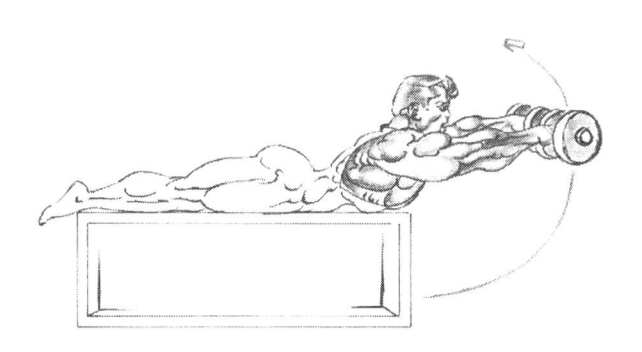

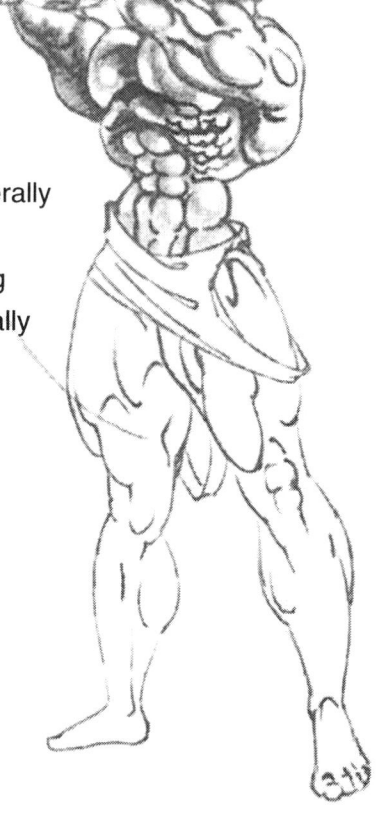

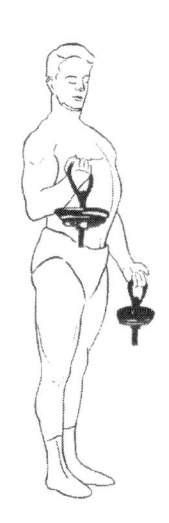

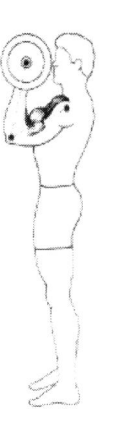

Light dumbbell training can also help healthy muscles maintain a structural homeostasis. That is the muscular relationship, one relative to another, in terms of size, length, position, strength, flexibility of body parts etc. In order to achieve such a state, it is important to follow a well-balanced training program that includes a wide-range of exercises for all of the different muscles and joints of the human body.

This is another reason for writing this book, to provide information relating to well-balanced dumbbell training, including choice of the the correct exercises, techniques and movement patterns.

A key to this structural balance is an equal pull by antagonistic muscles. Due to the attachments of muscles, any imbalance in the structural relationships between muscles can cause changes to the lever action(s) on the process and range of motion involved in movement.

Muscle imbalance can be due to several factors, including muscle strength, weakness, and the momentary degree of muscle tension/relaxation. When you add in any injuries to joints, tendons, bones etc; it is easy to see that maintaining a perfectly functioning structure is not always possible. And in fact it may not be desirable in every case.

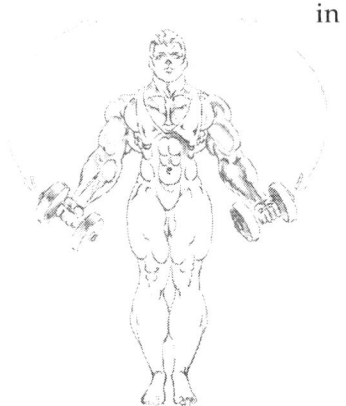

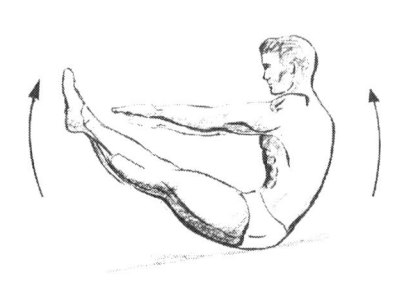

Nevertheless it seems clear that we should strive for muscle balance within our own body; so far as it is desirable, achievable and with respect to any other goals that we might have. It is worth noting that any athlete who wanted to achieve world-class level in a sport may perhaps have to forgo ideal muscle balance in favour of the specialist and abnormal capabilities that are the requirement of success in that particular sporting endeavour.

Even people who are natural athletes, with good general suppleness, flexibility, strength and skills; can have poor local and general muscle control. Muscle control refers to adequate balance, coordination, and control of one's body-parts and/or sufficient muscular strength to perform a given skill.

The lesson is that we all have something that we need to work on, and the aim should be balancing our physical capabilities; in order to create harmony and to engender a state of overall health and fitness. In other words, an ability to cope with the stresses and strains of every day life. Light dumbbell training may involve using 1 lb weights, even if you can bench press 400 lbs or more. Remember that light weights are heavy. Try this if you don't believe me. Stand up, grab a 2 lbs dumbbell, and whilst keeping your arm perfectly straight, perform a series of shoulder circles with the arm held out to the front/side of the body. Start with small circles - just a 2-3 inches, and move up to circles of 1 foot radius or more. Continue for 5-10 minutes if you can.

Notice how heavy the 2 lbs weight becomes, and how the whole shoulder area becomes engorged with blood. You will also find that if you perform similar movements regularly that you may experience improved joint ROMs and that any pains/aches that you previously experienced in the shoulder joint disappear. Plus your strength (in terms of joint stability) will in all likelihood increase at the same time.

And all from a 2 lbs dumbbell. Light really is sometimes heavy, and better even for strength building in some ways.

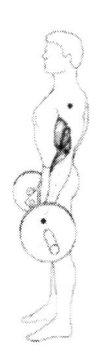

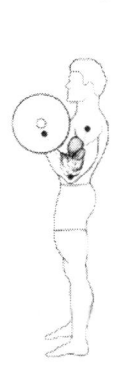

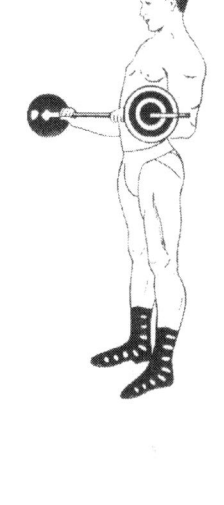

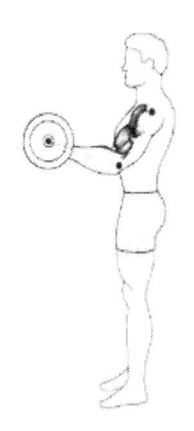

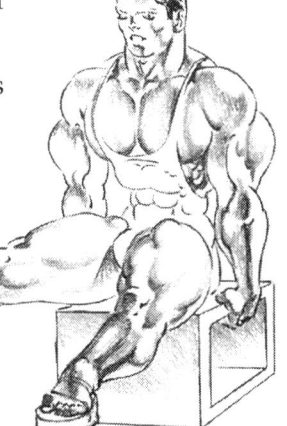

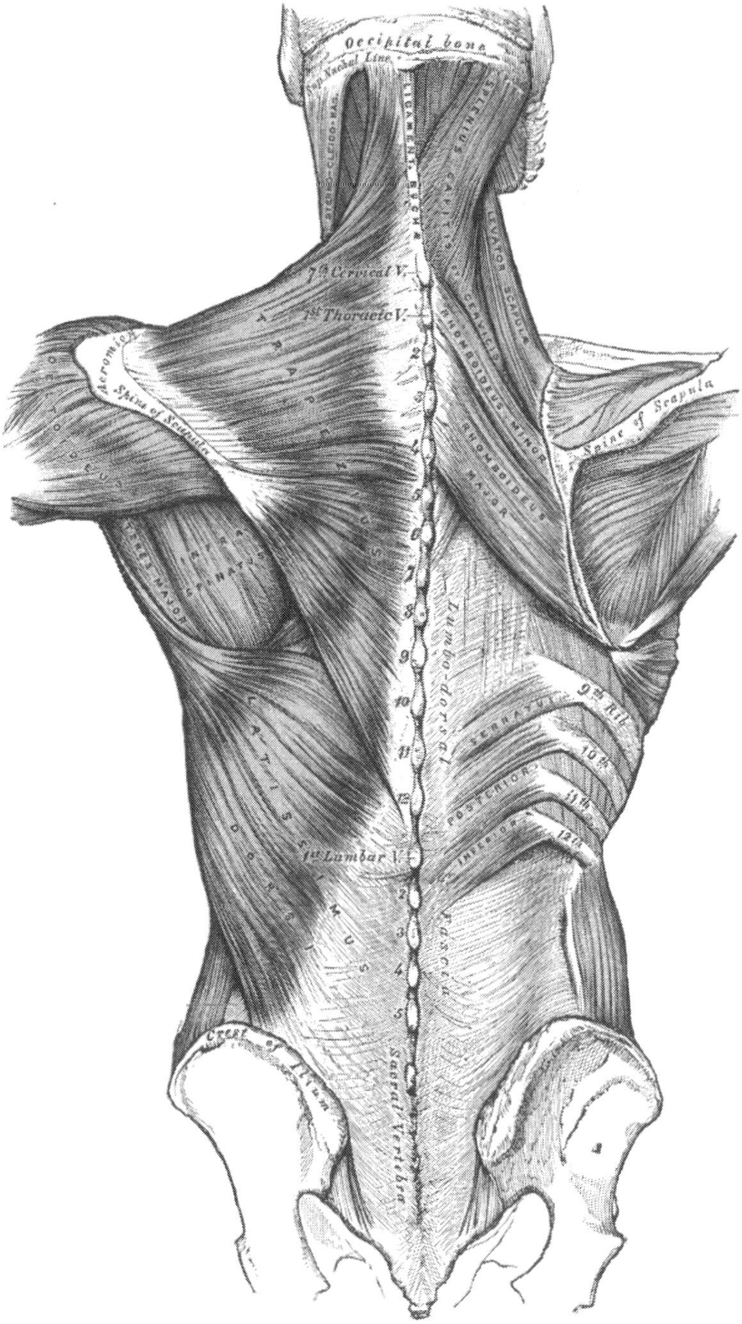
Occipital bone
Sup. Nuchal Line
SPLENIUS CAPITIS
LEVATOR SCAPULA
7th Cervical V.
1st Thoracic V.
RHOMBOIDEUS MINOR
RHOMBOIDEUS MAJOR
Acromion
Spine of Scapula
Spine of Scapula
TERES MAJOR
Lumbo-dorsal
9th Rib
10th
11th
12th
SERRATUS
POSTERIOR
INFERIOR
1st Lumbar V.
Fascia
Crest of Ilium
Sacral Vertebra

Safety

The following are the safety principles that should be observed when training with barbells / dumbbells. These principles are not necessarily the final word, but they do represent some important points to remember when undertaking a program of resistance training.

Given first are the general principles of safe dumbbell training. Remember, dumbbell training takes intelligence.

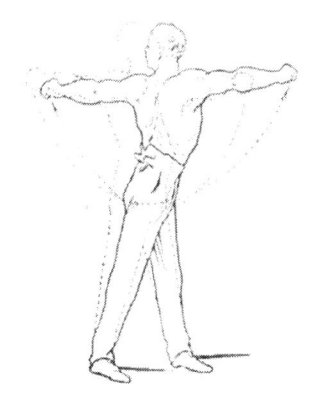

1. Safety

Safety always comes first. And this requires sufficient attitudes, skills, and knowledge about the control of potential hazards. A simple 4 step procedure is as follows: A) know the hazards, B) remove hazards when feasible, C) control those hazards that cannot be removed and D) create no additional hazards.

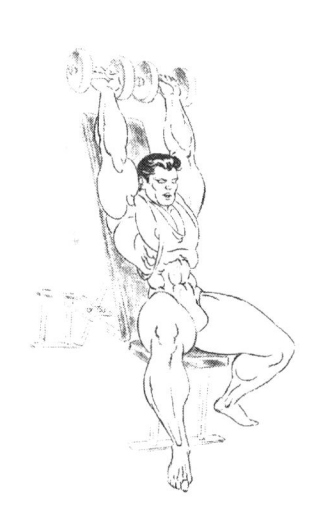

2. Medical Exam

Ideally, a medical examination should be obtained before undertaking any exercise program. Such an examination may reveal that certain types of dumbbell exercise are contra-indicated; due to the trainee's personal physical capabilities, limitations, diseases, structure and/ or general health and conditioning.

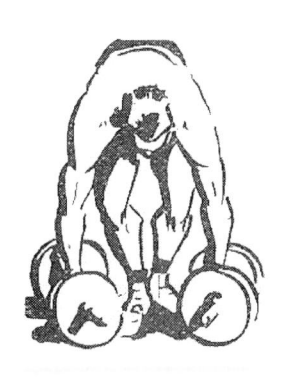

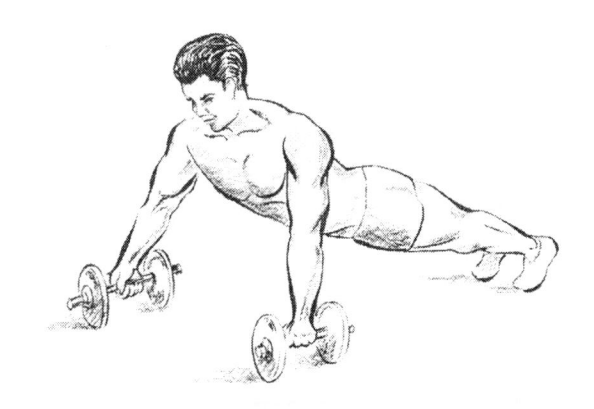

3. Identifiable Goals

You normally define your goals before you begin a dumbbell training program, and you should have an idea of the time it will take to reach your desired goals. Make sure, whatever your goals may be, that they are realistic.

4. Individualised Program

All dumbbell exercises should be designed to fit an individual's specific needs. Often a coach, instructor or other person expects the trainee to fit into their own conception of what a training program should be, without any real consideration whatsoever of the true needs of the individual. One has to be careful as a result, and only take advice/instruction from well-meaning and knowledgable people who proceed according to the needs, strengths and limitations of the individual trainee. It is beneficial to keep accurate records of training workouts, although not everyone likes to do this.

General Training Principles

We can identify a set of general training principles that can help anyone to train efficiently.

1   Listen to your own body - tune in - before you drop out!
2. Educate yourself about the exercises - form, tempo etc.

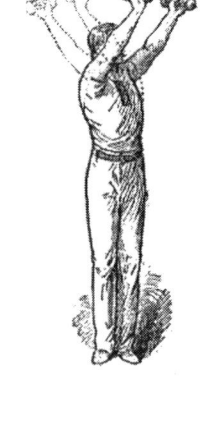

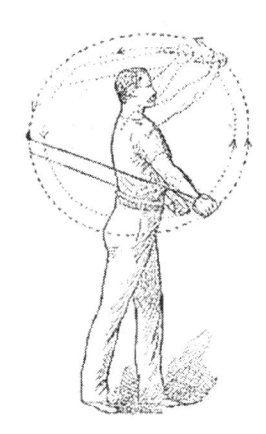

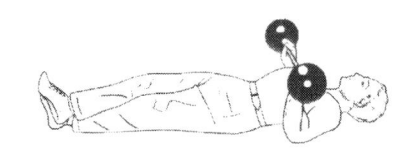

3. Learn from others - but remember that you are an individual and what works for them might not work for you and vice versa
4. Clothes and shoes - wear appropriate, loose fitting and / or easy-to-move in clothes
5. Do not attempt to compete with others - everyone is unique and has particular strengths and weaknesses
6. In general I would recommend exercising in the open air, and/or in a well-ventilated place
7. Mental set - maintain a positive mental attitude at all times, and don't spend time talking or chatting to people whilst training
8. Relaxation / tension - when lifting maintain a healthy balance between relaxation and tension. Do not over-strain or over-tense the body, and if you do then consider using lighter weights!

Always use the best (professional) equipment - and select high-quality barbells and dumbbells. A good-quality Olympic bar (7 feet long) is an essential tool for the clean and press, squats and dead-lifts etc. Eleiko, Leoko and York used to make some of the best Olympic bars and plates. Beware of imitations, and do not use poor or loose fitting plates. IronMind (USA) and Wolverson (UK) make the best dumbbells and kettle-bells; but there are many other excellent manufacturers. Try to get dumbbells with thicker handles (1.5-2 inches) and/or get ones with a "comfort" fatter-in-the-middle grip.

Dumbbell Practice

Pavel Tsatsouline, the famous kettle-bell instructor says that Russian lifters like to call training practice, and we shall follow suit here. General training considerations:

1. Always perform a general body warm up
2. Always warm up the joints / muscles to be worked
3. Warm up should not be with heavy resistance (weight)
4. Warm up should not involve deep stretching!
5. Start with light weights using a method and procedure to increase weight slowly (pyramiding weights is best)

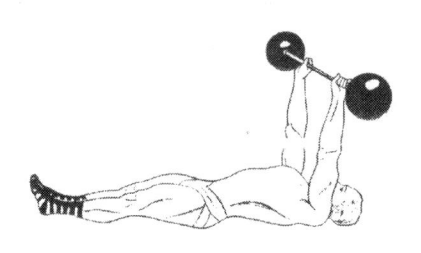

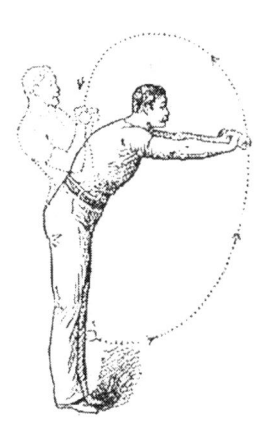

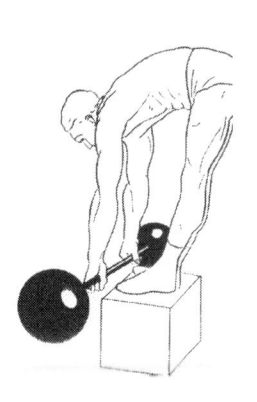

Zen Dumbbell Training

1. Use dumbbells over barbells or machines
2. Light weights are heavy - use full ROM
3. Pay attention to form - never cheat
4. Perform very light (ROM) dumbbell gymnastics daily
5. Choose standing exercises over seated/lying alternatives
6. Reduce rest between sets (10 - 30 seconds)
7. Always perform dips, chins, press-ups
8. Perform exercises for all 5 body regions (lots of movements)
9. Use static holds (up to minutes), rest-pause, burns, mid-range mini-reps, circular movement patterns, deep stretches
10. Perform lots of sets and the widest range of movements [around 50-60 sets in 40 minutes]

[SEE: CHAPTER 27 FOR 5 MOTTOS OF ZEN TRAINING]

I am going to try and convince you that you have to design your own routines, and use a far wider variety of exercises than you may be used to, and also that you must use very light (at least lighter) weights for some movements (ROM exercises). Lighter weights are heavier in a sense anyway. The individual muscles and joints of the body do not (in a real sense) know the difference between a light and heavy weight. But rather the muscles know that they are under strain - and if it exceeds or challenges current capacity or not.

My logic here is as follows: when you strain under a tremendous weight (one that is far too heavy), the larger joints/muscles take over in a load bearing capacity and the

> There is no singular way to perform any particular exercise. Often several correct performance styles are possible; and many incorrect styles. Some styles (movement patterns) may be more suited to a particular individual, and others less so. Sometimes (ROM training) one may benefit from experimenting with multiple movement patterns (performance styles) for an exercise.

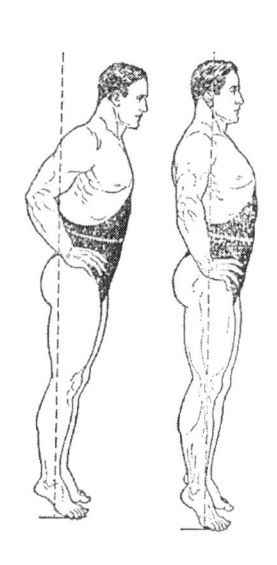

body distorts itself into a new shape or physical assembly in order to accommodate the extra stress. In such circumstances, the body becomes rigid in terms of the largest supporting structures, and so taking stress off many smaller muscles which just relax as a result.

Do not think of the body as a fixed assembly of parts, but rather as a set of machine parts which come-together and work in unison in response to environmental requirements and/or brain controlled instructions. Thus in order to use the body in its most natural form you should not overload it; letting the weight dictate the relationships between the parts - and hence structural shape of the body as a whole - but rather use weights which allow one's brain (and instincts) to determine (that is to choose) the appropriate overall (ideal) physical form of the body in response to any stress.

Do not be afraid to break with convention and try entirely new things, even methods nobody else has ever attempted. Especially "switch-things-up" once you have become adapted to one type of routine. Remember that you must (sometimes) surprise the body, by challenging it.

In the next sections we split the body into 5 main regions, and then look at the best exercises for the same. Unlike other muscle-building books we are concerned with bones, movement pattern optimisation plus joint ROMs. Do not be put-off by the apparent complexity of human anatomy. At the very least, become familiar with how three joint types in particular function: being the *spine, hip* and *shoulder (scapula)*; because one or the other are involved (to a greater or lesser degree) in almost every possible type of human movement.

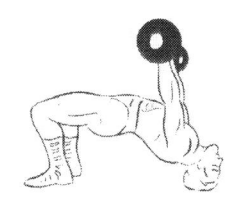

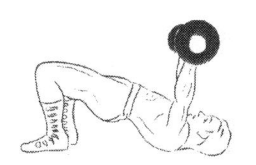

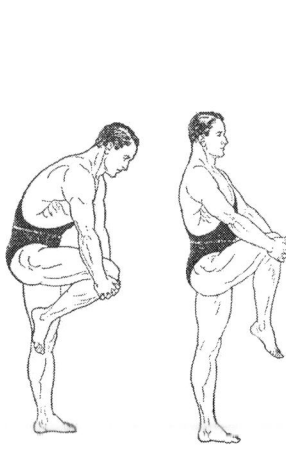

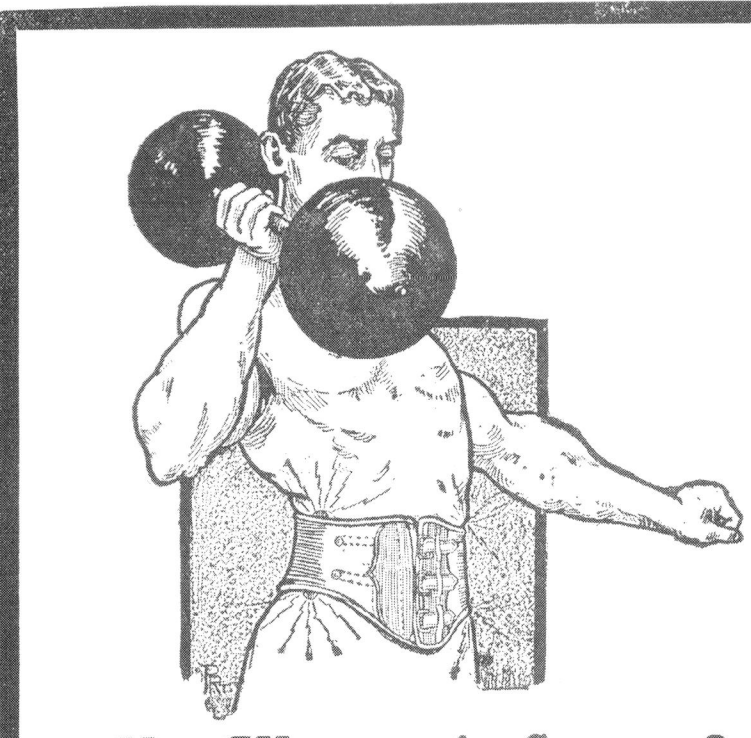

Do You Want to be Strong?

To feel as vigorous and healthy as you used to do? To enjoy life again? To get up in the morning refreshed by sleep and not more tired than when you went to bed? To have no weakness in the back or "come-and-go" pain? No Indigestion or Constipation? To know that your strength is not slipping away? To once more have bright eyes, healthy colour in your cheeks, and be confident that what other men can do is not impossible to you? In short, do you want to be a man among men?

There is nothing so penetrating, nothing so invigorating, nothing that will relieve weakness and pain as speedily and surely as the Pulvermacher Electric Belt. It assists Nature by a general reinforcement of the vital energy by infusing a mild, invigorating current of Electricity into the nerves, and by supplying the system with the very essence of nerve vigour and nerve strength.

THE PULVERMACHER ELECTRIC BELT

Cures Indigestion, Constipation, Biliousness, and all forms of Liver Complaint. Rheumatism, Gout, Sciatica, and Lumbago are speedily removed by its use. It proves an unfailing remedy for Kidney troubles, pain and weakness in the back. Its use revives health in delicate women, while for every kind of Nervous Weakness or Exhaustion and General Debility in Men and Women it is a sure and certain cure.

Thirty Days' Free Trial.

If you are a sufferer, write at once, in confidence, fully describing your case; when, in addition to the book, we will send a letter of advice, recommending the most suitable style of Belt for your case. To show our confidence in its curative powers, we will supply this Belt on Thirty Days' Trial. Then if you are not perfectly satisfied, return it to us. The trial will cost you nothing if you are not cured.

Get Pulvermacher's Great Book on Electro-Galvanism. It is sent FREE and post paid to all who write for it. Remember, it is not a mere catalogue of our goods, but a Standard Work on Electricity as a Curative Agent, and should be in the hands of every health-seeker.

WRITE OR CALL TO-DAY WITHOUT FAIL. Address your letter:

Superintendent, PULVERMACHER'S GALVANIC ESTABLISHMENT, 45, Vulcan House, 56, Ludgate Hill, London, E.C.

(Removed from 194, Regent Street, W.)   Established 1848.

Health and Strength Magazine - March 1904

CHAPTER SIX

Movement Anatomy

IN THIS Chapter we explore how the body moves; looking in detail at the various levers, joints and moving parts that make up the human body as whole. We take a different approach than any other weight-training book, in that we partition the body into 5 basic regions; being the trunk, shoulder, elbow, hip and knee, plus ankle and foot. In so doing we place emphasis on the mechanical actions of the various moving parts; and on the ways in which the body is "designed" to move, and especially in terms of joint ROMs.

Our approach is based on an analysis of the anatomy of movement, and in terms of the basic structure of the body and how the parts can, and do, move. We seek to discover natural movement patterns for the body as a whole.

The human body can be thought of as a type of machine, with systems of "hinged" parts and levers that afford movement. But if it is a machine, then the body is an intelligent one, and one that speaks to us directly. We must pay close attention to it's messages.

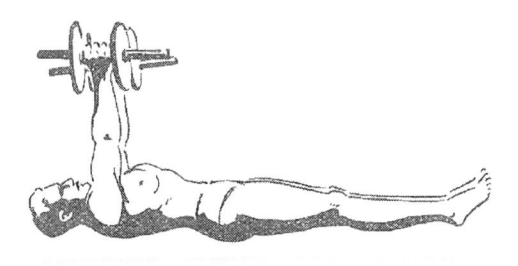

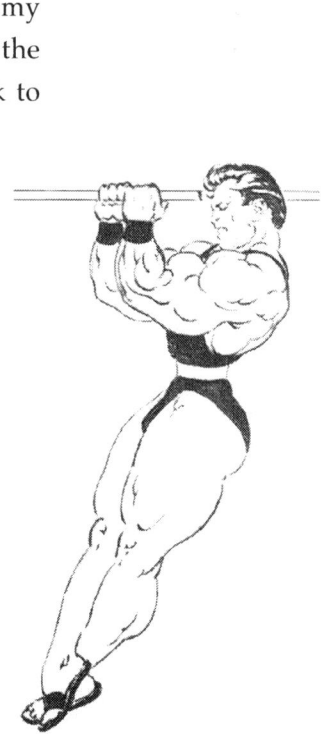

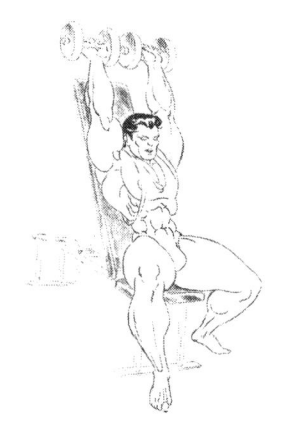

Anatomy

When the human body moves, it does so by interaction of three systems:

- the **bones** of the skeleton,
- linked together at the **joints**,
- are moved by action of the **muscles**.

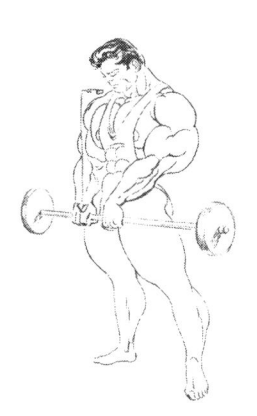

Therefore we are concerned with bones that move around joints; and as pulled by muscles. Other structures are involved as intermediaries also, including ligaments and tendons etc. Explanation of body movements is a difficult topic, because the various parts of the body can move in many different directions. Often several body parts move at once, and more than one joint is involved.

To aid analysis, we follow convention and identify:

- begin by considering each joint in isolation
- three perpendicular planes are used for reference
- movements are described in relation to the standard "anatomical position". This is where the body is standing upright, the feet are parallel, the arms hanging by the side, and the palms and face are directed forward.

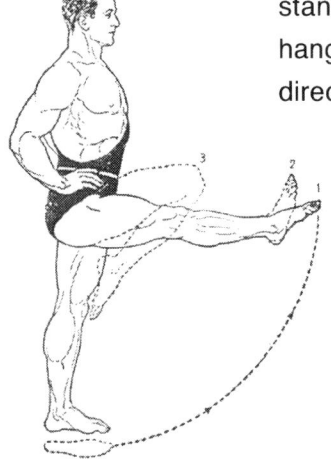

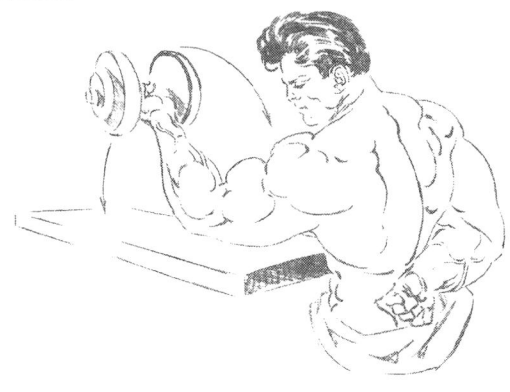

MOVEMENT ANATOMY   109

Flexion / Extension
of the shoulder

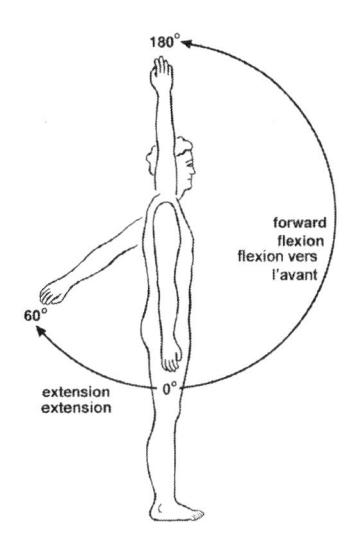

180°
forward flexion
flexion vers l'avant
60°
extension
extension
0°

Abduction / Adduction
of the Shoulder

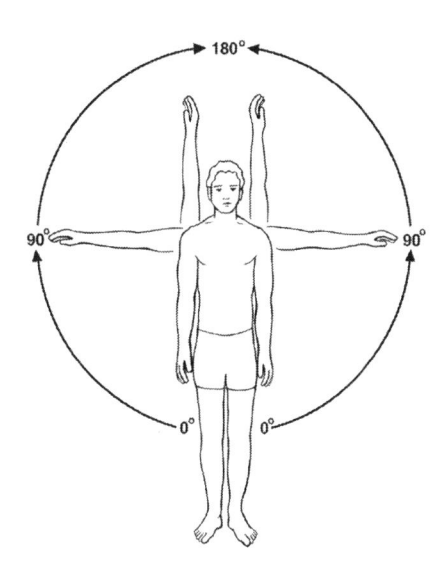

180°
90°   90°
0°   0°

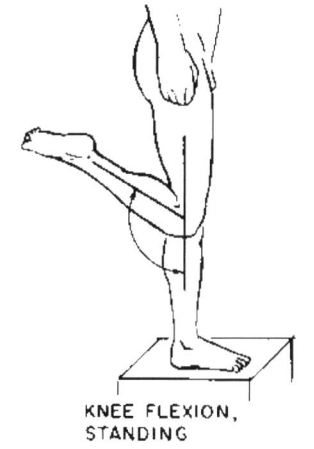

KNEE FLEXION,
STANDING

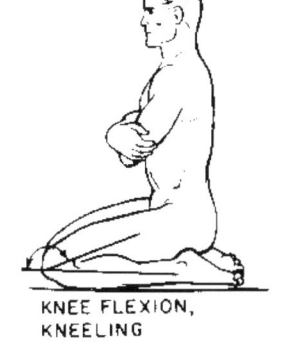

KNEE FLEXION,
KNEELING

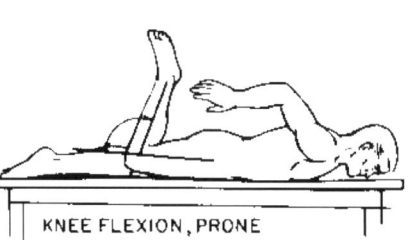

KNEE FLEXION, PRONE

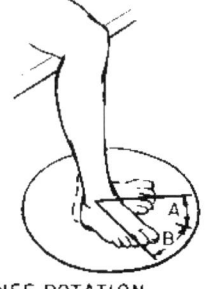

KNEE ROTATION,
MEDIAL (A),
LATERAL (B)

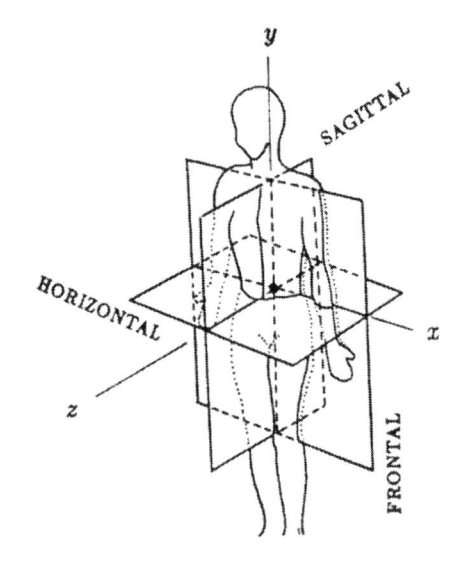

Planes of Movement

The **left/right plane** divides the body into symmetrical right and left halves. Any plane parallel to the median plane is called a **sagittal plane**.

A movement in a sagittal plane which takes a part of the body forward from anatomical position is called **flexion**. A movement in the sagittal plane which takes a part of the body backward from the anatomical position is called **extension**. N.B. Sagittal plane moves are seen from the side.

There are a few exceptions to this naming convention. Flexion of the knee is when you move the lower leg closer to the buttocks, and extension of the knee is when you move the leg towards a straightened position. Likewise extension of the ankle is when you bring the foot in line with the leg, and flexion is when you bend the ankle maximally.

A coronal or **frontal plane** is any plane perpendicular to the median plane. It divides the body into anterior and posterior parts. A movement in the frontal plane which takes a part of the body toward the median plane is called **adduction**. The opposite type of movement (away from the median plane) is called **abduction**. For the trunk or neck, movement in the frontal plane away from the median plane is called **lateral flexion** or **side-bending**.

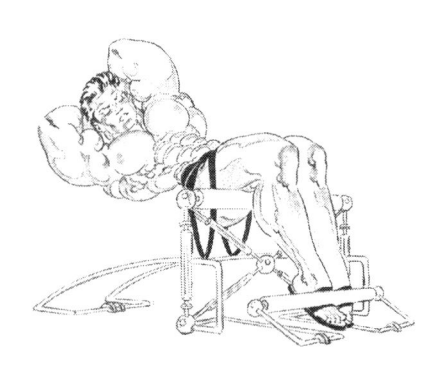

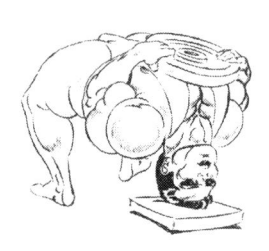

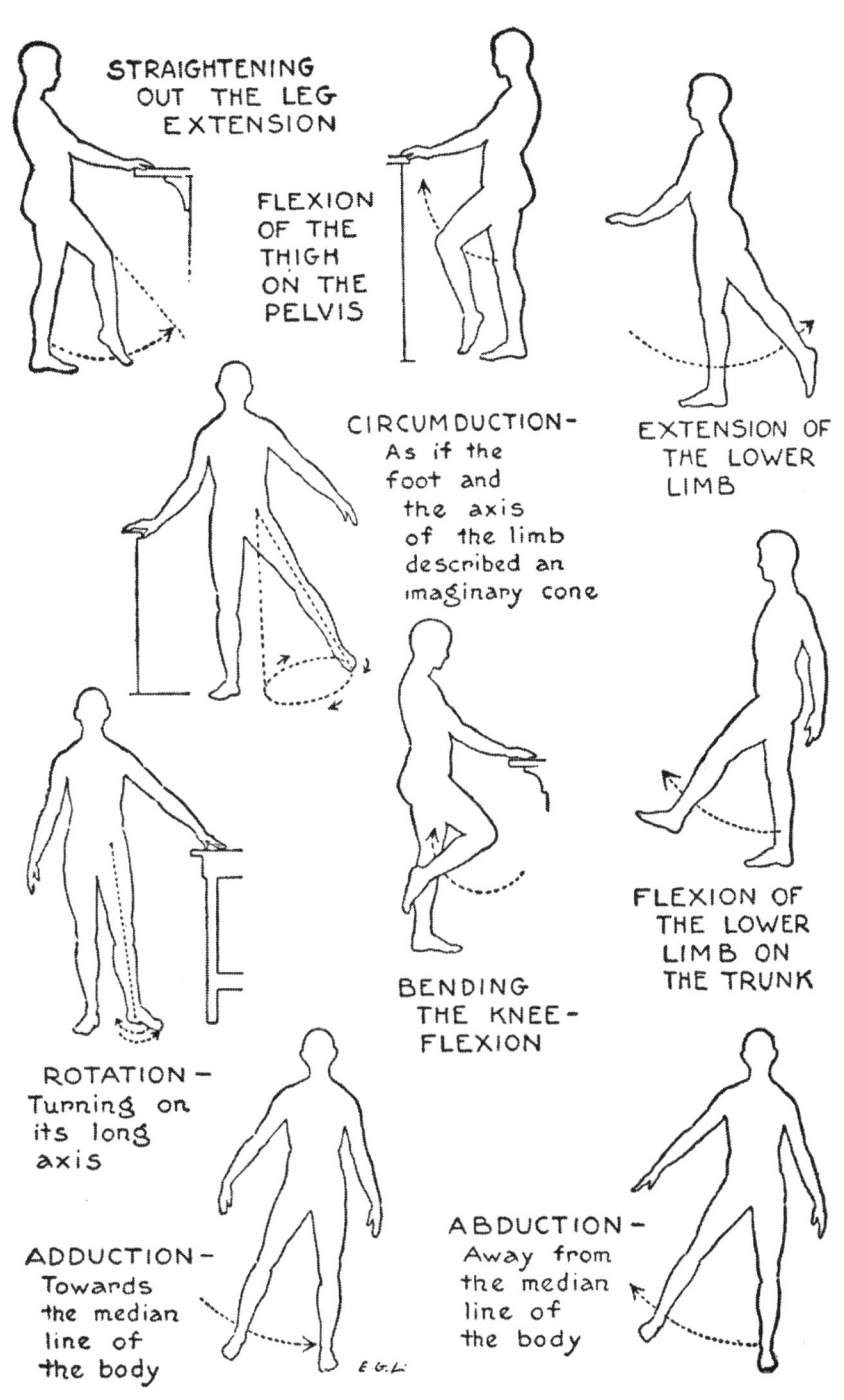

MOVEMENTS OF THE LOWER LIMB.

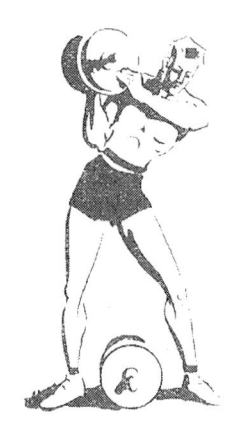

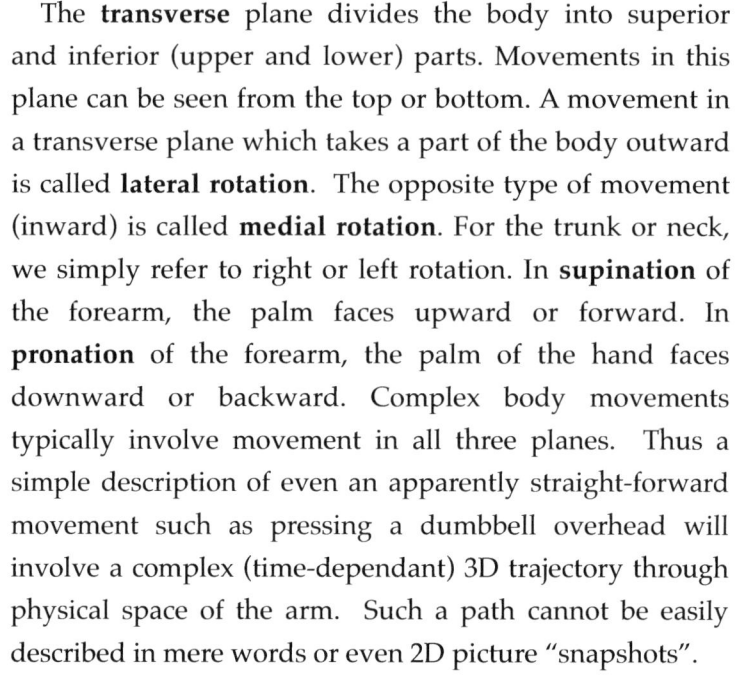

The **transverse** plane divides the body into superior and inferior (upper and lower) parts. Movements in this plane can be seen from the top or bottom. A movement in a transverse plane which takes a part of the body outward is called **lateral rotation**. The opposite type of movement (inward) is called **medial rotation**. For the trunk or neck, we simply refer to right or left rotation. In **supination** of the forearm, the palm faces upward or forward. In **pronation** of the forearm, the palm of the hand faces downward or backward. Complex body movements typically involve movement in all three planes. Thus a simple description of even an apparently straight-forward movement such as pressing a dumbbell overhead will involve a complex (time-dependant) 3D trajectory through physical space of the arm. Such a path cannot be easily described in mere words or even 2D picture "snapshots".

We can conclude that human movement is best captured in video form, and also should be viewed from multiple directions or perspectives. This fact is why weight-training (or any movement based sport) is really not something one can simply read about to learn. One has to actually practice, and in order to learn the 3D movement patterns involved, and normally (at first) under the supervision of an expert coach.

It is important to realise that usually one moves in several different planes to move a limb; which involves the action of multiple joints and many muscles etc. Overall, there is no need to remember the names and classification of each different type of movement; but rather it is useful to be able to "picture" in your head the way that each particular joint moves.

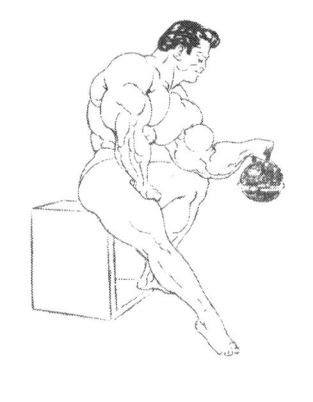

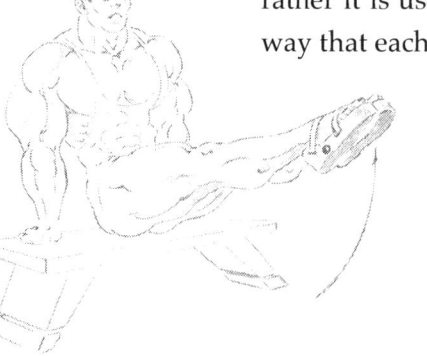

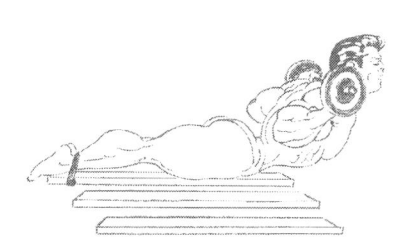

MOVEMENT ANATOMY 113

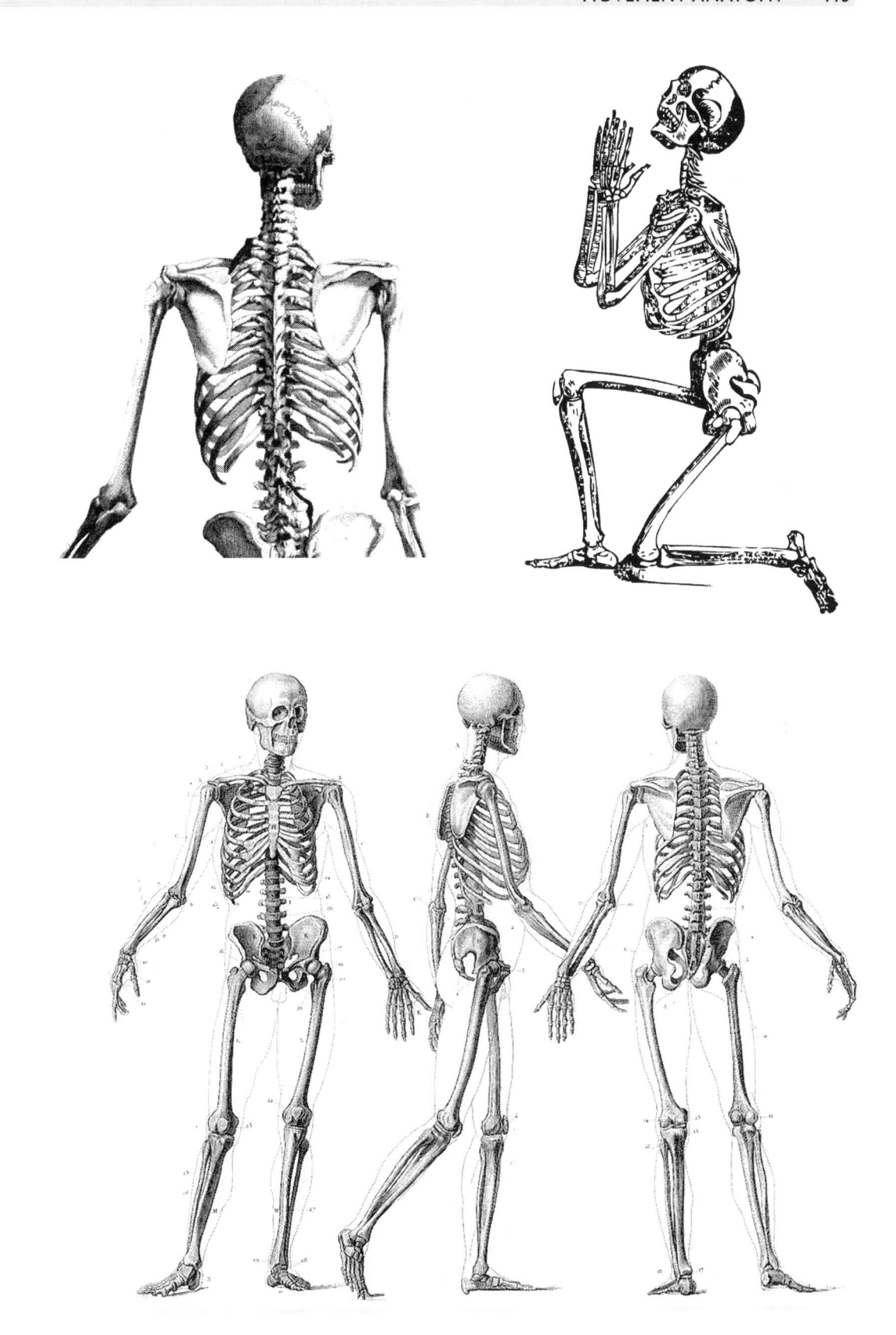

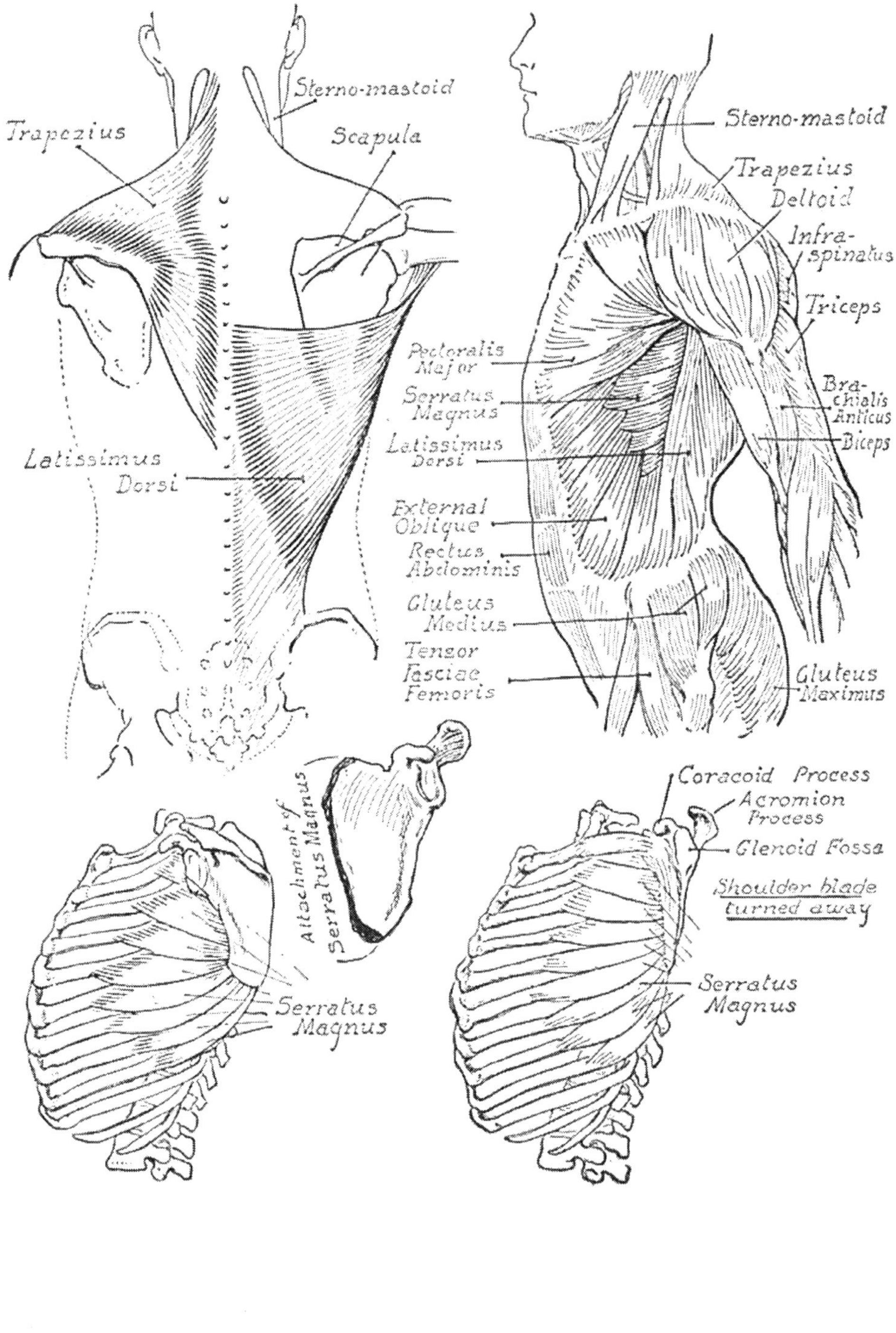
Sterno-mastoid
Trapezius
Scapula
Latissimus
Dorsi
Sterno-mastoid
Trapezius
Deltoid
Infra-
spinatus
Triceps
Pectoralis
Major
Serratus
Magnus
Latissimus
Dorsi
Bra-
chialis
Anticus
Biceps
External
Oblique
Rectus
Abdominis
Gluteus
Medius
Tensor
Fasciae
Femoris
Gluteus
Maximus
Attachment of
Serratus Magnus
Serratus
Magnus
Coracoid Process
Acromion
Process
Glenoid Fossa
Shoulder blade
turned away
Serratus
Magnus

Muscle Movements

Muscles come in many different forms and types. In fact, there are around 650 muscles in the human body and over 200 individual bones. When we speak of a particular movement, the muscle which produces it is called the **agonist**, and the muscle which produces the opposite movement is called the **antagonist**.

Note that mutually opposing muscles often function together to fix or stabilise a bone. Different muscles which cooperate to produce the same action are called **synergistic**.

When a muscle contracts, it tends to draw its origin and insertion points closer together. Anything which opposes this tendency is called **resistance**. For example, the brachialis and the biceps brachii are the major flexors of the elbow. Their action can be opposed by several types of resistance; including "curling" motions and "pulling" motions. When a muscle contracts, a movement occurs. However the movement may be caused by forces other than the muscle itself. Sometimes gravity and other forces "help" or "oppose" movement.

Whenever you make any type of movement with an arm or leg, literally dozens of muscles contract in order to achieve the limb articulation. There is no such thing as an "isolated" muscle contraction.

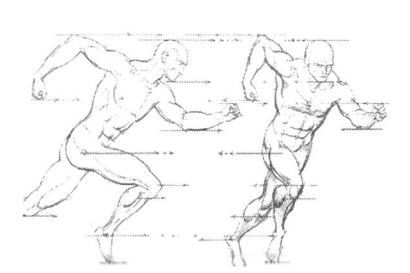

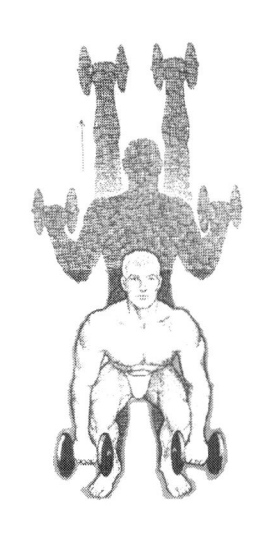

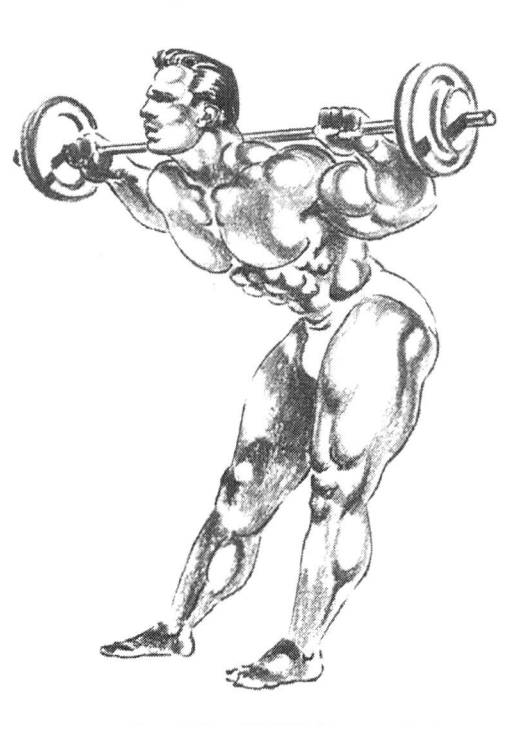

116   ZEN OF DUMBBELL TRAINING

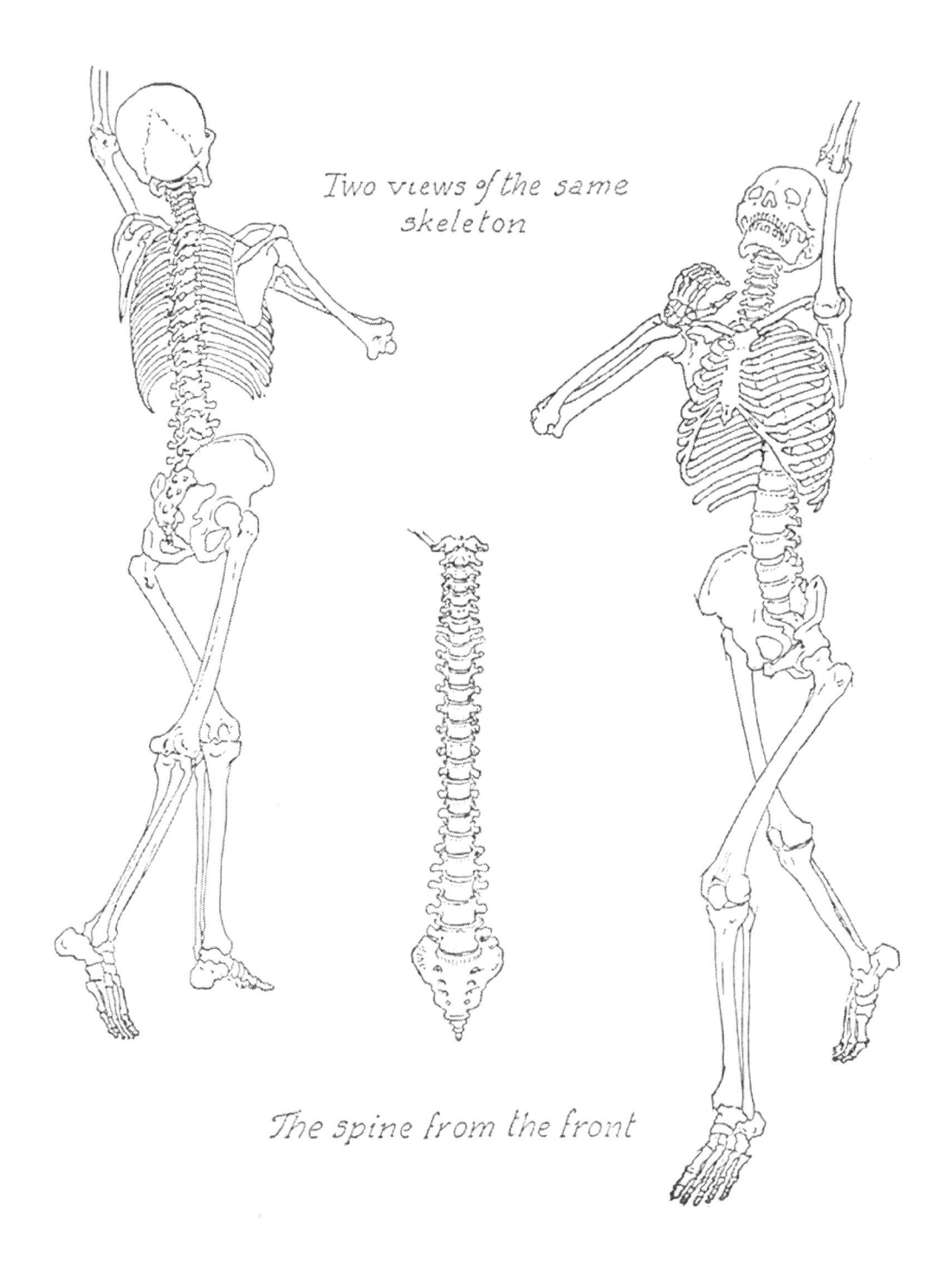

Two views of the same skeleton

The spine from the front

Even delicate finger movements normally require simultaneous contraction of multiple stabilising muscles in the arm and shoulder!

When you **flex**, you contract a specific muscle, creating a a force that attempts to "shorten" the muscle. When a movement occurs because of an active muscle, the muscle insertions are moved closer together. This type of contraction is called **concentric**. In some cases, a muscle works without initiating the action itself; instead, it "applies the brakes" to the action." Without the brakes of this muscle action, it would occur faster. If the muscles which oppose a movement apply the breaks, their contraction is called **eccentric**. This occurs during lengthening of muscles. It is possible that a muscle is contracted even though no movement is taking place. For example the thigh can be flexed and then held in this position (against gravity or other force).

In order to lift say, a heavy object, certain parts of the body must remain semi-rigid (often under semi-conscious control - whether you realise it or not) whilst other parts are allowed to move freely. The basis of all movement is a rigid base, which in the case of lifting an object overhead, often includes flexed (or semi-flexed) buttocks, firm leg muscles and flexed (firm) stabilising back and abdominal muscles. Thus the lower body and back (and associated skeleton and joints) must remain fairly "rigid" to lift something overhead.

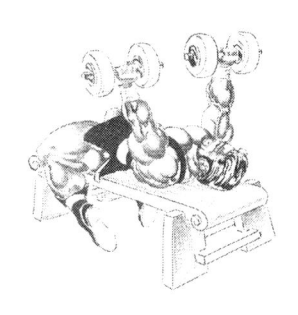

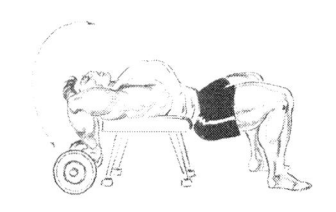

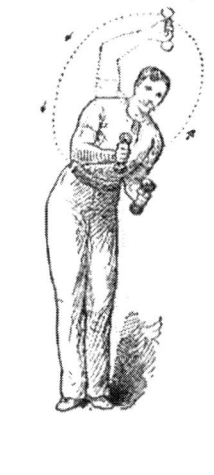

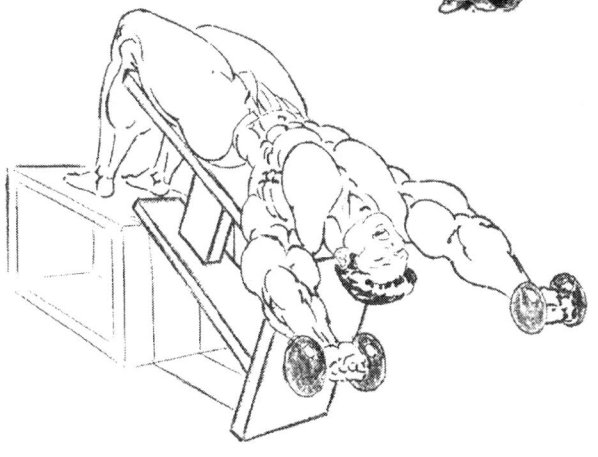

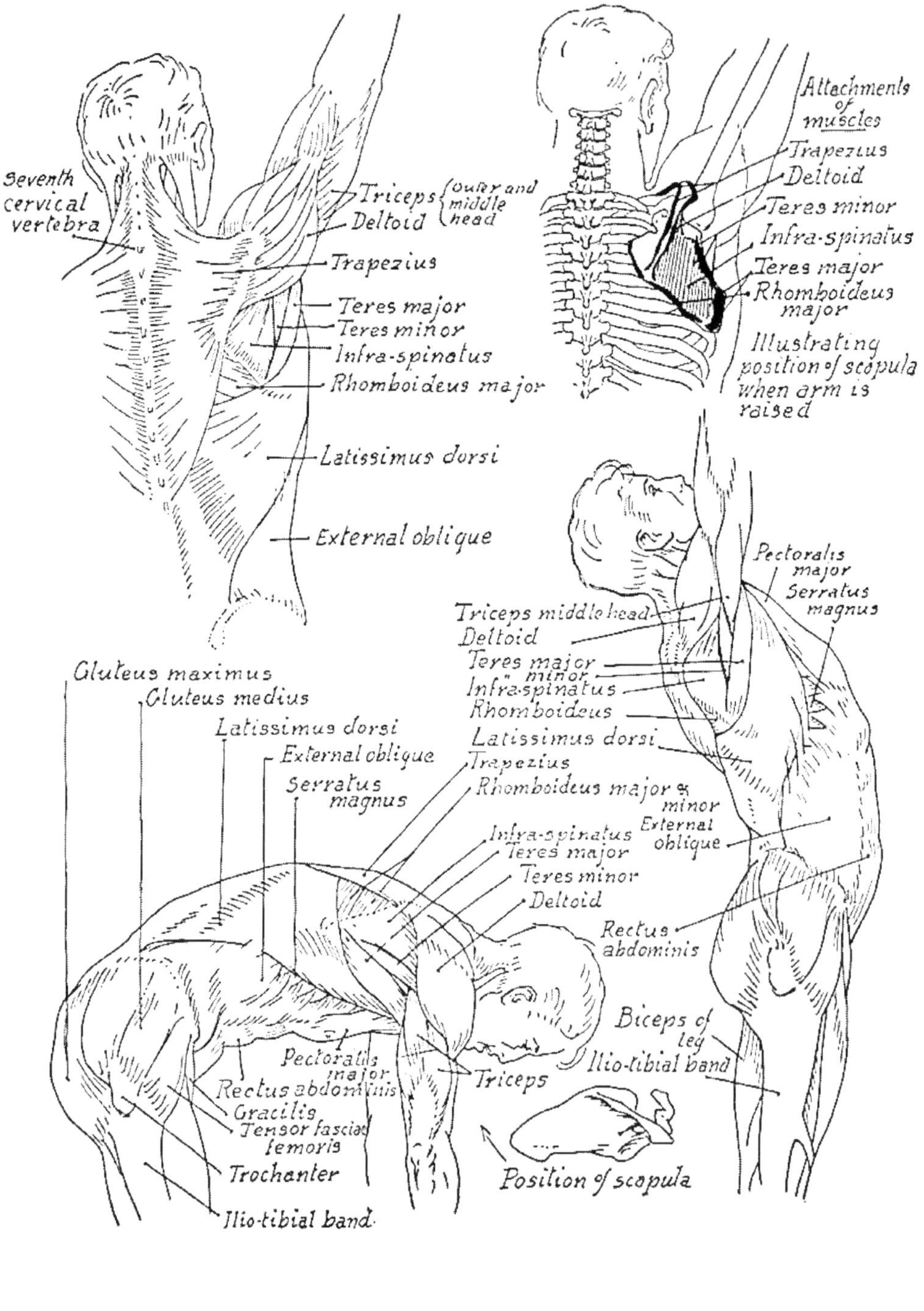
Seventh
cervical
vertebra
Triceps (outer and middle head)
Deltoid
Trapezius
Teres major
Teres minor
Infra-spinatus
Rhomboideus major
Latissimus dorsi
External oblique
Attachments of muscles
Trapezius
Deltoid
Teres minor
Infra-spinatus
Teres major
Rhomboideus major
Illustrating position of scapula when arm is raised
Pectoralis major
Serratus magnus
Triceps middle head
Deltoid
Teres major
" minor
Infra-spinatus
Rhomboideus
Latissimus dorsi
Gluteus maximus
Gluteus medius
Latissimus dorsi
External oblique
Serratus magnus
Trapezius
Rhomboideus major & minor
External oblique
Infra-spinatus
Teres major
Teres minor
Deltoid
Rectus abdominis
Biceps of leg
Ilio-tibial band
Pectoralis major
Rectus abdominis
Triceps
Gracilis
Tensor fasciæ femoris
Trochanter
Ilio-tibial band
Position of scapula

MOVEMENT ANATOMY 119

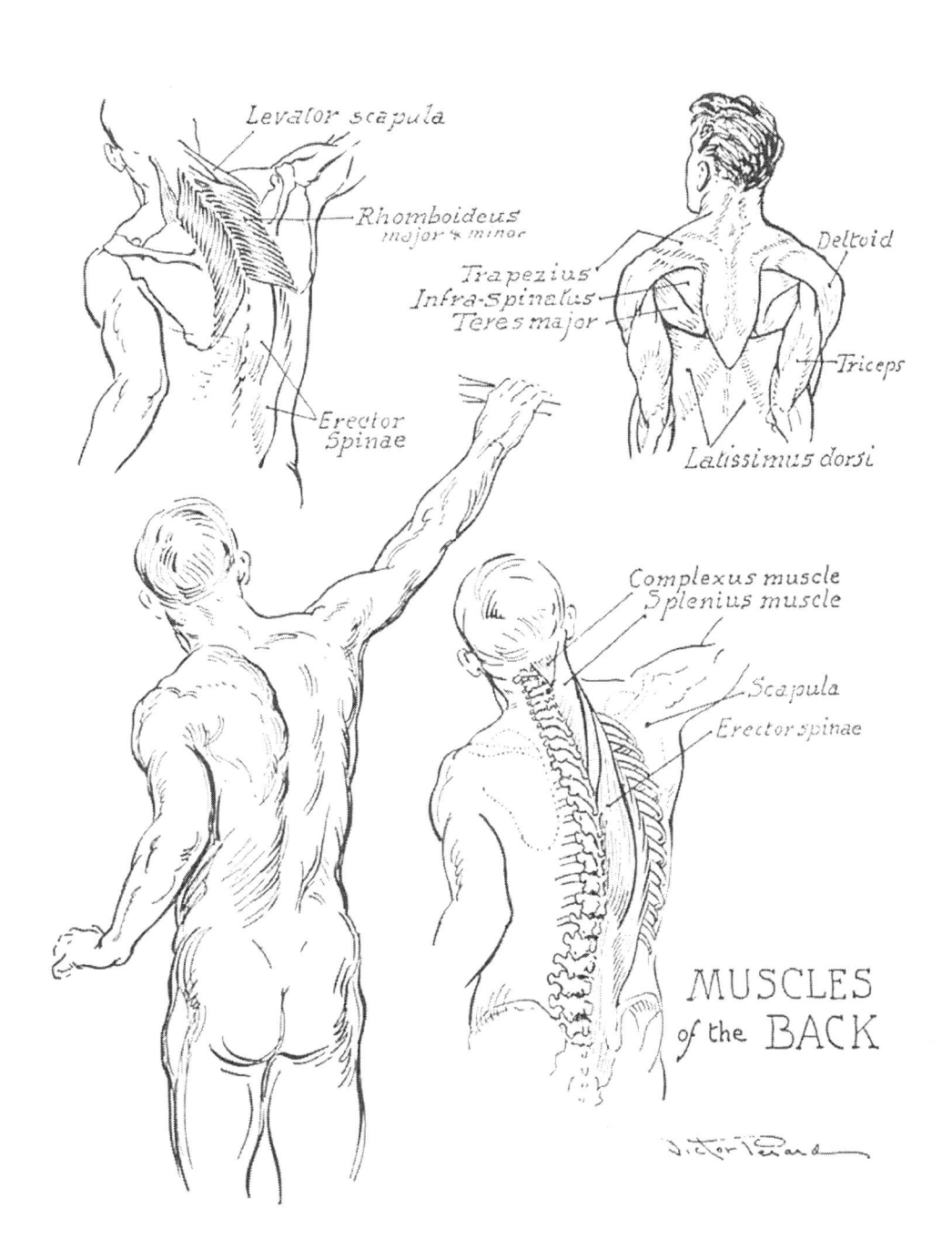

Levator scapula

Rhomboideus major & minor

Trapezius
Infra-spinatus
Teres major

Deltoid

Triceps

Erector Spinae

Latissimus dorsi

Complexus muscle
Splenius muscle

Scapula
Erector spinae

MUSCLES of the BACK

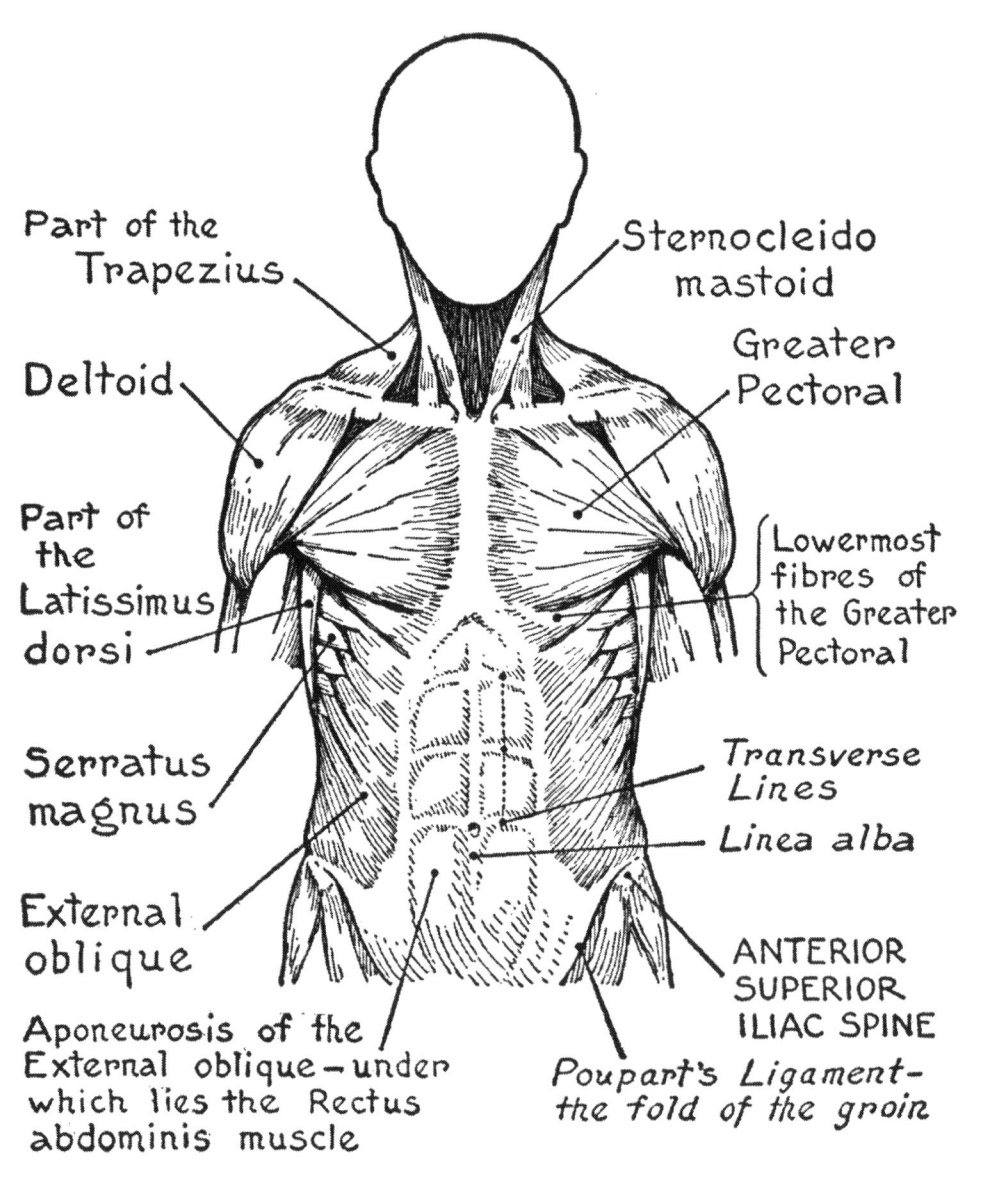

- Part of the Trapezius
- Sternocleido mastoid
- Deltoid
- Greater Pectoral
- Part of the Latissimus dorsi
- Lowermost fibres of the Greater Pectoral
- Serratus magnus
- Transverse Lines
- Linea alba
- External oblique
- ANTERIOR SUPERIOR ILIAC SPINE
- Aponeurosis of the External oblique – under which lies the Rectus abdominis muscle
- Poupart's Ligament – the fold of the groin

THE MUSCLES OF THE FRONT OF THE TRUNK.

CHAPTER SEVEN

The Trunk

THE TRUNK is the central part of the body. It serves a double function, firstly it can bend and perform curved movements not unlike those of a snake or measuring tape. This mobility is due to the flexibility of the vertebral column or spine, which has 26 articulation points.

Secondly the trunk must be able to align and stabilise the vertebral segments when the body is motionless, and especially when it is carrying a load. And because it contains a vital tunnel for nerves, the spinal cord and the nerve roots must be protected at all times - and the body structure attempts to do this at all costs.

The trunk contains a finely integrated system of muscles; which are either deep (composed of numerous small bundles) or superficial ones (usually arranged like broad sheets). We shall include the movements of the pelvis in this section because it is difficult to separate those from the movements of the vertebral column.

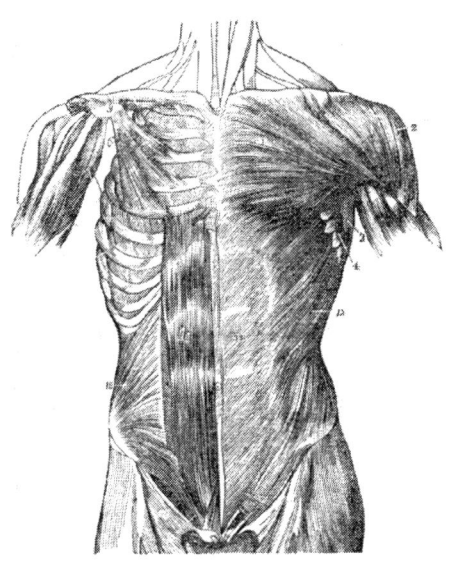

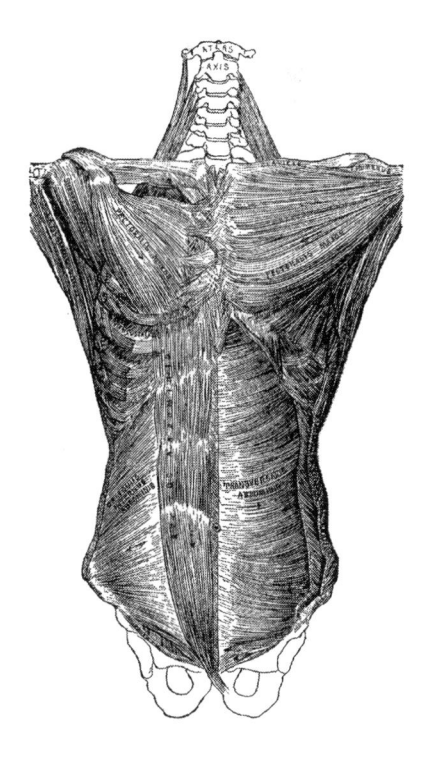

Due to the mobility of the vertebral column, the trunk can move in several directions. Range of movement varies depending on several factors including; shape of vertebrae, thickness of intervertebral discs (thicker discs = greater mobility), and variations due to the fact that the thoracic vertebrae articulate with the ribs which limits mobility.

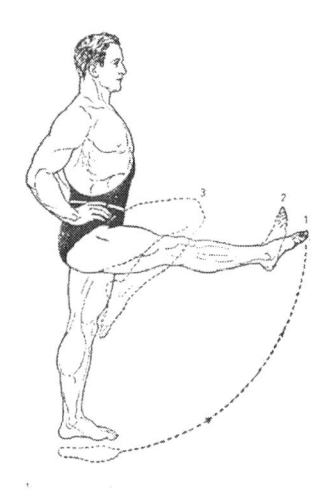

It is important to not confuse movements at the hip (i.e. flexion of the hip joint), with movement of the trunk (spine) itself. The trunk and hip can move independently of one another. The trunk provides a base for translation movements which involve sliding displacements of individual vertebrae; but the total resulting movement can be fairly large because of the many vertebrae involved.

The vertebral column, or spine, forms a mobile bony stem which constitutes a part of the skeleton of the trunk. Within each region, vertebrae are numbered sequentially from top to bottom. There are several characteristic curvatures of the vertebral column, and each person has curvatures that (naturally) vary from other people, and which are unique. Note that the external appearance of these curvatures can be affected by overlaying "soft" structures such as fat.

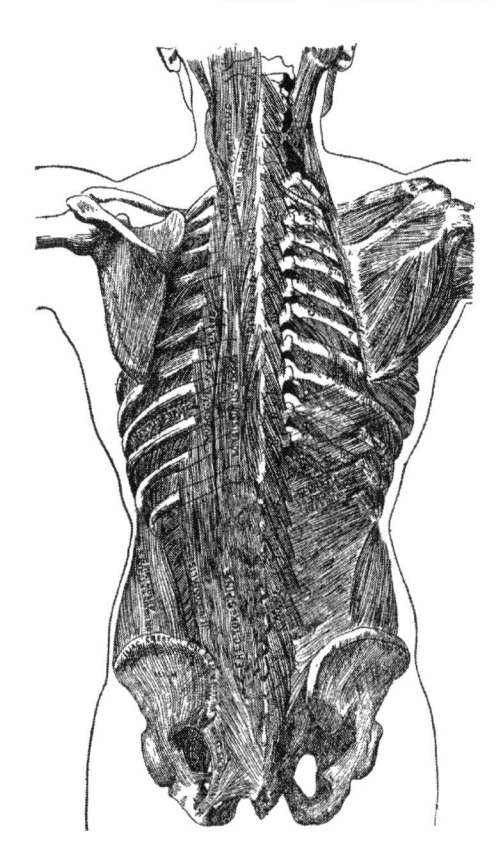

Put simply, the vertebral column consists of an arrangement of vertebra laid out in a particular structure or pattern.

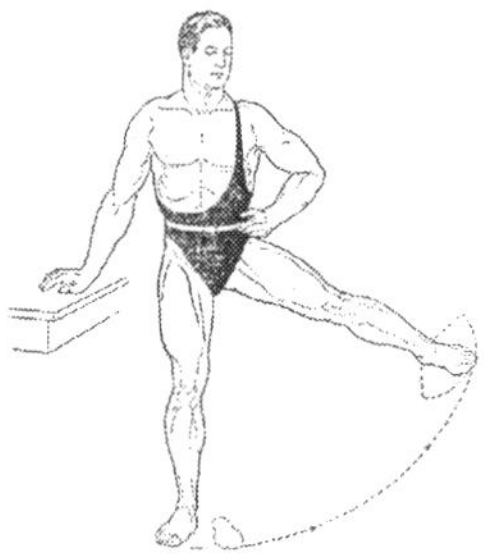

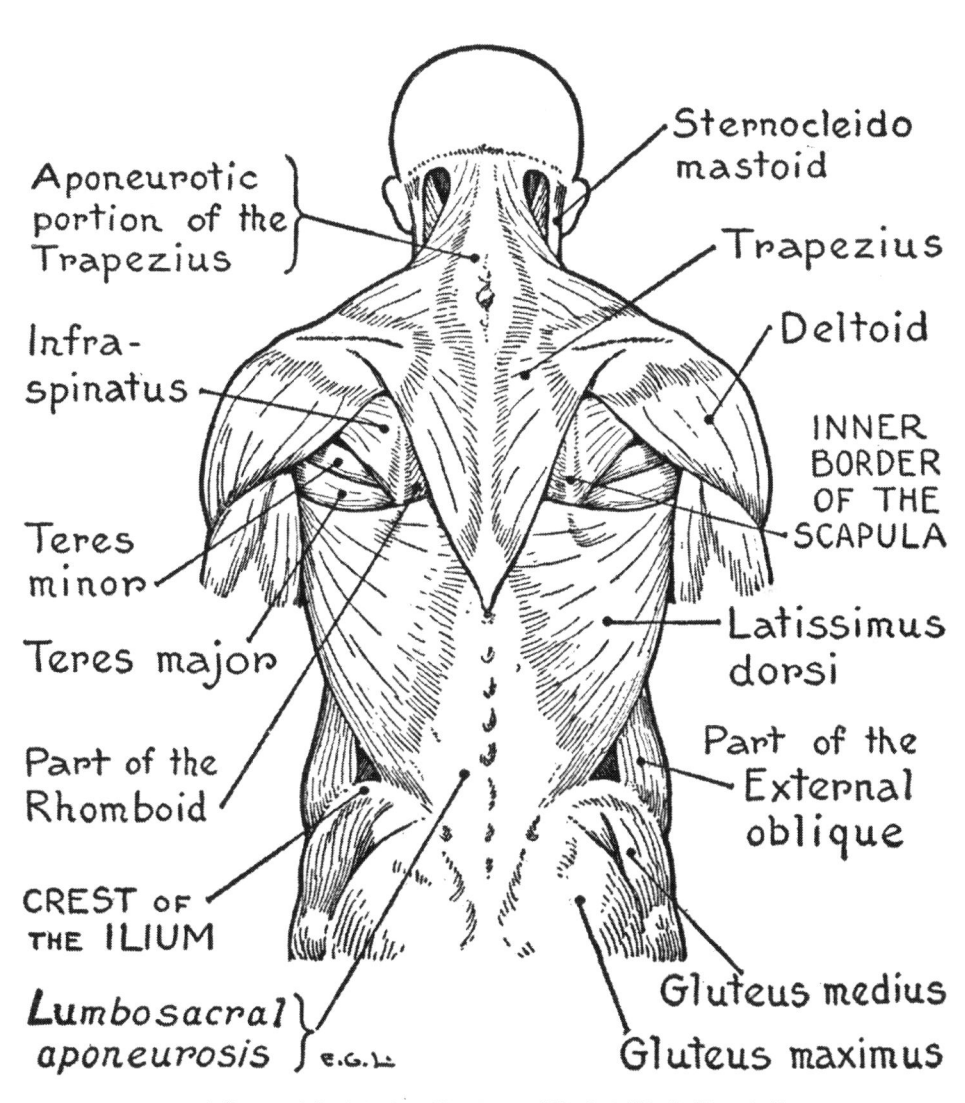

THE MUSCLES OF THE BACK OF THE TRUNK.

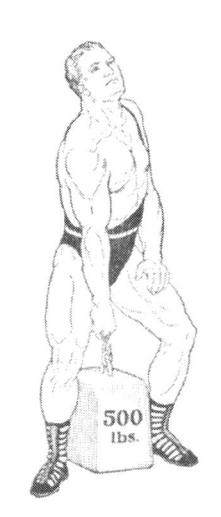

Each vertebra consists of 2 main parts; the massive **body** (anterior), and the **vertebral arch** (posterior)

In a wonderful miracle of nature, the vertebra fit together into a shape that both supports the weight of the body, and also allows movement of the spine itself. Individual vertebra are separated one from another by intervertebral discs; being a cushioning mechanism designed to allow the spine to absorb/bear weight, to allow movement vertically, and also to act as a shock absorber.

We can think of the vertebral column as a series of fixed segments (the vertebrae) having mobile connections (discs, ligaments). Movements of individual vertebrae are compounded such that the entire structure has considerable mobility in three dimensions.

In trunk flexion (spine bends forward), the disc is compressed anteriorly and expanded posteriorly, and the nucleus of the disc moves backwards slightly.

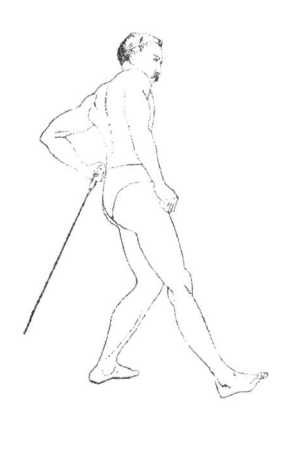

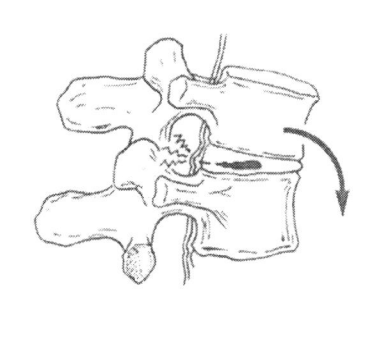

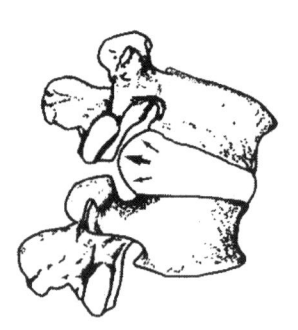

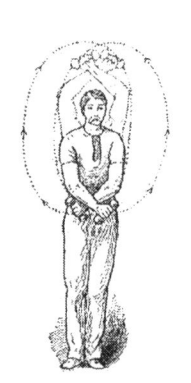

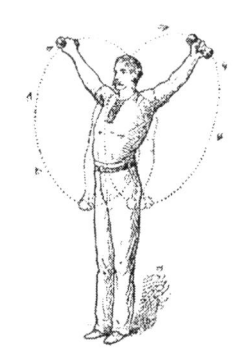

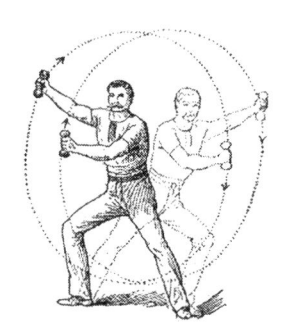

THE TRUNK 125

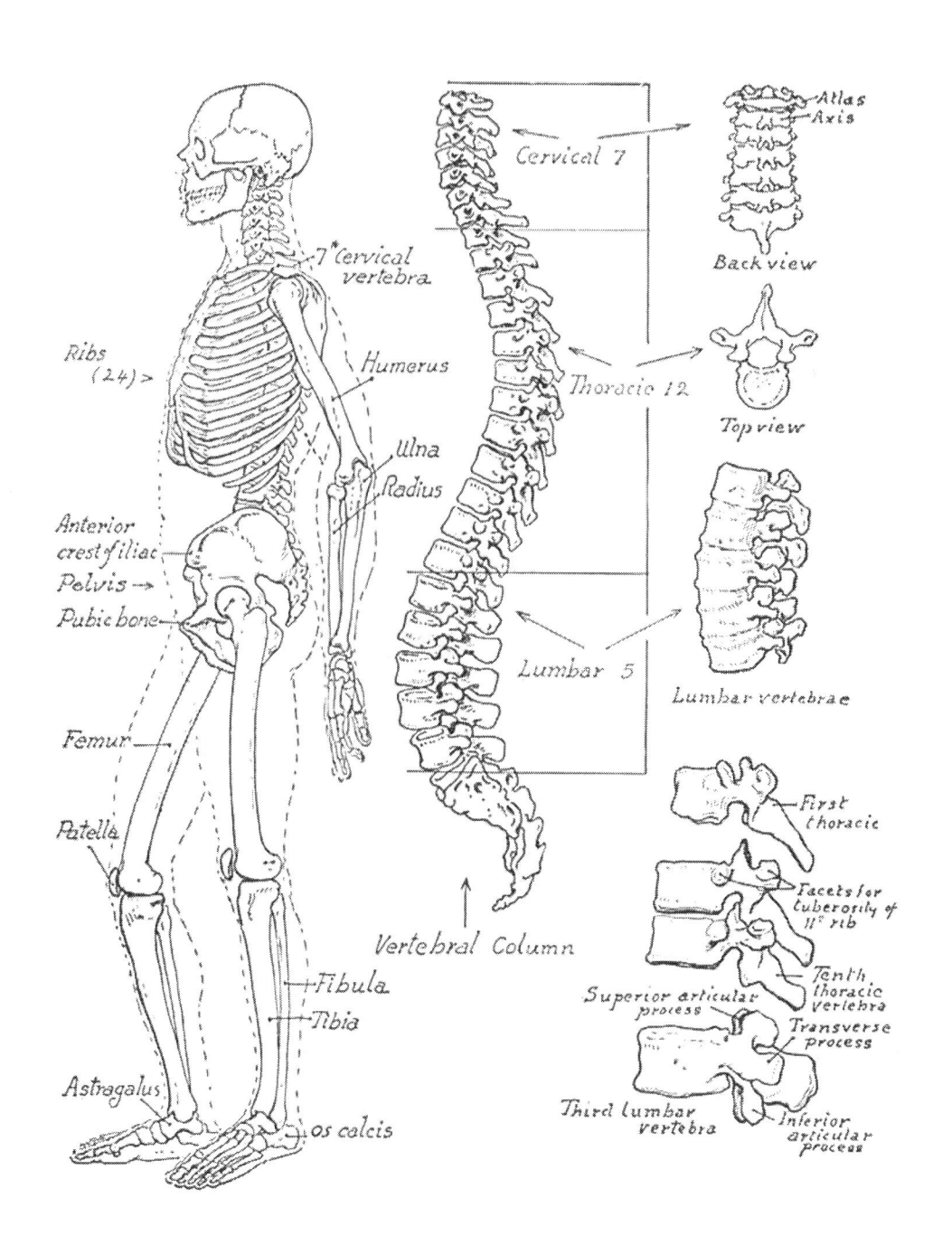

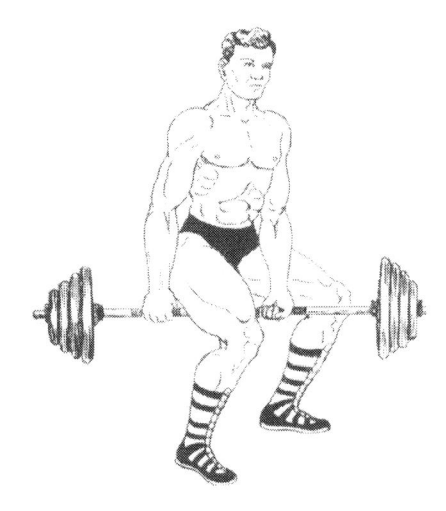

Due to ageing and/or excessive wear and tear, the disc may become partially damaged in this way. This condition is called herniated or ruptured disc, and it happens most commonly as a result of chronic flexion movements, during which the nucleus moves towards the back and fluid escapes. The fluid may then compress the nerve roots - causing pain.

To avoid these problems, it is important to avoid being "loaded" during vertebral flexion. Being loaded means flexing the lumber spine while lifting a heavy object. Instead, keep the spine straight (lumber arched) and flex at the hip and knee joint only when lifting heavy weights. In fact it is preferable to avoid loaded lumbar flexions in any type of physical exercise even if you are not lifting a heavy object (normally).

What we should really focus on is maintaining a concave shape to the lumber region (extended lower back) when lifting heavy objects. In other words the lumber should be fixed into a concave shape, and during the movement itself.

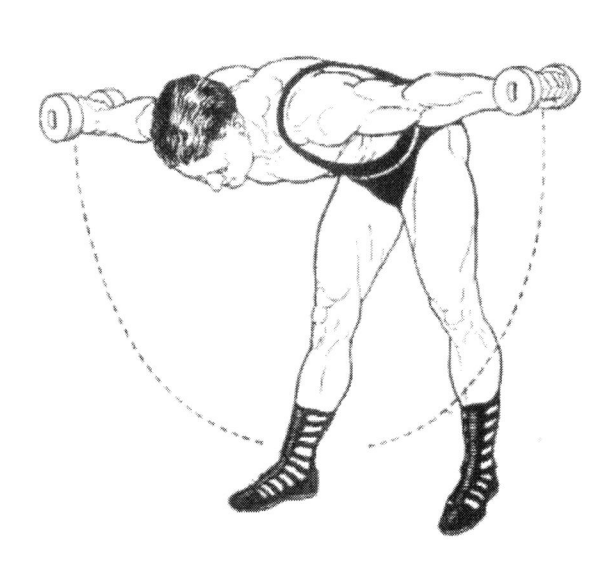

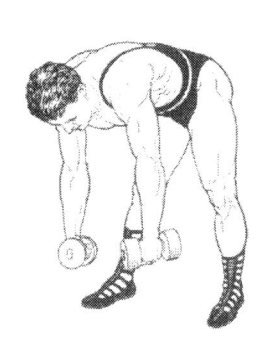

Athletes such as weightlifters, and other active people, naturally maintain this arch when lifting heavy weights (that is bending over and picking objects from the floor). Or rather they flex (contract) their lower back muscles to "arch" the lower back and so to maintain this position of strength throughout lifts such as the squat, clean or dead-lift. Remember, that once you loose the arched shape in the lumber region (whilst lifting), then you are doing something wrong because that is not how the back is designed to work when lifting heavy objects, that is with a "flat" back or less than concave shape (see exceptions below).

I know this all seems a bit complex, but "arching your lower back" (lower spine extension) really is a fundamental factor in vigorous athletic activity. And perhaps it is the fundamental athletic posture that we all must learn to perform in order to excel in our respective physical activities.

It seems strange that when you see someone performing a forward bend (apparently a flexion of the spine - but not in fact); that if done properly (when lifting heavy objects) this movement would not involve any movement (or minimal movement at least) in the lower vertebrae structure (that is the lumber). Rather we must bend at the hip (when lifting heavy weights), and this is the hinge that allows our back to maintain strength and avoid injury during any type of bending forward motion. Another way to "remember" the lower back arch, is to avoid collapsing the spine, that is to not let the spine collapse from the lumber region into a flexion, which is in fact the weakest position for the spine as a whole because the lumber is supposed to maintain a concave shape to support resistance. We must avoid *loading* the spine, or flexion of the lower back in particular (flexion whilst lifting).

Up to this point our discussion has concerned itself with heavy weightlifting exercises and back usage. However sometimes one might actually want to perform movements especially to exercise the flexion movement of the spine (torso crunching forward movement).

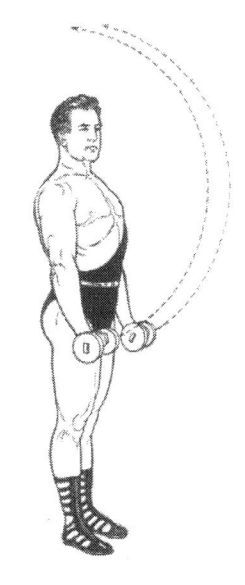

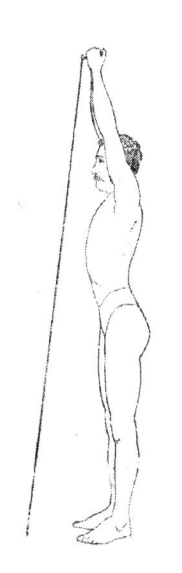

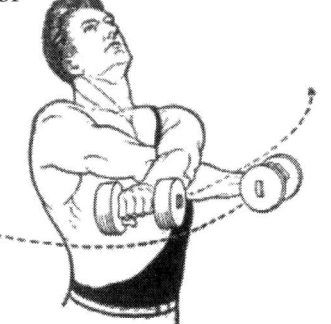

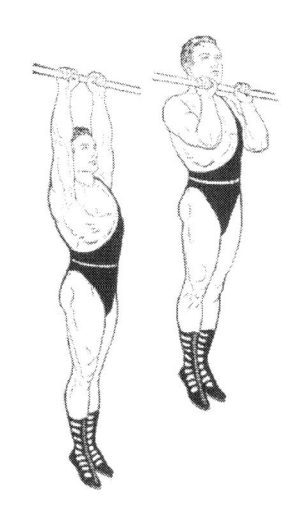

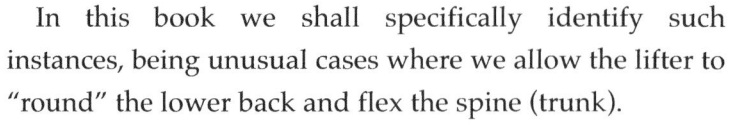

In this book we shall specifically identify such instances, being unusual cases where we allow the lifter to "round" the lower back and flex the spine (trunk).

There are four paired muscles in the abdominal wall. The deep transverse abdominis is involved in coughing functions and reduces the size of the abdomen in other situations. The internal and external oblique are involved in side-bending, whilst the rectus abdominis moves the sternum towards the pelvis, and it is the most direct flexor of the trunk.

There are many other moving structures present in the trunk area, which articulate the region in a large number of different ways. We have avoided discussion of how these structures work, largely because we want to focus on external movements from the perspective of exercises and joint ROMs.

Spinal health is key to maintaining our fitness as we age. As long as we keep the spine straight and aligned (with its normal curvatures), the load is evenly distributed through each disc at each level, which is an ideal shock absorbing and load-bearing condition. Basically the spine should not normally be flexed or "loaded" when standing upright.

Anatomy teaches us that the deep muscles and structures of the trunk are often "engaged" or working even when we are just standing still. Here we are fighting gravity to maintain our posture, and we must do so because our body is composed of an assemblage of parts that basically can move freely one relative to another.

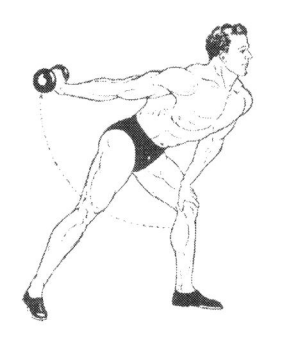

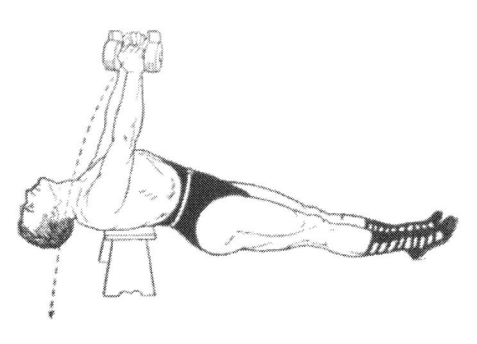

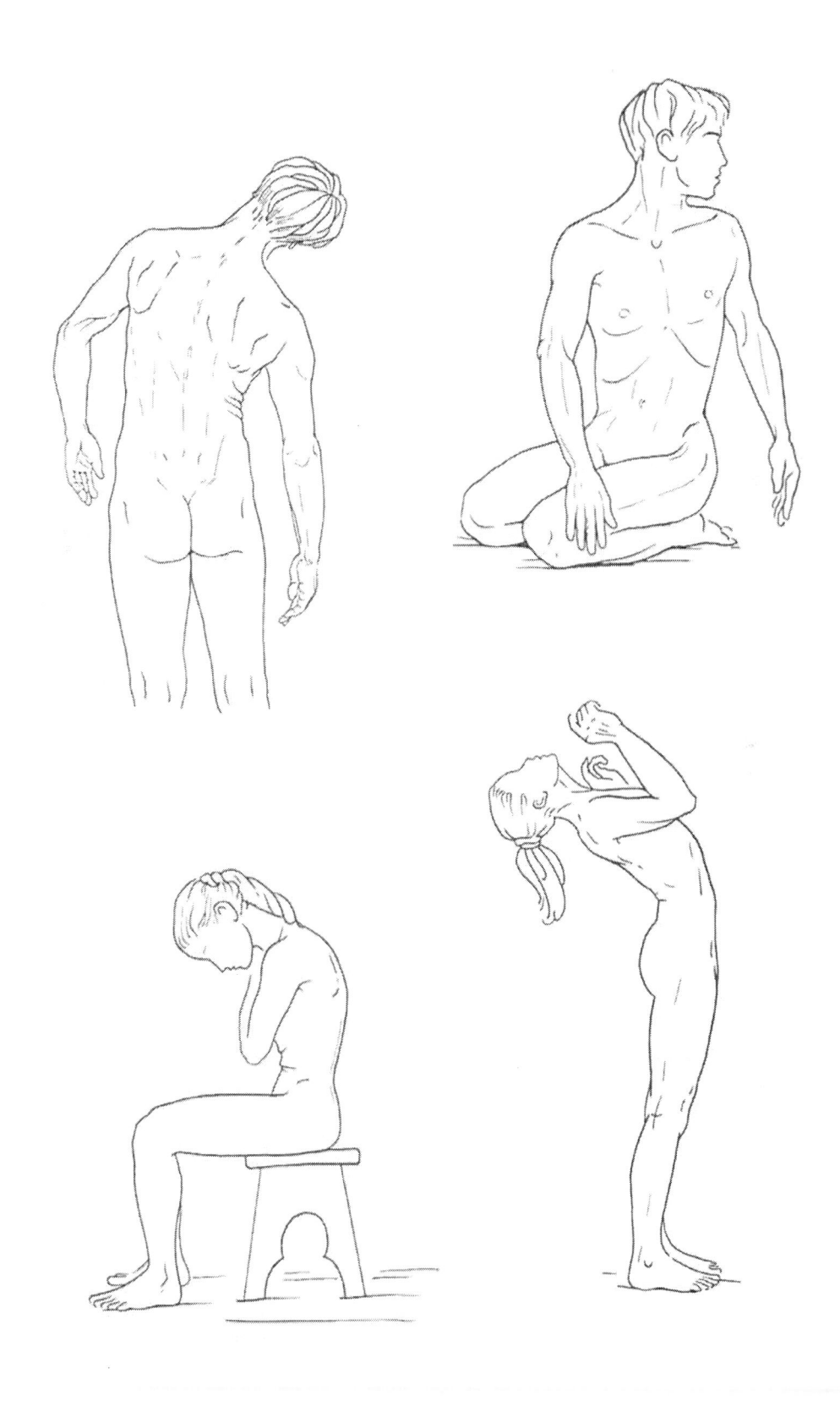

THE TRUNK

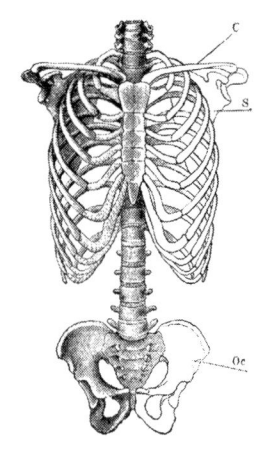

The deep muscles of the trunk help us to maintain an erect or upright posture even when the body's centre of gravity is altered, such as when you raise an arm or tilt the head. These muscles are "close to the bone". When you practice exercises directed at them, i.e. vertical alignment of the spine; expect a sensation of very slight muscular contraction.

For strengthening the deep muscles we are not necessarily looking to increase ROM (in contrast to flexibility exercises), but to stimulate and contract as many muscles and muscle fibres as possible.

Another important point relates to the different types of exercises used and required by the torso as a unit. It is important to remember that lighter weights are sometimes best for development of flexibility because of the previously mentioned tendency of the body to semi-contract many muscles and to fix joint positions in response to a heavy stimulus. Whereas the body as a structure becomes rigid in response to an overall load-bearing function when lifting very heavy weights. Thus in such situations where heavy loads are used, the tendency is to restrict range of motion due to this rigidity that is the bodies natural response to lifting a heavy load.

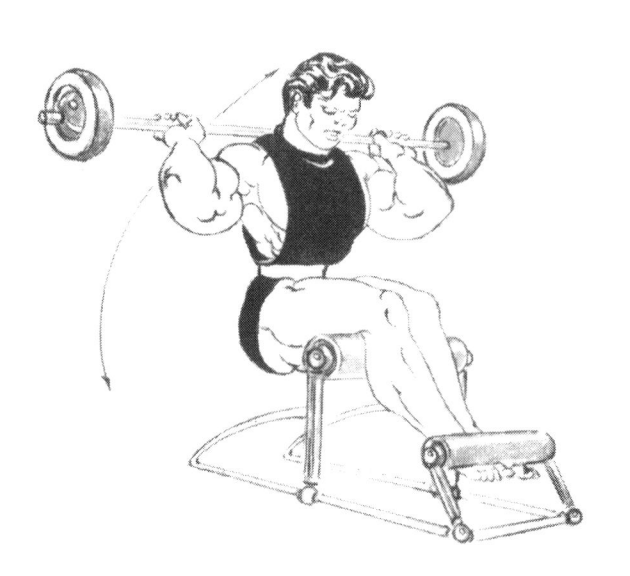

Take it from me, and use light, medium and (fairly) heavy weights on all strength exercises and combine all types into the same workout. In a sense, when using a very light weight, you are in effect performing a different exercise than when using a heavier weight. Try it for yourself, and perform some squats with a heavy weight and then a much lighter one. You will notice how the feeling (and range of motion) of the various muscular motions changes dramatically, to say nothing of the overall body position (often) being considerably different in each case.

Note that I do not believe in exercising the neck muscles (directly), at least in terms of strength building exercises. This is because the neck muscles receive sufficient stimulation and work along with everything else. That said, I do believe in stretching the neck muscles, if necessary, and where it seems natural to do so. In particular I think that maintaining correct head position on exercises like the bench-press, dead-lift, squat, and overhead press will develop the neck muscles to their fullest potential (my own neck is 18.5 inches).

It is important to have some idea of how the torso actually works in a mechanical sense. Remember here, do not confuse hip flexion with flexion of the trunk. For example in the dead-lift one normally does not flex the trunk but moves at the hip whilst maintaining a fixed (arched) lower spine.

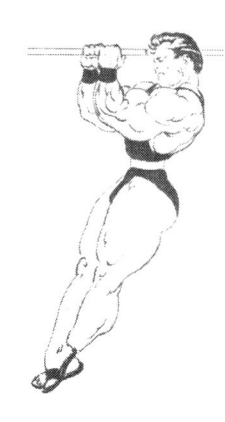

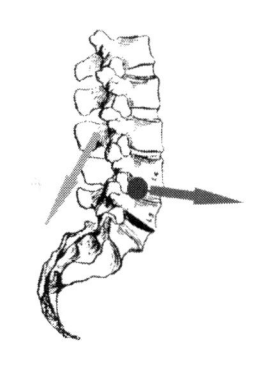

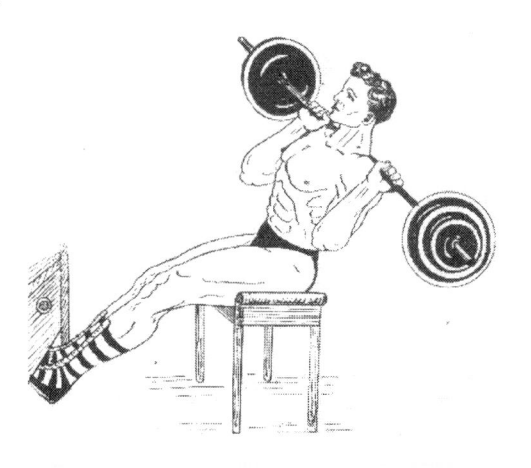

As far as range of motion (ROM) of the torso, we are really talking about the flexibility of the spine. We do know that this will vary from person to person. Remember that individual vertebrae move only a small amount, but that when combined together the overall deviation of the trunk (e.g. at the head) becomes fairly large. Referring to the movements of the trunk, a trunk extension of around 30 degrees is normal when standing, and 20 degrees when lying. Some people can do allot more (40-50 degrees), but unless you are a yoga specialist or contortionist it is not advisable or necessary.

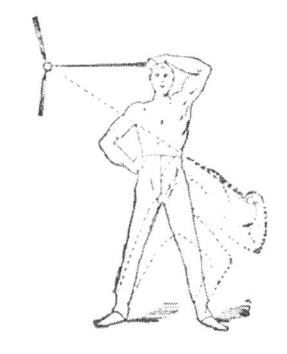

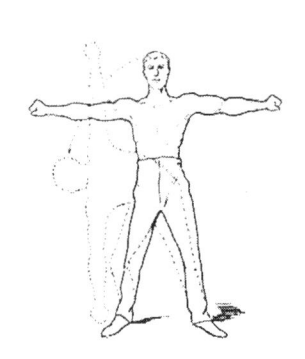

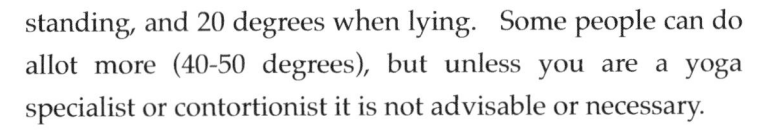

In terms of a flexion of the trunk, determining (and visualising) ROM is more difficult. This is because we often confuse such a movement with flexion of the hip. For example when we bend over to touch the toes, "bending" happens largely at the hips as opposed to an overall movement of the spine. In fact (normal) maximum flexion ROM of the spine is around 15-20 degrees. If you remember nothing else - remember this fact - that the spine can only actually bend forward by about 20 degrees! Bending over (more than this) always involves bending at the hip joint.

As mentioned earlier, in terms of weight-training (at least in the most load-bearing exercises such as the deadlift, squat or when handling heavy-weights overhead), we do not ever want to a perform a full trunk flexion. Only in the lying abdominal "crunch" and related movements would such a full-range flexion of the spine take place. This is because trunk flexion takes place almost exclusively in the lumber region, and places the spine in a very weak and (somewhat) unnatural position in structural terms.

The thing about forward bending is that you can bend forward from the spine or the hips or, often, a combination of both. Because the hips are more mobile, people tend to bend forward from the hips, and only try to move the spine when the pelvis won't move anymore. This is because the muscles on the backs of their legs are so stretched the pelvis will not move further, especially if the knees are kept straight.

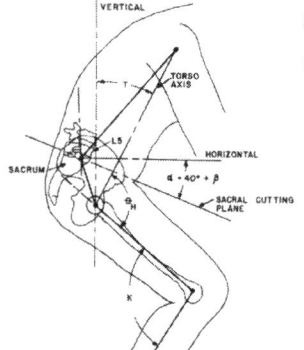

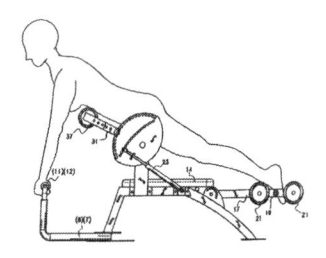

THE TRUNK 133

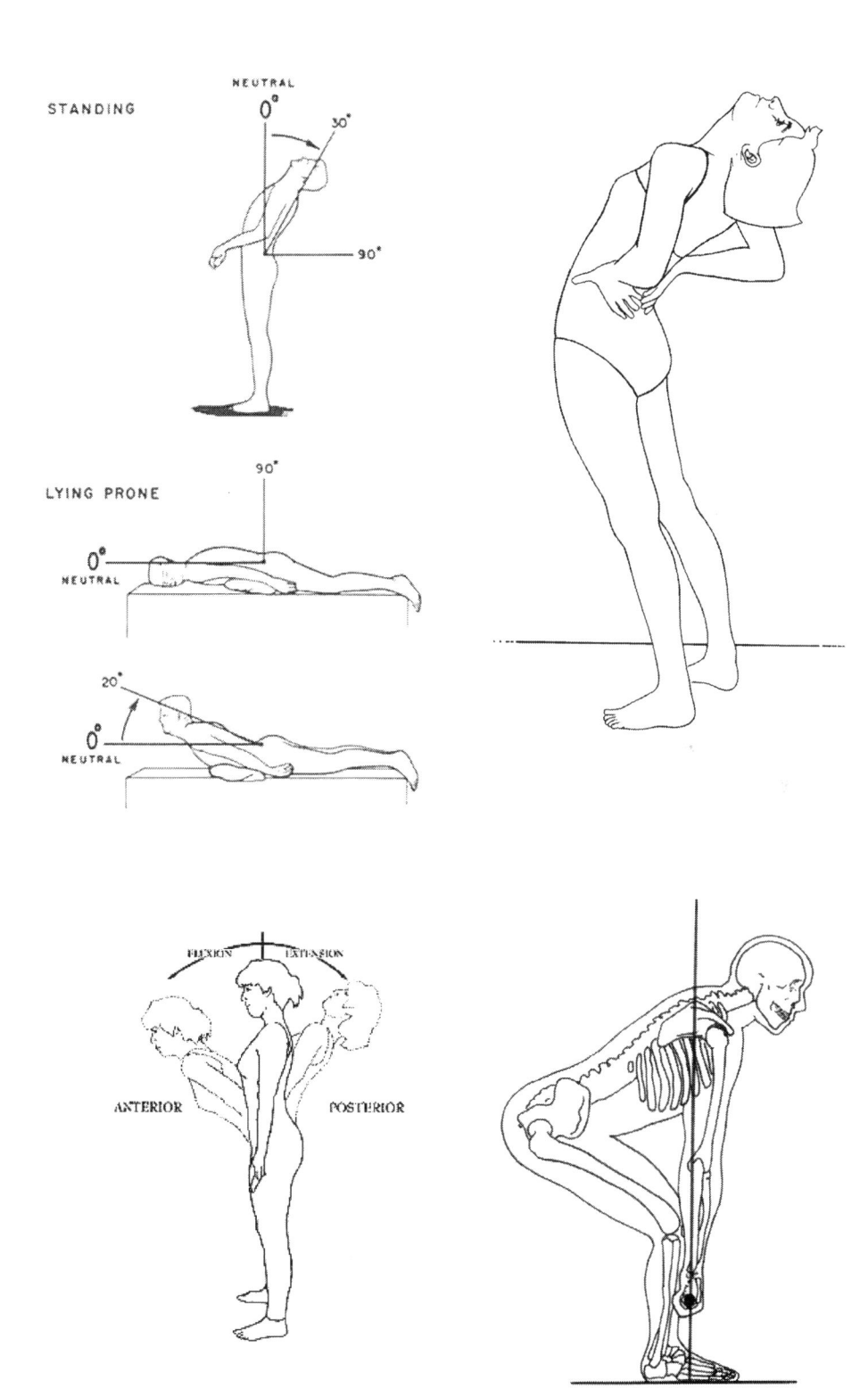

STANDING

LYING PRONE

FLEXION — EXTENSION

ANTERIOR — POSTERIOR

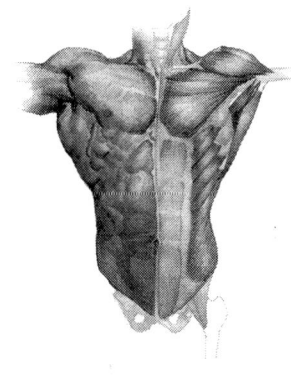

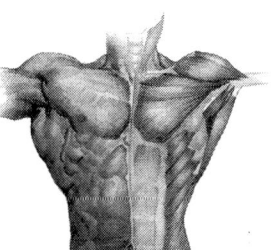

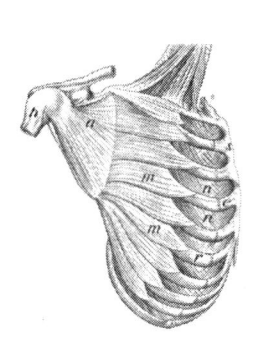

What can end up happening is that the backs of the legs stretch until the pelvis won't move any more and, in an effort to reach the floor or the toes, the spine starts rounding and stretching as well.

One of the rules I stick to is: do not stretch the hamstrings and the back of the spine at the same time. That is, in general, you do one or the other, but not both. An exception to this is when we are performing exercises where we wish to work spine flexion - for example as in the stiff legged dead-lift and similar exercises. Note that we shall explicitly say in this book which type of bending we are aiming at with particular exercises; stating hip flexion, spine flexion, or hip and spine flexion.

Note that in situations where you wish to perform a bending movement at the waist by flexion of the spine, then it is best to keep your knees slightly bent. The act of bending the knees allows the spine to move more freely.

Remember, here I am emphasising that (normally and unless specifically directed to); you do not want to feel the back of the spine stretching at the same time as the back of the legs (bend the knees to help). Remember also to never "collapse" the back whilst lifting *heavy weights* - that is do not fix your spine into a position of flexion and then attempt to lift with it so set. Rather your spine must be extended (arched lower back) when lifting heavy objects.

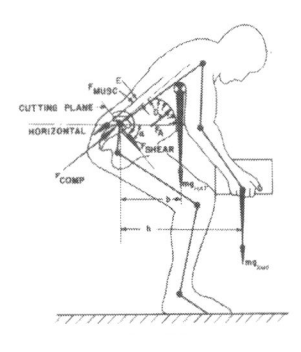

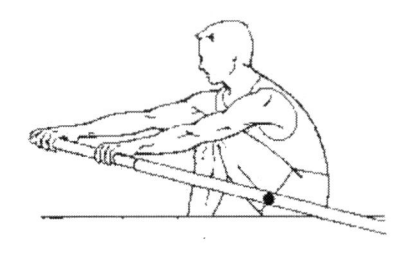

If you are going to bend to the floor from standing you definitely will not reach it just by bending forward from the spine. The spine does not really bend very much at-all (15-20

degrees in flexion). So, you will need to bend at your hips, and perhaps, for most people, your knees as well (slightly).

To summarise, forward bending does have a ROM of 90 degrees or more, but this is composed of a maximum spine flexion of 20 degrees combined with 70 or more degrees of hip flexion. Be aware of which type of flexion you are aiming for in any exercise; be it one or the other - or a combination of both types of bending (rare).

Shown below are three kinds of bending at the waist. In image A, we see bending at the waist with normal lumber and hip flexion. In image B we see limited hip flexion with excessive lumber flexion. In image C we see limited lumber flexion with excessive hip flexion.

How we should actually bend at the waist, will depend upon the nature of the task at hand, and also upon the flexibility and movement ROMs of the various hip and lumber flexors. With heavy weights, one normally wants to limit lumber flexion and use mostly hip flexion as in C.

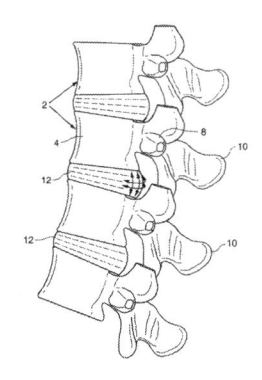

FIG. 1B

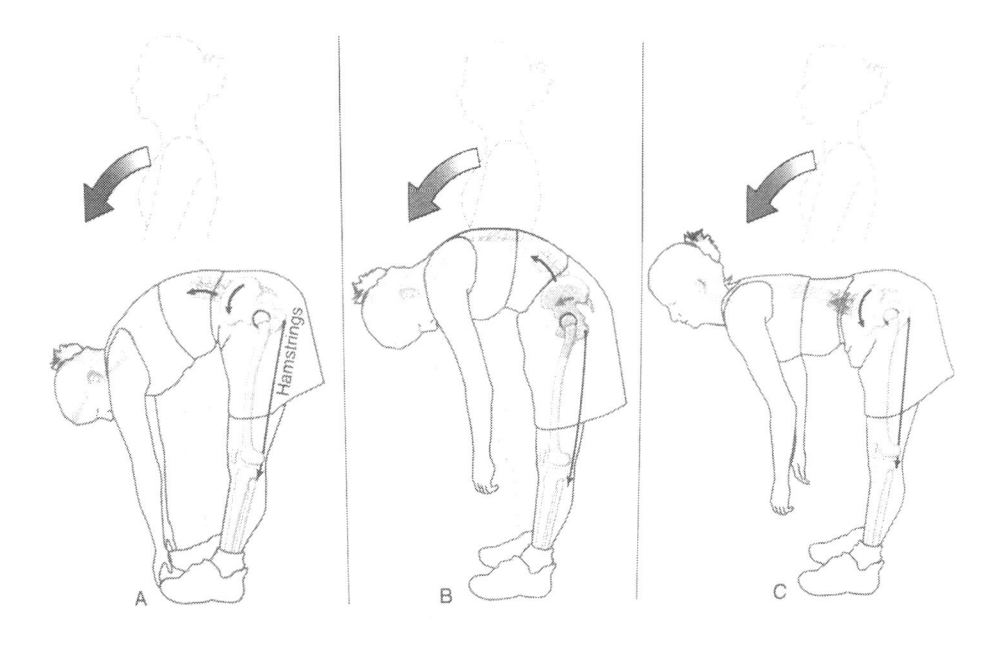

A

B

C

ASANA POSITION

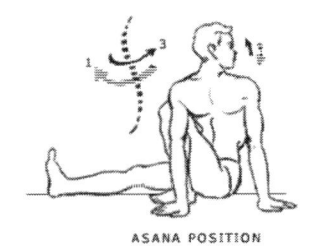

Now let us turn our attention to side-bending movements of the torso. Here things become quite a bit simpler because you only have to consider movement of the spine itself. Basically the spine has a ROM laterally of around 25-35 degrees. Note that here we refer to a movement purely in the lateral plane, with no forward bending component. If you do combine the movement with forward bending, then by definition you bring in one or both of the hip and/or forward spine flexion type of movement(s). Hence range of motion of the bend increases as you bend more to the front of the body.

Turning our attention to the twisting movements of the torso, we find that anything from 30 to 80 degrees (or more) is normal for a torso twist in either direction. The only point worth remembering is to isolate hip rotation from spinal rotation, or at least to be aware that these are separate movements in principle. Often we can do both together to achieve a practical twist of the body, unless we are attempting to isolate some specific muscle or function. Note that twisting motions of the torso (spine + hip), are more common than we may think, and happen in everyday activities such as walking. It is useful to be aware of these.

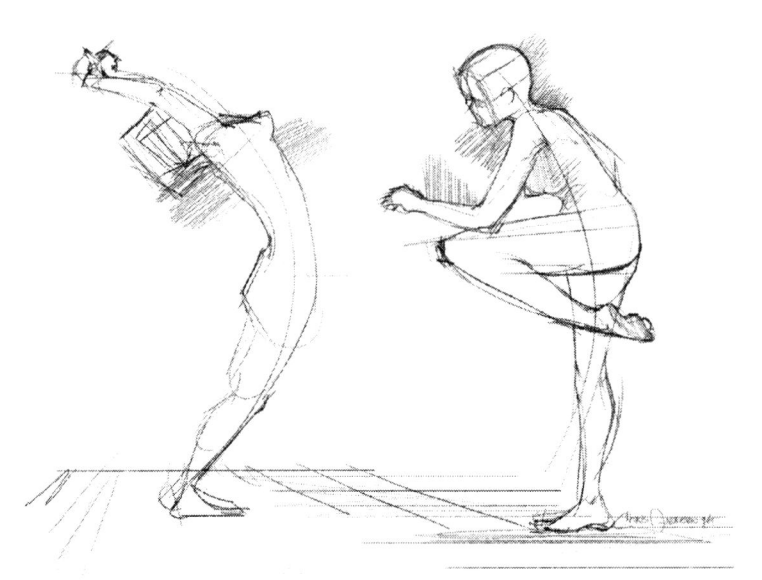

We now go on to provide a list of recommended exercises for the torso. Note that these are not the only ones that are beneficial or even possible, but they are the ones that are most effective, safe and those that produce the best results. We list some variations of each movement, but the different indicated performances are by no means comprehensive. Note the exercises are numbered, and so that we can refer to specific movements throughout the book.

Another point relates to the body areas/muscles being exercised in each movement. As discussed previously it is difficult to isolate the muscles/body-parts; and normally many regions of the body will be affected by any particular movement or exercise. In this section we present exercises mainly for the torso, but we must recognise that these movements will affect other body-parts (joints +muscles) as well.

Note that we do not claim that all of these exercise will be suitable (or even safe) for everyone to perform. Certain individuals will need to eliminate specific exercises altogether for reasons of injury and/or in relation to personal capability and/or due to any physical limitations.

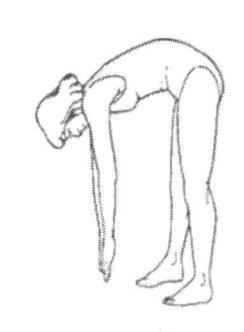

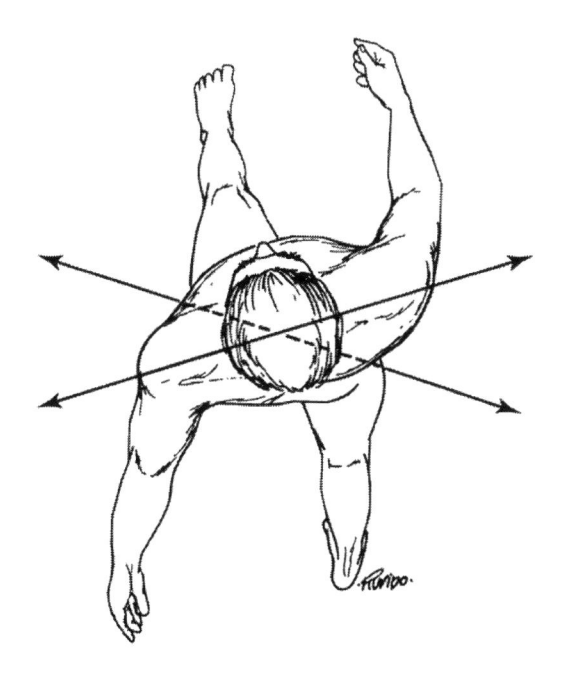

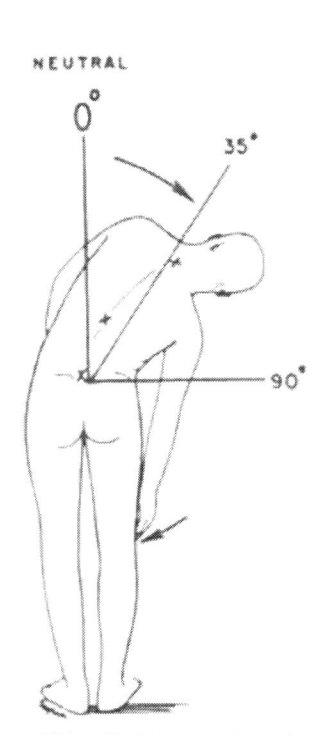

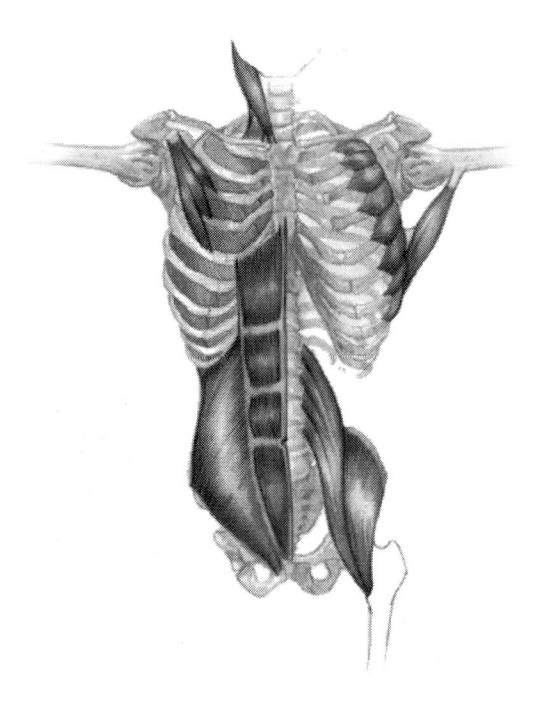

Torso Joint(s) - Exercises

1. The Swing
2. Lean Forward / Back
3. Body / Trunk Circles
4. Toe Touching
5. Lean-Overs
6. The Twist
7. Twisting Lean-Back
8. Side Bends
9. Windmill
10. Forward Bend
11. Dead-lift
12. Stiff-leg dead-lift
13. Stiff-leg dead-lift (to feet)
14. Clean
15. High Pull
16. Good Morning
17. Hyperextension
18. Sit-up (fixed legs)
19. Sit-up (dumbbells overhead)
20. Incline Sit-up
21. Crunch
22. Leg Raise

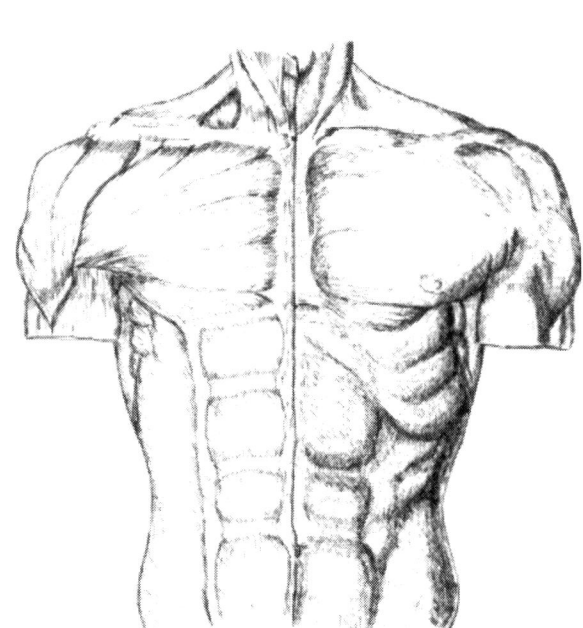

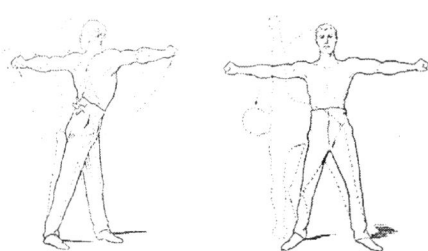

23. Seated Knee-in
24. Leg Raise + Torso Raise [Jack Knife]
25. Seated Leg Raise
26. Side-Lying Crunch
27. Roman Chair Sit-Up

I find it useful to think of the torso as the basic column against which everything else is related and/or moves. Often the torso must be "fixed" in position (with stable hips, knees, ankles etc). If your torso was not to some degree "braced", what would you push and/or pull "against", or else "towards"? Once again I would like to draw your attention to the importance of holding certain parts of the body in a rigid position, and in order to allow other parts to move with strength and confidence. In a sense one cannot be told how to lift weights, but rather it is something that you must learn yourself. And perhaps (in a sense) it is not only the conscious mind that learns in this respect.

And thats about it for our (relatively brief) discussion of the moving anatomy of the trunk. What have we learned? Perhaps that movement is complex. And that there is allot more going on whenever you move than your conscious mind can control, and in terms of the movements/rigidity of multiple body-parts. Recognise therefore that movement requires constant learning and re-learning, and with both the conscious and unconscious mind. In the exercises that follow, the spine and hip positions refer to flexion/extension in the sagittal plane (and not to twisting movements in the frontal plane).

Note the two different uses of the term "flex" when used in relation to the torso/back. When we speak of a flexion movement of the torso we are referring to spinal flexion whereby we move the torso forward from the anatomical position in a crunching movement. Flexing the lower back muscles, on the other hand, refers to producing a concave (arched) lumbar and extending the spine from the anatomical position. Thus flexing the spinal erector "muscles" results in lower back (spine) extension and a concave lumbar.

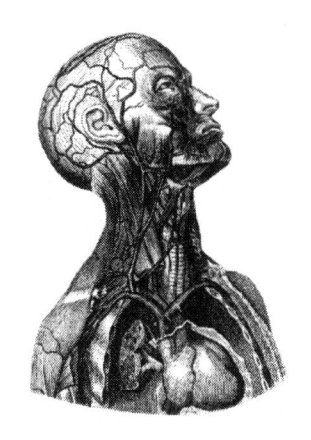

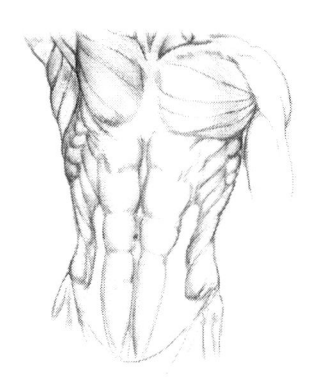

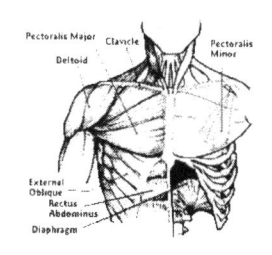

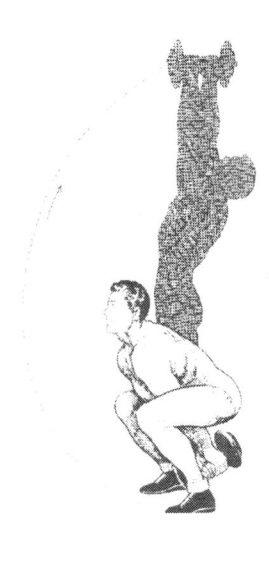

1. The Swing

Equipment: single / double - kettle-bell / dumbbell
Effect: Strength / conditioning of entire body
Resistance : Light / Medium [fast movement / ballistic]
Hip position: Hip Hinge - Flexion and Extension
Spine position: Neutral / fixed (arched) throughout
Scapula position: Neutral / locked (rotation if above head)
Muscles: gluteus maximus (buttocks), erector spinae, internal / external oblique, rectus femoris, hamstrings, quadriceps, latissimus dorsi, rectus abdominis, hip structure
Typical Poundage: 8-16 kg kettle-bell (women); 12-24 kg (men)
Joints: Hip, knee, ankle, neck, shoulder, rib-cage, vertebrae

Some experts proclaim the swing to be the greatest resistance training exercise of them all (and so it may be) - providing significant muscular stimulation for the entire body. You can perform it with a single or twin kettle-bells, and one or two dumbbells. Form is very important, and to some extent this must be learned with constant practice. It is a fast movement and the muscles work hard to provide acceleration to, and also to decelerate, the weight at various points in the movement. Stand upright with legs apart and the kettle-bell between your feet. Bend forward and pick up the kettle-bell. You start by swinging the kettle-bell down between your legs and then you swing the bell up to chest level by exploding with your hips while tightening your core by locking out your knees, pull up your thighs, tighten your gluts and your abs. Snap or thrust hips forward to generate power. Swing the kettle-bell back down between your legs and repeat. Swing the weight to shoulder level or overhead etc. Switch hands between sets.

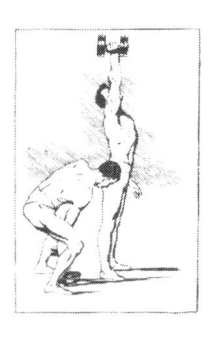

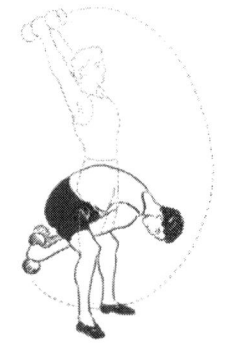

The swing can be used in various ways and for different effects. The russian "Girevoy" sport is performed with kettle-bells, and the swing is a core part of that fitness training system. They measure kettle-bell weights in terms of a 1-pood (16 lbs) increment, with 1, 1.5 and 2 pood kettle-bells etc. Often (in Girevoy sport) the trainee would perform many repetitions of the swing exercise, and in order to build combined strength and stamina. Other weight-lifters such as Thomas Inch and John Grimek set swing records whereby over 200 lbs would be lifted into an overhead position.

THE TRUNK 141

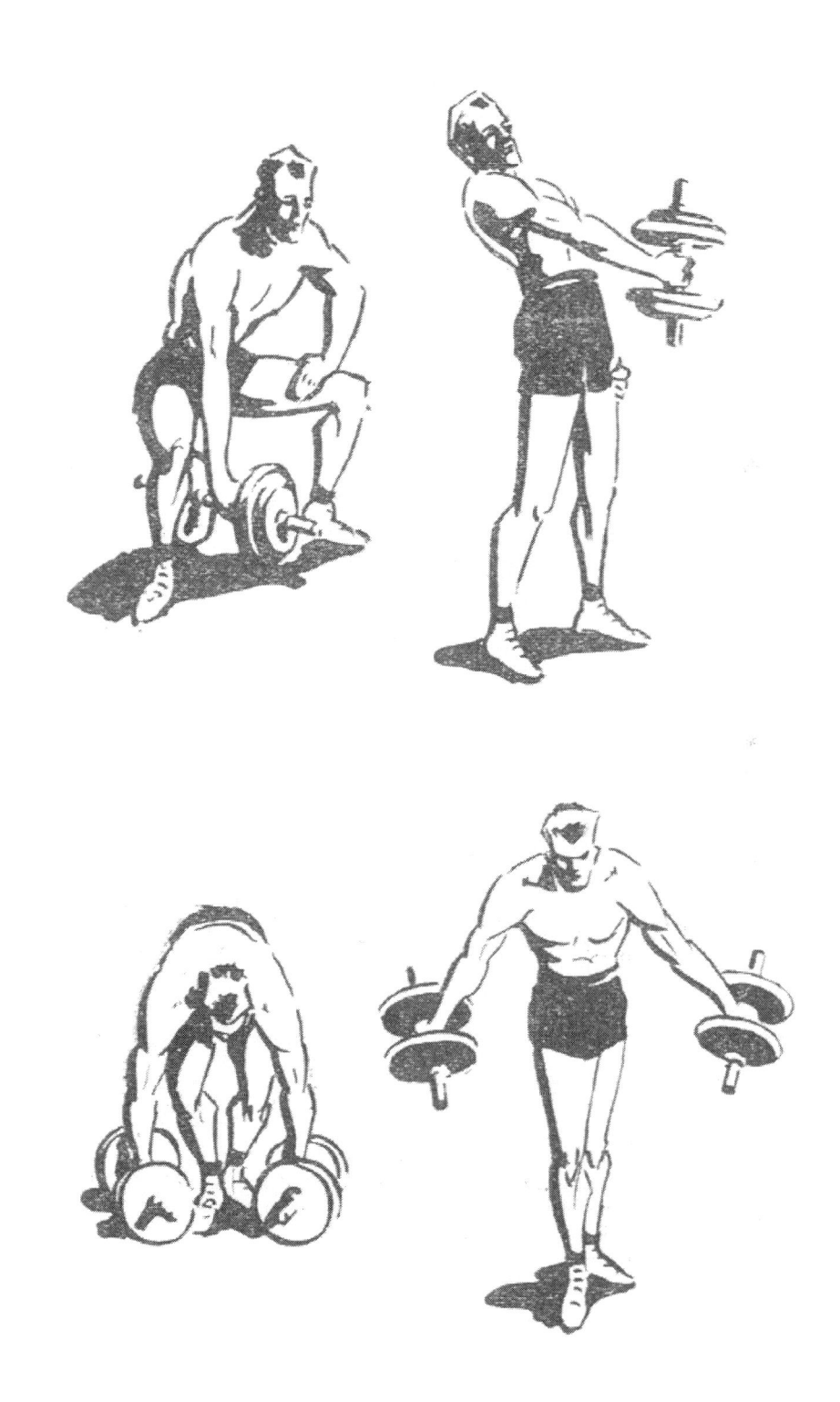

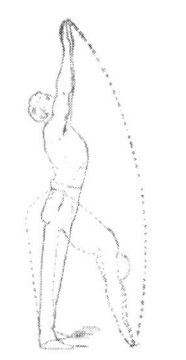

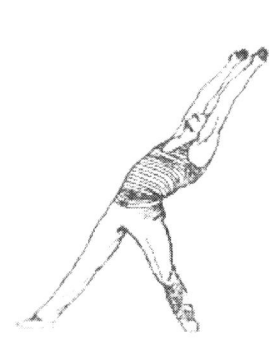

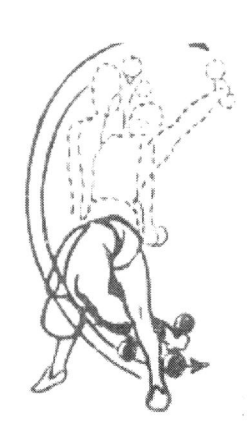

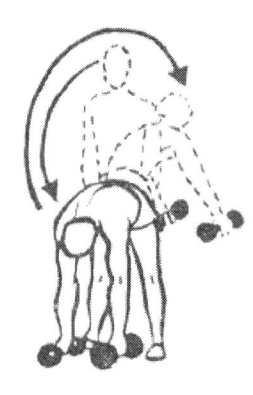

2. Lean Forward / Back (ROM)

Equipment: twin dumbbells / nothing [perform daily]
Effect: Warm up torso, hips, shoulder, lower-back, neck etc
Resistance : Light / Medium [slow / medium speed]
Hip position: Flexion and Extension
Spine position: Neutral / slight flexion (bending forward), slight extension (when reaching backwards)
Scapula position: Neutral / natural rotation at end
Muscles: gluteus maximus, hamstrings, erector spinae, internal / external oblique, rectus abdominis, hip structure
Typical Poundage: 1-2 kg dumbbells (women); 2-5 kg (men)
Joints: Hip, shoulder, neck, ankle, rib-cage, vertebrae

This a warm-up movement that stretches all of the muscles and structures of the hip and torso. It is performed with or without resistance, and with one or two dumbbells.

At the top / bottom you can hold the dumbbells together or far apart. You can vary the degree of lean-back at the top, and likewise for the degree of forward bend. Engage the spine as desired, and a slight flexion when bending forward would be acceptable as long as it is gentle and within personal capacity. You may wish to extend the stretch at the top by extending the spine (curving low back), and by also looking backwards and reaching as far backwards as possible. You can also take a step backwards with one foot as you move the dumbbells overhead.

In this movement you mostly bend forwards at the waist, but some slight flexion of the spine is acceptable for stretching purposes. The hip extensors (gluteus maximus, biceps femoris) are contracted at the top also.

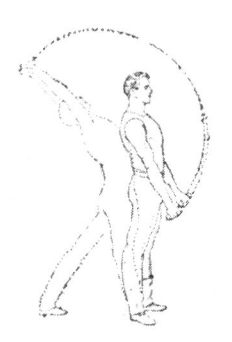

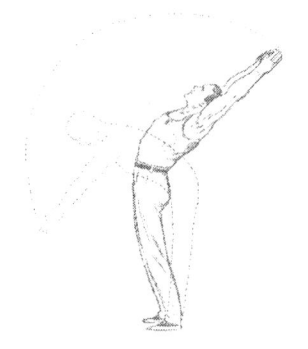

Holding a Dumbbell

You might think that the simple task of holding a dumbbell would be relatively straightforward, however as with all matters physical, there are right and wrong ways to do so. Let me take you through the correct method.

Firstly grab a light dumbbell - say 2-3 lbs. Hold it in one hand and notice if you have a central grip with respect to the "bells" or handle edges. Normally you want to have a centralised grip, but this is not always the case. Sometimes, as in a biceps curl or else when pressing you might want to have an off-centre grip in order to enhance muscle contractions / stretches. A grip towards the outside of the dumbbell is sometimes useful in order to make supination more difficult to achieve (curls) or else you can load the dumbbell with extra plates on the inside. Likewise you can experiment with the effects of an off-centre grip in presses etc. Although generally you want to have a centralised grip.

Another important point relates to the angle of the wrist during exercise performance (flexion / extension). Normally you want to have a neutral wrist angle whereby the handle sits firmly into the meat of the hand; and then your wrist takes its natural position with the hand slightly bent upwards (very slight extension), thus balancing the weight centrally over the palm. However sometimes - as in curls you may want to drop the wrist back (partial extension) somewhat at the top position, and in order to fully contract the biceps. Also on preacher curls and wrist-curls you may want to unwrap the wrist (full extension) at the bottom. Sometimes you also want to slightly extend the wrist upwards - for example on reverse curls.

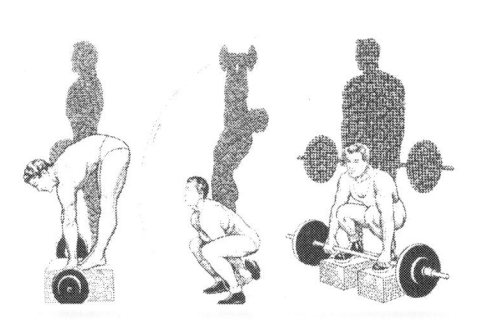

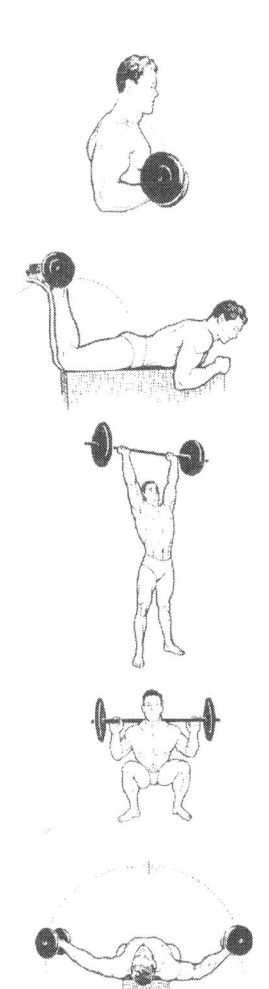

3. Body / Trunk Circles (ROM + Strength)

Equipment: twin dumbbells / nothing
Effect: Twist and warm up spine / hip mobility
Resistance : Light / Medium [slow speed]
Hip position: Neutral + slight flexion / extension
Spine position: Neutral + slight flexion / extension
Scapula position: Neutral / natural rotation
Muscles: erector spinae, internal / external oblique, rectus abdominis, hip structure, gluteus maximus & medius
Typical Poundage: 1-3 kg dumbbells (women); 2-5 kg (men)
Joints: Hip, shoulder, rig-cage, vertebrae (slight/full)

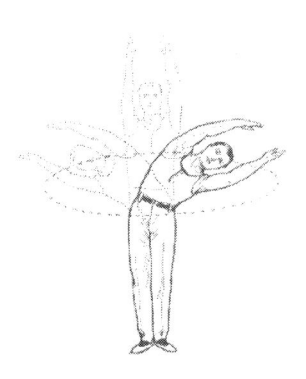

Grab twin dumbbells and lift them overhead with arms straight. Next begin circling the body - small circles at first and increase if desired. Hips may move in a counter-motion to the circular movement of the arms at the top. Keep your knees locked or slightly bent but firm throughout. Perform in both directions, and increase movement ROM slowly.

A second (very unusual) type of body circle is shown below. This is a completely different exercise from the above; and it is for strengthening the arms and shoulders. Hold a barbell out to the front of the body (under-hand, over-hand or mixed grip) - and curl the bar into a mid-position. Next twist the barbell (slowly) by raising one hand (+ elbow) upwards, whilst lowering the other hand (+ elbow) at the same time (body remains stationary). Thus the bar moves in a semi-circle in front of the body, and the biceps, forearms and shoulders experience very strong muscle contractions.

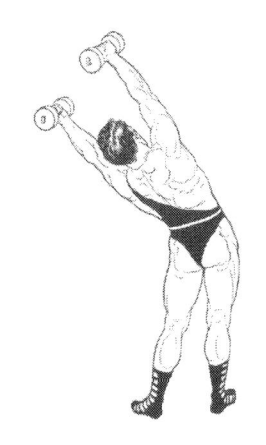

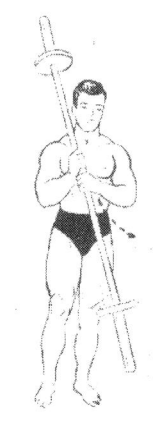

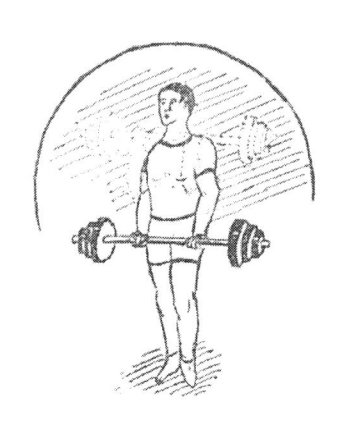

The objective here (above) is to warm up all of the muscles / joints in the spine and hip region, plus to stretch all of the moving parts of the lower part of the torso; including both abdominals and lower vertebrae. This is a truly fantastic movement - and it can really help you to develop superior flexibility in the entire hip region. With no weights, or else very light weights, you can perform the movement with gradually increasing radii of curvature and so increase ROM. You can also perform the movement with slightly heavier weights and in order to work the inner structures more intensely.

4. Toe Touching (ROM)

Equipment: twin dumbbells / nothing
Effect: Twist and warm up spine / abdominals / shoulder
Resistance : Light [medium / slow speed]
Hip position: Hip Hinge - Flexion
Spine position: Neutral throughout
Scapula position: Neutral / locked
Muscles: hamstrings, erector spinae, internal / external oblique, rectus abdominis, hip structure, shoulder / neck structure, hip flexors
Typical Poundage: 1-3 kg dumbbells (women); 2-5 kg dumbbells (men)
Joints: Hip, shoulder, vertebrae (slight/full)

Grab twin dumbbells and hold the arms outstretched to the sides, and then bend over at waist. Next begin circling the body in a wide-arc, alternately touching the toes. Perform in both directions, for one toe and then the other. This movement has a beneficial effect on the entire abdominal region and also the lower / upper spine. Perform daily.

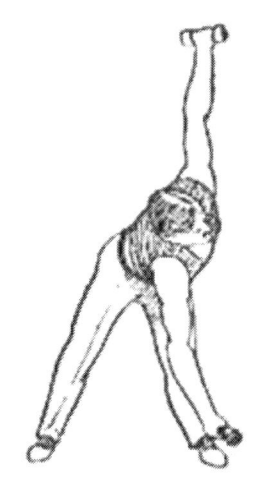

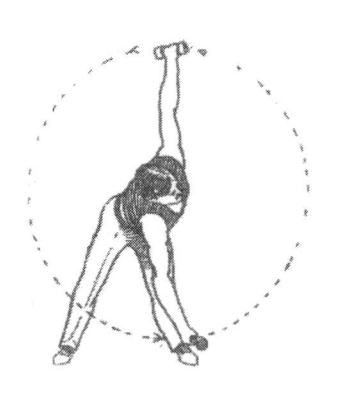

To obtain a torso like a greek god; perform all kinds of sit-ups, side bends, forward bends and twisting moves. Pay close attention to the muscles of the spine also, and perform dead-lifts, stiff-leg dead-lifts and all types of rowing motions. The human torso is (when fully developed) an incredibly powerful assembly of bony supports, joints, muscles, ligaments and tendons. Many of these different parts are designed to work together, and it is a mistake to just perform a few isolation movements and then expect to obtain full and complete development in these areas.

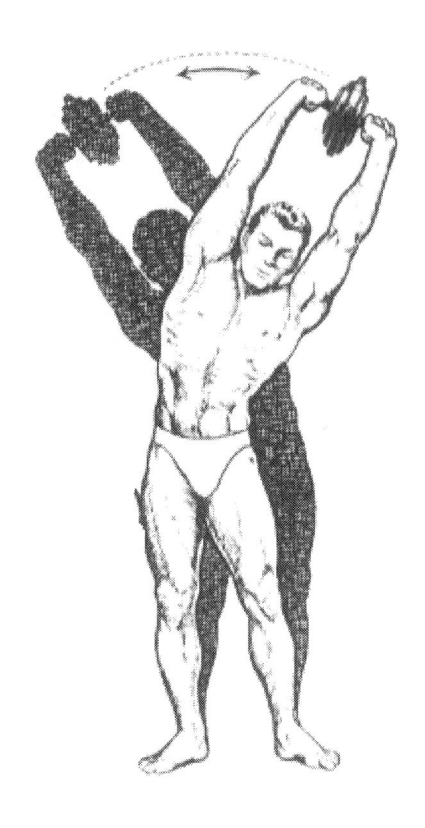

5. Lean Overs (ROM)

Equipment: twin dumbbells / swing-bell
Effect: Twist and warm up spine / waist
Resistance : Light [slow / medium speed]
Hip position: N/A
Spine position: Neutral throughout
Scapula position: Neutral / natural rotation
Muscles: erector spinae, internal / external oblique, rectus abdominis, gluteus medius
Typical Poundage: 1-3 kg dumbbells (women); 2-5 kg dumbbells (men)
Joints: Hip, shoulder, neck, rib-cage, vertebrae (slight/full)

Grab twin dumbbells and hold the arms at the sides. Next circle one arm in wide-arc right overhead and across the body behind the opposite shoulder. During the movement twist at the waist and bring the dumbbell as far backwards as possible upon completion of the arc. Perform in both directions and with both arms, one at a time. The goal is to really twist the entire torso to its maximum extent, and to warm up the shoulder structures at the same time. Do not move fast at any stage.

Perform daily.

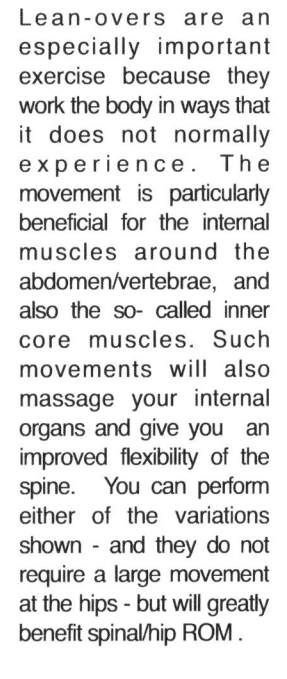

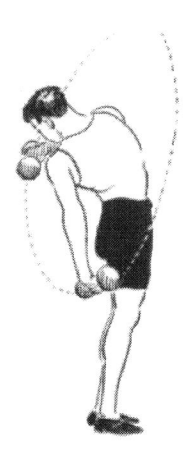

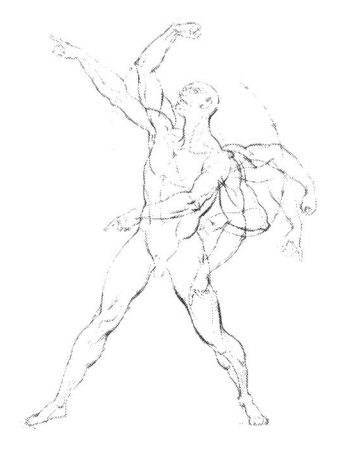

Lean-overs are an especially important exercise because they work the body in ways that it does not normally experience. The movement is particularly beneficial for the internal muscles around the abdomen/vertebrae, and also the so-called inner core muscles. Such movements will also massage your internal organs and give you an improved flexibility of the spine. You can perform either of the variations shown - and they do not require a large movement at the hips - but will greatly benefit spinal/hip ROM.

6. The Twist (ROM)

Equipment: twin dumbbells / barbell
Effect: Twist and warm up spine / waist
Resistance : Light [slow / medium speed]
Hip position: N/A
Spine position: Neutral throughout
Scapula position: Neutral
Muscles: erector spinae, internal / external oblique, rectus abdominis
Typical Poundage: 1-3 kg dumbbells (women); 2-5 kg dumbbells (men)
Joints: Hip, shoulder, vertebrae (slight/full)

Grab twin barbell/dumbbells and outstretch these overhead / out to sides. Next perform a torso twist to each side alternately. Try to twist slowly and to the maximum extent, reach as far back as possible. In a variation hold dumbbells at sides / waist.

Perform daily (can perform with barbell behind head). Twists, side-bending and crunches can also be performed with a cable machine (below).

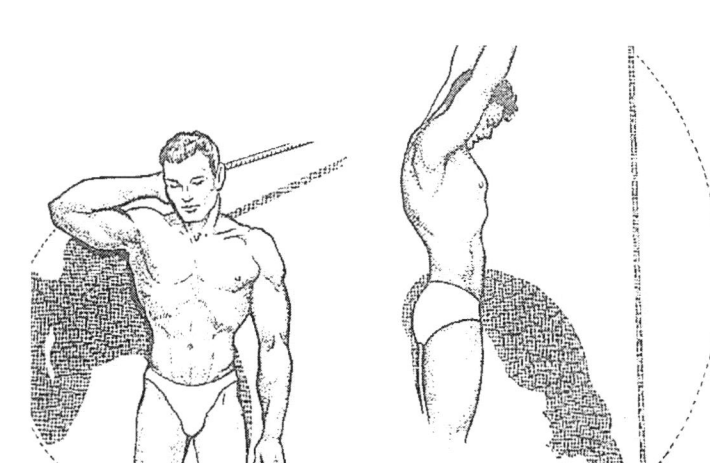

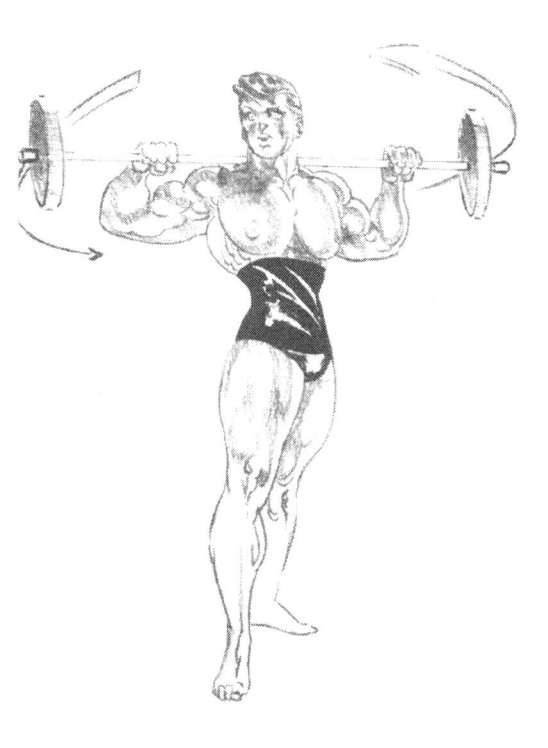

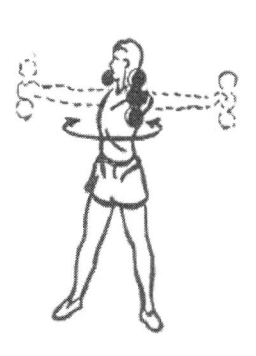

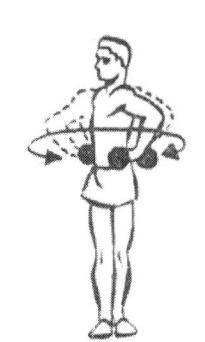

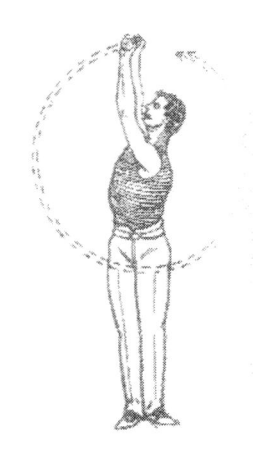

7. Twisting Lean Back (ROM)

Equipment: twin dumbbells
Effect: Twist and warm up spine / waist
Resistance : Light [slow speed]
Hip position: Slight extension at movement end
Spine position: Neutral / slight extension
Scapula position: Neutral / natural rotation at end
Muscles: gluteus maximus & medius, erector spinae, internal / external oblique, rectus abdominis, hip structure / extensors
Typical Poundage: 1-3 kg dumbbells (women); 2-5 kg (men)
Joints: Hip, ankle, neck, rib-cage, vertebrae (slight/full)

Twisting lean-backs are an important exercise because once again they work the body in ways that it does not normally experience. The movement is particularly beneficial for the internal muscles around the vertebrae and rib-cage, and also works the shoulders. Such movements will also massage your internal organs and give you an improved flexibility of the spine and rib-cage. You can perform either of the variations shown.

Grab twin dumbbells, and lift together into an overhead position. Next slowly and in a controlled manner twist the torso to either side (and backwards in a simultaneous lean-back), with the dumbbells all-the-time facing each other. Alternative version shown at top left.

Remember to lean back fully at the top of the movement and so to fully stretch both the rib-cage and the lower back/ shoulders. This move is really unlike any other, and if it were possible to perform a twisting lying pullover exercise; then this would be (in a way) the standing equivalent.

Do not move fast or use momentum. Perform daily.

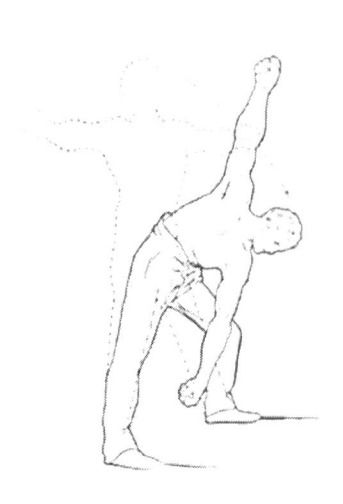

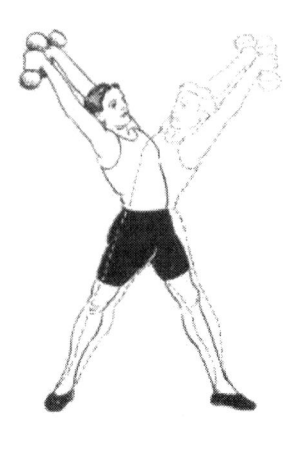

8. Side Bends (ROM)

Equipment: twin dumbbells
Effect: Bend and warm up spine / waist
Resistance : Light / Medium [slow / medium speed]
Hip position: N/A normally (+ flexion if you move the dumbbell forward from feet)
Spine position: Neutral throughout (possible slight flexion if you move the dumbbell(s) forward)
Scapula position: Neutral
Muscles: erector spinae, internal / external oblique, rectus abdominis, gluteus medius
Typical Poundage: 1-3 kg dumbbells (women); 2-5 kg dumbbells (men)
Joints: Hip, shoulder, rib-cage, vertebrae (slight/full)

Grab twin (or single) dumbbell(s), hold at sides, and then alternatively bend to each side and bring the dumbbell furthest away from the motion direction towards the shoulder. Keep knees unmoving and firm throughout, and keep your torso in sagittal plane. Often better to use only one dumbbell. If you do move the dumbbell somewhat forward from your feet, you gain greater ROM in terms of reaching lower, and the hip flexors become involved. Perform daily.

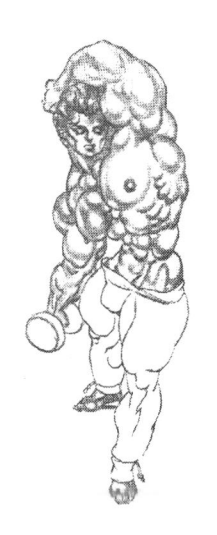

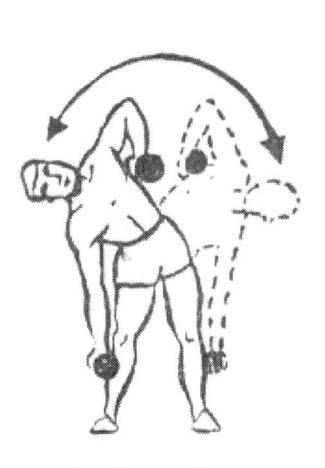

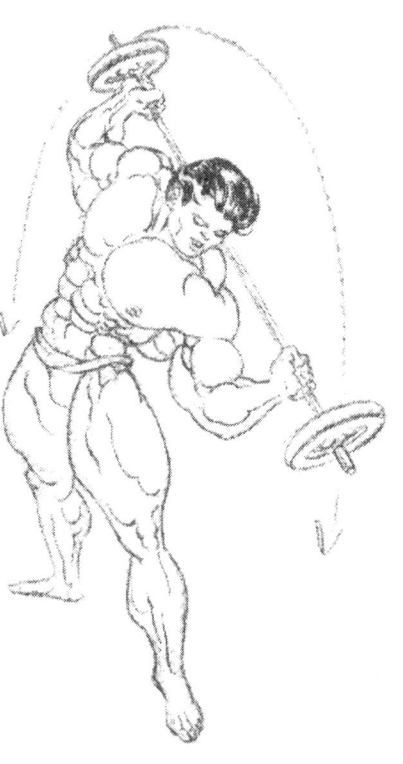

Side-bends are another especially important exercise because once again they work the body in ways that it does not normally experience. The movement is particularly beneficial for the internal muscles around the vertebrae and abdominals, and also works the oblique muscles. Such movements will also massage your internal organs and give you an improved flexibility of the spine. You can perform any of the variations shown.

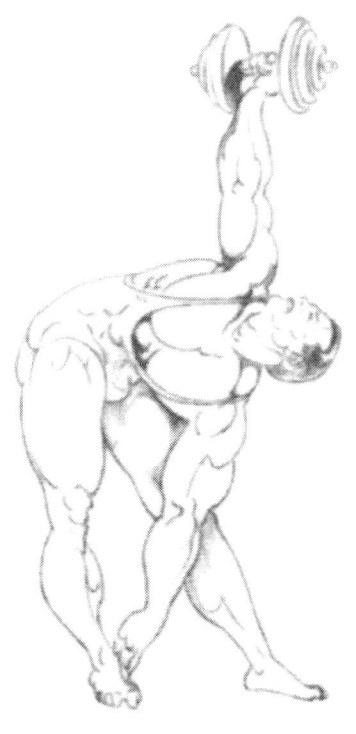

9. Windmill (ROM + Strength)

Equipment: single kettle-bell or dumbbell
Effect: Spine / abdominals / waist
Resistance : Light / Medium [very slow speed]
Hip position: Hip-Hinge - flexion / extension
Spine position: Neutral throughout
Scapula position: Neutral / natural rotation raised arm
Muscles: gluteus maximus & medius, erector spinae, internal / external oblique, rectus abdominis, entire hip structure, hip flexors / extensors, hamstrings
Typical Poundage: 3-8 kg dumbbell (women); 8-16 kg (men)
Joints: Hip, shoulder, ankle, neck, rib-cage, vertebrae

Grab a kettle-bell, and stand upright with legs apart. Hold kettle-bell overhead. Next turn one leg outwards (opposite side from hand holding the weight) and bend over very slowly to the same side (or other leg) whilst looking at the weight. Return to the upright position and repeat. In a variation you can take the lower arm towards the opposite foot - causing a very tight contraction of the abdominal muscles. Perform approx. two times weekly. Can also perform a reverse (twisting) windmill with opposite shoulder to opposite leg (corner image).

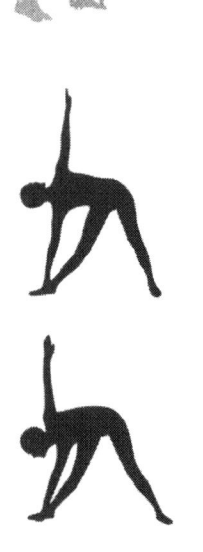

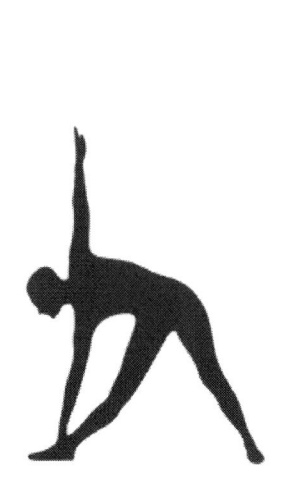

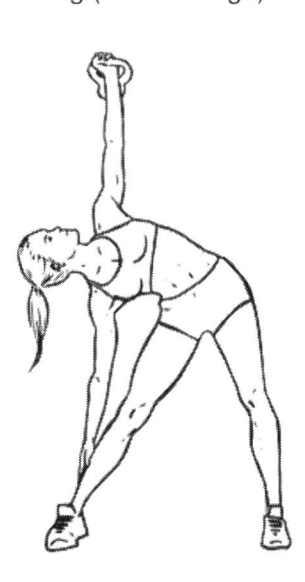

10. Forward bend (ROM)

Equipment: twin dumbbells
Effect: Strengthen lower back, shoulders, spine / waist
Resistance : Light / Medium [slow speed]
Hip position: Hip Hinge - Flexion + Extension
Spine position: Neutral / arched throughout
Scapula position: Neutral / natural rotation
Muscles: erector spinae, rectus abdominis, shoulders, gluteus maximus, hip structure, hip flexors / extensors
Typical Poundage: 1-3 kg dumbbell (women); 2-5 kg (men)
Joints: Hip, hand, knee, ankle, shoulder, vertebrae (slight/full)

Grab a pair of dumbbells, and stand upright with dumbbells overhead. Next lean forward slowly whilst keeping knees slightly bent but firm. Stop when dumbbells are at waist level and hold the contraction for a second or two, repeat for a number of repetitions. Legs (feet) can be separated in a sprinting position, or together. This movement is a bit odd - since it would appear to be designed to work the shoulders (holding the dumbbell in an out-stretched arm position) at the same time as the hips / lower-back. However such is the charm of this (older) exercise.

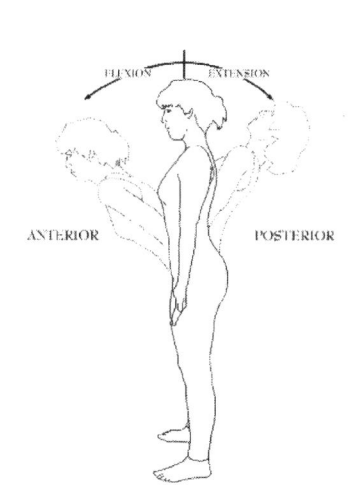

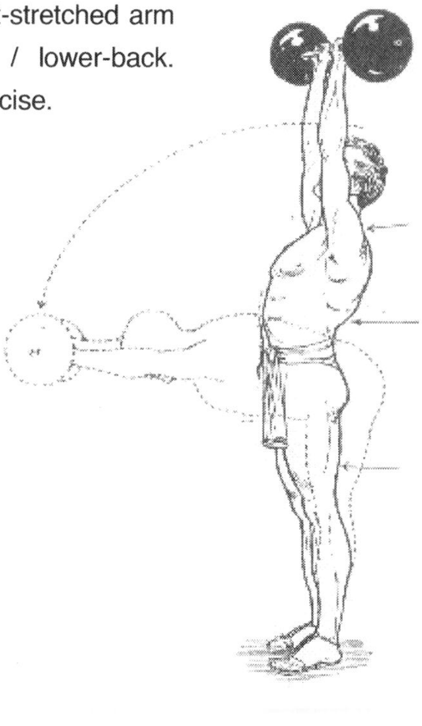

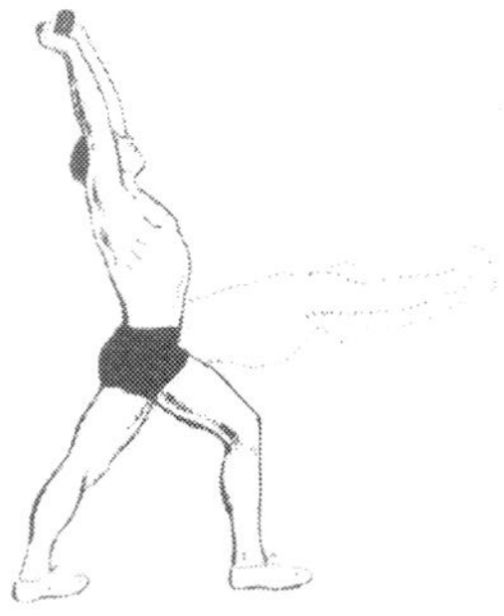

11. Dead-lift

Equipment: barbell, feet / barbell blocks (possibly)
Effect: Strengthen lower back, buttocks, leg-biceps, spine / waist, trapezius, grip
Resistance : Light / Medium / Heavy [Slow]
Hip position: Hip Hinge - Flexion / Extension
Spine position: Arched lumbar throughout (extension)
Scapula position: Neutral / natural position throughout
Muscles: gluteus maximus, erector spinae, hamstrings, rectus abdominis & aponeurosis, trapezius, quadriceps, external oblique, splenius capitis, levator scapulae, calves [look up at end]
Typical Poundage: 10-60 kg barbell (women); 60-200 kg barbell (men) - poundage varies depending upon style / goals.
Joints: Hip, hand, knee, ankle, neck, vertebrae

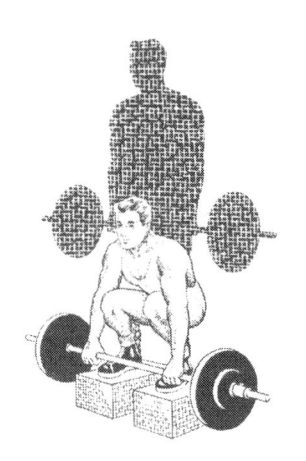

On lifts such as the squat, dead-lift and clean; it is acceptable to use a weight-lifting belt in order to support the spine / lower back on those sets which are your heaviest lifts; but do not wear one normally on training sets because such a practice can actually weaken your back structure over time.

Walk up to a loaded barbell, and place your feet behind it close to the bar but not touching it, being about 2-3 inches away. The dead-lift means to take a barbell from the floor to hip level. Place your hands about shoulder width apart, usually the right overhand and the left underhand, and lift the bar by pushing your legs through the floor, while maintaining your chin up (face directly in the mirror) and chest up. Use feet blocks for extra stimulation.

Do not, sway your back or lift the bar off the floor by locking out your legs so your back is bent over the bar. Maintain the erect position, chin up, and chest up and out, pulling all the way up till you are at arms length and the bar is stopped at thigh level. Do not "shrug" or lean backward. Repeat for reps.

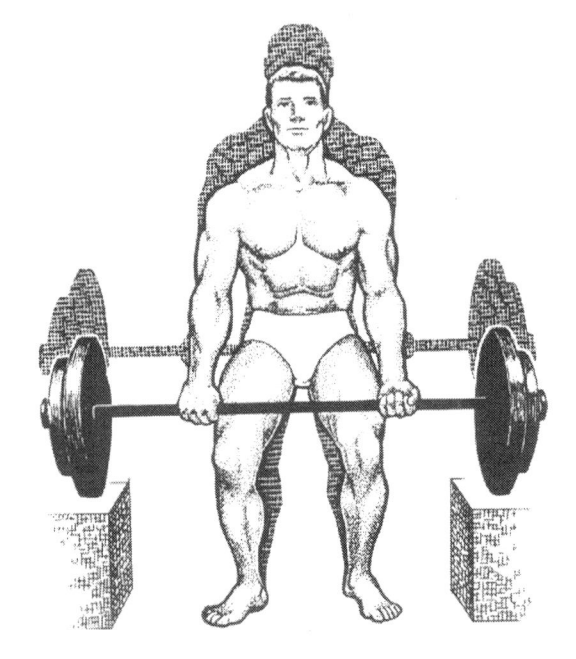

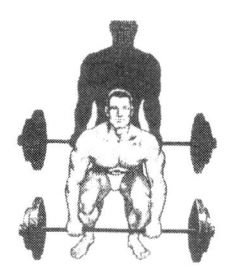

12. Stiff-leg Dead-lift (ROM + Strength)

Equipment: twin dumbbells (or barbell) plus feet blocks
Effect: Strengthen lower back, buttocks, leg-biceps, spine / waist
Resistance : Light [Very Slow] Start with 6 lbs dumbbells for a man
Hip position: Hip Hinge - Flexion / Extension
Spine position: Neutral lumbar / slight flexion at bottom
Scapula position: Neutral / slight protraction at bottom
Muscles: erector spinae, gluteus maximus, hamstrings (biceps femoris etc), rectus abdominis, semitendinosus, semimembranosus
Typical Poundage: 2-16 kg dumbbells (women); 3-24 kg dumbbells (men) - stay very light and stick to 10-12 repetitions
Joints: Hip, neck, vertebrae (medium/full)

Begin by standing upright with twin dumbbells at your sides. You want to have your feet straight ahead or even angled out to the sides slightly (perhaps feet closer together than with ordinary dead-lift - maybe 12 inches apart here). Make sure your feet stay flat on the floor at all times. You want to make sure that your head follows your body. The weight should be on your heels. It is best to keep your knees just slightly bent throughout the movement. As you bring the weight off of the floor, you should be bringing the weight up using your hamstrings. It should feel as if you are driving your hips forward. Make sure that your shoulders and hips are ascending together, if they aren't then you know you are using more of your lower back rather than your hamstrings. Bring the weight all the way up until you are standing straight up. Repeat for necessary repetitions. Note that the movement is performed at a very pace slow up and down (3-5 seconds each way). Do not deliberately flex the spine (this may happen naturally), but rather maintain spine neutrality - at least mentally.

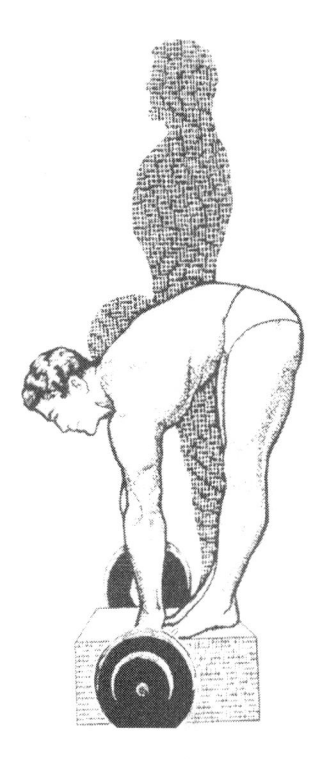

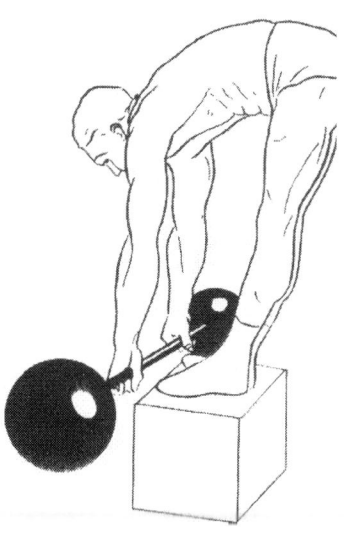

The dead-lift and stiff-legged dead-lift are two of the best (i.e. most beneficial) exercises that you can perform. I would perform these two movements (along with the squat and clean and press with a barbell/dumbbells) over any other movement. Some people believe that stiff legged dead-lifts are potentially dangerous for the lower back - but I believe this to be false so long as you use strict form, slow speed and employ a very light weight.

13. Stiff-leg Dead-lift (to feet) (ROM)

Equipment: twin dumbbells, barbell
Effect: Strengthen lower back, spine / waist, buttocks, leg-biceps
Resistance : Light [Very Slow]
Hip position: Hip Hinge - flexion / extension
Spine position: Arched lumbar (slight flexion at end if desired)
Scapula position: Neutral / slight protraction at bottom
Muscles: erector spinae, gluteus maximus, hamstrings, rectus abdominis, internal / external oblique, semitendinosus, semimembranosus
Typical Poundage: 4-16 kg dumbbells (women); 8-24 kg dumbbells (men) - stay very light and stick to 10-12 repetitions
Joints: Hip, neck, vertebrae (medium/full)

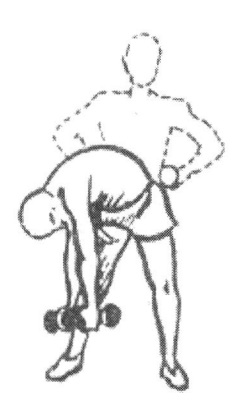

The stiff-legged dead-lift to alternate feet is one of the best moves you can perform in the gym. It has a really beneficial affect on the muscles at the back of the thigh, and all the structures of the spine and also the buttocks; plus it is especially beneficial to the abdominals including giving a massage to all of the internal organs etc. Perhaps best performed after ordinary dead-lifts or stiff-legged dead-lifts are completed, this exercise will see you bending over and touching your toes in no time. After just a few weeks spent using this movement, picking objects off the floor will seem so easy and natural that you won't believe it.

Pick up a pair of light dumbbells, and spread your legs out wider than shoulder width. Keep legs straight or slightly bent throughout. Stand upright, next slowly lower both the dumbbells to one foot as in the stiff-legged dead-lift. Raise up again, and perform the same to the other foot. Repeat for necessary repetitions. Maintain a neutral or arched lumber (spine extension) throughout, but it may be acceptable to perform a slight flexion stretch of the spine at the bottom position (if natural and desired).

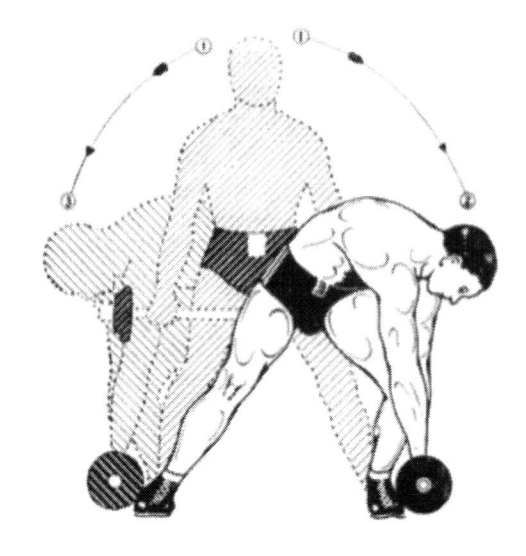

14. Clean

Equipment: barbell, single or twin dumbbells
Effect: Strengthen lower back, upper back, spine / waist, trapezius, buttocks, leg-biceps
Resistance : Light / Medium / Heavy [fast]
Hip position: Hip Hinge - Flexion / Extension
Spine position: Ached lumbar throughout (extension)
Scapula position: Neutral
Muscles: erector spinae, gluteus maximus, hamstrings, rectus abdominis, trapezius, latissimus dorsi, rhomboids, calves, biceps (end)
Typical Poundage: 10-60 kg barbell (women); 60-140 kg (men)
Joints: Hip, hand, knee, ankle, elbow, shoulder, vertebrae (slight/full), ribcage, wrist (greater involvement if thick bar)

Stand over a barbell with balls of feet positioned under the bar pointing forward, hip width apart or slightly wider. Squat down and grip bar with over hand grip slightly wider than shoulder width (thumbs length from ends of knurling on Olympic bar). Position shoulders over bar with back arched tightly. Arms are straight with elbows pointed along bar. Pull bar up off floor by extending hips and knees. As bar reaches knees vigorously raise shoulders while keeping barbell close to thighs. Jump upward extending body. Shrug shoulders and pull barbell upward with arms, allowing elbows to flex out to sides, keeping bar close to body. Aggressively pull body under bar, rotating elbows around bar. Catch bar on shoulders while moving into a squat position (semi or full). Hitting bottom of squat, stand up immediately. Repeat. The muscular action of the up-motion of the "power" clean; can be thought of as a type of "jumping squat" - because you "jump" against gravity using the quads, hamstrings, glutes and lower back muscles.

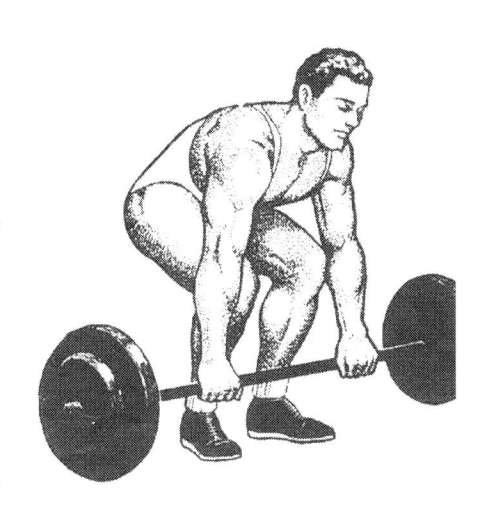

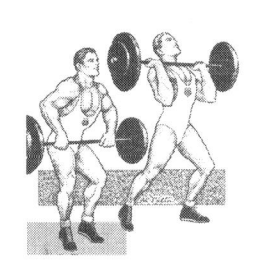

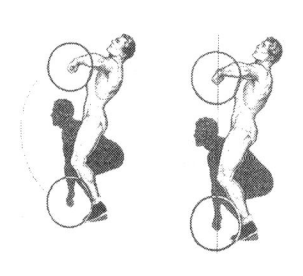

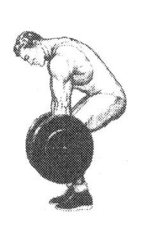

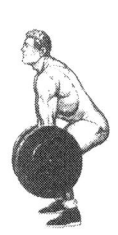

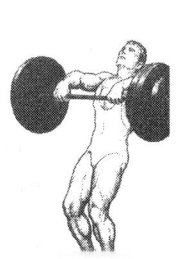

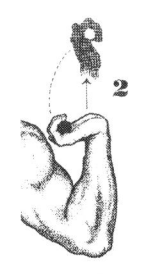

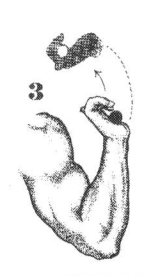

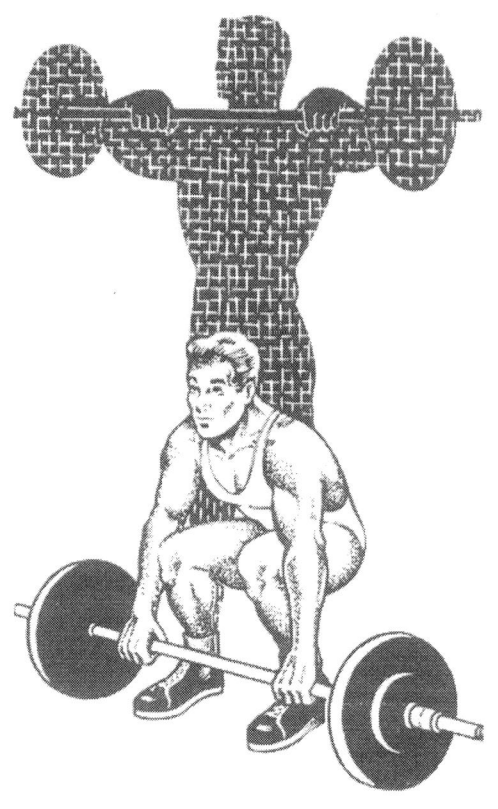

15. High Pull

Equipment: barbell
Effect: Strengthen lower back, trapezius, hip extensors, spine / waist
Resistance : Light / Medium / Heavy [fast]
Hip position: Hip Hinge - Flexion / Extension
Spine position: Arched lumbar throughout
Scapula position: Neutral
Muscles: erector spinae, gluteus maximus, hamstrings, rectus abdominis, trapezius, anterior, posterior and middle deltoid, splenius, sternocleidomastoid, calves
Typical Poundage: 10-60 kg barbell (women); 60-140 kg barbell (men)
Joints: Hip, neck, knee, ankle, elbow, shoulder, vertebrae, wrist

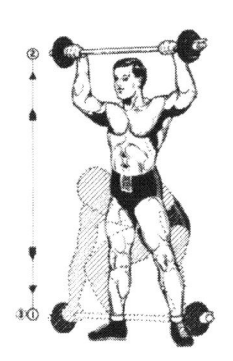

Walk up to a loaded barbel, and place your feet behind it close to the bar but not touching it, being about 2-3 inches away. Next grab the bar and contract the lower back muscles and whilst holding them in the arched (extended) position throughout, raise the bar rapidly to waist level and then continue pulling until the bar reaches approximately chest / eye height. Immediately lower (do not resist motion on way down) and repeat. Since this is a fast move, and there is a tendency to "fight" the weight to make it move high enough, but you must maintain a spine extension throughout (arched lumbar).

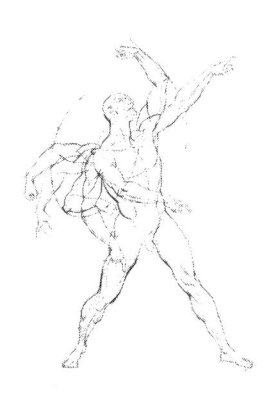

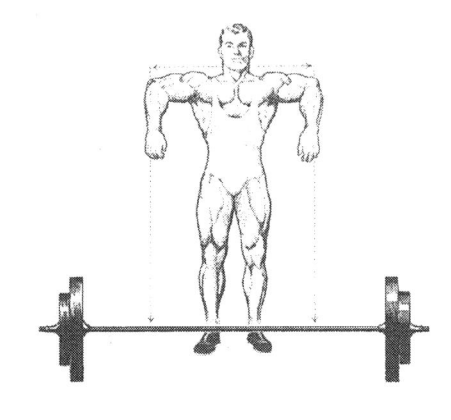

16. Good Morning (ROM + Strength)

Equipment: barbell
Effect: Strengthen lower back, spine / waist
Resistance : Light / Medium / Heavy [slow]
Hip position: Hip Hinge - Flexion / Extension
Spine position: Extended / arched lumbar throughout
Scapula position: Neutral / slight retraction throughout
Muscles: erector spinae, gluteus maximus, hamstrings, semimembranosus, semitendinosus, quadratus lumborum, neck muscles, quadratus lumborum, iliocostalis lumborum
Typical Poundage: 5-15 kg barbell (women); 10-40 kg (men)
Joints: Hip, neck, vertebrae, hamstrings

POTENTIALLY DANGEROUS EXERCISE - ONLY PERFORM IF YOUR SPINE IS IN PERFECT HEALTH AND YOU ARE WILLING TO ACCEPT THE RISK OF DAMAGING YOUR LOWER BACK

Position barbell on back of shoulders and grasp bar to sides. Keeping back straight, bend hips to lower torso forward until parallel to floor. Raise torso until hips are extended. Repeat. Begin with very light weight (10 lbs for a man) and add additional weight gradually. Throughout lift keep back and knees straight. Do not lower weight beyond mild stretch through hamstrings. Full range of motion will vary from person to person depending on flexibility. Never use more than 80-90 pounds (men), and 10-30 pounds should be enough in general.

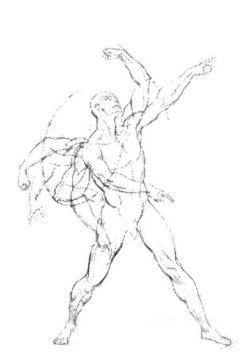

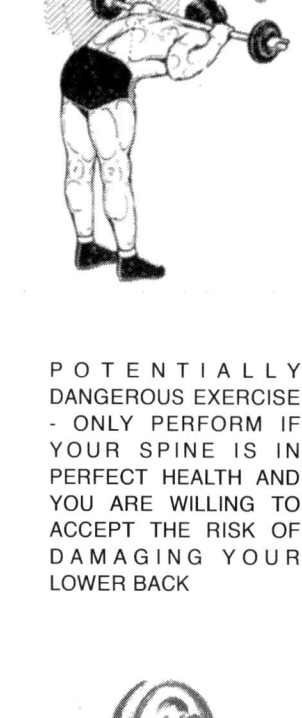

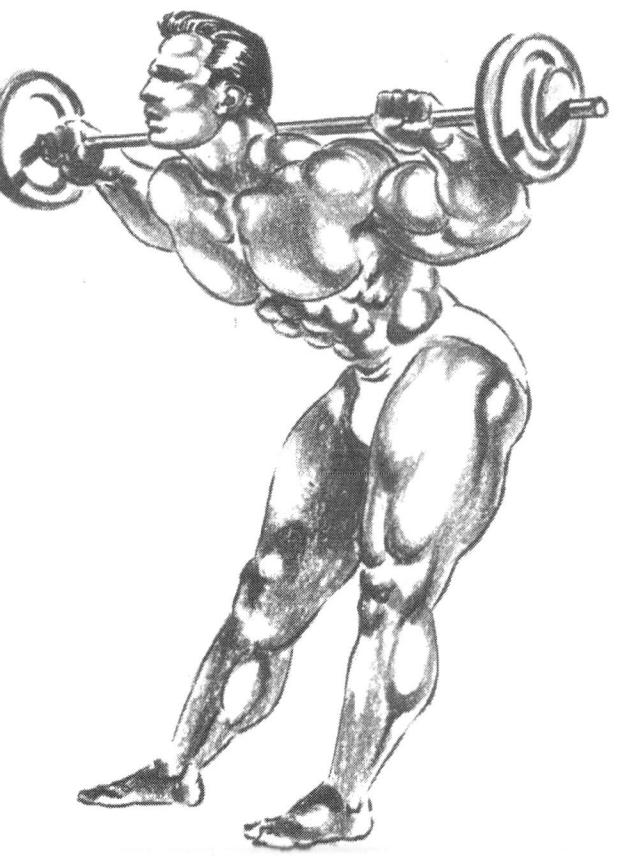

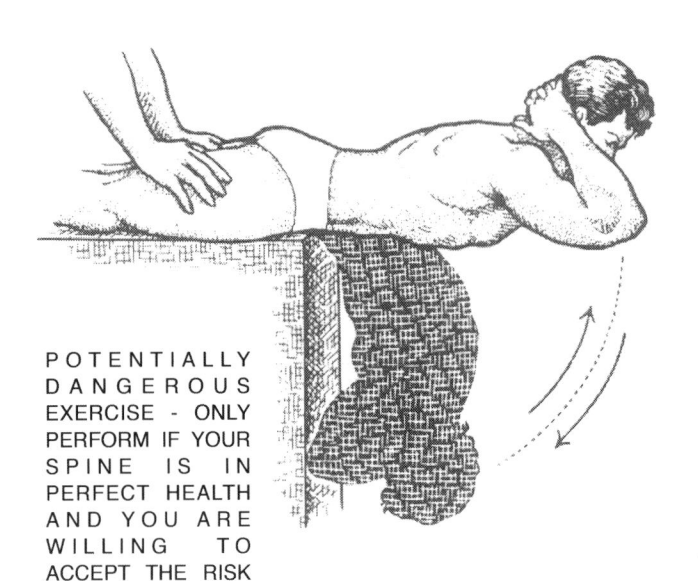

17. Lying Hyperextension

POTENTIALLY DANGEROUS EXERCISE - ONLY PERFORM IF YOUR SPINE IS IN PERFECT HEALTH AND YOU ARE WILLING TO ACCEPT THE RISK OF DAMAGING YOUR LOWER BACK

Equipment: nothing / barbell
Effect: Strengthen lower back, spine / waist
Resistance : Light / Medium / Heavy [slow speed]
Hip position: Hip Hinge - Flexion / Extension
Spine position: Neutral / extended / arched lumbar throughout (no flexion)
Scapula position: Neutral
Muscles: erector spinae, gluteus maximus, hamstrings, semimembranosus, semitendinosus, quadratus lumborum, neck muscles, quadratus lumborum, iliocostalis lumborum, spinalis thoracis, longissimus thoracis, iliocostalis thoracis
Typical Poundage: 5-15 kg barbell (women); 10-40 kg (men)
Joints: Hip, neck, vertebrae. [use only very light weights]

The hyperextension is a controversial exercise. I believe it is without a doubt one of the most beneficial exercises you can do for improving the health, function and strength of the lower back region. You must be careful when using a machine or hypertension bench to make certain that the bench does not hurt your knees and/or other vulnerable parts.

Performed either lying flat on floor / bench, or on a special hyperextension bench. Place barbell on back of shoulders and grasp bar to sides. Raise upper body until hip and waist are fully extended. Lower body (slowly) by bending hips and waist until fully flexed. Repeat. Some people advise not going (much) beyond parallel at the end of the exercise (i.e. no hip / spine extension); and perhaps it is best to avoid so doing to an excessive degree. NEVER USE A MACHINE (MOVING PARTS) FOR THIS EXERCISE

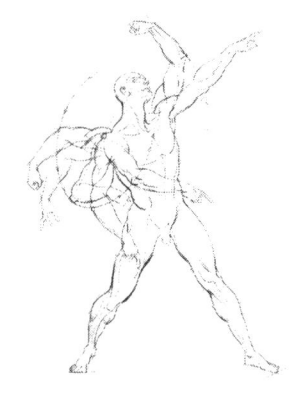

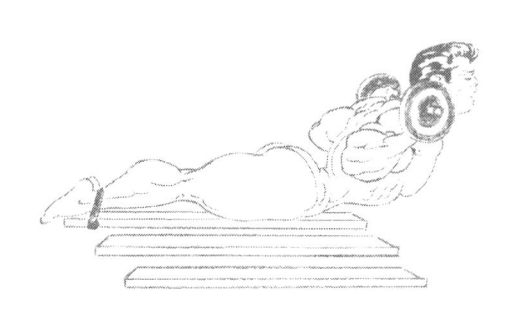

18. Sit-up

Equipment: nothing / barbell / dumbbells
Effect: Strengthen waist
Resistance : Light [Slow / Medium]
Hip position: Hip Hinge - flexion / extension
Spine position: Neutral (be aware if you do flex the spine at the end - this could be dangerous)
Scapula position: Neutral
Muscles: rectus abdominis, external oblique, hip flexors, quadriceps rectus femoris, tensor fasciae latae
Typical Poundage: none / 5 kg (women); 10 kg (men)
Joints: Hip, vertebrae (slight) - SHOULD NOT INVOLVE NECK!

To be effective, sit-ups must pull the torso upward from a lying position toward the knees using largely the abdominal group. Often, however, other, more powerful, muscles (those that flex the legs and hips) do much of the work (normally). This is especially true with straight-leg sit-ups. Bending the knees during sit-ups helps to neutralise the action of the hip flexors and makes the abdominal muscles work more. Even so, the abdominal group tends to be involved only in the initial phase of the sit-up, after which the hip flexors take over. Raising slowly only part way works the abdominal muscles best. Twisting (right elbow to left knee and vice versa) at the top of the sit-up places rotational stress on the lower back that may lead to injury.

It is not necessary to interlace the fingers of your hands behind your head as this may place a strain on the neck - instead place your hands on either side of the head.

The sit-up has been the topic of much debate. Some people proclaim that you should never perform it at-all - because (they claim) it can damage the lower back and/or neck. I do not believe that these concerns are a worry for most people. I think that the sit-up - if performed without jerking - is a very beneficial exercise indeed.

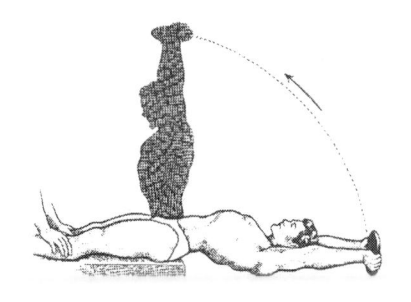

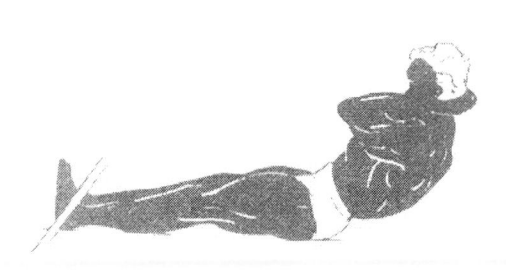

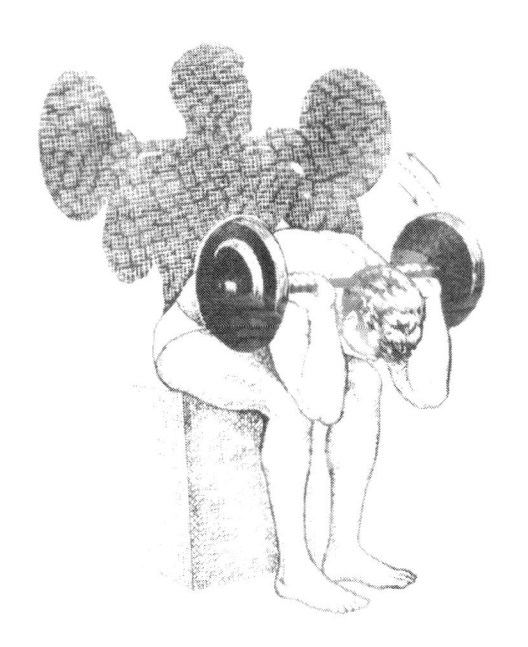

19. Sit-up (dumbbell(s) overhead)

Equipment: twin dumbbells/ barbell
Effect: Strengthen waist
Resistance : Light [Slow]
Hip position: Hip Hinge - Flexion / Extension?
Spine position: Neutral (dumbbells overhead)
Scapula position: Neutral
Muscles: rectus abdominis, external oblique, hip flexors, quadriceps rectus femoris, tensor fasciae latae
Typical Poundage: 1-3 kg dumbbells (women); 3-6 kg dumbbells (men)
Joints: Hip, shoulder, vertebrae (none/full)

The sit-up whilst holding dumbbells overhead is an advanced exercise that can really strengthen the entire stomach region.

The seated sit-up with a dumbbell/barbell behind the head whereby you crunch forward really works and massages the internal organs and abdomen.

CRUNCHING FORWARD (FLEXION) OF SPINE WITH WEIGHT IS A DANGEROUS MOVEMENT

Simply lie down on the floor with a pair of light dumbbells, place them overhead and then perform slow sit-ups. Keep the arms overhead throughout. Advanced exercise with high degree of difficulty. Can also perform a version with weight behind head (VERY DANGEROUS - NOT RECOMMENDED BY THE AUTHOR). Latter move may have a slight crunching forward movement (spine flexion) to work/massage internal structure/organs (warning: only perform with due care because the spine could be loaded under flexion here and so get a Physician's advice before attempting).

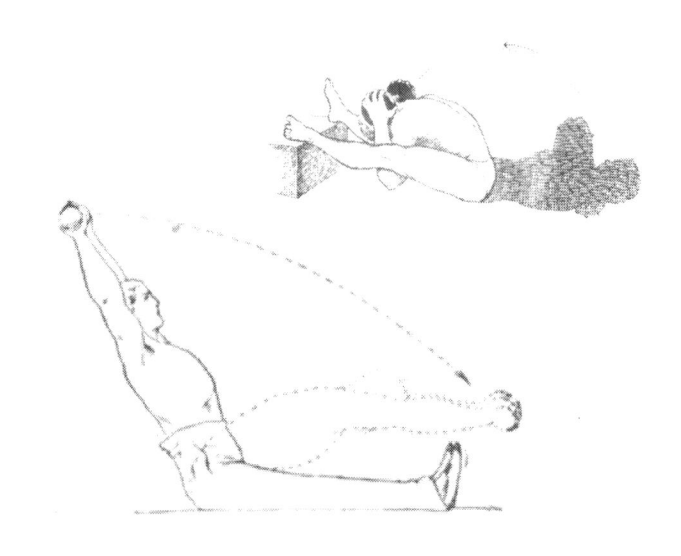

20. Incline Sit-up

Equipment: N/A
Effect: Strengthen waist
Resistance : N/A [Slow]
Hip position: Hip Hinge - Flexion
Spine position: N/A (do not flex spine at end)
Scapula position: Neutral
Muscles: rectus abdominis, external oblique, quadriceps, rectus femoris, tensor fasciae latae, hip flexors
Typical Poundage: none / 1-3 kg dumbbells (women); 3-6 kg (men)
Joints: Hip

Simply lie down on an incline bench and perform sit-ups as desired. Hook feet under supports or do not. Hold hands behind your head or do not. Keeping the legs slightly bent is best and do not jerk the body when starting and/or during the movement. Do not flex the spine at any point.

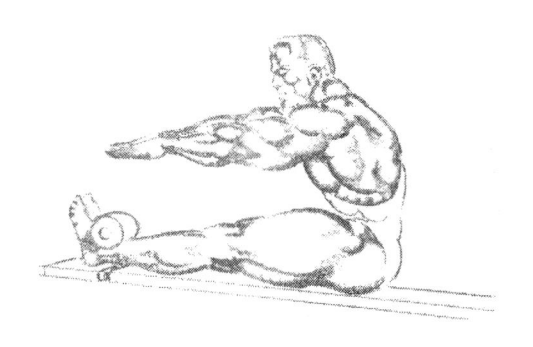

THE INCLINE SIT-UP IS A POTENTIALLY DANGEROUS EXERCISE - ONLY PERFORM IF YOUR SPINE IS IN PERFECT HEALTH AND YOU ARE WILLING TO ACCEPT THE RISK OF DAMAGING YOUR LOWER BACK

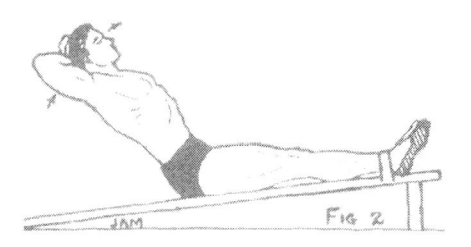

The incline sit-up is a supreme strengthening exercise for the abdominals. You can also hold a weight plate or dumbbell behind the head and/or on chest to make the exercise more difficult and effective.

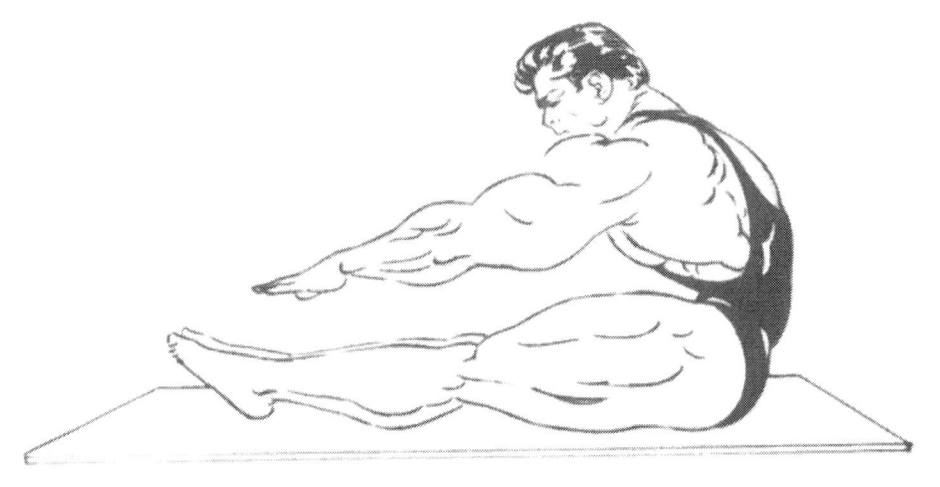

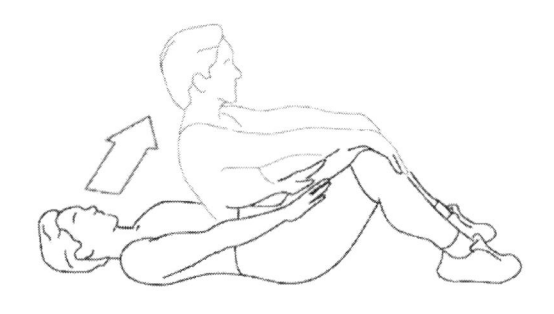

21. Crunch

Equipment: Nothing / Exercise Ball
Effect: Strengthen waist
Resistance : N/A [Slow]
Hip position: Hip Hinge - flexion /extension
Spine position: Deliberate flexion
Scapula position: Neutral
Muscles: rectus abdominis, external oblique, tensor fasciae latae, quadriceps, rectus femoris
Typical Poundage: none / 2-4 kg dumbbell (women); 3-5 kg (men)
Joints: Hip, vertebrae (slight/full)

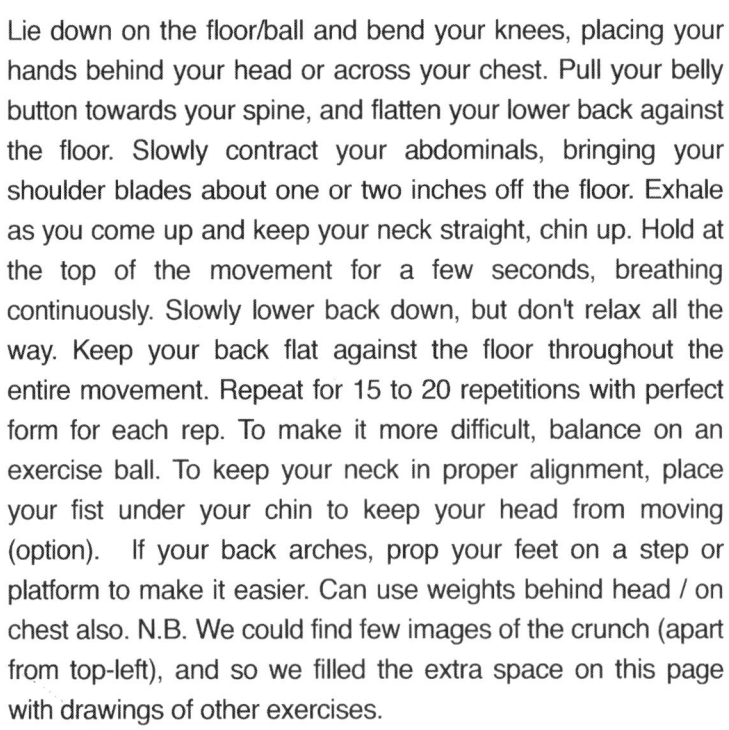

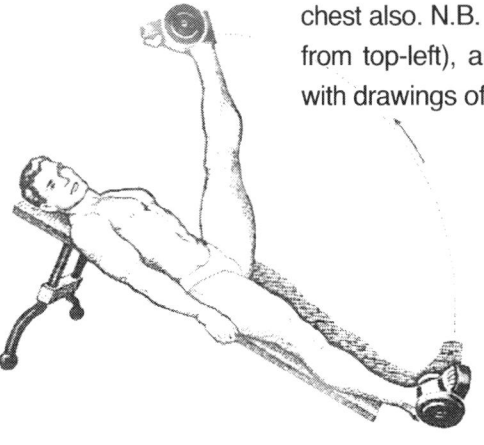

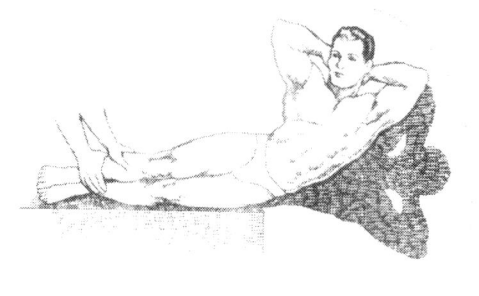

Lie down on the floor/ball and bend your knees, placing your hands behind your head or across your chest. Pull your belly button towards your spine, and flatten your lower back against the floor. Slowly contract your abdominals, bringing your shoulder blades about one or two inches off the floor. Exhale as you come up and keep your neck straight, chin up. Hold at the top of the movement for a few seconds, breathing continuously. Slowly lower back down, but don't relax all the way. Keep your back flat against the floor throughout the entire movement. Repeat for 15 to 20 repetitions with perfect form for each rep. To make it more difficult, balance on an exercise ball. To keep your neck in proper alignment, place your fist under your chin to keep your head from moving (option). If your back arches, prop your feet on a step or platform to make it easier. Can use weights behind head / on chest also. N.B. We could find few images of the crunch (apart from top-left), and so we filled the extra space on this page with drawings of other exercises.

22. Leg-Raise

Equipment: Nothing / Leg-bell
Effect: Strengthen waist
Resistance : N/A [Slow / Medium]
Hip position: Hip Hinge - flexion / extension
Spine position: Neutral / Slight flexion at end ?
Scapula position: Neutral
Muscles: rectus abdominis, hip flexors, external oblique, quadriceps, rectus femoris, tensor fasciae latae
Typical Poundage: none / 2-4 kg leg-bell (women); 3-5 kg (men)
Joints: Hip

Lie on the floor/mat on your back. Keep lower back in contact with the floor, feet and legs straight and together. Place hands to sides or under lower-back/bottom for support. Keeping legs straight and together, back flat, lift legs upward until they are straight above hips. Lower down to starting position slowly and with control (but do not allow feet to touch the ground between reps) to complete one rep. Make sure the back stays flat on floor and abs are tight (pull navel in towards spine) - but you may also perform a more advanced version where you raise the lower back at the movement end. May add weights to feet.

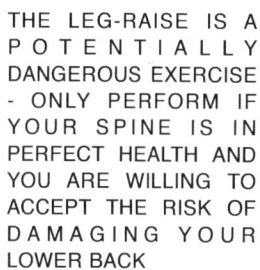

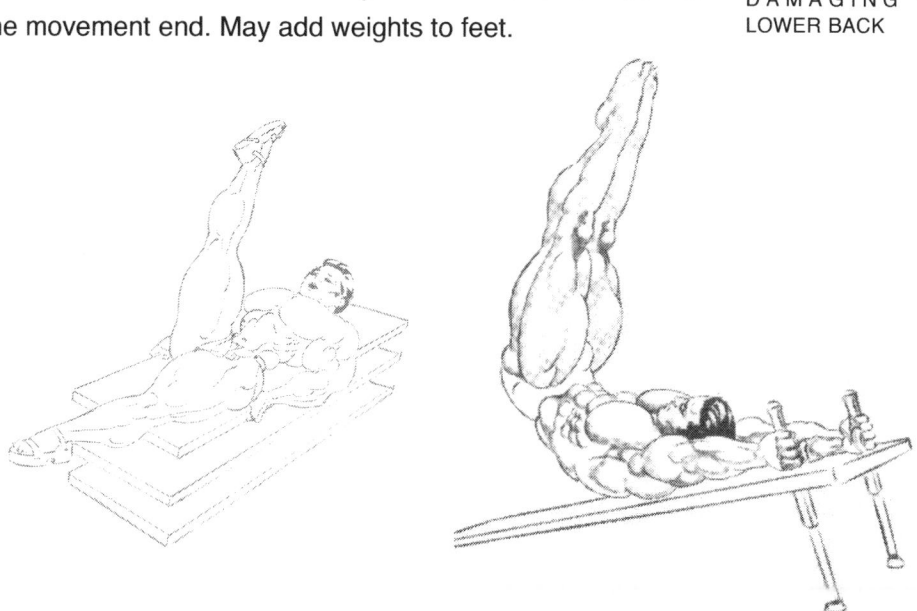

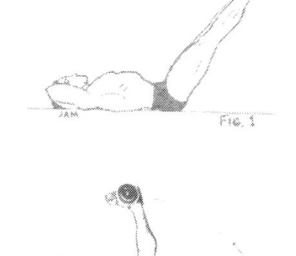

THE LEG-RAISE IS A POTENTIALLY DANGEROUS EXERCISE - ONLY PERFORM IF YOUR SPINE IS IN PERFECT HEALTH AND YOU ARE WILLING TO ACCEPT THE RISK OF DAMAGING YOUR LOWER BACK

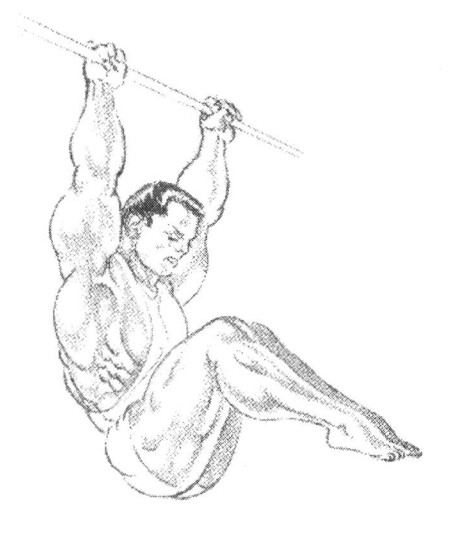

23. Seated Knee-In / Knee-Tucks

Equipment: Nothing or chin-up/leg-raise bar
Effect: Strengthen waist
Resistance : N/A [Slow]
Hip position: Hip Hinge - flexion / extension
Spine position: Neutral or flexion (hanging version)
Scapula position: Neutral
Muscles: rectus abdominis, hip flexors, external oblique, quadriceps, rectus femoris, tensor fasciae latae
Typical Poundage: none
Joints: Hip, knee

The seated or hanging knee-in is a superb exercise for the abdominals/ hip flexors. It is very easy to perform and can be combined with sit-ups or other types of leg raises to really make the abs burn.

THE KNEE-IN IS A POTENTIALLY DANGEROUS EXERCISE - ONLY PERFORM IF YOUR SPINE IS IN PERFECT HEALTH AND YOU ARE WILLING TO ACCEPT THE RISK OF DAMAGING YOUR LOWER BACK

Sit on a sturdy chair with your hands holding the front of the chair for support. Lean back in the chair and draw your bent legs up. Move your legs out into a pike position. Extend them as far and high as possible with stability. Return and repeat. Can also perform hanging from a bar and possibly with a "reverse crunch" at the end of the movement in such a case (spine flexion).

This movement is a super one for the entire front abdominal region, and I suggest that you perform it whenever you train your abdominals. You can use a dumbbell between the feet for extra resistance, or else use leg-bells or iron boots etc. It is also fun to combine the exercise into a super-set with various sit-ups and other kinds of leg raises and leg swings.

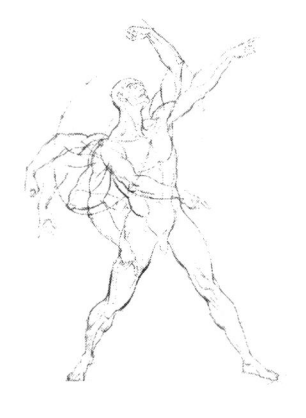

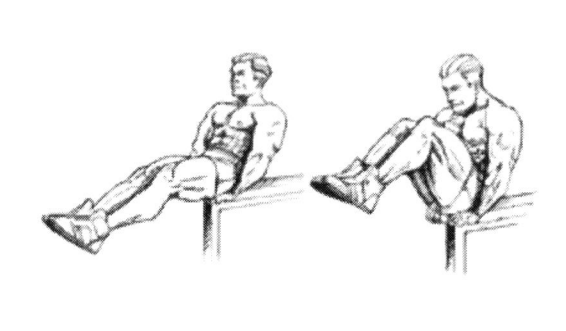

24. Leg Raise + Torso Raise (Jack Knife)

Equipment: Nothing / exercise ball
Effect: Strengthen waist
Resistance : N/A [Medium]
Hip position: Hip Hinge - flexion / extension
Spine position: N/A / slight flexion
Scapula position: Neutral
Muscles: rectus abdominis, hip flexors, external oblique, quadriceps, rectus femoris, tensor fasciae latae
Typical Poundage: none
Joints: Hip, knee, vertebrae (slight)

Lie on your back, with your legs and arms extended. Keeping your knees and elbows locked, simultaneously raise your upper body while trying to touch your fingers to your toes as you raise your legs up off the ground and towards your upper body. You can perform a slight crunch at the end with corresponding spinal flexion.

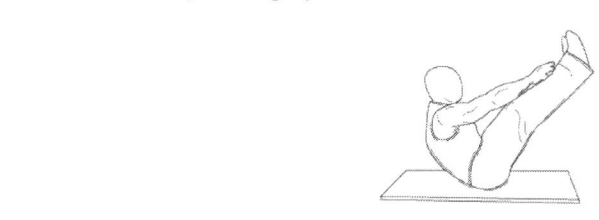

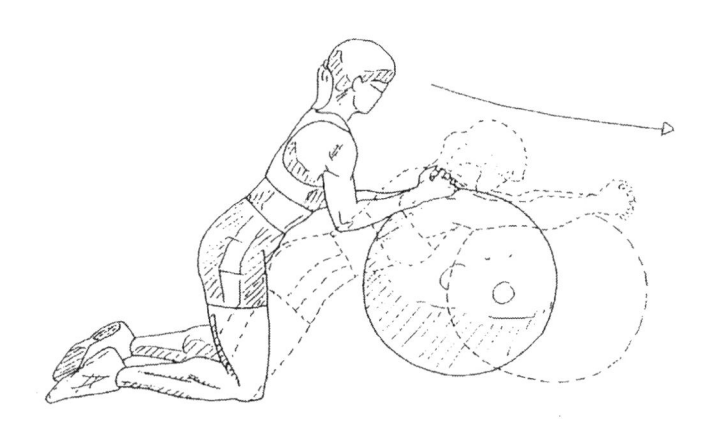

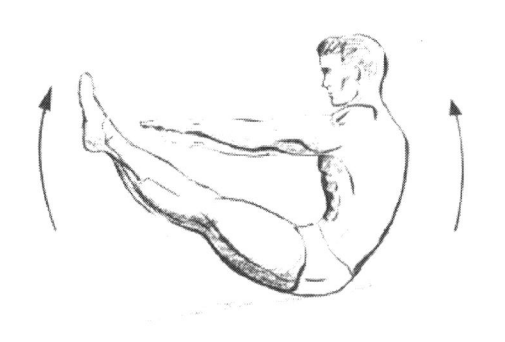

The leg-raise + torso raise is another superb exercise for the abdominals. It is quite difficult to perform and can be classified as an advanced exercise.

Another similar but useful exercise is shown at left - and is the dumbbell / wheel / or exercise ball roll-out. This exercise strongly works the abdominals and is a truly beneficial (and slightly safer) way to work in the same manner as in the jack-knife.

THE LEG RAISE PLUS TORSO RAISE IS A POTENTIALLY DANGEROUS EXERCISE - ONLY PERFORM IF YOUR SPINE IS IN PERFECT HEALTH AND YOU ARE WILLING TO ACCEPT THE RISK OF DAMAGING YOUR LOWER BACK

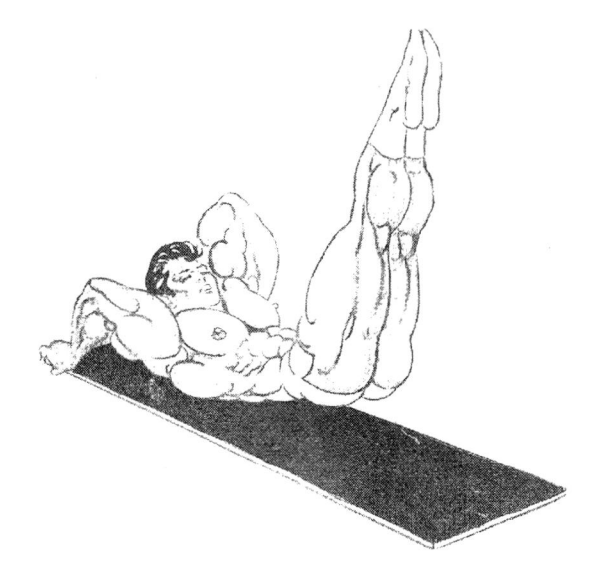

25. Seated Leg Raise

Equipment: Nothing / bench
Effect: Strengthen waist
Resistance : N/A [Slow]
Hip position: Flexion / extension
Spine position: N/A / flexion (end)
Scapula position: Neutral
Muscles: rectus abdominis, hip flexors, external oblique, quadriceps, rectus femoris, tensor fasciae latae
Typical Poundage: none
Joints: Hip, knee

The seated or lying straight leg-raise is a superb exercise for the abdominals. It is very easy to perform and can be combined with sit-ups or other types of leg raises to really make the abs burn.

THE STRAIGHT-LEGGED LEG RAISE IS A POTENTIALLY DANGEROUS EXERCISE - ONLY PERFORM IF YOUR SPINE IS IN PERFECT HEALTH AND YOU ARE WILLING TO ACCEPT THE RISK OF DAMAGING YOUR LOWER BACK

Sit on a bench, arms close to your sides, palms down, and grab onto the bench for support. Extend your legs outward, with your heels about 3 inches above the bench. Now raise each of your legs upwards whilst keeping them straight at the knee (either move both legs at the same time or each one individually) - and repeat for reps. Can perform a slight back-lift at the end, and/or crunch abdominals at the end (slight spinal flexion).

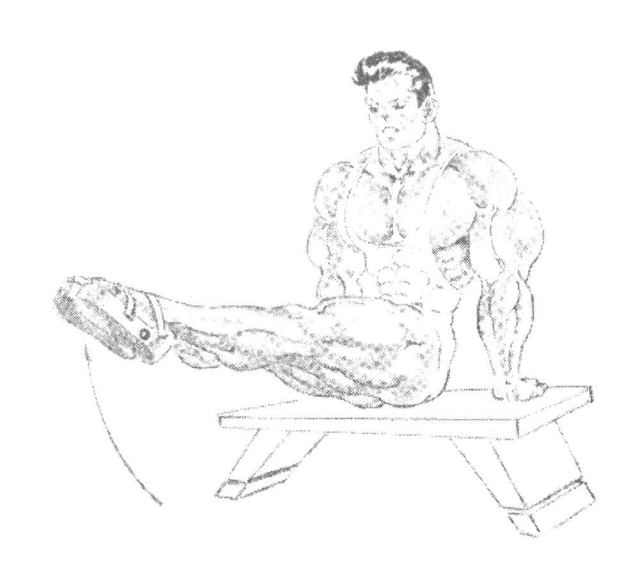

26. Side-Lying Crunch

Equipment: Nothing / bench + partner
Effect: Strengthen waist
Resistance : N/A [Slow]
Hip position: Neutral / flexion + extension
Spine position: Deliberate spine flexion (possibly)
Scapula position: Neutral
Muscles: rectus abdominis, hip flexors, external oblique, quadriceps, rectus femoris, tensor fasciae latae
Typical Poundage: none
Joints: Hip, vertebrae (slight/full)

Lie on a mat on your side with your knees bent at a right angle and twisted to the left. Can hold a small barbell plate up to your chest. Curl up your upper body, lifting your shoulders off the floor a few inches. Pause at the top of the contraction and slowly lower back down.

Note that the side crunch is classified as an advanced move, and you will soon tire because your oblique muscles are not (typically) that strong compared to your rectus abdominis. Your range of motion when lying by yourself and twisting sideways will be quite small, so make certain that you don't try to jerk yourself higher.

The side-lying crunch is a superb exercise for the obliques/ abdominals. You don't always need a partner (as seen here) but you can simply lie down on the floor and start side crunching.

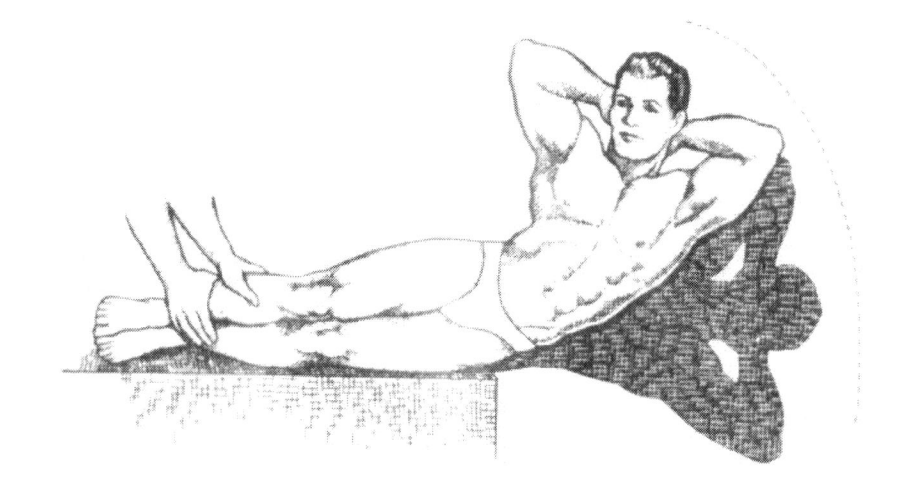

27. Roman Chair Sit-Up

Equipment: Bench plus barbell (feet wrest) or exercise ball or roman chair bench (could be dangerous if used with weights due to loaded spine flexion)
Effect: Strengthen waist
Resistance : N/A / Light [Slow]
Hip position: Hip Hinge - flexion / extension
Spine position: Neutral / flexion (end)
Scapula position: Neutral
Muscles: rectus abdominis, hip flexors, external oblique, quadriceps, rectus femoris, tensor fasciae latae
Typical Poundage: none / 4-8 kg (women); 8-20 kg barbell or plate (men)
Joints: Hip, vertebrae (slight/full)

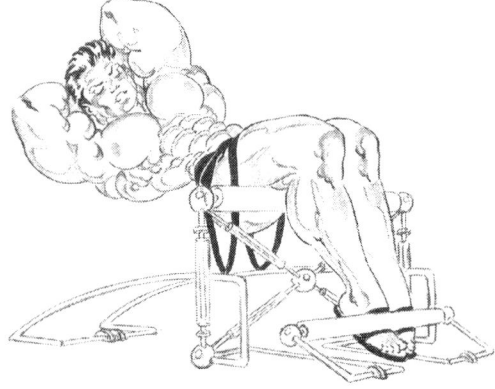

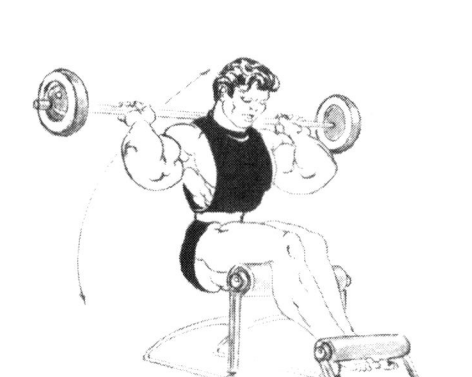

THE ROMAN CHAIR SIT-UP IS A POTENTIALLY DANGEROUS EXERCISE - ONLY PERFORM IF YOUR SPINE IS IN PERFECT HEALTH AND YOU ARE WILLING TO ACCEPT THE RISK OF DAMAGING YOUR LOWER BACK

Sit on a chair, bench or exercise ball, with lower leg secured under low over hang or heavy bar. Place hands on waist, chest, neck, or head depending upon desired difficulty. Lower body back until hips are almost extended. Raise body by flexing hips until torso is upright. Repeat. Feet must be propped securely to prevent injury. Rectus Abdominis and Obliques only contract dynamically if actual waist flexion occurs. With no waist flexion, Rectus Abdominis and External Oblique will only act to stabilise pelvis and waist during hip flexion. You can use waist (spine) flexion at end if so desired. Watch out here for the danger of lifting with a loaded (i.e. flexed spine) - use intelligence.

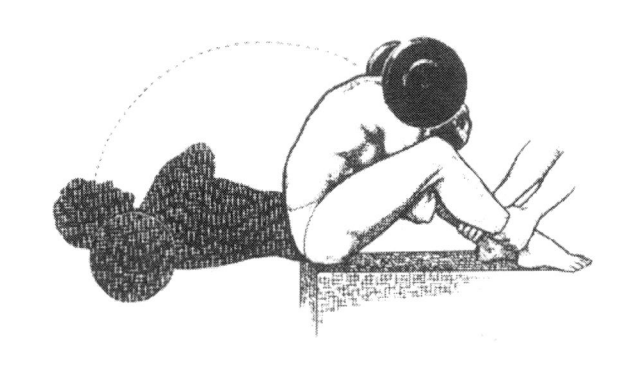

THE TRUNK 169

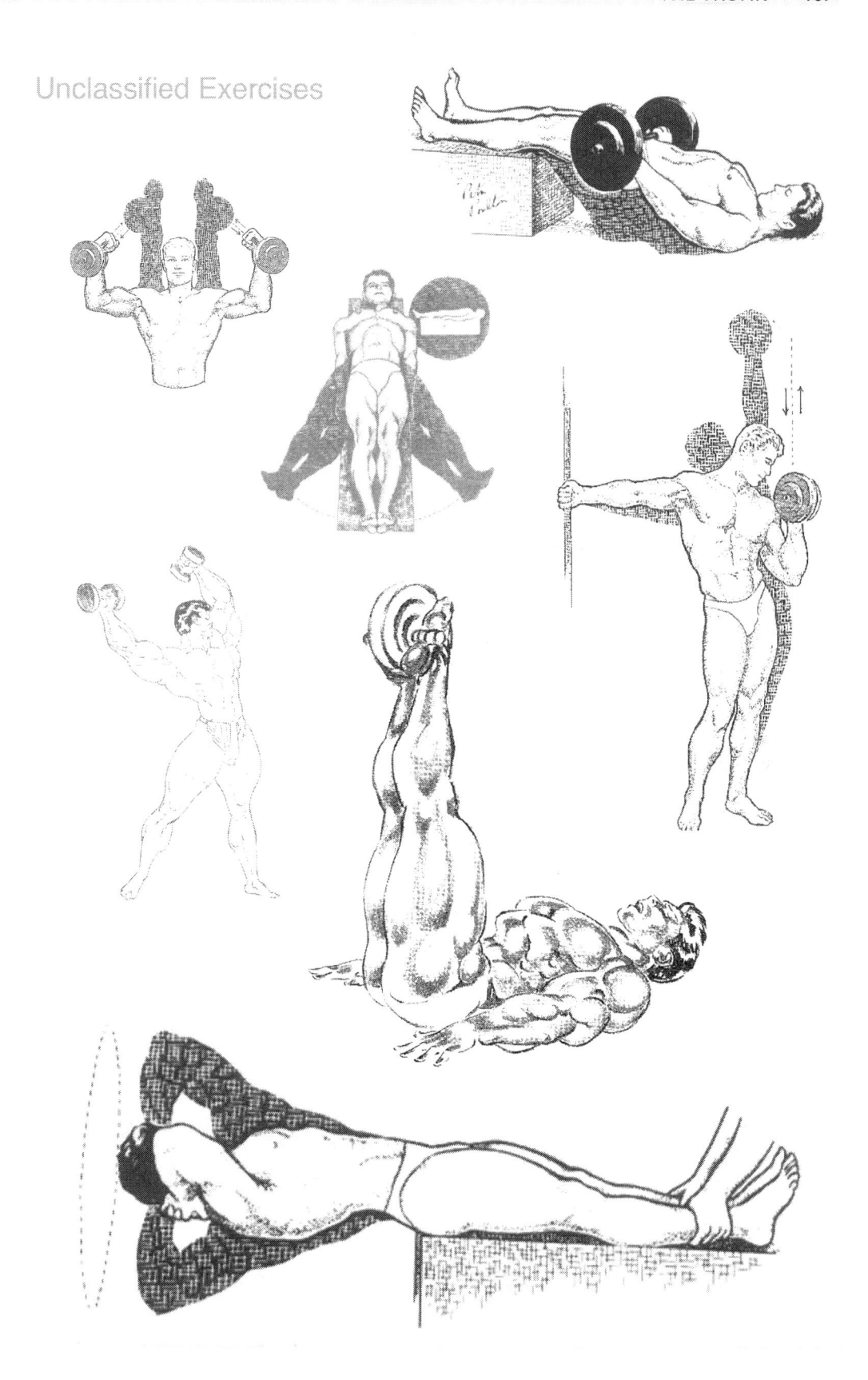

Unclassified Exercises

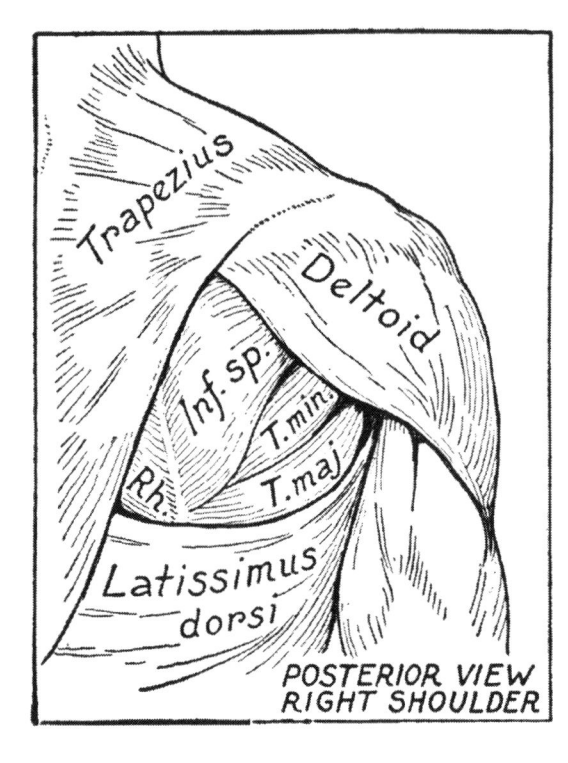

Inf. sp.
Infraspinatus

T. min.
Teres minor

T. maj.
Teres major

Rh. Rhomboid

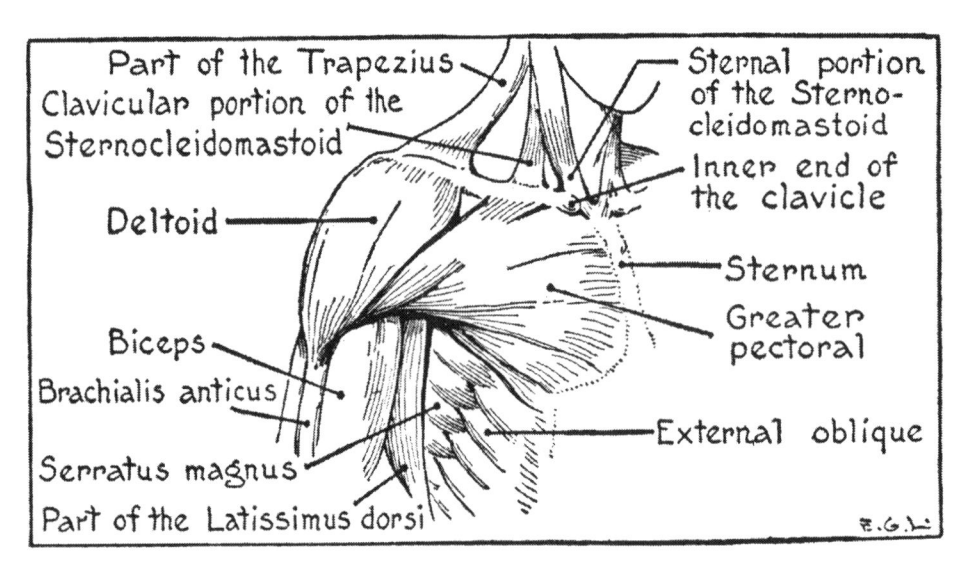

THE MUSCLES OF THE RIGHT SHOULDER AND ADJACENT REGIONS.

CHAPTER EIGHT

The Shoulder

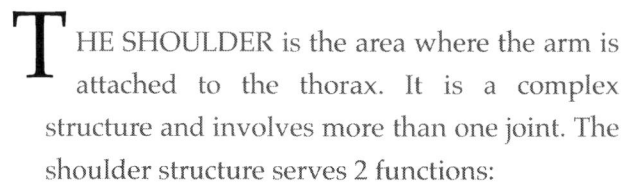

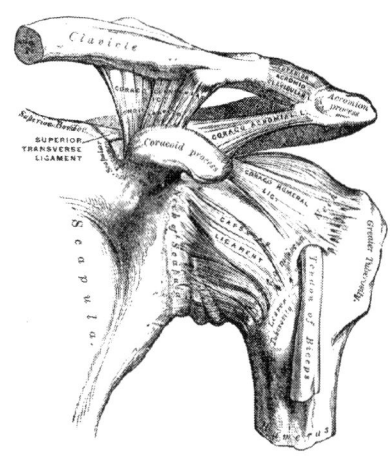

THE SHOULDER is the area where the arm is attached to the thorax. It is a complex structure and involves more than one joint. The shoulder structure serves 2 functions:

1. It must be very flexible, to allow the hand and arm the huge range of motion which they require.

2. It must provide a strong, stable and fixed point for certain actions (lifting a heavy object with the arms, pushing against resistance, etc).

The shoulder comprises three joints, plus important gliding planes.

There are two types of movement of the shoulder, and the two functional areas work individually or else together to make them possible.

The first type of movement, as shown below, concerns how the shoulder moves on the thorax. Thus the shoulder can experience translation; as scapula **elevation, depression, abduction** (move away from spine), **adduction** (move close to spine). And there is secondly rotation of the shoulder. Here we have first **medial rotation** (tilting by moving the inferior

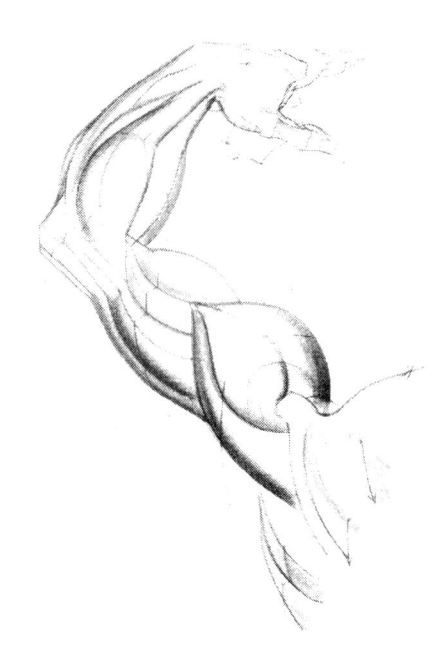

The way I sometimes imagine a movement of the arm; is in terms of first fixing the position (and angle) of the shoulder joint (plus scapula) relative to the torso, prior to then making movements of the arm whilst normally the shoulder joint (scapula may rotate) remains mostly stationery (at least on pressing/curling moves). However when performing pulling / rowing movements with the arms, you perform a scapula protraction (shoulder joint moves forward) at the start with the arms outstretched and a scapula retraction (shoulder joint moves backwards) at the end when the bar comes close to the body. Sometimes also when performing "hugging" pec type motions the scapula would be protracted.

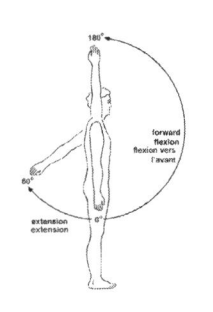

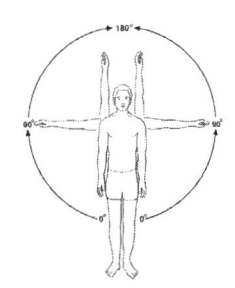

angle of the scapula toward the midline. Plus there is **lateral rotation** (tilt by moving the inferior angle away from the midline). Note that we can also refer to shoulder abduction as scapula protraction; and to shoulder adduction as scapula retraction.

We can think of these various positions as the movements (and positions) of the scapula without movement of the arms. There is also a second type of movement of the shoulder in which we see combined actions of the scapula and arm that allow the arm to move in many different ways. These are the normal case when moving the arm into different positions in space.

Flexion of the arm by the shoulder moves it forward and upwards at first, but once the arm reaches beyond shoulder height the arm starts to move backwards. One can also perform an extension by moving the shoulder backwards which has a much smaller range of motion. Lateral abduction is where you move your arm out to the side and then up towards the midline by moving the arm overhead.

Next there is movement medially (adduction) where the arm moves closer to the body. Here you can move your arm either in-front or behind the body.

Another type of movement is where you rotate the humorous on its axis, either inwards or outwards.

Now that we have a basic overview of shoulder movements, it is useful to examine range of motions (ROMs); to further our knowledge of the different types of shoulder exercises that are possible.

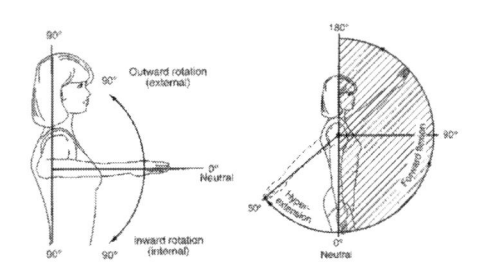

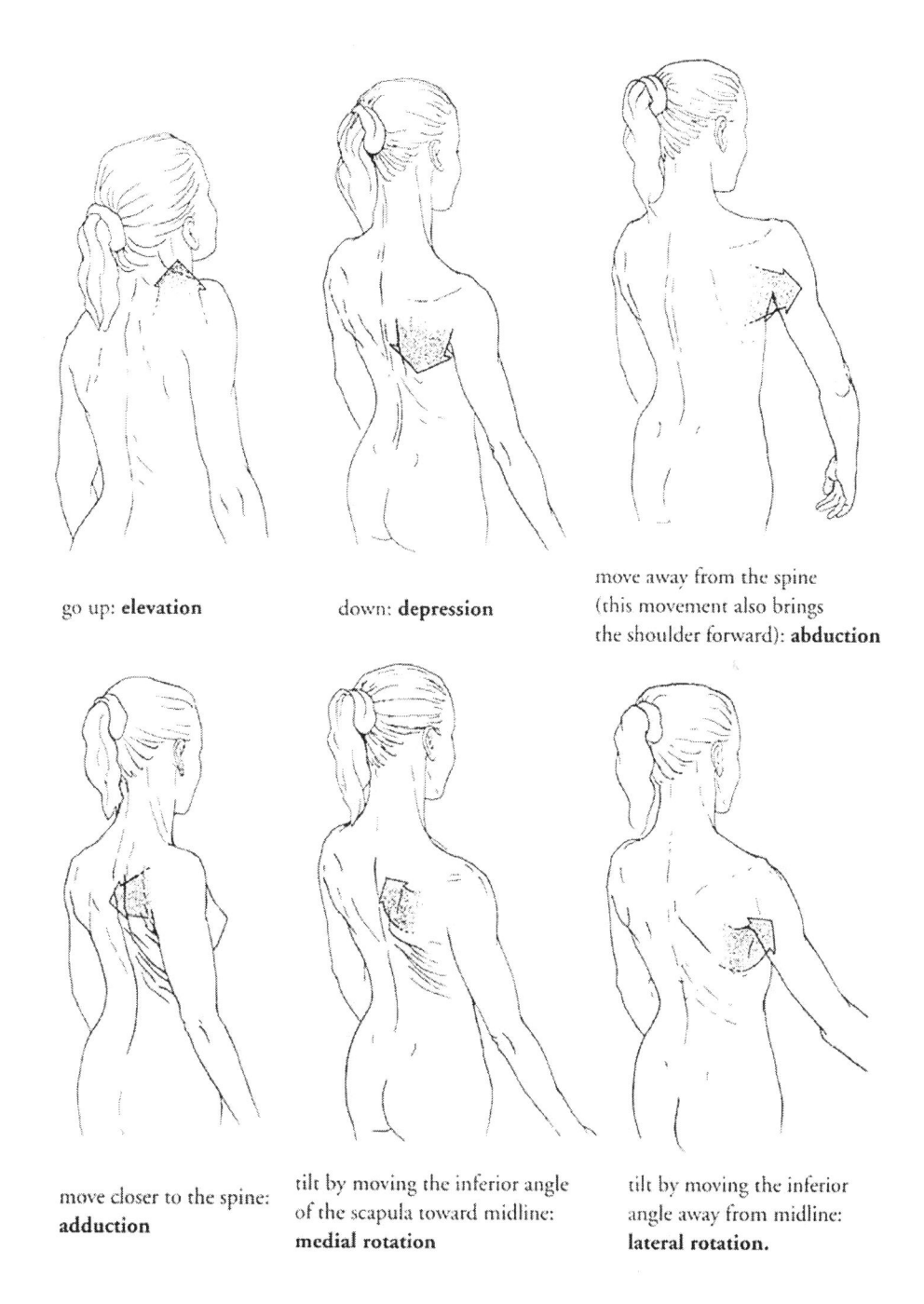

THE SHOULDER 173

go up: **elevation**

down: **depression**

move away from the spine (this movement also brings the shoulder forward): **abduction**

move closer to the spine: **adduction**

tilt by moving the inferior angle of the scapula toward midline: **medial rotation**

tilt by moving the inferior angle away from midline: **lateral rotation.**

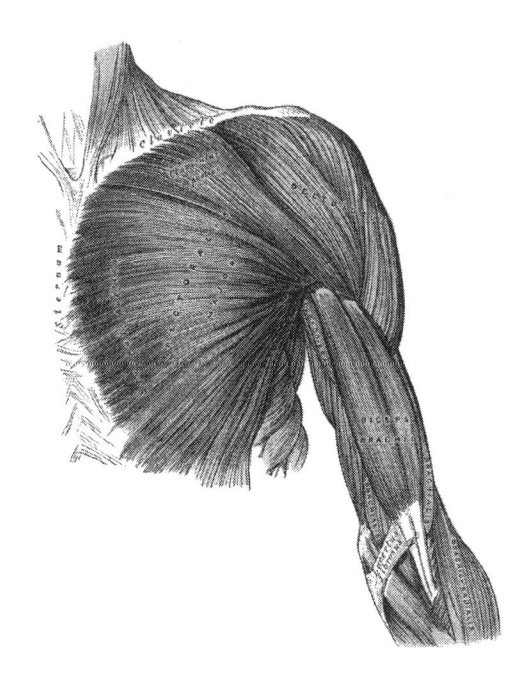

In this book we have not attempted to closely examine the nature of the various muscle actions involved in the different body movements. We have done so because to some extent such knowledge would be redundant; and also because isolation of the different muscles is nearly impossible because you always find that the different muscles work together to achieve almost any possible movement.

Our philosophy in this respect is the opposite of most exercise books, because here we place emphasis on joint ROMs and movement patterns (as opposed to muscles). Plus we are not going to describe the movement anatomy of the neck, because we do not believe in performing specific resistance exercises for that area alone. We shall however mention neck/head position where we think that it is non-obvious in the exercise descriptions that follow.

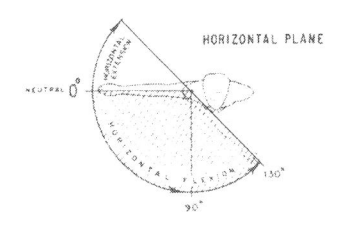

We now turn our attention to ROM in terms of specific shoulder movements. Note that we shall include discussion (in terms of ROM); of the basic movements and positions of the scapula, including elevation, depression, adduction, abduction and medial and lateral rotations. Unlike other "muscle" focussed books, we think that the actual set-positions (conscious shoulder starting/ending positions) are more important than knowledge of moving muscle anatomy (at least for the beginner).

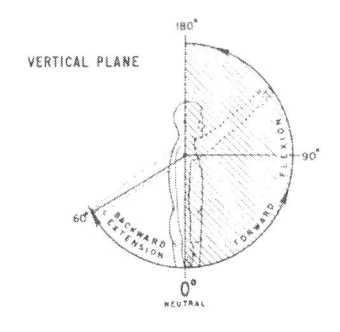

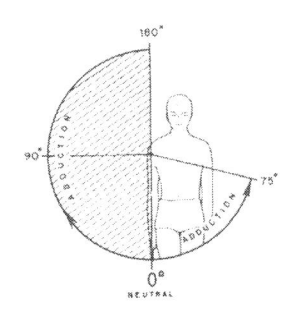

Name	Description	Muscles
Scapula Retraction	The scapula is moved posteriorly and medially along the back, moving the arm and shoulder joint posteriorly. Retracting both scapulae gives a sensation of "squeezing the shoulder blades together."	rhomboideus major, minor, and trapezius
Scapula Protraction	The opposite motion of scapula retraction. The scapula is moved anteriorly and laterally along the back, moving the arm and shoulder joint anteriorly. If both scapulae are protracted, the scapulae are separated and the pectoralis major muscles are squeezed together.	serratus anterior (prime mover), pectoralis minor and major
Scapula Elevation	The scapula is raised in a shrugging motion.	levator scapulae, the upper fibres of the trapezius
Scapula Depression	The scapula is lowered from elevation. The scapulae may be depressed so that the angle formed by the neck and shoulders is obtuse, giving the appearance of "slumped" shoulders.	pectoralis minor, lower fibres of the trapezius, subclavius, latissimus dorsi
Arm Abduction	Arm abduction occurs when the arms are held at the sides, parallel to the length of the torso, and are then raised in the plane of the torso.	True abduction: supraspinatus (first 15 degrees), deltoid; Upward rotation: trapezius, serratus anterior
Arm Flexion	The humerus is rotated out of the plane of the torso so that it points forward (anteriorly).	pectoralis major, coracobrachialis, biceps brachii, anterior fibres of deltoid.
Arm Extension	The humerus is rotated out of the plane of the torso so that it points backwards (posteriorly).	latissimus dorsi and teres major, long head of triceps, posterior fibres of the deltoid

Table 4: Muscular Actions of the Shoulder

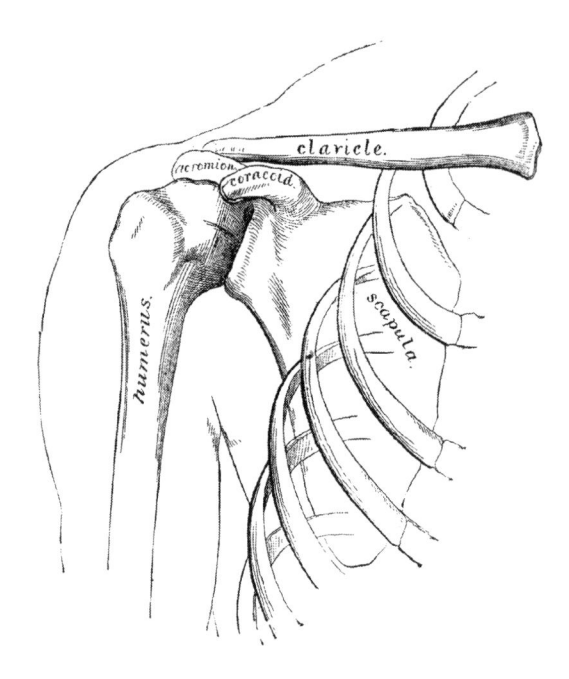

In the table above we see an explanation of common movements of the shoulder. Missing from the table are medial and lateral rotation of the arm along the axis of the humorous, and arm circumduction.

Below we see the side abduction of the shoulder, labelled from 0 to 180 degrees. Note that we can (and often do) combine such a movement with other movements of the shoulder by starting at less than 0 and going beyond 180 degrees (as for example with front wide-arc shoulder circles).

Of-coarse it is often possible (and normal) to combine several types of movements into one.

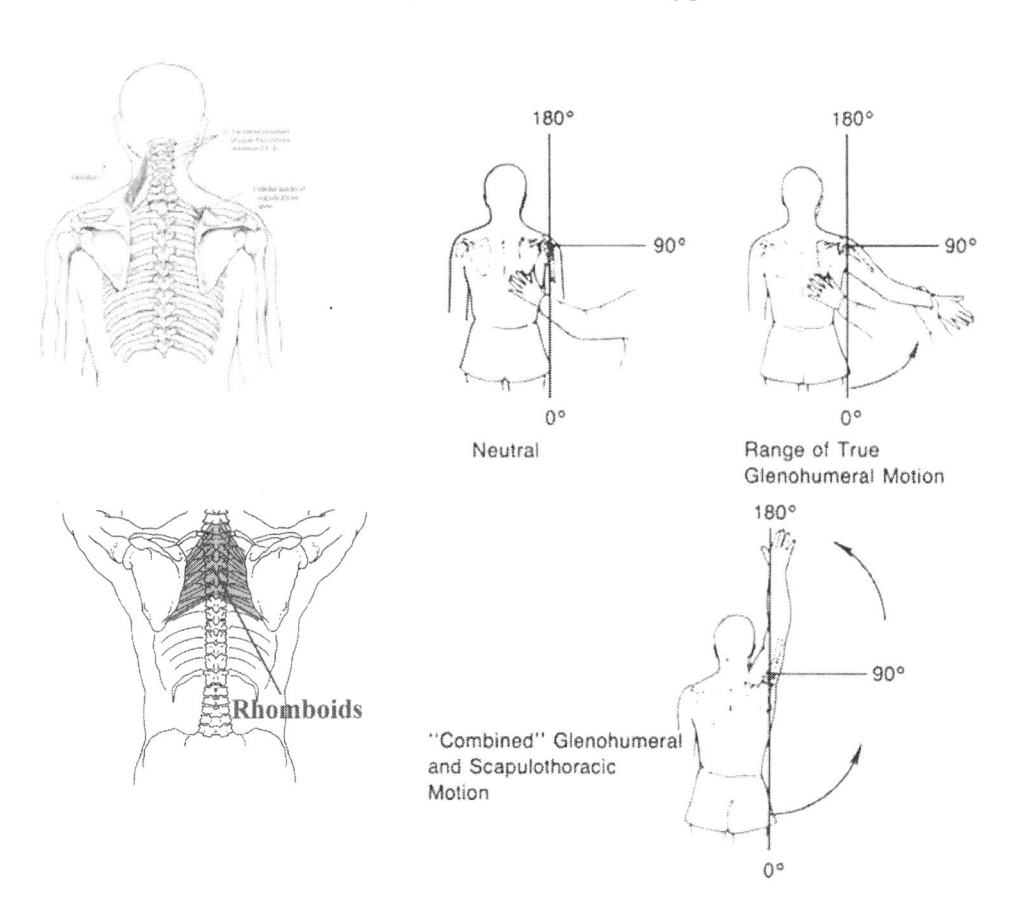

Neutral

Range of True Glenohumeral Motion

Rhomboids

"Combined" Glenohumeral and Scapulothoracic Motion

THE SHOULDER

Shoulder Joint(s) - Exercises

28. Overhead Lateral
29. Top Lateral
30. Front Lateral
31. Horizontal Shoulder Circle
32. Crucifix
33. Side Shoulder Circles
34. Front Shoulder Circles
35. Front / Side Lateral Raise
36. Upright Row
37. Press
38. Round The World
39. Hang
40. Pullover
41. Parallel Bar Dip
42. Bench Press
43. Incline Bench Press
44. Fly (Bent Arm)
45. Fly (Straight Arm)
46. Lying (Lateral) Circles
47. Chin-Up
48. Rowing
49. Cable Rowing

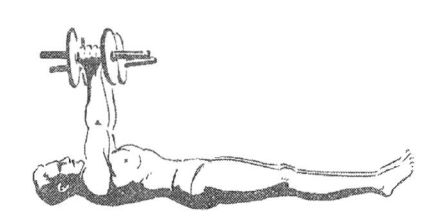

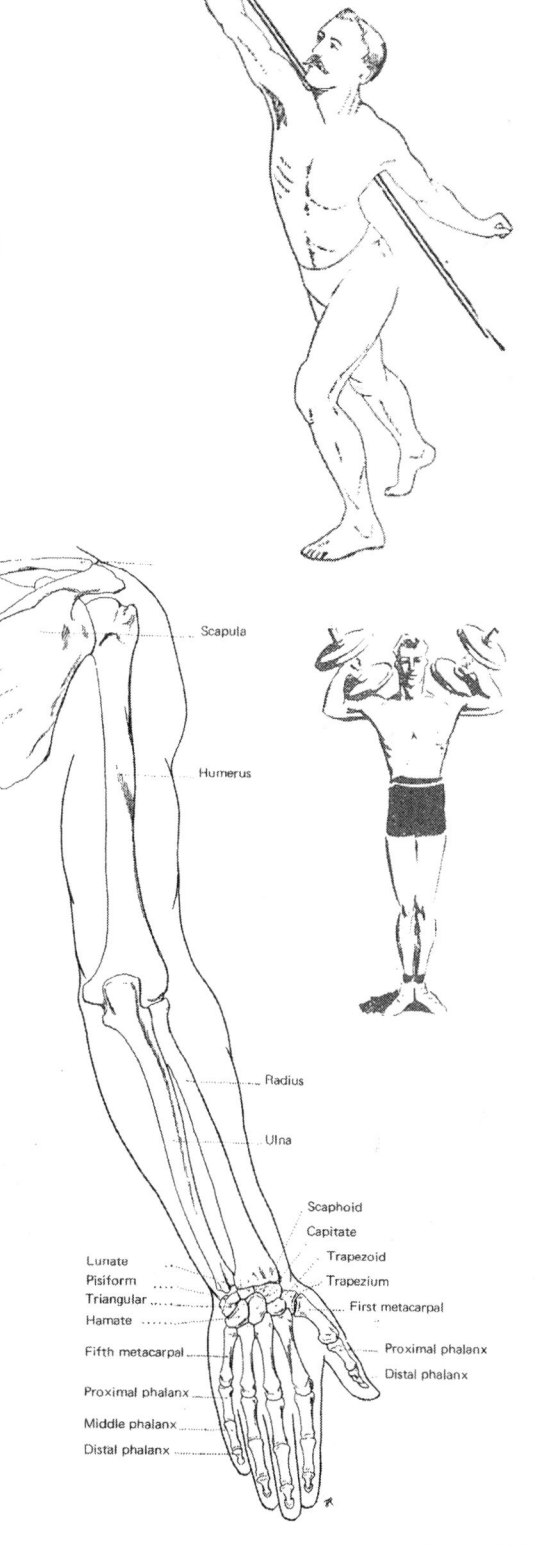

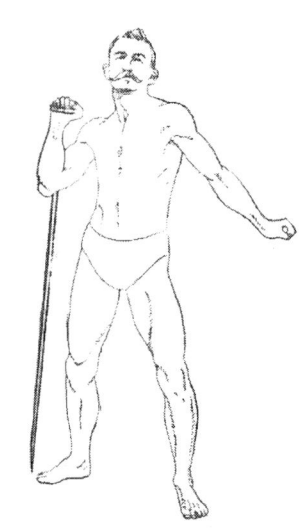

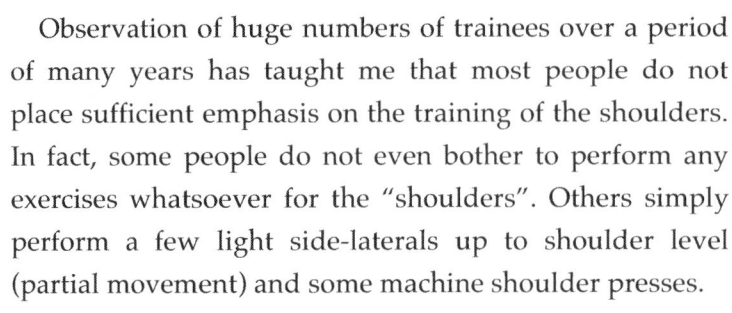

Observation of huge numbers of trainees over a period of many years has taught me that most people do not place sufficient emphasis on the training of the shoulders. In fact, some people do not even bother to perform any exercises whatsoever for the "shoulders". Others simply perform a few light side-laterals up to shoulder level (partial movement) and some machine shoulder presses.

Our shoulders can be (potentially) a super strong joint, with flexibility, stability and full musculature all evident. However, the shoulders are complex in terms of anatomy, and in terms of the number and diversity of movements that are possible. It is my belief that trainees should practice the vast majority of movements that are listed here. Experience tells me that if you do exercise the shoulders in such a comprehensive manner, then you will enjoy a new degree of flexibility in the upper body generally, and you will also experience a far greater degree of freedom of movement in terms of all the upper limb articulations as well.

Try using very light weights (1-3 lbs) for ROM exercises and as a warm-up/cool-down and prior to / after the heavier lifts, and also on a daily basis. That said, take it easy with shoulder training; and strengthen the entire structure together and slowly, and do so using lighter weights performed with full concentration. Stop doing anything that causes pain.

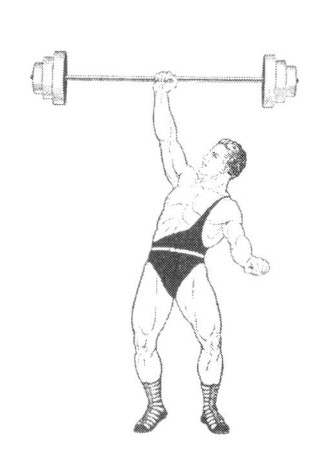

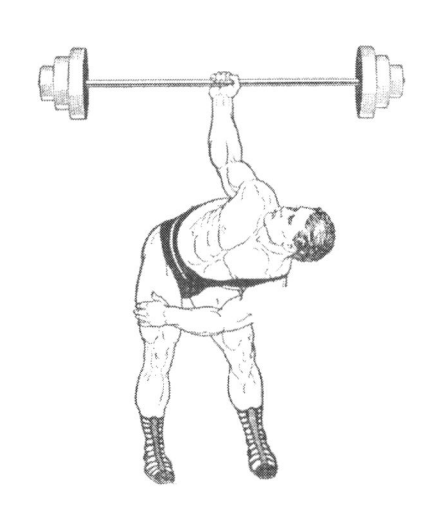

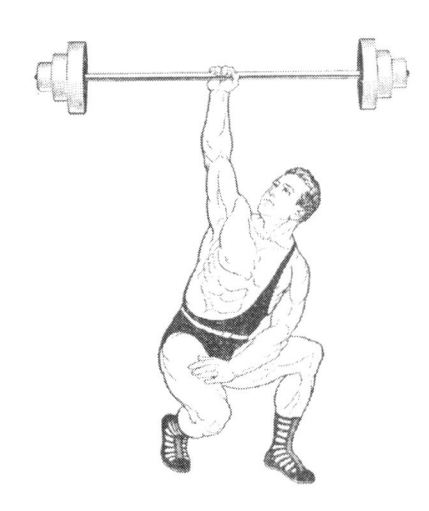

28. Overhead Lateral / Triceps Circle (ROM)

Equipment: twin dumbbells
Effect: Strengthen / ROM for deltoids, trapezius, triceps
Resistance : Light / Medium [Slow]
Hip position: N/A
Spine position: N/A
Scapula position: Neutral / natural rotation at end
Muscles: anterior, posterior, middle deltoid, trapezius, splenius, levator scapulae, triceps (if dumbbells held to rear as in a triceps circle)
Joints: Shoulder (use very light weight - 2-8 lbs for men)

Grab a pair of light dumbbells, and hold at your sides. Stand upright with head looking forward. Next, whilst keeping the arms straight, and elbows locked (almost), raise the dumbbells in a wide-arc out to the sides and then all the way overhead. Repeat for reps. This is a very slow and controlled movement, and you may turn the dumbbells in any way that feels natural, either twisting them as the rep executes, or keeping the dumbbells facing one direction. Do what comes naturally with respect to static holds also (perhaps at a mid-point between the shoulder and overhead levels).

You may want to start with the dumbbells behind the back at the bottom position and then extend the dumbbells as far behind you (with straight arms) throughout the rep, culminating in the dumbbells being slightly behind the head at the overhead position (this version is named a triceps circle if the arms are held well to the rear throughout - see middle diagram on right).

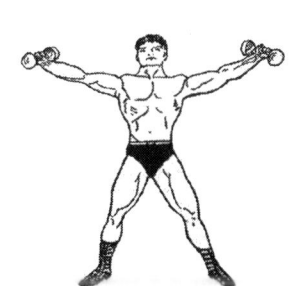

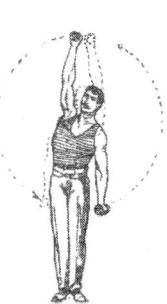

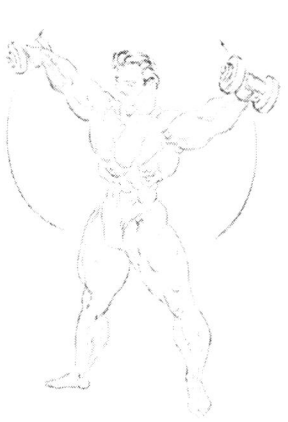

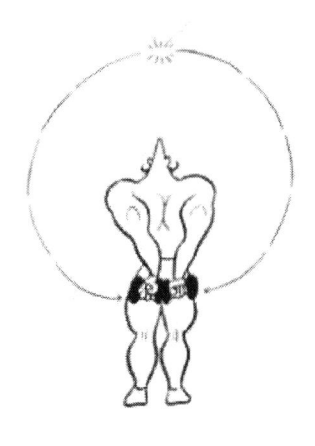

29. Top Lateral (ROM)

Equipment: twin dumbbells
Effect: Strengthen / ROM for deltoids, trapezius
Resistance : Light / Medium [Slow]
Hip position: N/A
Spine position: N/A
Scapula position: Natural rotation throughout
Muscles: anterior, posterior, middle deltoid, trapezius, splenius, levator scapulae
Typical Poundage: 2-6 kg dumbbells (women); 4-10 kg (men)
Joints: Shoulder

Perform a similar movement to the side or overhead lateral, except that you only perform the top half of the movement - finishing at the shoulder outreach - or arms at shoulder height point and repeating. You can also perform this movement on an incline bench as shown below.

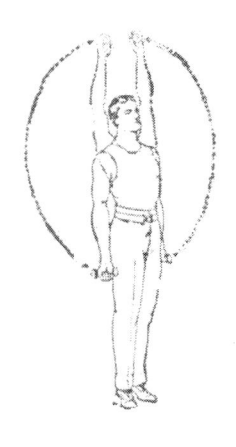

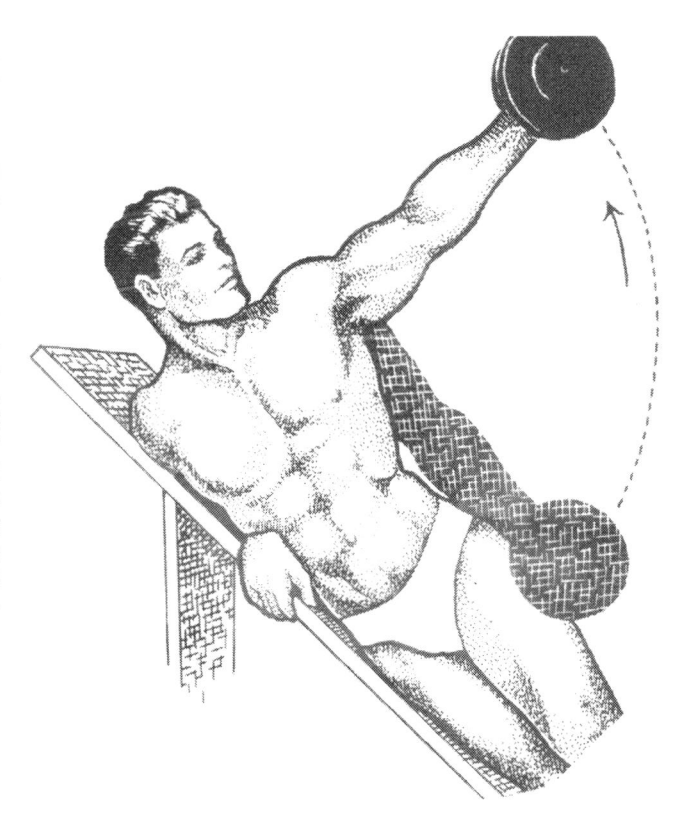

We could not find any pictures of the top-lateral exercise. The closest is on the right - which shows the dumbbell in the start position for a top lateral raise. Note here that we recommend side-lateral motions where the dumbbell moves above the shoulder level, whereas in bodybuilding normally one only goes up to shoulder level; however whilst that works the deltoids (to a lesser degree) sometimes for full ROM you need to go well above shoulder level and in order to work the whole shoulder region fully.

WE NORMALLY RECOMMEND THAT YOU PERFORM LATERAL RAISES FROM A STANDING POSITION. WHEN PERFORMED AS SHOWN GRAVITY MAINTAINS TENSION ON THE DELTOID THROUGHOUT THE MOVEMENT AS LONG AS YOU DONT RAISE THE DUMBBELL TOO HIGH - EXPERIMENT

30. Front Lateral (ROM)

Equipment: twin dumbbells
Effect: Strengthen / ROM for front deltoids, trapezius
Resistance : Light / Medium [Slow]
Hip position: N/A
Spine position: N/A
Scapula position: Neutral / natural rotation at end
Muscles: deltoids (front-side), trapezius, splenius, levator scapulae, pectoralis major
Typical Poundage: 2-6 kg dumbbells (women); 4-10 kg (men)
Joints: Shoulder

Grab a pair of light dumbbells, and hold at your sides. Stand upright with head looking forward. Next, whilst keeping the arms straight, and elbows locked, raise the dumbbells in a wide-arc out to the front and then all the way overhead. Repeat for reps. This is a very slow and controlled movement, and you may turn the dumbbells in any way that feels natural, either twisting them as the rep executes, or keeping the dumbbells facing one direction. Do what comes naturally with respect to static holds (perhaps at the shoulder level) also.

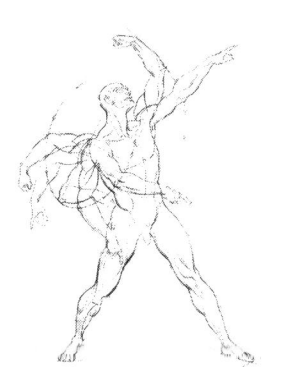

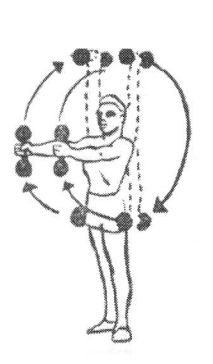

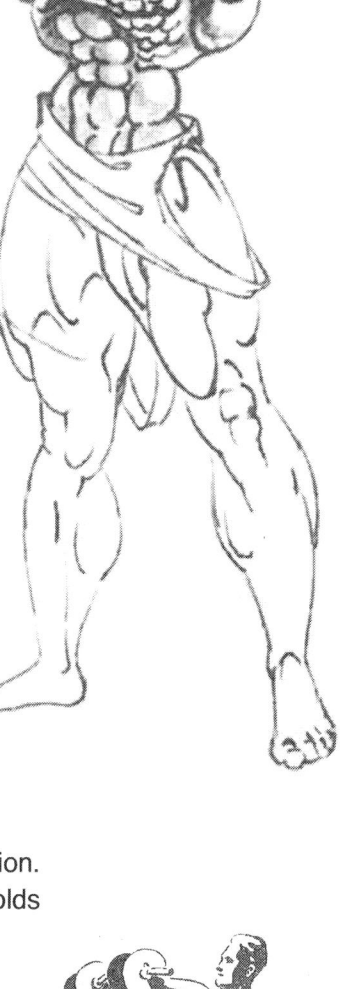

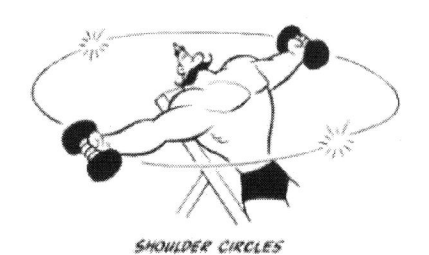

31. Horizontal Shoulder Circle (ROM)

Equipment: twin dumbbells
Effect: Strengthen / ROM for front deltoids, trapezius
Resistance : Light / Medium [Slow]
Hip position: N/A
Spine position: N/A
Scapula position: Neutral

Muscles: deltoids, trapezius, splenius, levator scapulae, pectoralis major (slight involvement)
Typical Poundage: 2-6 kg dumbbells (women); 4-10 kg (men)
Joints: Shoulder, rib-cage

SHOULDER CIRCLES

If you bring the dumbbells right back so they touch behind you - then this exercise becomes a superb ROM exercise for the entire shoulder region.

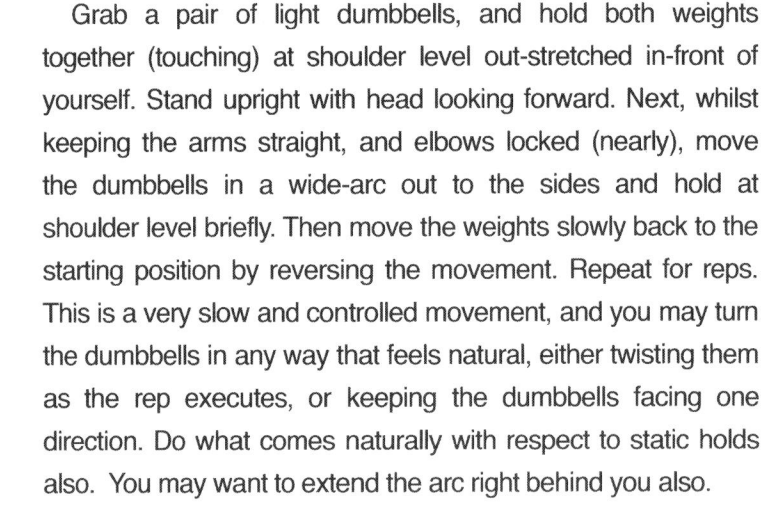

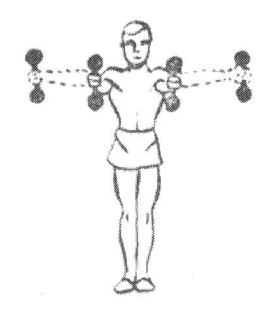

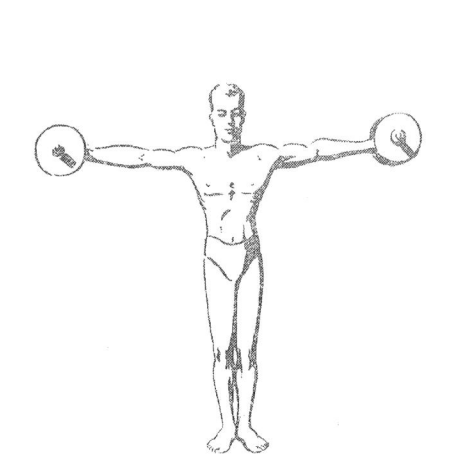

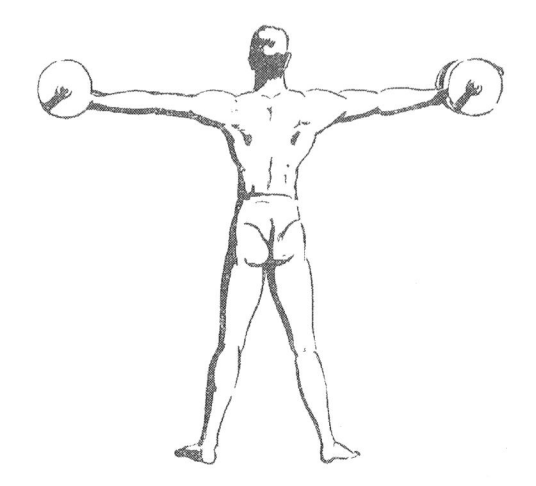

Grab a pair of light dumbbells, and hold both weights together (touching) at shoulder level out-stretched in-front of yourself. Stand upright with head looking forward. Next, whilst keeping the arms straight, and elbows locked (nearly), move the dumbbells in a wide-arc out to the sides and hold at shoulder level briefly. Then move the weights slowly back to the starting position by reversing the movement. Repeat for reps. This is a very slow and controlled movement, and you may turn the dumbbells in any way that feels natural, either twisting them as the rep executes, or keeping the dumbbells facing one direction. Do what comes naturally with respect to static holds also. You may want to extend the arc right behind you also.

32. The Crucifix

Equipment: twin dumbbells
Effect: Strengthen / ROM for front deltoids, trapezius
Resistance : Light / Medium [Slow]
Hip position: N/A
Spine position: N/A
Scapula position: Neutral
Muscles: front deltoids, trapezius, splenius, levator scapulae
Typical Poundage: 2-8kg dumbbells (women); 4-25 kg (men)
Joints: Shoulder, rib-cage

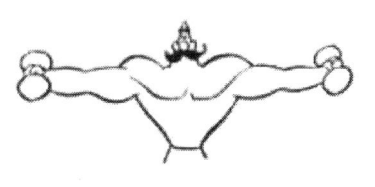

The crucifix is a superb test of strength, and many weightlifters can use 70-90 lbs in this exercise for 1 repetition with practice.

Grab a pair of light dumbbells, and hold both weights overhead. Stand upright with head looking forward. Next, whilst keeping the arms straight, and elbows locked (almost), lower the dumbbells in a wide-arc out to the sides and hold at the shoulder level for 20-60 seconds.

Repeat for reps (or stop at 1 rep). This is a very slow and controlled movement, and you may turn the dumbbells in any way that feels natural, either twisting them as the rep executes, or keeping the dumbbells facing one direction.

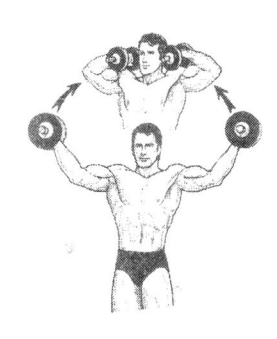

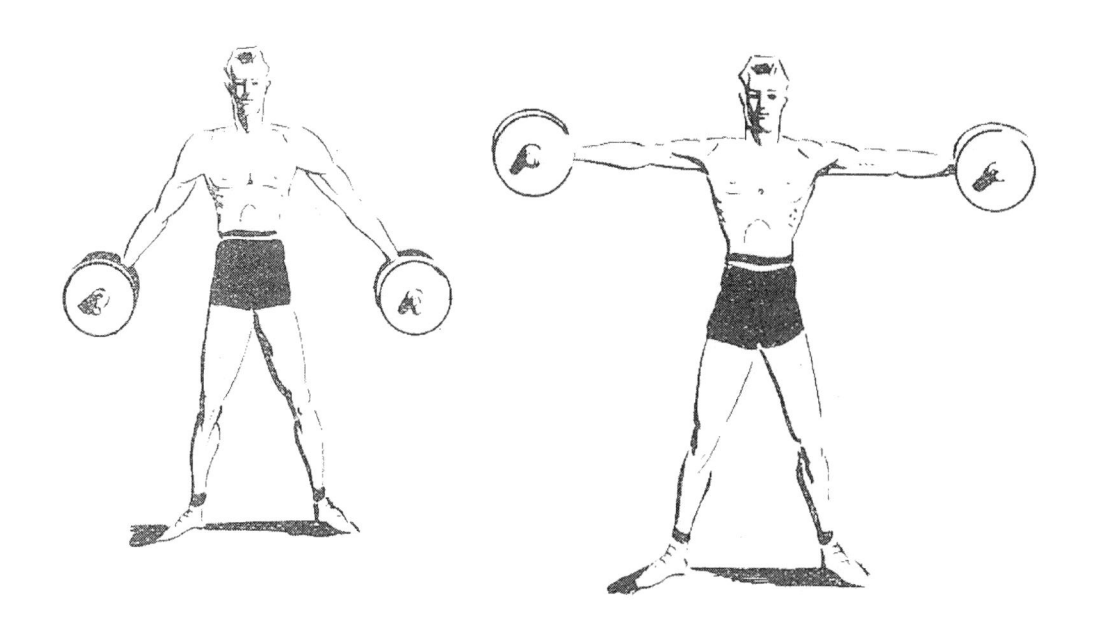

33. Side Shoulder Circles (ROM)

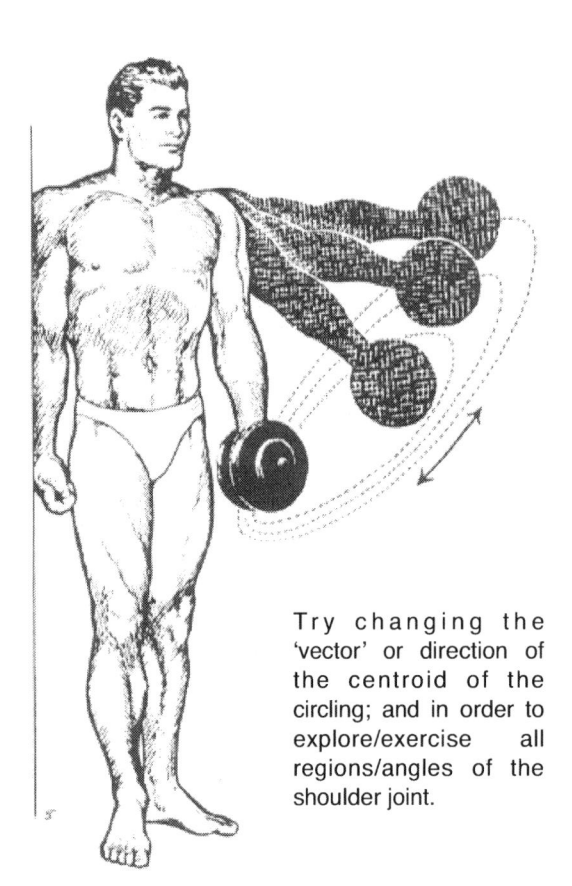

Equipment: single dumbbell
Effect: Strengthen / ROM for front deltoids, trapezius
Resistance : Light / Medium [Slow]
Hip position: N/A
Spine position: N/A
Scapula position: Neutral / rotation if arms go above shoulder level at any point
Muscles: deltoids, trapezius splenius, levator scapulae
Typical Poundage: 2-5kg dumbbells (women); 3-8 kg (men)
Joints: Shoulder

Try changing the 'vector' or direction of the centroid of the circling; and in order to explore/exercise all regions/angles of the shoulder joint.

Grab a light dumbbell, and hold at the sides. Stand upright with head looking forward/sideways. Next, whilst keeping the arms straight, and elbows locked (almost), raise the dumbbell to shoulder level, and then move in repeating circular motions (of small/large, constant or varying radii) around the out-stretched central position. Repeat the circles in both directions - and with the other arm. This is a very slow and controlled movement, and you may turn the dumbbells in any way that feels natural, either twisting them as the rep executes, or keeping the dumbbells facing one direction. Do what comes naturally with respect to static holds (perhaps at shoulder level) also.

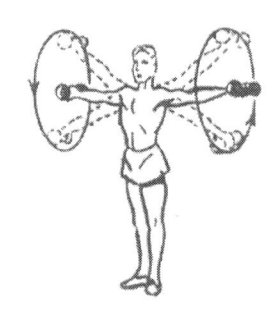

Other kinds of "circle exercises" are possible. Hand circles involve standing with the dumbbells hanging at the sides, and "circling" the hand in a 360 degree movement.

"Arm circles" are where you circle the wrist (with/without supinating the elbow) by turning the humorous in it's socket along the axis of the arm. These can be performed by holding a dumbbell and with the upper arm at various (fixed) positions relative to the body (i.e. arms at sides/raised-up etc).

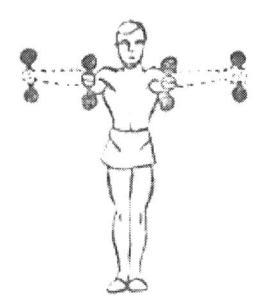

THE SHOULDER 185

34. Front Shoulder Circles (ROM)

Equipment: single dumbbells
Effect: Strengthen / ROM for front deltoids, trapezius
Resistance : Light / Medium [Slow]
Hip position: N/A
Spine position: N/A
Scapula position: Neutral / rotation if arms go above shoulder level at any point
Muscles: front deltoids, trapezius, splenius, levator scapulae, pectoralis major (slight involvement)
Typical Poundage: 2-5kg dumbbells (women); 3-8 kg (men)
Joints: Shoulder

Perform as in Side-Circles but with the dumbbell held out to the front, and the centre of circular motion being at the shoulder level and directly to the front of the torso.

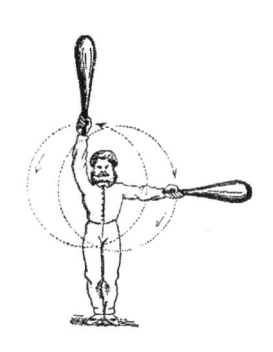

We could find no pictures of front circles, but since they are so similar to side-circles simply copy the exercise to the left - only perform with the arm outstretched to the front. Image below is unrelated and shows seated side/forward lateral raise.

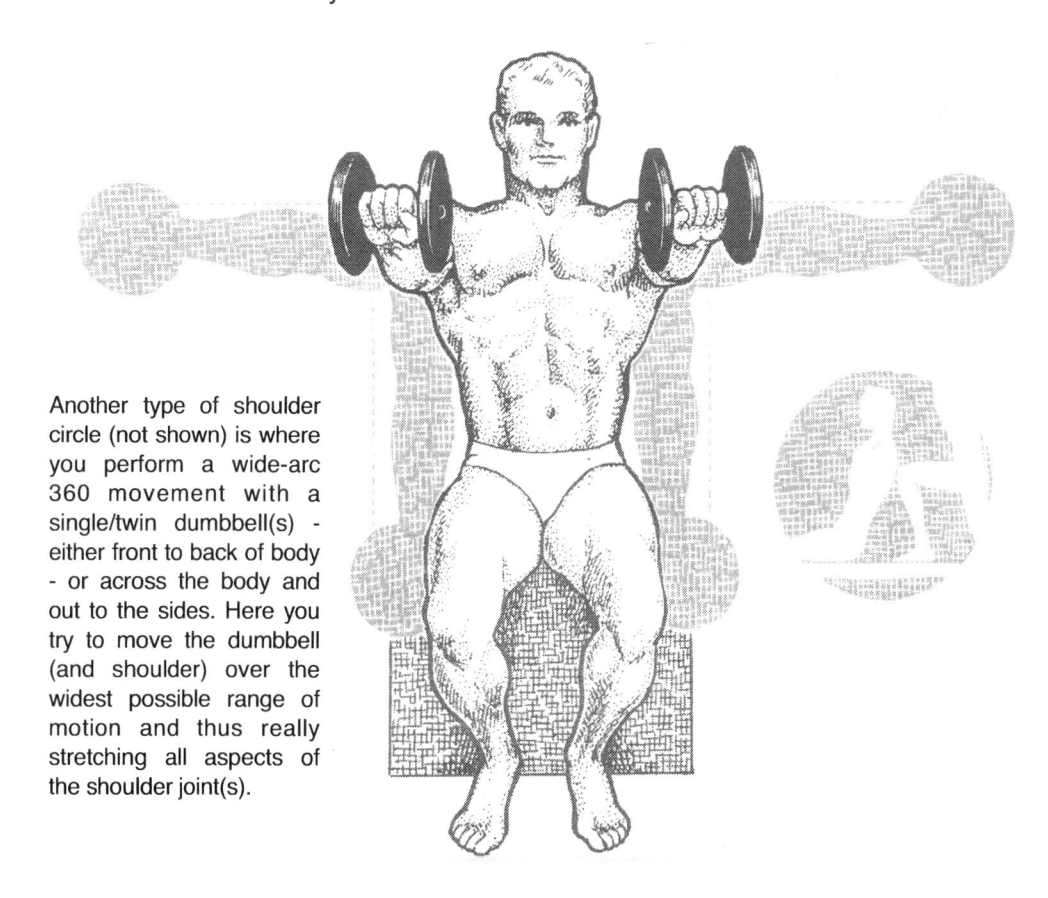

Another type of shoulder circle (not shown) is where you perform a wide-arc 360 movement with a single/twin dumbbell(s) - either front to back of body - or across the body and out to the sides. Here you try to move the dumbbell (and shoulder) over the widest possible range of motion and thus really stretching all aspects of the shoulder joint(s).

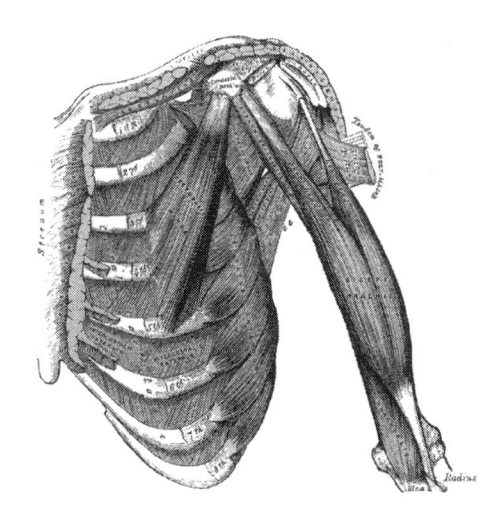

35. Front / Side Lateral Raise

Equipment: dumbbells
Effect: Strengthen / ROM for front deltoids, trapezius
Resistance : Light / Medium [Slow]
Hip position: N/A
Spine position: N/A
Scapula position: Neutral
Muscles: deltoids (front -side), trapezius, splenius, levator scapulae, pectoralis major (slight involvement)
Typical Poundage: 4-8kg dumbbells (women); 8-20 kg dumbbells (men)
Joints: Shoulder (N.B. it is often better to perform the top-lateral)

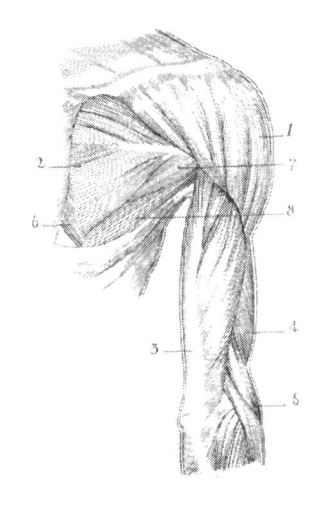

Grab a pair of light dumbbells, and hold at the sides. Stand upright with head looking forward. Next, whilst keeping the arms straight, and elbows locked (almost), raise the dumbbells (simultaneously) to front shoulder level, hold for a second or two and then move out to sides and hold, before lowering to start once again. Repeat for reps. Try to really stretch outwards (in all directions) as you perform the movement in the widest possible arc.

This is a very slow and controlled movement, and you may turn the dumbbells in any way that feels natural, either twisting them as the rep executes, or keeping the dumbbells facing one direction. Do what comes naturally with respect to static holds also. DO NOT GO TOO HEAVY AND NEVER SWING AND HEAVE THE WEIGHTS AROUND

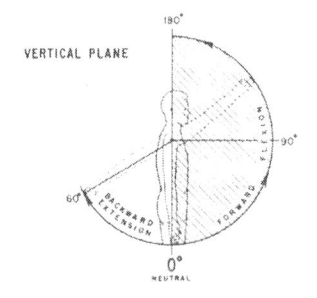

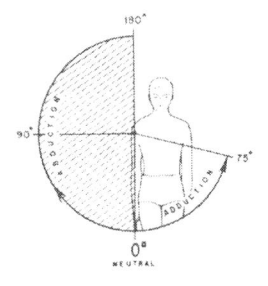

36. Upright Row

Equipment: twin dumbbells / barbell
Effect: Strengthen / ROM for front deltoids, trapezius
Resistance : Light / Medium [Slow]
Hip position: N/A
Spine position: N/A
Scapula position: Neutral / rotation at end
Muscles: front deltoids (all heads), trapezius
Typical Poundage: 8-12kg dumbbells (women); 12-30 kg dumbbells (men)
Joints: Shoulder, wrist, elbow, hand

Stand next to a bar, and grasp the bar with shoulder width or slightly narrower overhand grip - next pick it up and hold at waist level. Pull bar to neck with elbows leading. Allow wrists to flex as bar rises. Lower and repeat. Best performed with twin dumbbells to improve shoulder flexibility.

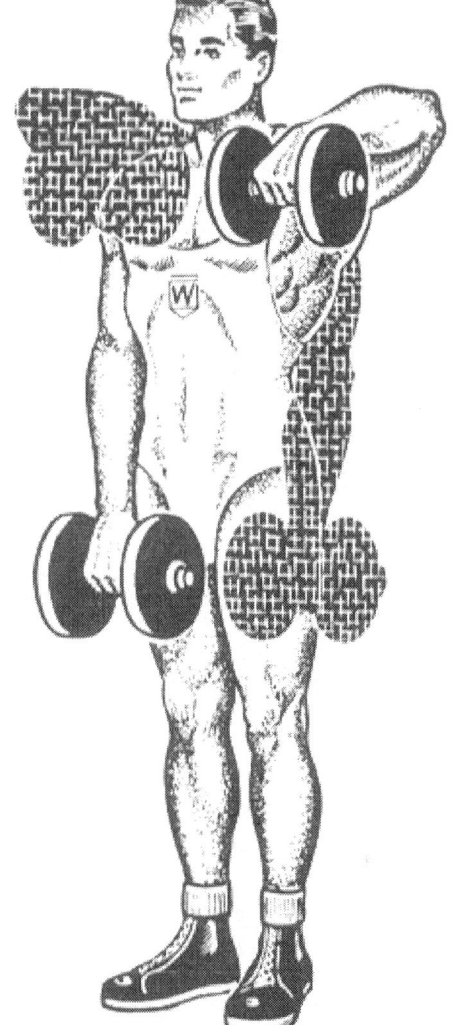

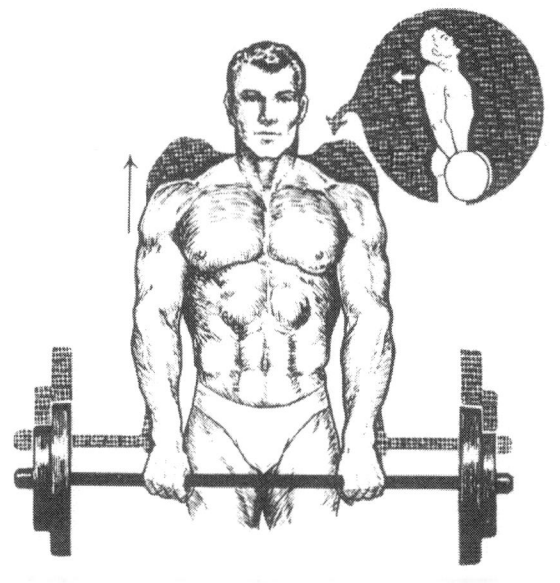

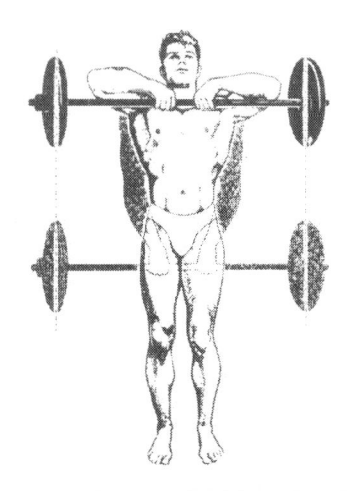

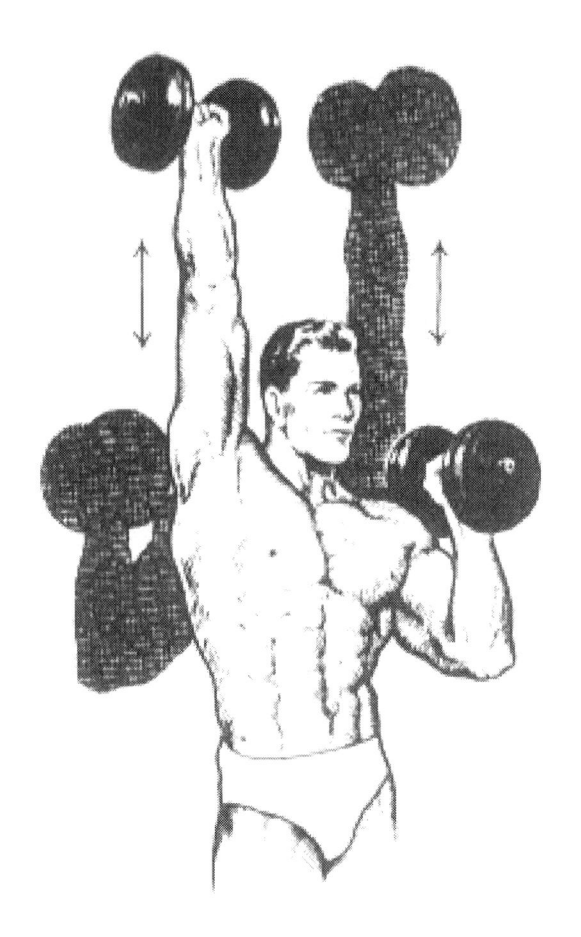

37. Press

Equipment: twin dumbbells / kettle-bells / barbell
Effect: Strengthen shoulders
Resistance : Light / Medium / Heavy
[Slow speed throughout]
Hip position: N/A
Spine position: N/A
Scapula position: Neutral / rotation
Muscles: deltoids (all heads), triceps brachii (all heads), supraspinatus, pectoralis major (if touching deltoid)
Typical Poundage: 6-15kg dumbbells (women); 15-40 kg dumbbells (men)
Joints: Shoulder, elbow, hand

Standing upright, first grab a pair of dumbbells. Next position dumbbells to each side of shoulders with elbows below. Flair lats, depress scapula. Press dumbbells upward until arms are extended overhead. Lower to shoulders and repeat. There are several different styles of movement performance. In one style you start with the dumbbells facing each other and resting almost on top of the clavicles, next you push the dumbbells upwards and twist the dumbbells (slightly) until they face the front. This seems to be the most natural style. In another one you start higher up and with the dumbbells facing the front at all times. Sometimes it is good to perform mid-range reps and/or to perform "top-only" reps once you are tired and in order to really work the deltoids. It is a good idea to sometimes perform the press with just a single dumbbell.

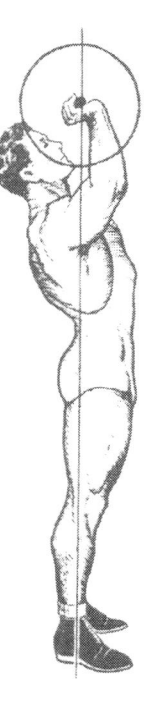

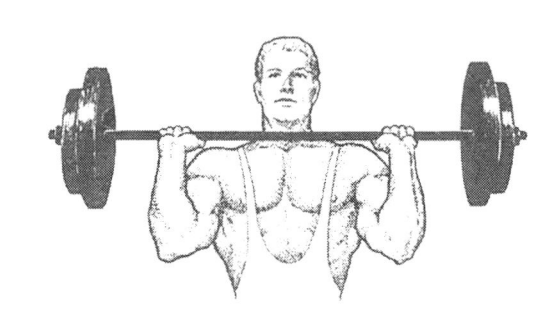

38. Round The World (ROM)

Equipment: Twin dumbbells, flat bench, exercise ball
Effect: Stretch shoulders / lats / scapula / ROM
Resistance : Light [Slow / Medium]
Hip position: N/A
Spine position: N/A
Scapula position: Neutral / rotation + some retraction
Muscles: pectoralis major, serratus anterior, deltoid, lats
Typical Poundage: 1-6kg dumbbells (women); 2-10 kg (men)
Joints: Shoulder, hand, rib-cage

This is a super exercise for the entire shoulder girdle. It will stretch everything to an unbelievable degree - but you must be careful and go very, very light; 1-2 lbs to begin). Grab a par of dumbbells, and lie down on a flat bench. Next beginning with the dumbbells at the sides, and with the arms straight or rigid, move the arms out to the sides, and in a very wide-arc until they are in a position with dumbbells together and outstretched overhead. Repeat for reps. The movement is a bit like overhead laterals performed lying down. It is normal to move very slowly, and to stop at certain positions and just let the dumbbells hang - as in the hang.

This exercise is one of the best for improving shoulder flexibility and ROM. I suggest that you always do it in your shoulder routine - and perform it once the other exercises are finished. After a few weeks of doing it you will be amazed at how flexible your shoulders will become - and you will be able to move in all kinds of new ways - at least that is my experience. Try performing static holds at various points in the lift (for even a few minutes). Also try performing tiny circles along the axis of the arm with the dumbbells at the fully extended position.

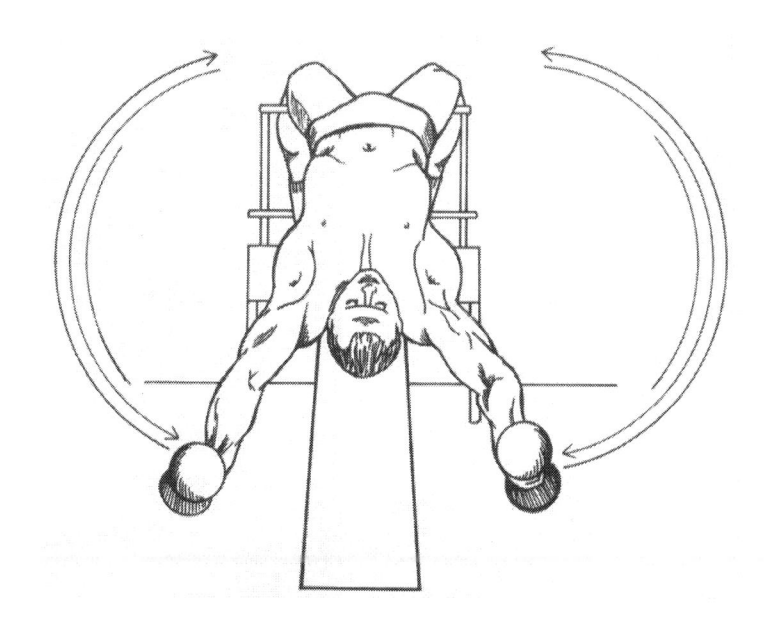

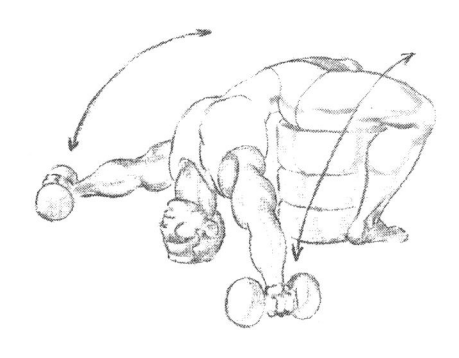

39. Hang (ROM)

Equipment: Twin dumbbells, flat bench, exercise ball
Effect: Stretch shoulders / lats / scapula / ROM
Resistance : Light [Slow / Medium]
Hip position: N/A
Spine position: N/A
Scapula position: Neutral / rotation + retraction
Muscles: pectoralis major, serratus anterior, deltoid, teres major, serratus anterior, lats
Typical Poundage: 2-6kg dumbbells (women); 4-8 kg (men)
Joints: Shoulder, rib-cage

Perform this exercise along with the round-the-world (at the end of). I suggest that you always do it in your shoulder routine - and perform it once the other exercises are finished. This will really greatly improve shoulder flexibly.

Similar to the round-the-world movement. But you just let the dumbbells hang (or hold them static) at various positions in the movement. Try and hold the dumbbells for even as long as several minutes in the same position. The dumbbells will gradually fall lower as the stretch improves and as you hold it for longer. Look well back and overhead at the end. Note that the Hang and Pullover can both be performed quite nicely on an exercise ball - but only if you are using fairly light weights. I would suggest that both movements are essential to maintaining shoulder joint health - and especially if you perform lots of barbell bench-presses.

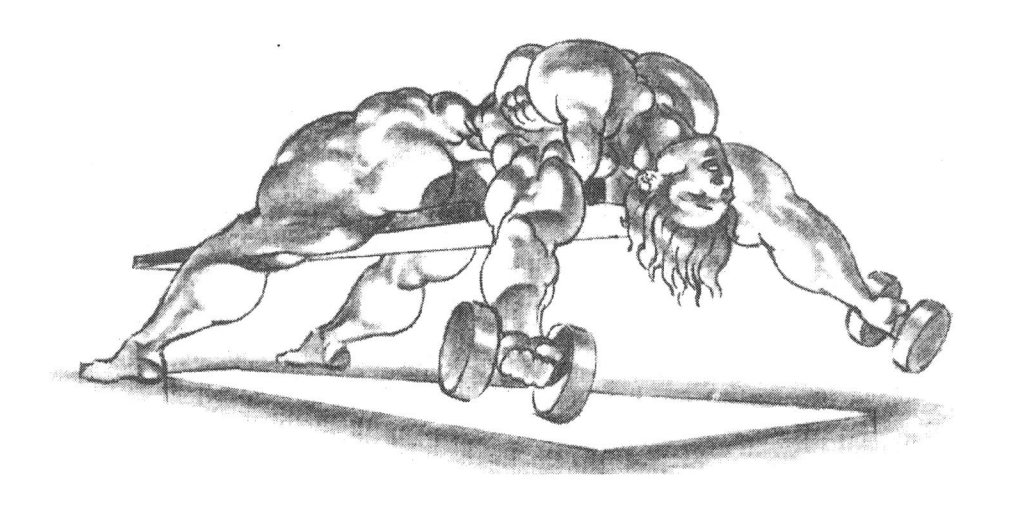

THE SHOULDER   191

40. Pullover (ROM + Strength)

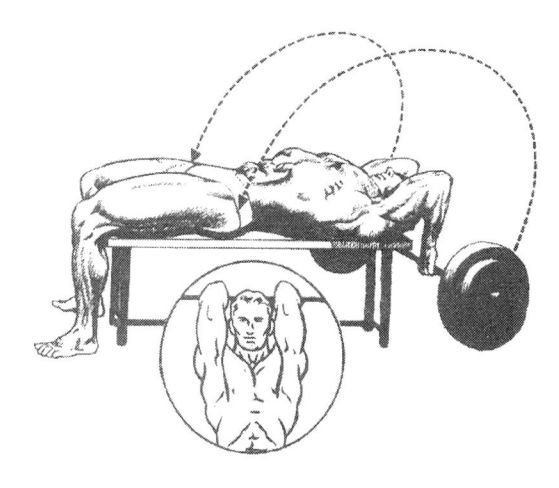

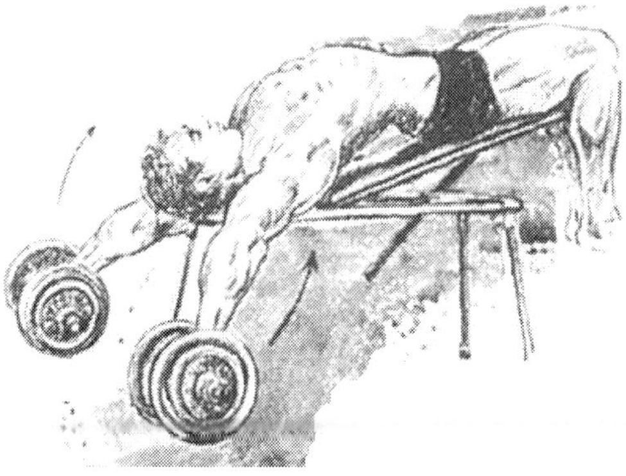

Equipment: Dumbbells, barbell, bench, ball

Effect: Stretch chest, shoulders, lats

Resistance : Light [Slow / Medium]

Hip position: N/A

Spine position: N/A

Scapula position: Neutral / rotation + retraction

Muscles: pectoralis major, serratus anterior, deltoid, lats, teres major, serratus anterior, triceps brachii (long head)

Typical Poundage: 4-8kg dumbbells (women); 8-15 kg (men)

Joints: Shoulder, rib-cage

I will explain the straight-arm style dumbbell pullover. Grab a pair of dumbbells, and lie down on a flat bench. Lie perpendicular to the bench (torso across it as in forming a cross) with only your shoulders lying on the surface. Hips should be below the bench and legs bent with feet firmly on the floor. The head will be off the bench as well. Hold the dumbbells straight over your chest at arms length. This will be your starting position. While keeping your arms straight, lower the weights slowly in an arc behind your head while breathing in until you feel a deep stretch on the chest. At that point, bring the dumbbells back to the starting position using the arc through which the weights were lowered and exhale as you perform this movement. Repeat. It is good to hold the weights also at the fully stretched position. Excellent movement when performed with a barbell (straight-arm) using a variety of grip widths. You can also do the exercise with bent arms and with a single dumbbell / barbell if desired (for slightly different effects). Good on exercise ball also.

This exercise is excellent, and in the past it was sometimes performed on a moon-bench. I prefer to do it with a dumbbell or twin dumbbells across a bench, and to arch my hips very low and so to create an exaggerated arch to the entire body - and then perform the pullovers with a deep rib-cage stretch at the bottom.

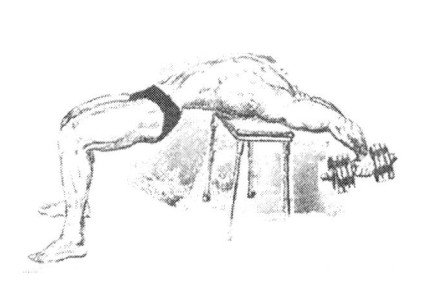

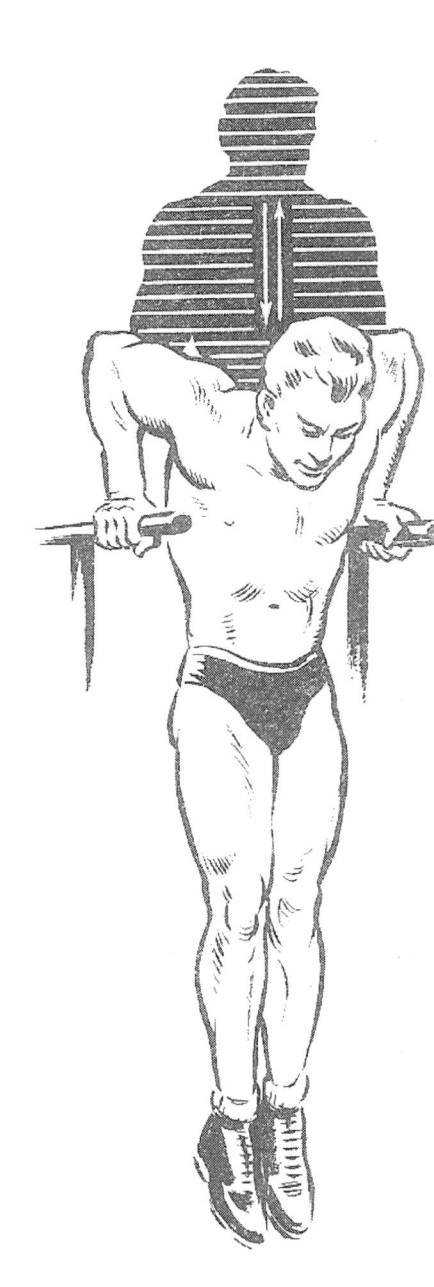

41. Parallel Bar Dip

Equipment: Dipping bars / belt / weight
Effect: Strengthen chest, shoulders, triceps
Resistance : Light / Medium / Heavy [Slow / Medium speed]
Hip position: N/A
Spine position: N/A
Scapula position: Neutral
Muscles: Pectoralis major, triceps (all heads), anterior deltoid, anconeus
Typical Poundage: 5-10kg (women); 10-30kg (men)
Joints: Shoulder, elbow, hand

You can perform dips by grasping two parallel bars that are approximately shoulder-width apart. Raise yourself up to an initial position with your arms extended and supporting the entire weight of your body. Next, lower yourself to a final position where your elbows are bent and your shoulders are mildly stretched, and then use your arms to push yourself upwards to the initial position.

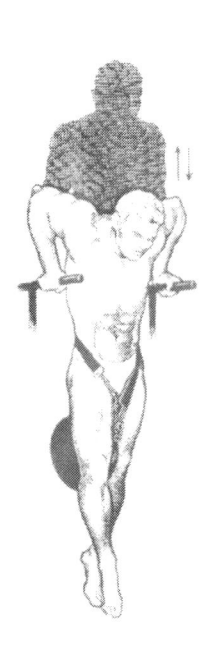

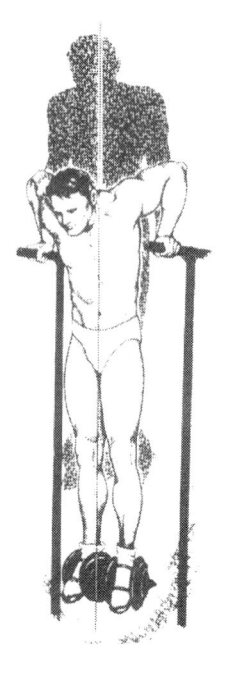

THE SHOULDER 193

42. Bench Press

Equipment: Barbell / dumbbells, flat bench
Effect: Strengthen chest, shoulders, triceps
Resistance : Light / Medium / Heavy
[Slow / Medium]
Hip position: N/A
Spine position: N/A
Scapula position: Partial / full retraction
Muscles: Pectoralis major, triceps (all heads), anterior deltoid
Typical Poundage: 10-20kg dumbbells (women); 20-50 kg (men)
Joints: Shoulder, elbow, hand

Lie supine on bench. Dismount barbell from rack over upper chest using wide oblique overhand grip. Lower weight to mid-chest. Press bar upward until arms are extended. Repeat. Range of motion will be compromised if grip is too wide. Use a spotter with heavy weights!

On heavier (standing) lifts such as the dead-lift, and the clean and press etc; it is acceptable to (sometimes) use gripping aids such a chalk (magnesium carbonate); but my advice is to not rely on such techniques and in order to make-up for having a weak grip. Everyone needs chalk sometimes, but nobody needs it all of the time and/or on lighter exercises like rows, curls, stiff-legged dead-lifts etc.

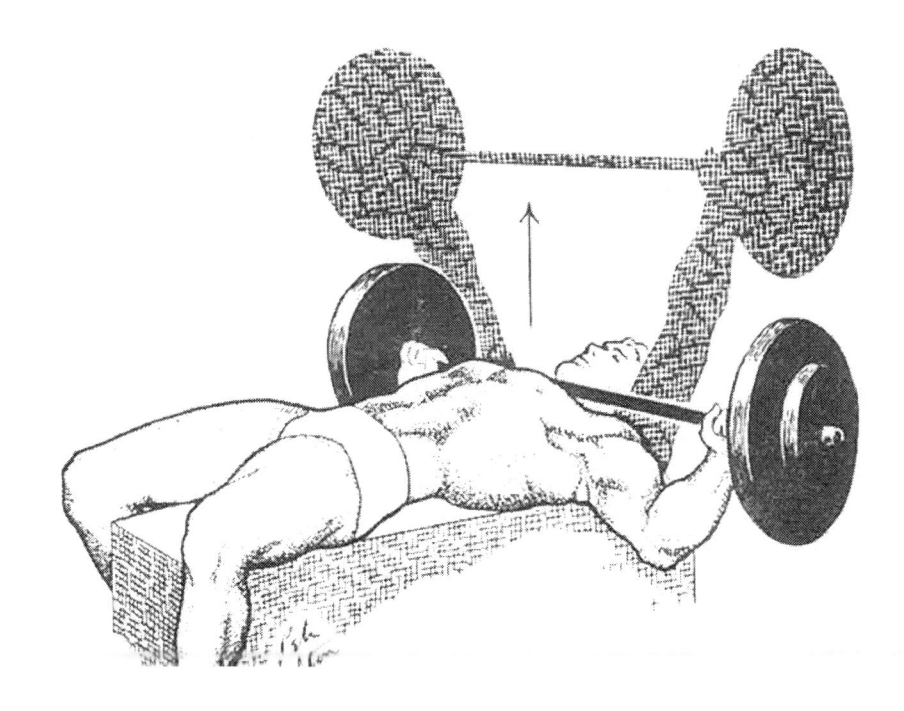

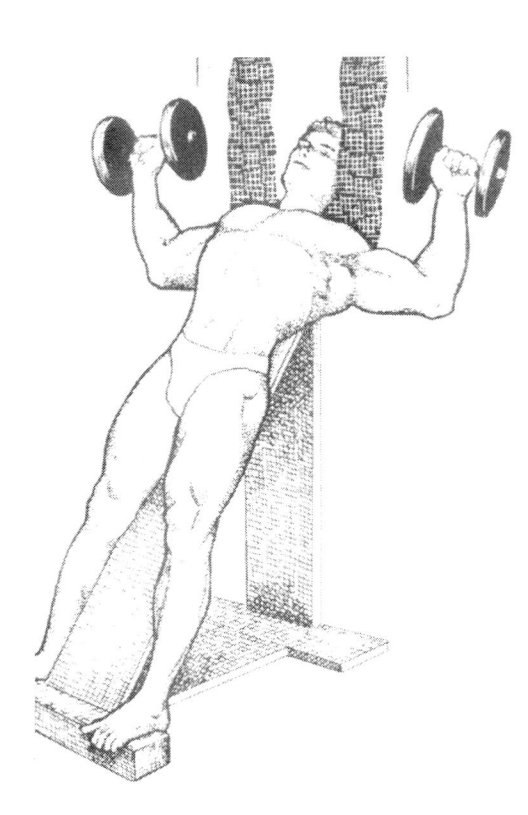

43. Incline Bench Press

Equipment: Twin dumbbells, incline bench
Effect: Strengthen chest, shoulders, triceps
Resistance : Light / Medium / Heavy [Slow / Medium speed]
Hip position: N/A
Spine position: N/A
Scapula position: Neutral / rotation + retraction at end
Muscles: Pectoralis major, triceps (all heads), anterior deltoid
Typical Poundage: 10-20kg dumbbells (women); 20-50 kg dumbbells (men)
Joints: Shoulder, elbow, hand

On this exercise you should make an effort to take the dumbbells wide out to the sides at the bottom position - which will create a nice exaggerated stretch for the pectoral muscles.

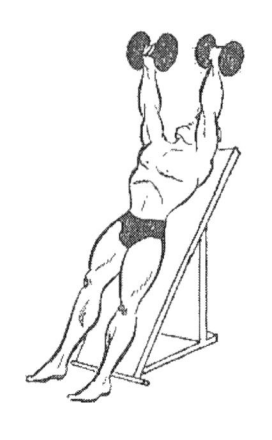

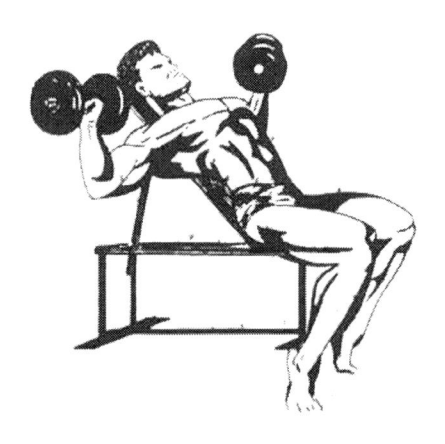

Sit down on an incline bench with dumbbells resting on lower thigh. Kick weights to shoulders and lean back. Position dumbbells to sides of chest with upper arm under each dumbbell. Press dumbbells up with elbows to sides until arms are extended. Lower weight to sides of upper chest until strong stretch is felt in chest or shoulder. Repeat. Dumbbell should follow slight arched pattern, above upper arm and between elbow and chest at bottom, and traveling inward over each shoulder at top. It is best to bring the dumbbells somewhat outward at the bottom in order to fully stretch the pectorals.

44. Fly (Bent Arm) - Bent Arm Laterals (ROM + Strength)

Equipment: Twin dumbbells, flat bench
Effect: Strengthen chest, shoulders
Resistance : Light / Medium [Slow / Medium]
Hip position: N/A
Spine position: N/A
Scapula position: Neutral / some retraction
Muscles: Pectoralis major (all heads)
Typical Poundage: 10-15kg dumbbells (women); 15-25 kg dumbbells (men)
Joints: Shoulder, hand

Lie on the bench. Hold weights over the chest with the palms facing each other. Keeping the elbows slightly bent, lower the arms out to the sides and down until they're level with (or below) the chest. Keep the elbows in a fixed position and avoid lowering the weights too low. Squeeze chest to bring the arms back up as though you're hugging a tree. Repeat for reps.

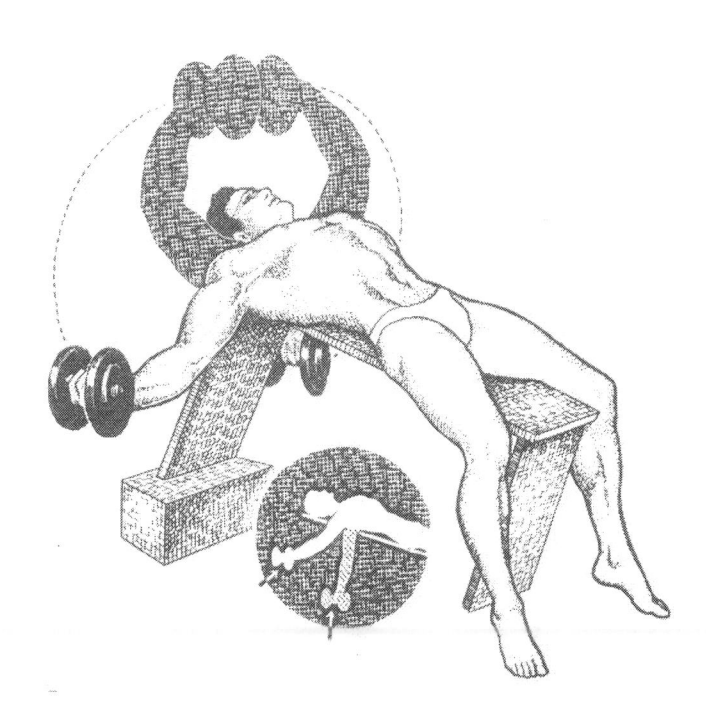

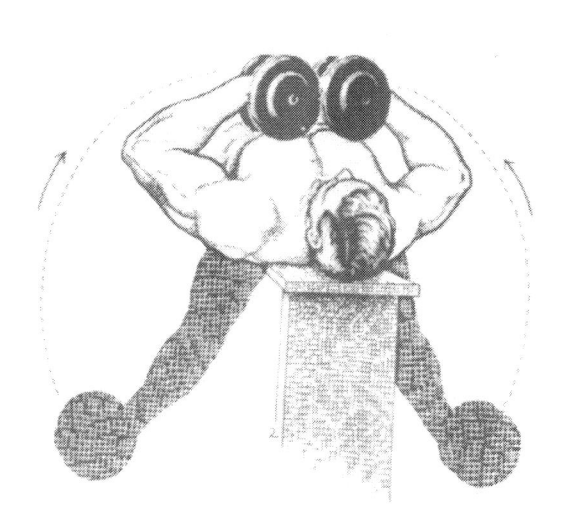

On this exercise it does not matter how low you actually take the dumbbells (in terms of pectoral function) - but rather you should take the elbows both deep and wide to fully engage the pectorals. You can adjust the dumbbell direction in the hand - try with palms facing different directions at the start / end.

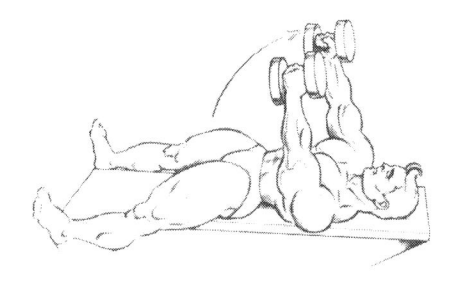

45. Fly (Straight Arm) - Lying Lateral Raise (ROM)

Equipment: Twin dumbbells, flat bench
Effect: Strengthen chest, shoulders
Resistance : Light [Slow / Medium]
Hip position: N/A
Spine position: N/A
Scapula position: Neutral / some retraction
Muscles: Pectoralis major (all heads)
Typical Poundage: 1-5kg dumbbells (women); 2-8 kg (men)
Joints: Shoulder, elbow (bicep stretch as you lower dumbbells)

This exercise is excellent, but it is rarely performed today. It is similar to a normal fly or lateral raise whilst lying down - only the difference is that you keep your arms straight and locked (or close to locked) throughout. You will get a fantastic stretch of the entire pectoral region. You do not need to use much weight at-all, in fact 5-7 lbs is enough for almost everyone.

Lie on the bench. Hold weights over the chest with the palms facing each other. Keeping the elbows locked (close to) and arms very straight, lower the arms out to the sides and down until they're much deeper than the chest. Keep the elbows in a fixed position and lower the weights as low as possible. Squeeze chest to bring the arms back up as though you're hugging a tree. Repeat for reps. Use a very light weight - and even as low as 3 lbs to begin with for men!

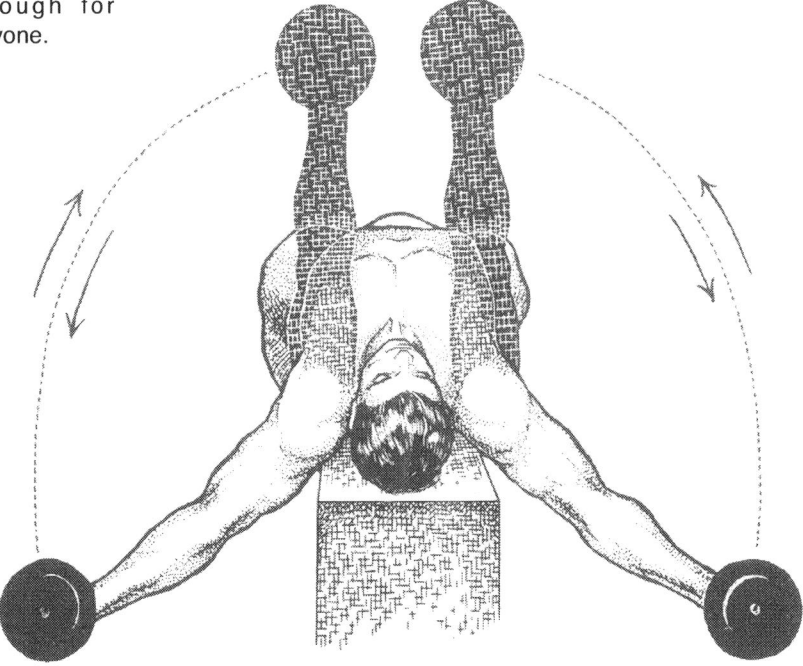

THE SHOULDER 197

46. Lying (Lateral) Circles (ROM)

Equipment: Twin dumbbells, flat / incline bench
Effect: Strengthen chest, shoulders
Resistance : Light [Slow]
Hip position: N/A
Spine position: N/A
Scapula position: Neutral / some rotation depending on height above shoulder level + some retraction
Muscles: Pectoralis major (all heads)
Typical Poundage: 2-4 kg dumbbells (women); 5-8 kg (men)
Joints: Shoulder

Lie on the bench. Hold weights out to the side and in-line with the shoulders. Keeping the elbows locked (almost) and arms straight, move the weight in small circular articulations. Keep the elbows in a fixed position and use varying sized circles. Repeat for as many "circles" as you like.

I could not find a picture of this exercise which is similar to side circles (above) only performed whilst lying down. The picture below shows the dumbbell roll-out which is good for the shoulders / pectoral muscles also.

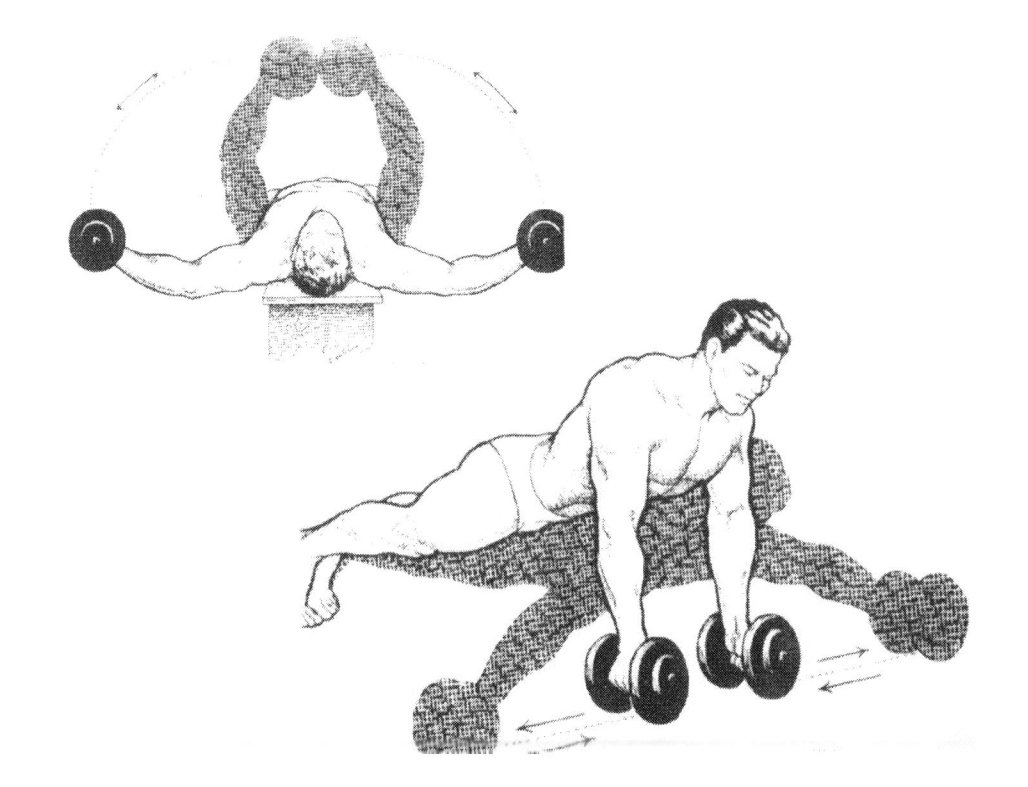

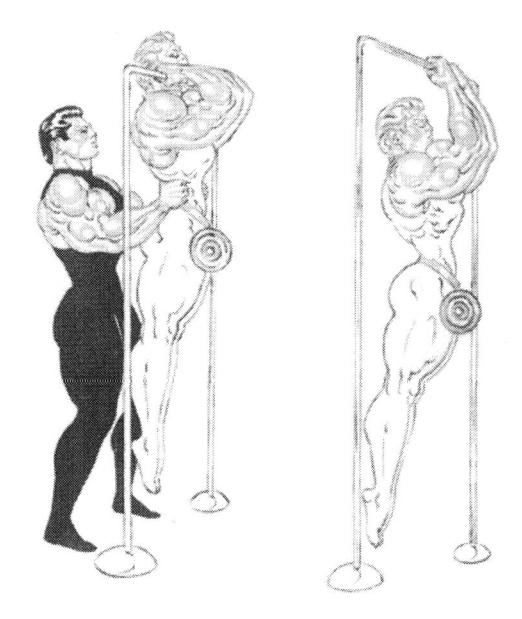

47. Chin-Up

Equipment: Chin-up bar + weights
Effect: Strengthen upper back, biceps
Resistance : Light / Medium / Heavy [Slow]
Hip position: N/A
Spine position: N/A
Scapula position: Outward rotation + elevation on way down, inward rotation and depression on way up
Muscles: Latissimus dorsi, rhomboid major, rhomboid minor, teres major, brachioradialis, biceps brachii, brachialis, trapezius (lower)
Typical Poundage: None / 5-10 kg (women); 10-40 kg (men)
Joints: Shoulder, elbow, hand

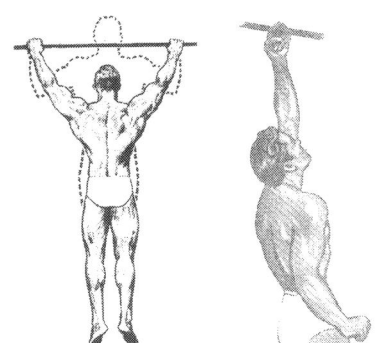

Begin from a dead hang: arms fully extended, hands about shoulder width apart (palms facing out for pull-ups, facing you for chin-ups), elbows straight, chest up, shoulders back and tight, eyes trained on the bar above. Pull yourself up toward the bar, leading with the chest and keeping your eyes focused on the bar. Drive your elbows toward the floor. Clear the bar with your chin if you can. Lower yourself in a controlled fashion, then repeat. Stay honest when you clear the bar. Don't lift your chin and strain your neck just so you can say you cleared it. You run the risk of pinching a nerve and cutting off muscular power. Keep your body neutral. Don't swing with your hips to generate momentum. Keep those shoulder blades tight/retracted. Pulling with a loose shoulder girdle can lead to rotator cuff problems. Retract scapula back/downwards at top! (my own record is 33 non-stop chins)

One of the greatest strength + flexibility exercises that you can ever do. There are many versions including weighted chins, swinging from side to side and one-arm versions. To learn how to perform a one-arm chin simply start doing 2-arm chins with weights around your waist. Once you can chin with 150 - 200 lbs for 1 rep with 2 arms, you might be then strong enough to do a 1 arm chin-up which is one of the greatest feats of strength.

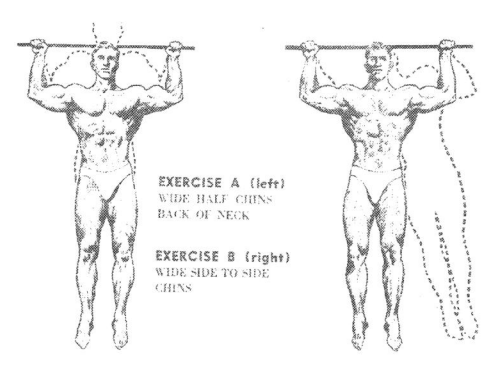

EXERCISE A (left)
WIDE HALF CHINS
BACK OF NECK

EXERCISE B (right)
WIDE SIDE TO SIDE
CHINS

48. Rowing

Equipment: twin dumbbells / barbell
Effect: Strengthen upper / lower back
Resistance : Light / Medium / Heavy [Slow]
Hip position: Hip Hinge - fixed position
Spine position: Extended / arched lumbar
Scapula position: Protracted when arms extended to retracted at end when arms close to body (scapula close in together)
Muscles: Latissimus dorsi, rhomboid major, erector spinae, teres major, teres minor, infraspinatus, posterior deltoid, trapezius, brachioradialis, biceps brachii, brachialis
Typical Poundage: 8-15 kg dumbbells (women); 10-40 kg (men)
Joints: Shoulder, elbow, hand

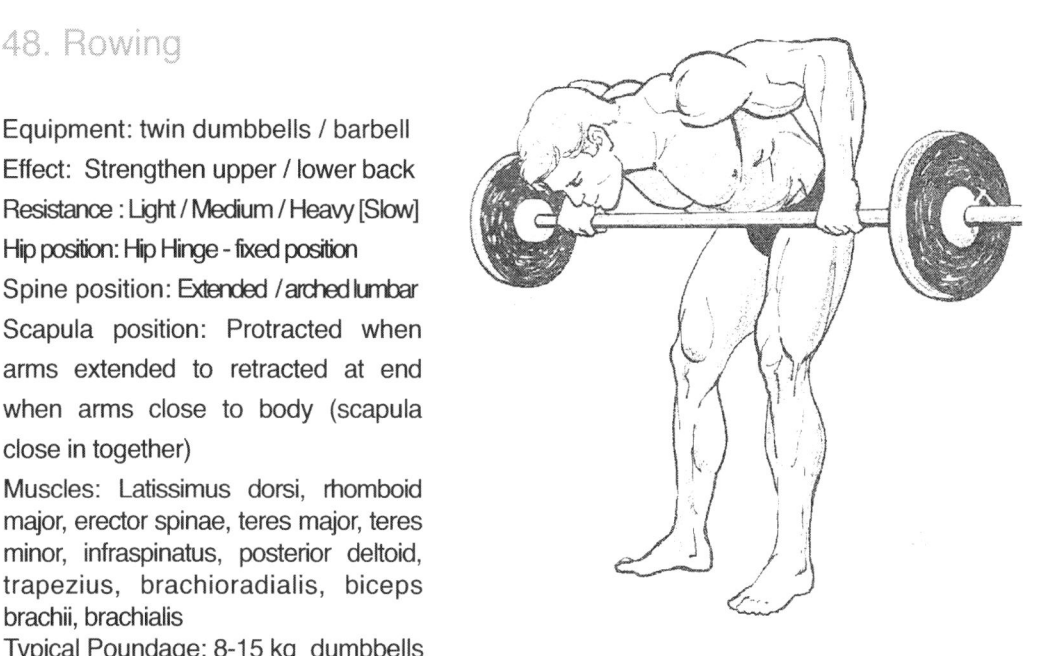

Gab a barbell. Bend knees slightly and bend over bar with back straight. Grasp bar with wide overhand grip. Pull bar to upper waist or nipple area. Return until arms are extended and shoulders are stretched downward. Repeat. Although the barbell version is acceptable, I prefer to use a single dumbbell for rows because you get a better stretch at the bottom and also a better (higher) movement at the top. An unusual version of the dumbbell row is performed as follows. Stand with feet well part - bend over with a single dumbbell, and row from the opposite foot to the top position using the dumbbell. Other hand holds onto opposite knee. You should really get a fantastic stretch of the lat in this way, and also a good contraction of the lat when you pull the dumbbell high up at the top position.

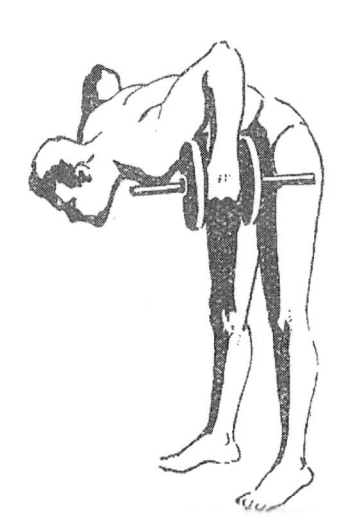

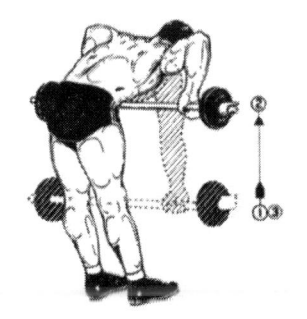

One of the best exercises for the lats or latissimus dorsi muscles of the upper back. There are several different styles of performance, including with barbell and one or two dumbbells. You can try spreading your feet and rowing to either foot. Also you can bring the bar to the chest at the top, or else to the waist (chest is probably best). Lately it has become fashionable to hold the torso at a 45 degree angle whilst performing rows, but I prefer the classic version with the torso held parallel throughout. It is a good idea to protract the scapula (as you go forward) and then retract the scapula at the top position.

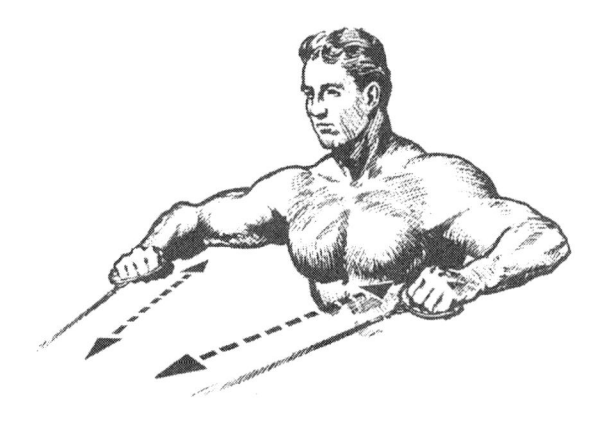

49. Cable Rowing

Equipment: Low cable machine
Effect: Strengthen upper / lower back
Resistance : Light / Medium / Heavy
[Slow speed]
Hip position: Hip Hinge - fixed position
Spine position: Neutral
Scapula position: Protracted when arms extended to retracted at end when arms close to body (scapula close in together) (do not arch back excessively at end)
Muscles: Latissimus dorsi, rhomboid major, erector spinae, teres major, teres minor, infraspinatus, posterior deltoid, trapezius, brachioradialis, biceps brachii, brachialis
Typical Poundage: 10-30 kg (women); 20-80 kg (men)
Joints: Shoulder, elbow, hand

A great exercise for the lats or latissimus dorsi muscles of the upper back. There are several different styles of performance, including with one or two handles attached to the cable machine. You can bring the bar to the chest at the top, or else to the waist (waist is probably best). You can also round the back slightly at the end (spine flexion) - but only if you think that this is safe for your lumbar region.

Sit slightly forward on seat or bench and grasp cable attachment. Place feet on vertical platform. Slide hips back positioning knees with slight bend. Pull cable attachment to waist while straightening lower back. Pull shoulders back and push the chest forward while arching back - as you finish with bar at waist. Return until arms are extended, shoulders are stretched forward, and lower back is flexed forward. Repeat. Do not pause or bounce at bottom of lift. Full range of motion through lower back will vary from person to person.

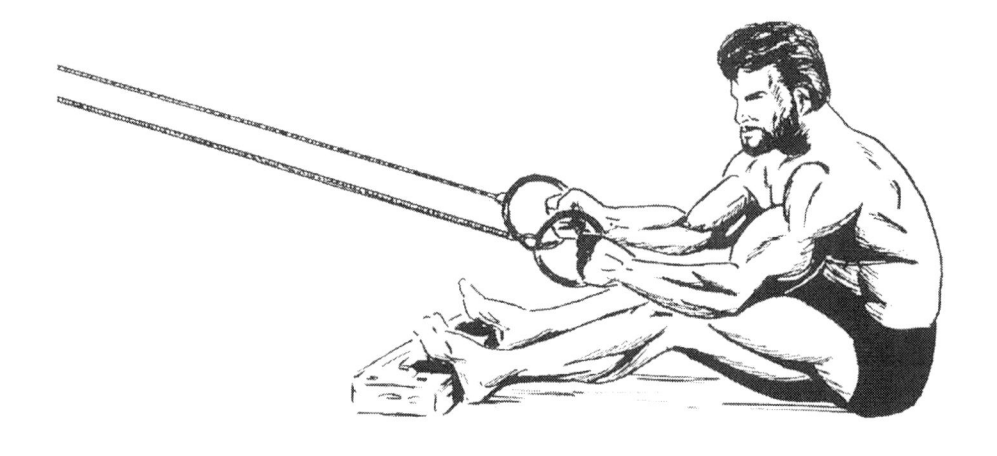

Unclassified Exercises

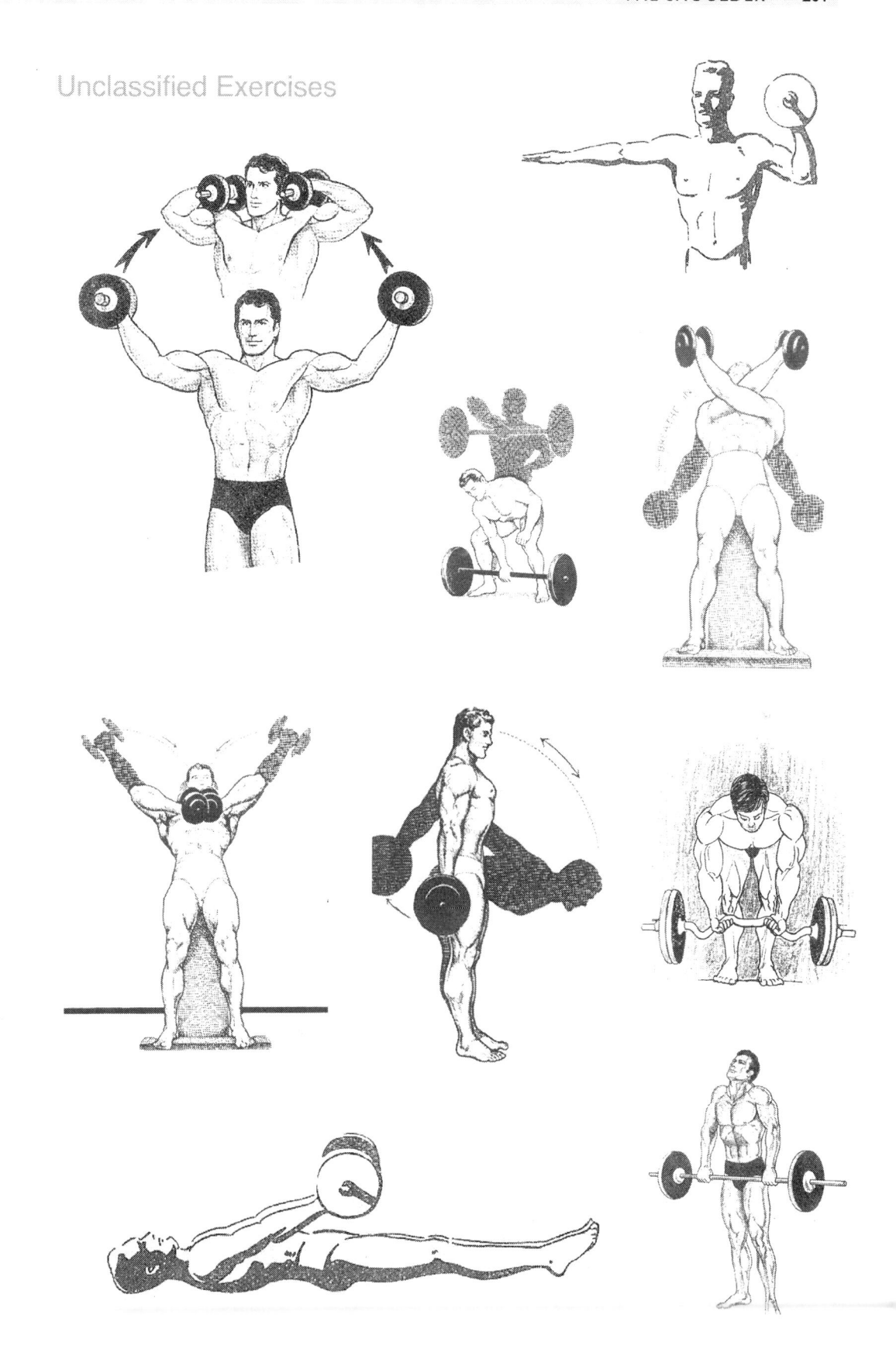

202   ZEN OF DUMBBELL TRAINING

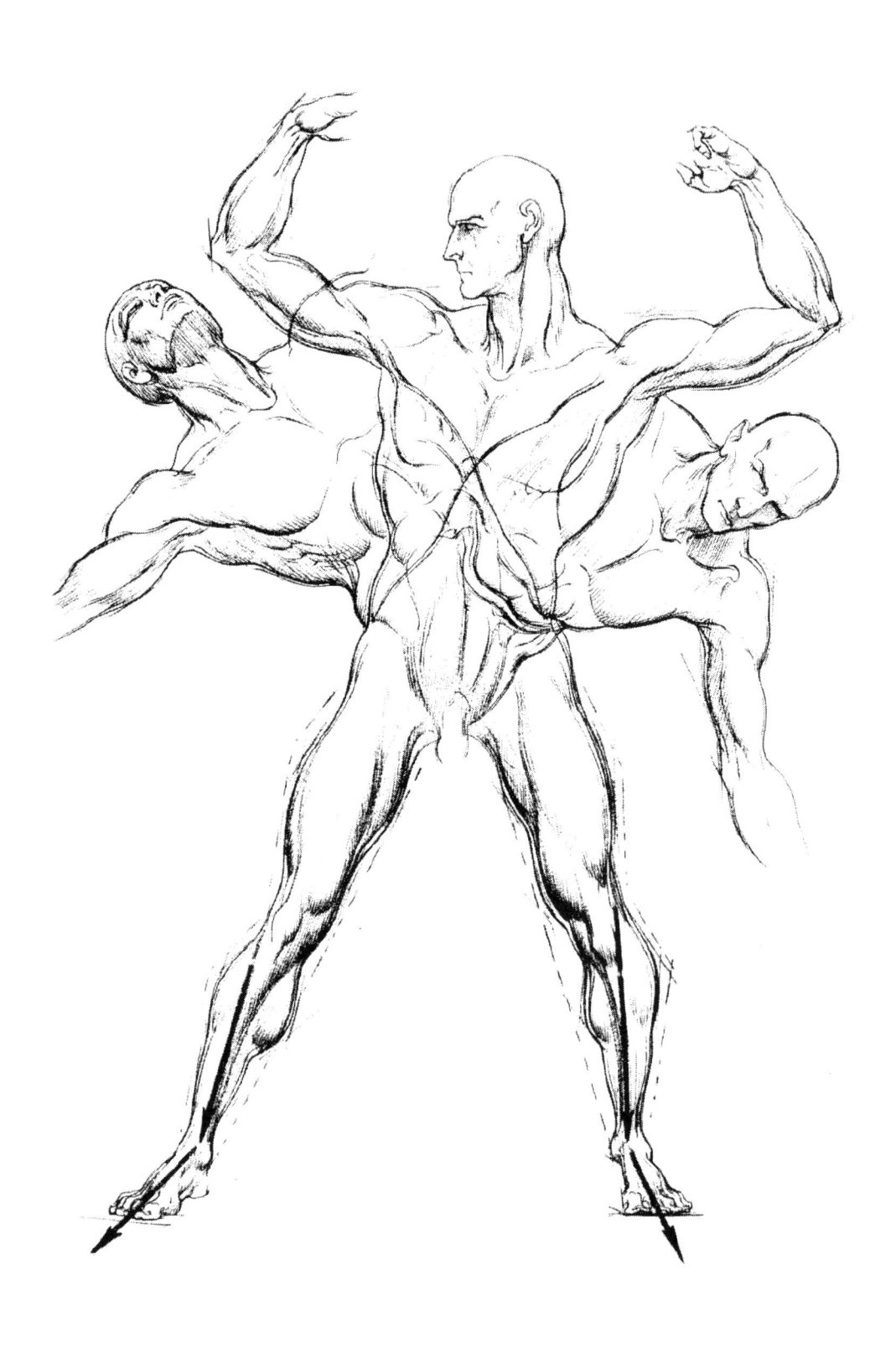

CHAPTER NINE

The Elbow

THE ELBOW serves two functions; first it allows the upper limb to fold on itself and to extend, so that the distance between the shoulder and the hand can be shortened and lengthened. This is the flexion-extension action of the elbow.

Second, the elbow also participates in rotating the forearm around its longitudinal axis, multiplying the possible positions of the hand. This is the pronation-supination action of the elbow.

Flexion of the elbow can be defined as a movement that decreases the angle between the anterior surfaces of the arm and forearm. In active flexion, the movement is limited by contraction between the bodies of the muscles involved. Extension of the elbow is a return from flexion to anatomical position. In other words, an increase in the angle between the arm and forearm.

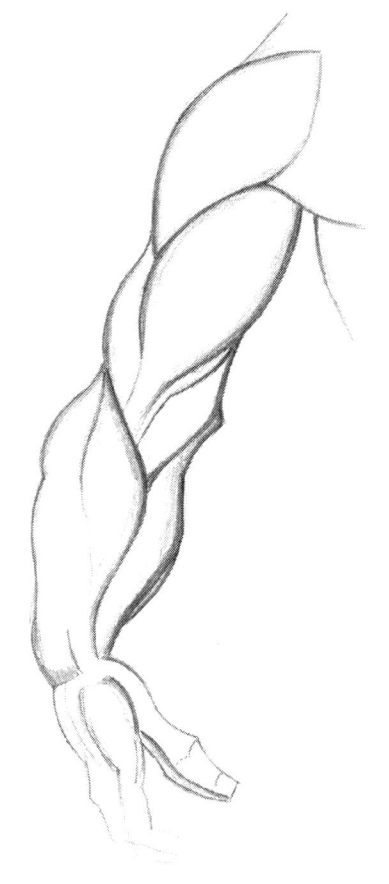

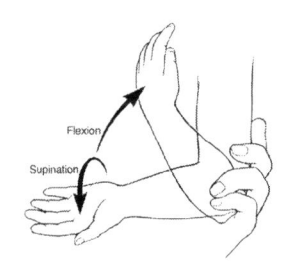

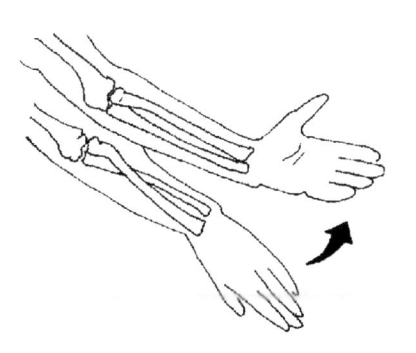

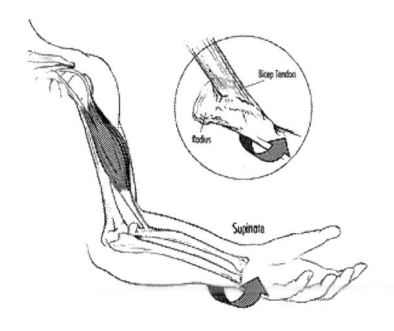

The flexor muscles of the elbow include the biceps brachii, being the long and short heads which have a shared attachment at the elbow, but attach at different points at the shoulder. The triceps brachii have three heads and extend the elbow. Once again we shall avoid all talk of the details of muscle actions and concentrate on actual limb movements; and in order to illustrate basic movements.

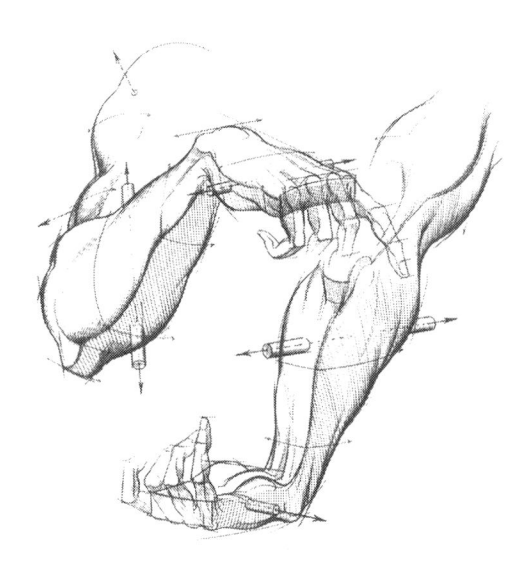

We shall now explain ROM details for the elbow region. Here we see quite a simple set of movements when compared to the far more complex movements of the shoulder region. Normal flexion/extension ROM goes from 0 to around 150 degrees. Supination/pronation ROM is normally from 0 to 90 degrees in either direction.

If you think about it, the elbow is a very important joint. For example, moving the hand into different spatial positions cannot be easily performed without the use of the elbow. And when the elbow becomes injured, as it does in a so-called golf or tennis-elbow, it can be a very bothersome and annoying injury.

One might think that exercise - and care - of the elbow would be a primary concern as a result, however people never seem to think in such terms, but rather speak of building up the biceps or triceps (for example). And the elbow is also important for lifting anything overhead, and for picking objects off the floor etc. All-in, the elbow is a vital part of the body, and one that gets exercised on every occasion that you move a limb in almost any way whatsoever. Avoidance of over-training here is vital.

I would like to stress that you should not (in general) perform any exercise listed here (or elsewhere), or probably any movement for that matter, that causes you pain.

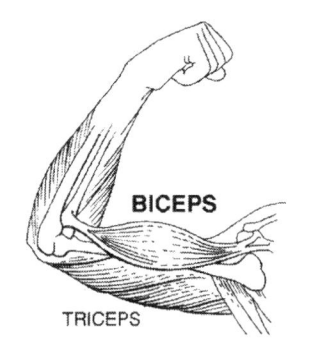

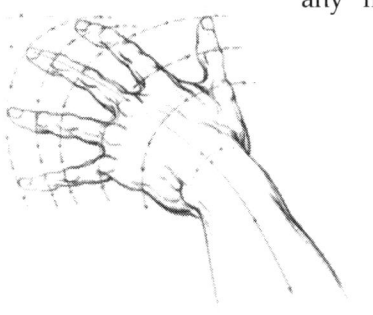

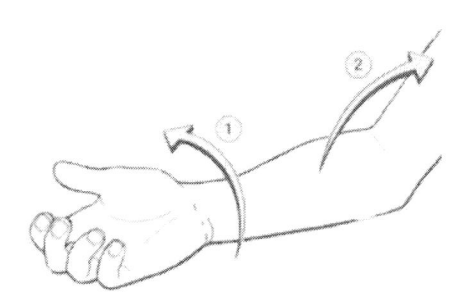

Sometimes during rehabilitation or just out of pure necessity, you must move despite feeling pain. But if a particular exercise seems to aggravate an injury - or to be the actual cause of pain - then you should cease its performance at once. Now I have noticed that some exercises are quite "hard" on the elbow joint in particular.

One is the overhead single-triceps extension, another is preacher curls, and yet another is lying triceps extensions. You may find other exercises that hurt your elbow, and you should not perform such movements, unless they form part of a carefully planned therapeutic course of exercise. And for some people certain exercises should not ever be performed.

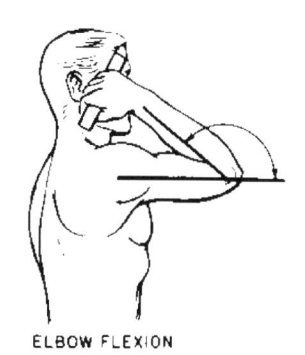

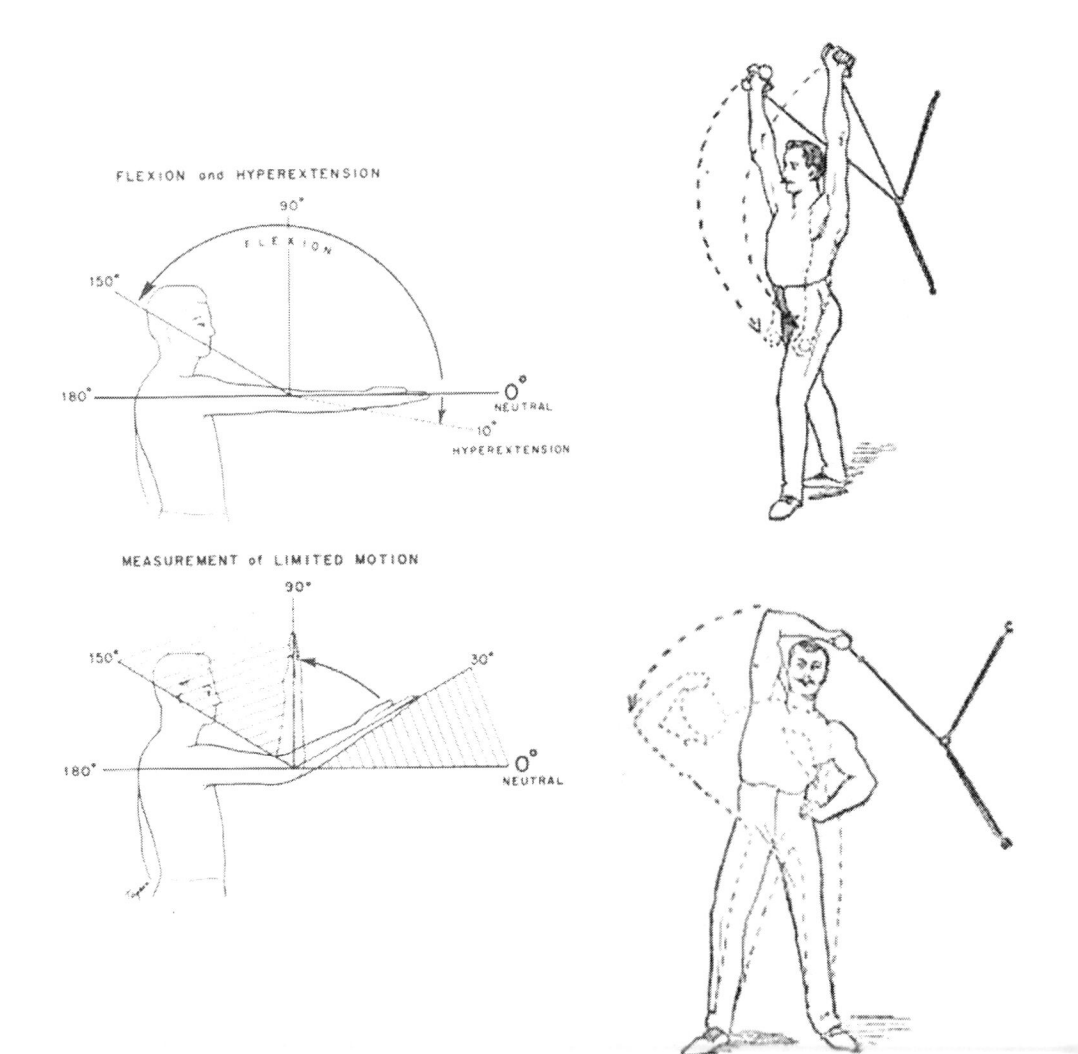

ELBOW FLEXION

FLEXION and HYPEREXTENSION

MEASUREMENT of LIMITED MOTION

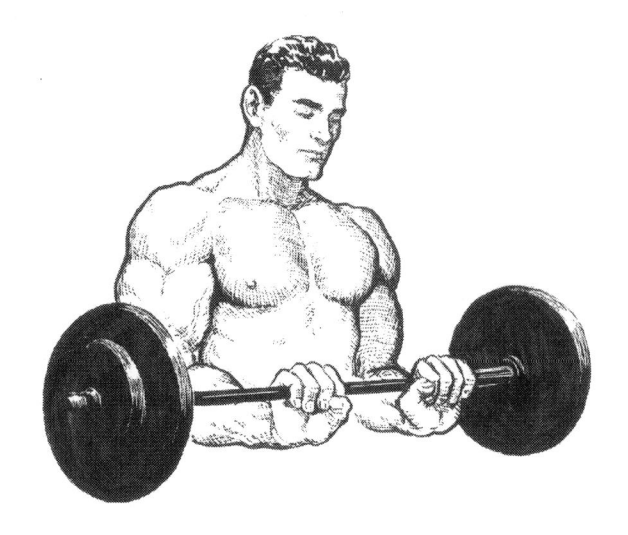

Elbow Joint Exercises

50. Curl
51. Supination Curl
52. Incline Curl
53. Preacher Curl
54. Reverse Curl
55. Hammer Curl
56. Curl Behind Neck
57. Bent-Over Curl
58. Face Down Curl
59. Lying Triceps Extensions
60. Standing Triceps Extensions
61. Cable PushDowns
62. Cable Overhead Extensions
63. Close Grip Bench Press
64. Press Up
65. Bent Over Extensions
66. Bench Dips

A few words on exercise selection may be useful at this point. As stated in the beginning of this book, it is my belief that appropriate selection of exercises is the first rule of any properly planned and executed training schedule or program. I have attempted to give you what I consider to be the very best

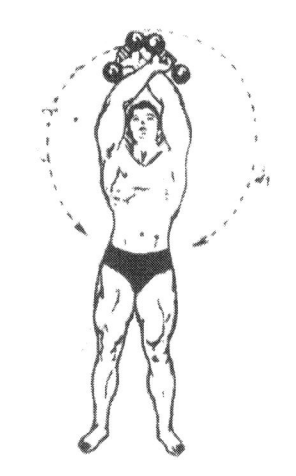

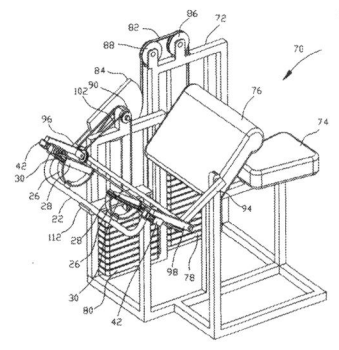

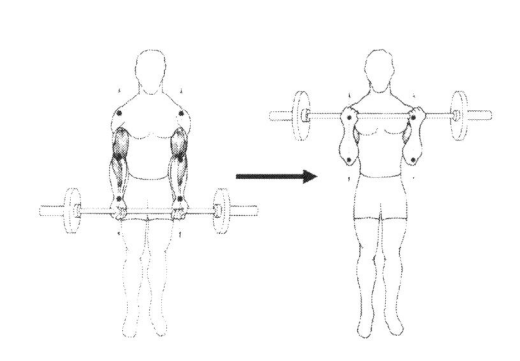

FIG. 8

weight-training exercises here, and listed are around 80 movements. Most people could not perform all of these different movements in their training program, even within an entire one month training cycle. Rather it is up to you to select particular exercises that seem to offer beneficial routes to where you are attempting to get to in terms of personal fitness.

Given in later chapters are example training programs for specific purposes. In your own program, you must select appropriate lifts, and it is vital to not miss out any muscle groups, or else to perform too many movements for smaller muscles at the expense of larger muscles which need more work and which can provide greater overall benefits (in stimulation), and in terms of improved overall fitness levels and development.

Here in this section we provide (for example) 9 different types of exercise for the biceps. However no-body would perform all 9 movements in any one routine because the biceps is a small muscle group and it would be over-trained by such a procedure. Similarly one might not need all of the different types of shoulder raise (and circular movements) that are listed in the previous chapter. At least one might not want to perform all of these in a standard routine or else in a single training workout. At all times, use common sense.

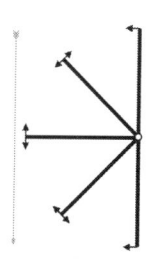

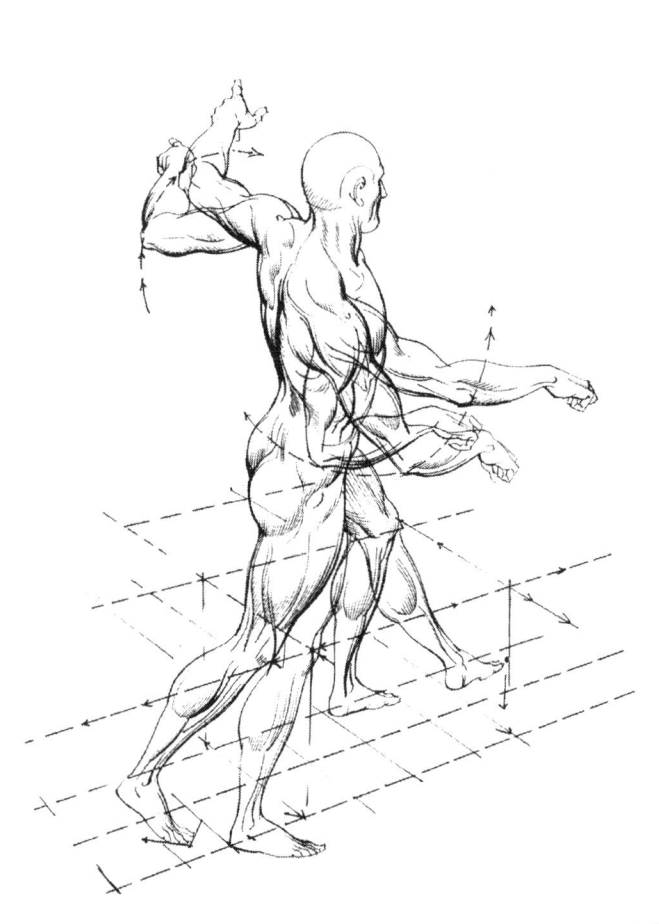

50. Curl

Equipment: twin dumbbells / barbell (not easy-curl bar)
Effect: Strengthen biceps, brachialis, brachioradialis
Resistance : Light / Medium / Heavy [Slow]
Hip position: N/A
Spine position: N/A
Scapula position: Neutral / locked
Muscles: Biceps (long and short heads), brachialis, brachioradialis
Typical Poundage: 8-16 kg dumbbells (women); 12-35 kg (men)
Joints: Elbow, wrist, hand [flex biceps at the top position]

Stand upright, and position two dumbbells at the sides, palms facing in, arms straight. Raise one dumbbell and rotate forearm until forearm is vertical and palm faces shoulder (supinate the hand). Lower to original position and repeat with the opposite arm. Continue to alternate between sides. Biceps may be exercised alternating (as described), simultaneous (both dumbbells raised together), or in simultaneous-alternating fashion. You may also keep the arms in the face-front position (largely supinated) throughout the movement.

If you hold the elbows back at the top, you may get a better contraction at the top, because the biceps are held under tension from gravity. Also to improve the ability to contract at the top, hold the weight in the hand in such a way whereby the hand drops backwards slightly at the wrist. The resistance is zero at the start and end of the curling movement, and so it is sometimes a good idea to perform only the mid-range part of the movement for reps - and in order to maintain constant tension on the biceps (as in "21s").

A tip to make bicep supination more difficult - is to load the inside of the dumbbell with more weight (plates)!

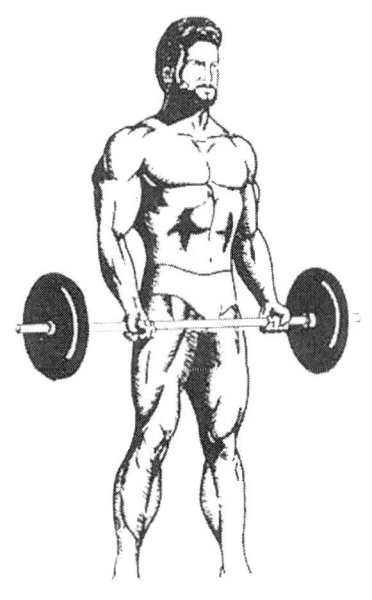

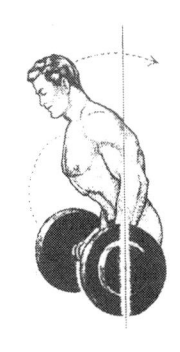

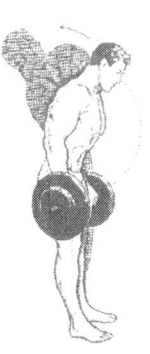

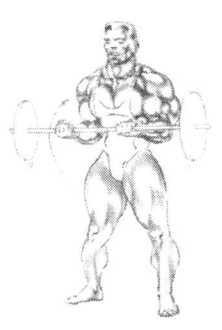

Some people believe (when performing curls) in cheating quite a bit. They use momentum from the body in order to get the weight up to the top position - normally after a few stricter reps have been completed. Other people believe that such training does not build muscle. However I think that (used moderately) cheating reps can and do build muscle. I think that it is best to use both approaches (strict and slight cheating reps) in the same workout for best results. Also try using an off-set grip - with hands-towards the outer edge of the handle - and so to make supination more difficult. Another trick is to lean forward slightly at the end (top point of the curl); instead of leaning backwards; which will more fully engage your biceps and make the final part of the curl very difficult to complete.

THE ELBOW 209

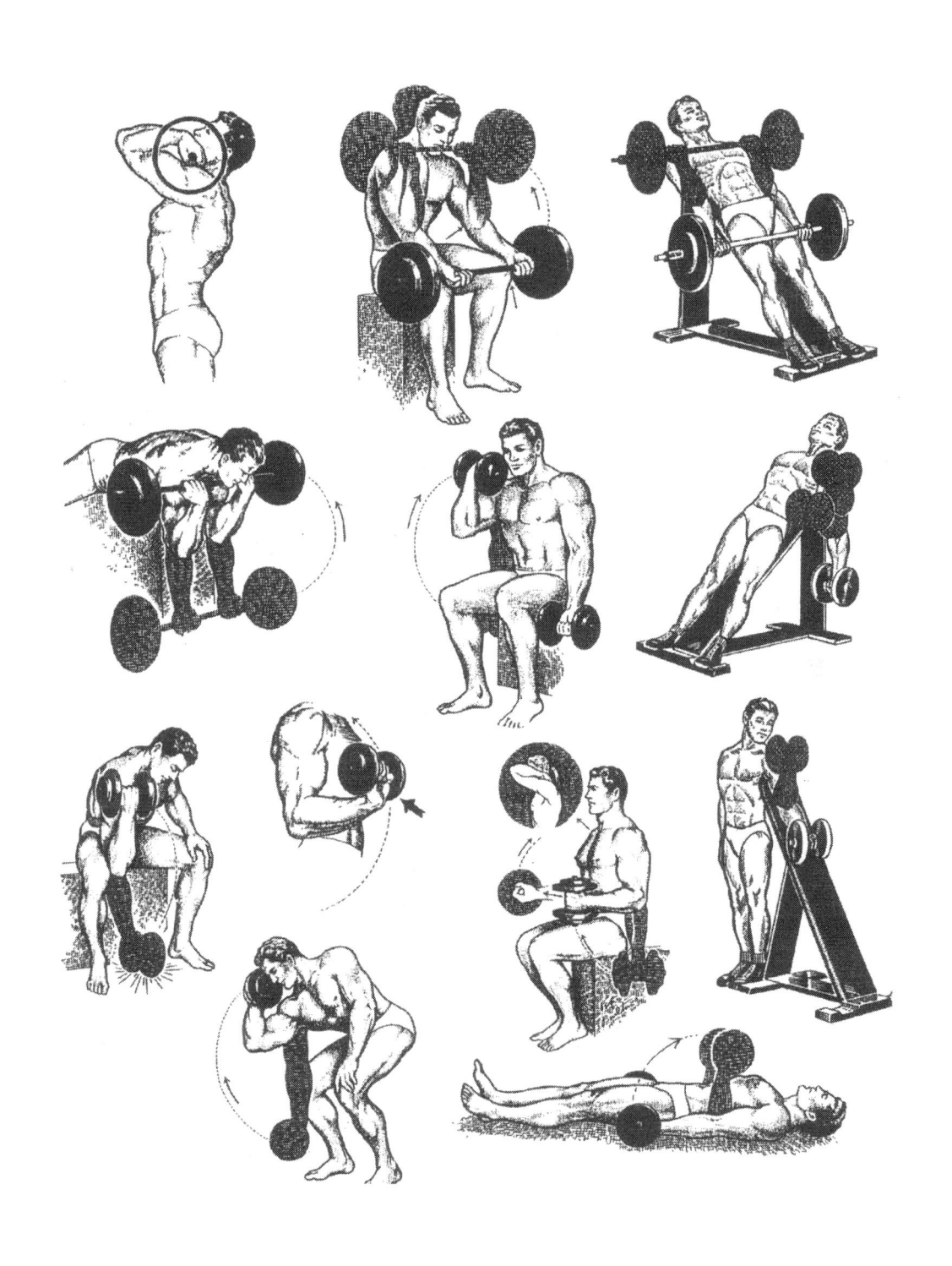

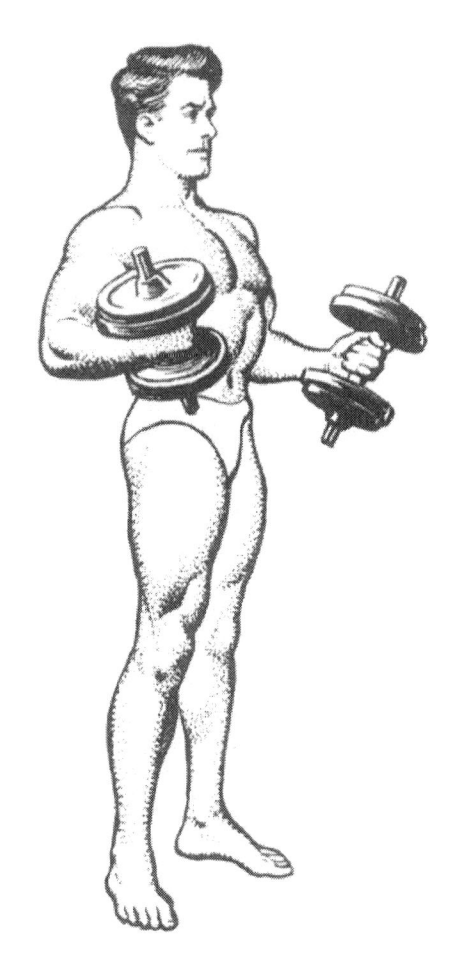

51. Supination Curl

Equipment: twin dumbbells
Effect: Strengthen biceps, brachialis, brachioradialis
Resistance : Light / Medium / Heavy [Slow]
Hip position: N/A
Spine position: N/A
Scapula position: Neutral / locked
Muscles: Biceps (biceps brachii), brachialis
Typical Poundage: 8-35 kg dumbbells (women); 12-35 kg dumbbells (men)
Joints: Elbow, wrist, hand

Perform as in the standard curl. But the more you twist the little finger inwards at the top (towards outer shoulder) - the greater will be the bicep contraction. Another tip is to load an extra plate on the inner side of each dumbbell making supination harder, and thus forcing the bicep to contract to a greater degree.

Contrary to popular belief, the biceps brachii is not the most powerful flexor of the forearm, a role which actually belongs to the deeper brachialis muscle. The biceps brachii functions primarily as a powerful supinator of the forearm (turns the palm upwards). So emphasise supination for biceps.

Never use a bent easy-curl bar for bicep curls - at least with the normal underhand grip - because this in fact holds your hand away from supination and prevents supination from happening - thus releasing stress from the biceps.

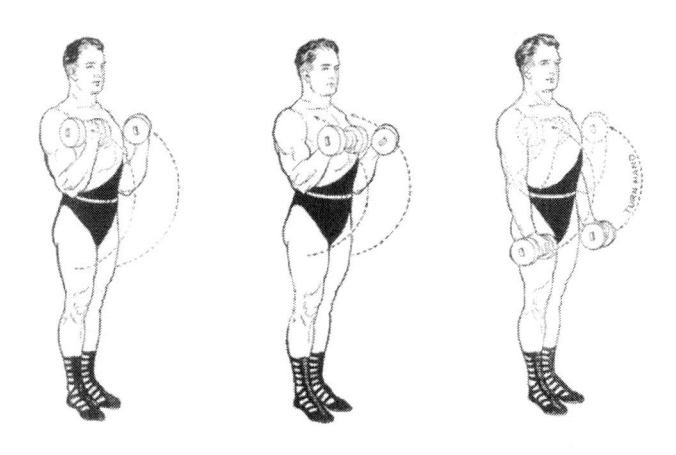

52. Incline Curl

Equipment: twin dumbbells
Effect: Strengthen biceps, brachialis, brachioradialis
Resistance : Light / Medium / Heavy [Slow]
Hip position: N/A
Spine position: N/A
Scapula position: Neutral / locked
Muscles: Biceps, brachialis
Typical Poundage: 8-16 kg dumbbells (women); 12-35 kg (men)
Joints: Elbow, wrist, hand

Sit back on a 45-60 degree incline bench. With arms hanging down straight, position two dumbbells with palms facing inward. With elbows back to sides, raise the dumbbells and rotate forearm until forearm is vertical and palm faces shoulder. Lower to original position and repeat. This exercise may be performed by alternating, simultaneous, or in simultaneous-alternating fashion. Supinate or do not supinate. Keeping the elbows back will help contraction at the top, and to maintain tension on the biceps all the way through the exercise. Plus some people like to keep the dumbbells facing forwards throughout (no supination).

A great exercise for the biceps which was a favourite of Steve Reeves. It is important to keep your elbows back throughout. Try to get a good stretch at the bottom position, and move the dumbbells very slowly throughout.

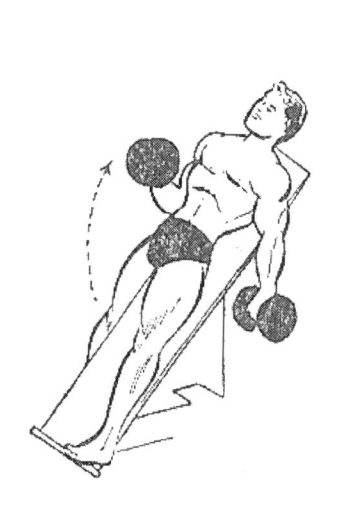

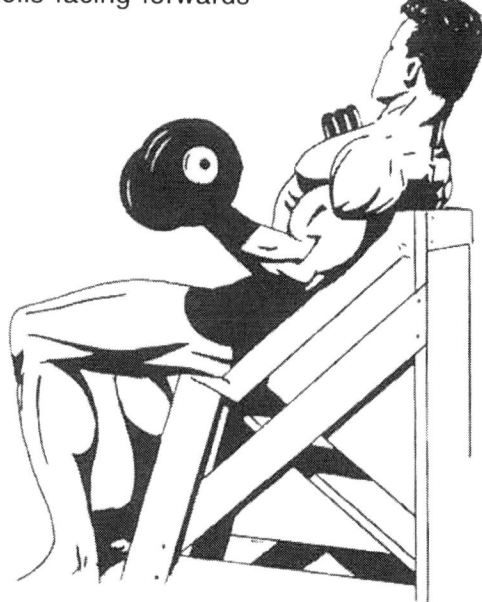

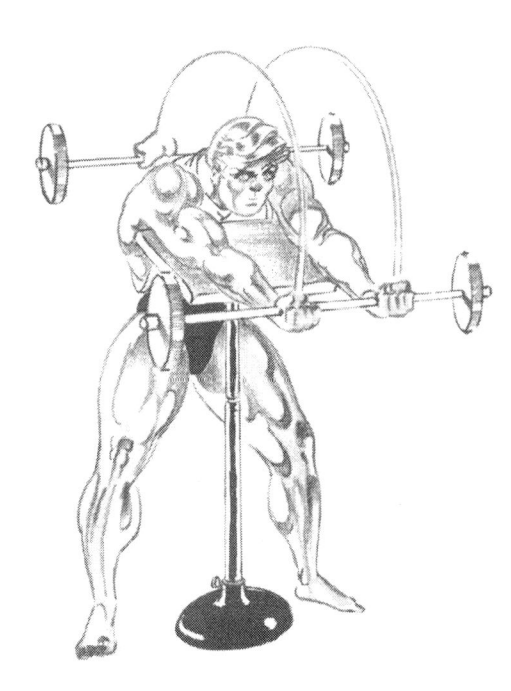

53. Preacher Curl

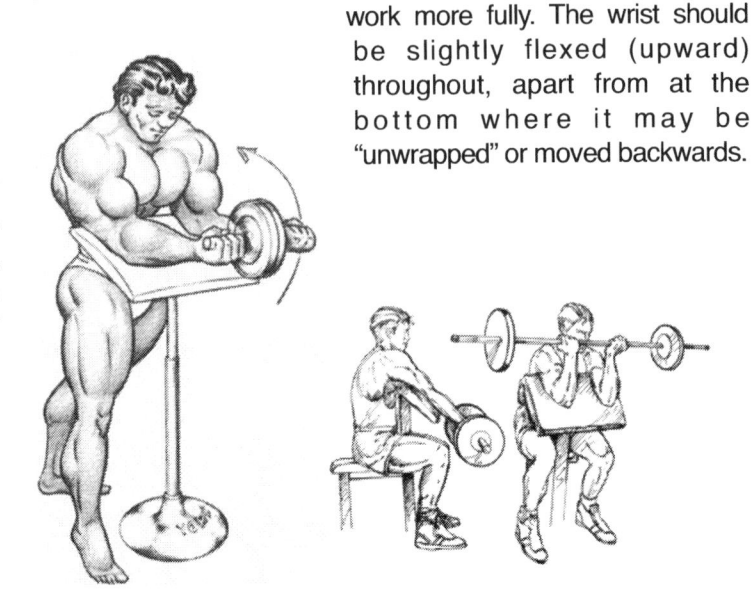

Equipment: dumbbells/barbell + preacher bench
Effect: Strengthen biceps, brachialis, brachioradialis
Resistance : Light / Medium [Slow]
Hip position: N/A
Spine position: N/A
Scapula position: Neutral / locked
Muscles: Lower biceps, brachialis, brachioradialis
Typical Poundage: 8-16 kg dumbbells (women); 12-30 kg dumbbells (men)
Joints: Elbow, wrist, hand

A "curved-face" preacher bench is the best for this exercise (see Larry Scott's book "Loaded Guns"). Although quite difficult to construct you will find that making such a device is worth it in the end, because the bench is very comfortable to use (due to the curved face). In fact you don't even really need to use any padding because the bench shape allows the elbows to bend in a totally free manner and without "digging-into" the bench. Elbow pain is thus eliminated and you can use much heavier weights as a result.

Sit on (or stand in-front of) the preacher curl bench and rest the backs of your arms on the pad. The seat should be adjusted so that your elbows are close to the top of the pad. Grasp the bar at about shoulder width apart. Slowly curl the bar up until your forearms are pointing towards the ceiling (slightly more than vertical). Pause for a second, contract biceps strongly, and lower the bar to the starting position. The preacher curl bench adjusts the resistance direction of gravity relative to the elbow hinge such that the bicep is placed under greater tension in the bottom half of the curl (see Chapter 13). Thus the bicep is placed under a great deal of a "stretch" tension and is forced to work more fully. The wrist should be slightly flexed (upward) throughout, apart from at the bottom where it may be "unwrapped" or moved backwards.

54. Reverse Curl

Equipment: straight / easy-curl barbell
Effect: Strengthen biceps, brachialis, brachioradialis
Resistance : Light / Medium / Heavy [Slow]
Hip position: N/A
Spine position: N/A
Scapula position: Neutral / locked
Muscles: Biceps, brachialis, brachioradialis, forearm extensors etc
Typical Poundage: 6-8 kg dumbbells (women); 8-20 kg dumbbells (men)
Joints: Elbow, wrist, hand

Best performed on a preacher bench, with a reverse grip on an easy-curl bar. Same movement as preacher bench curl, but with overhand grip.

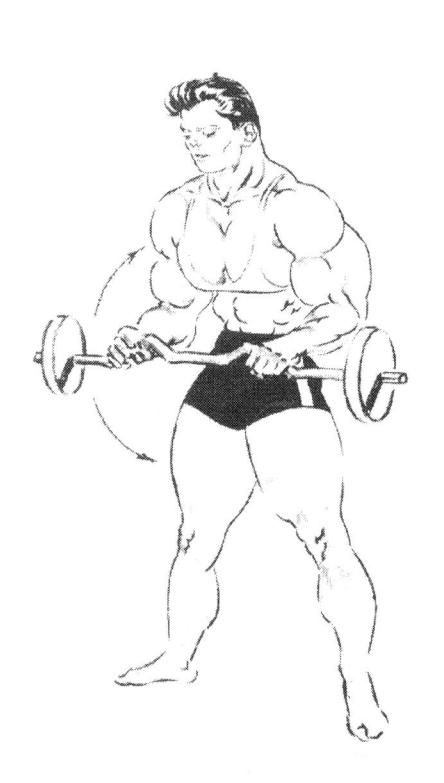

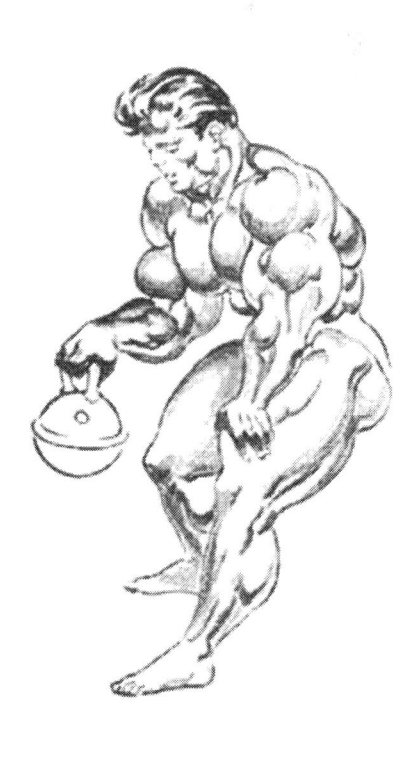

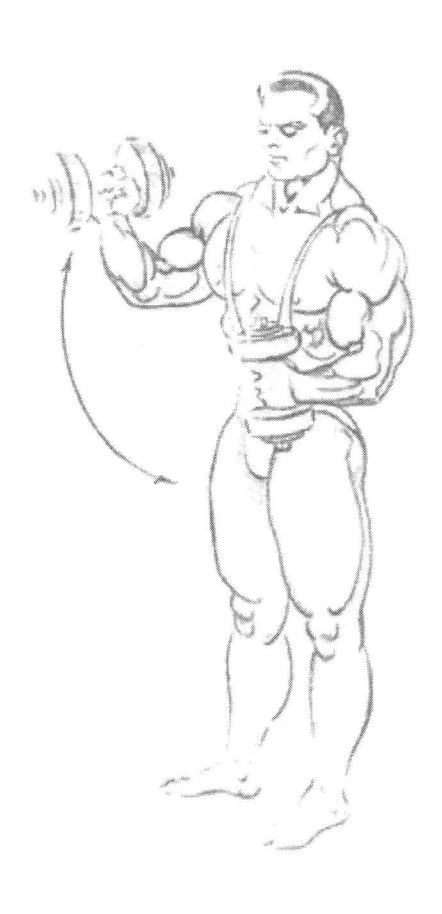

55. Hammer Curl

Equipment: twin dumbbells
Effect: Strengthen biceps, brachialis, brachioradialis
Resistance : Light / Medium / Heavy [Slow]
Hip position: N/A
Spine position: N/A
Scapula position: Neutral / locked
Muscles: Biceps, brachialis, brachioradialis, forearm extensors etc
Typical Poundage: 8-12 kg dumbbells (women); 12-24 kg dumbbells (men)
Joints: Elbow, wrist, hand

Position two dumbbells to the sides, palms facing in (throughout movement), arms straight. With elbows to sides, raise one dumbbell until forearm is vertical and thumb faces shoulder. Lower to original position and repeat with alternative arm. The biceps may be exercised alternating (as described), simultaneous, or in simultaneous-alternating fashion. When elbows are fully flexed, they can travel backwards slightly to enhance tension at the top of the movement.

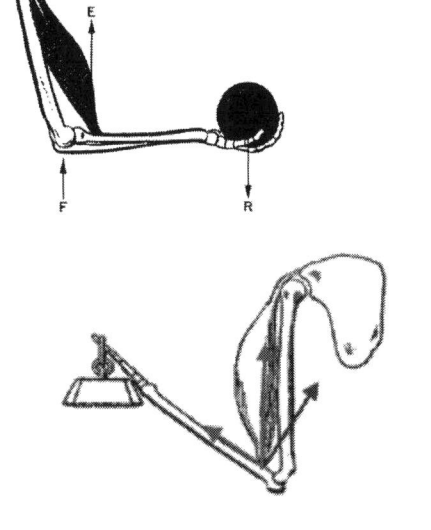

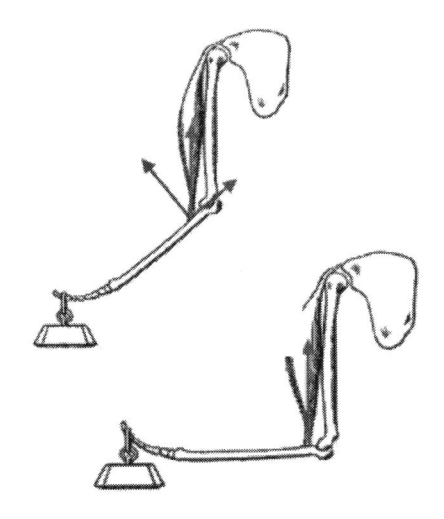

56. Curl Behind Neck / To Neck

Equipment: Cable machine
Effect: Strengthen biceps, brachialis, brachioradialis
Resistance : Light / Medium / Heavy [Slow]
Hip position: N/A
Spine position: N/A
Scapula position: Neutral / locked
Muscles: Biceps, brachialis
Typical Poundage: 12 -15 kg barbell (women); 20-30 barbell kg (men)
Joints: Elbow, shoulder, wrist, hand

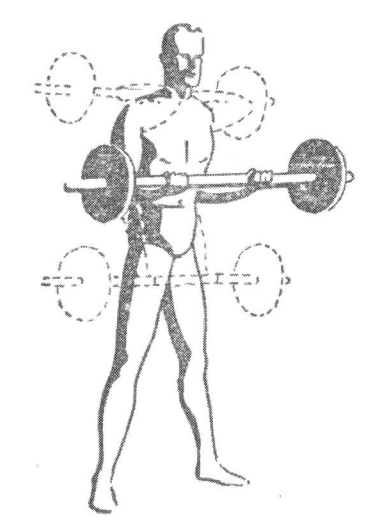

Lie / sit down in-front of a cable machine setup (use low pulley position). Perform curling motions whereby at the end of the movement the bar goes right behind the head for a very tight contraction of the biceps. Alternatives include those exercises shown here. Especially interesting is the (older-style) standing curl whereby you hold the elbows high at the end and bring the bar into the neck (top right).

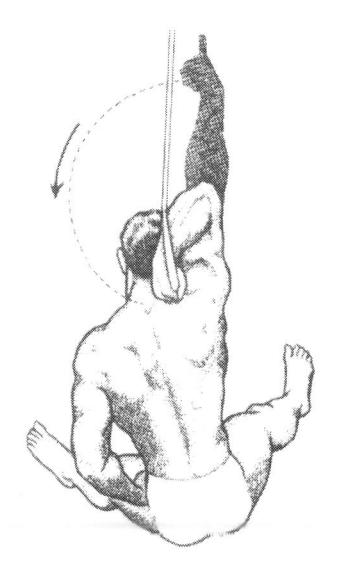

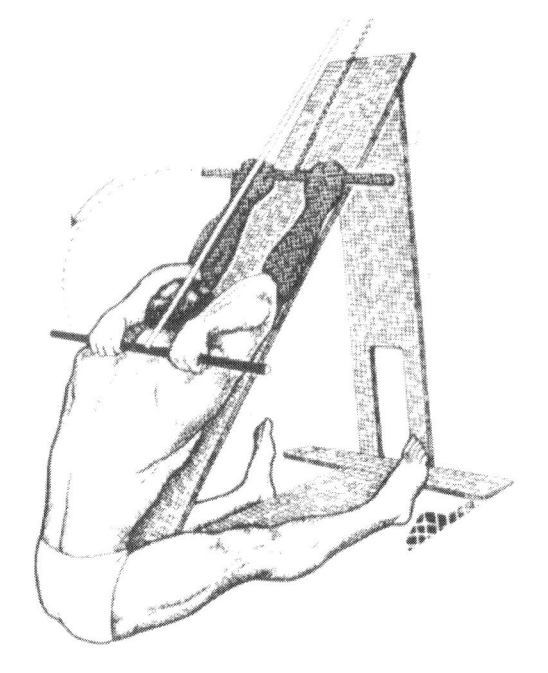

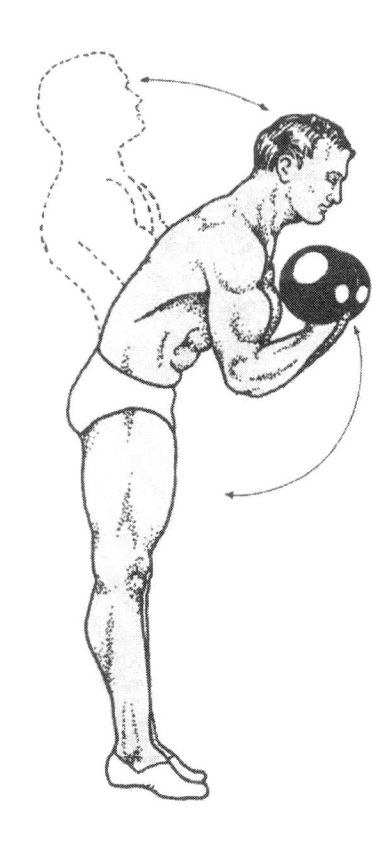

57. Bent-Over Curl

Equipment: single dumbbell
Effect: Strengthen biceps, brachialis, brachioradialis
Resistance : Light / Medium / Heavy [Slow]
Hip position: N/A
Spine position: N/A
Scapula position: Neutral / locked
Muscles: Biceps, brachialis
Typical Poundage: 8-12 kg (women); 12-20 kg (men)
Joints: Elbow, wrist, hand

Stand with your feet shoulder width apart for stability. Bend over (approx. 30 degrees) keeping your legs straight until the dumbbell hangs freely beneath you. Curl the dumbbell up squeezing your bicep at the top of the motion. Lower the dumbbell down in a slow, controlled manner not allowing you arm to fully lockout before starting the next rep as this will maintain pressure on the bicep muscle and increase the overall benefits of the exercise. Repeat with the other arm. Also perform the version shown being a one-arm concentration curl.

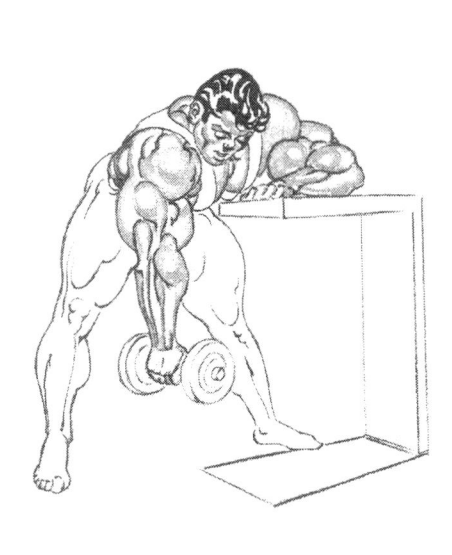

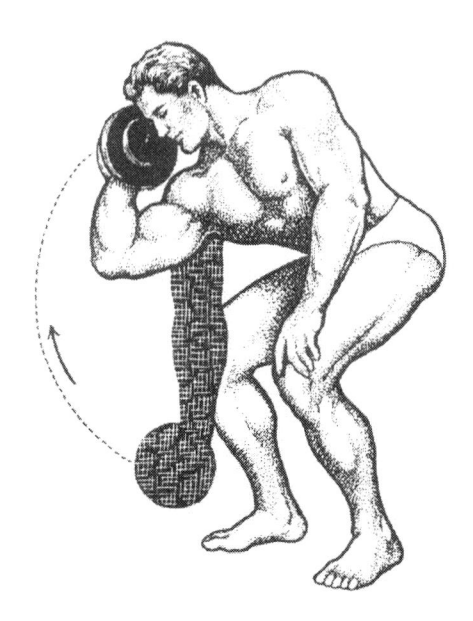

58. Face Down Curl

Equipment: twin dumbbells
Effect: Strengthen biceps, brachialis, brachioradialis
Resistance : Light / Medium / Heavy [Slow]
Hip position: N/A
Spine position: N/A
Scapula position: Neutral / locked
Muscles: Biceps, brachialis
Typical Poundage: 8-16 kg (women); 12-24 kg (men)
Joints: Elbow, wrist, hand

Lie face down on an incline or flat bench. Curl dumbbells from this position, whilst noticing a very tight contraction in the bicep due the elbow being in a raise position relative to the upper body placing the biceps in a good position to achieve full contractions.

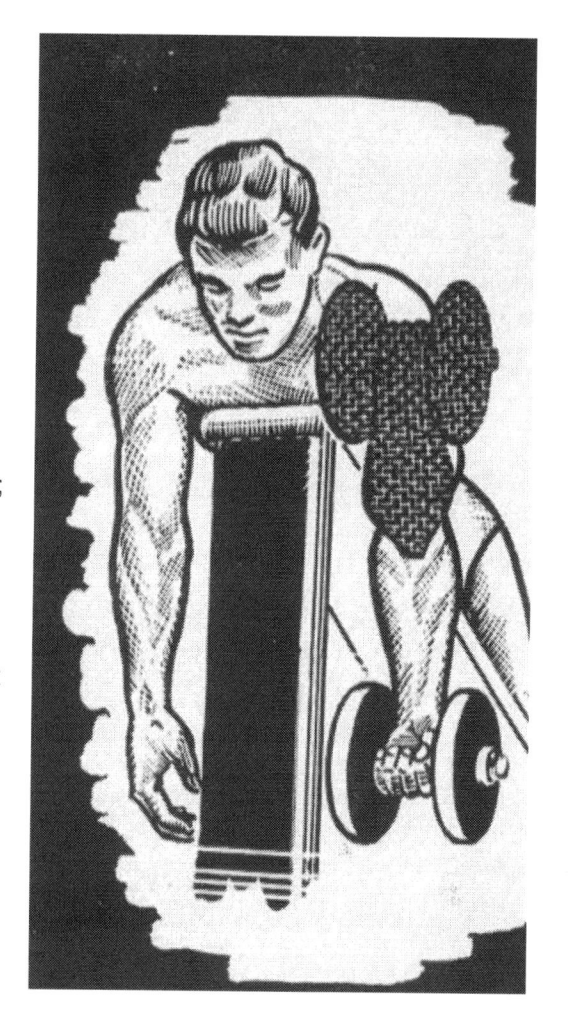

The table-top curl (shown below) is a good combinational movement for super-sets (stretch position resistance).

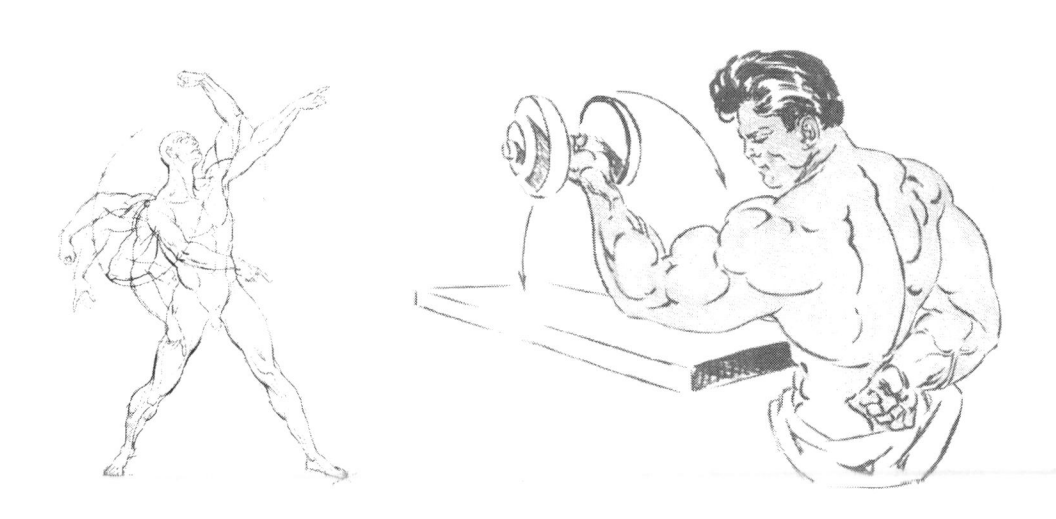

59. Lying Triceps Extensions

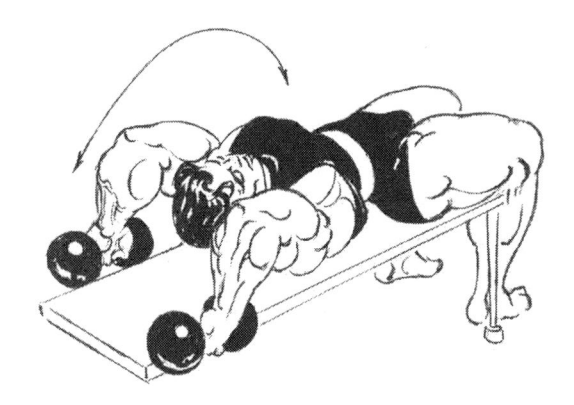

Equipment: twin dumbbells, barbell
Effect: Strengthen triceps
Resistance : Light / Medium [Slow]
Hip position: N/A
Spine position: N/A
Scapula position: Rotated / locked
Muscles: Triceps (all heads), anconeus
Typical Poundage: 5-8 kg dumbbells (women); 8-20 kg dumbbells (men)
Joints: Elbow, wrist, hand

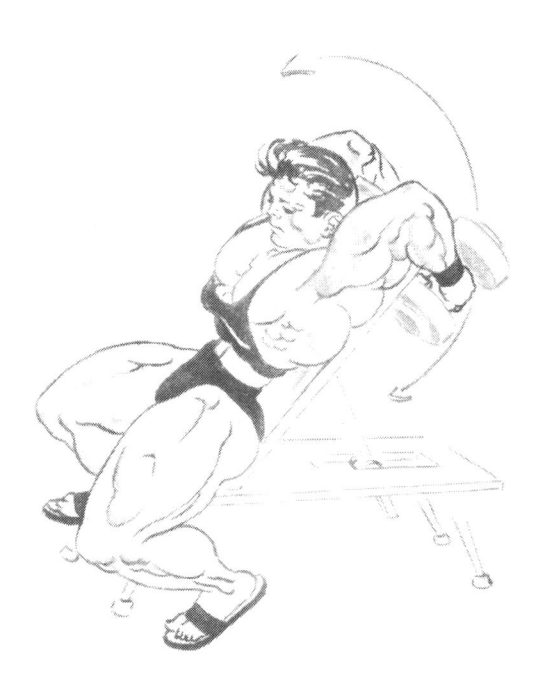

Lie on a bench and position dumbbells over-head with arms extended. Lower dumbbells by bending elbow until they are to sides of head. Extend arm. Repeat. To keep the tension on the triceps, do not lockout at the top, or else once finished immediately perform some close grip presses with the same weight - again in a non-lockout fashion.

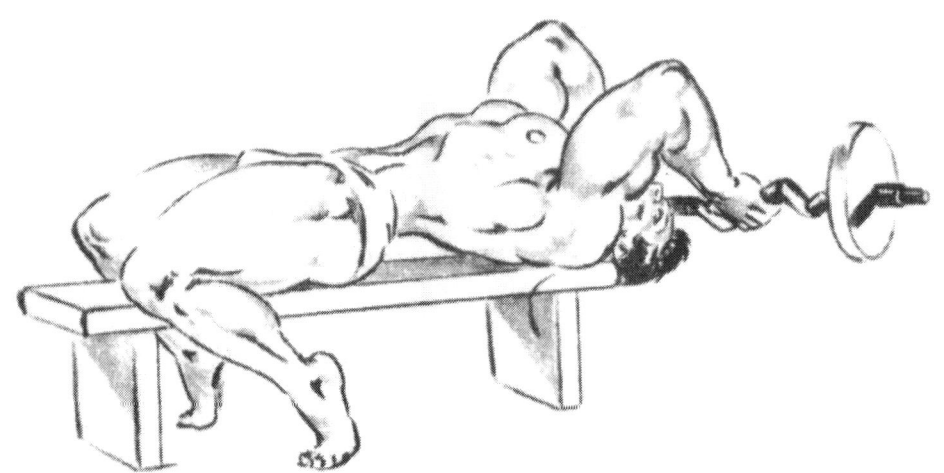

60. Standing Triceps Extensions

Equipment: single dumbbell / barbell
Effect: Strengthen triceps
Resistance : Light / Medium [Slow]
Hip position: N/A
Spine position: N/A
Scapula position: Rotated / locked
Muscles: Triceps (all heads), anconeus
Typical Poundage: 4-8 kg dumbbells (women); 8-15 kg dumbbells (men)
Joints: Elbow, shoulder, wrist, hand

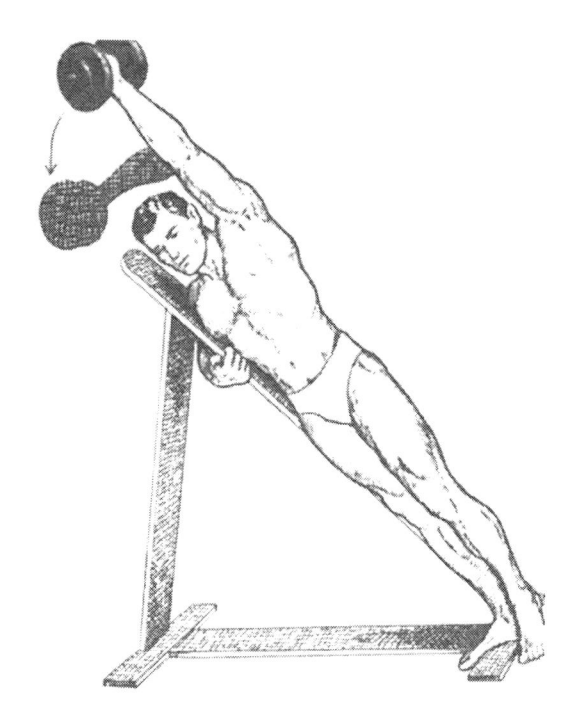

To begin, stand up with a dumbbell held by one hand. Lift it over your head until arm is fully extended. The palm of the hand should be facing up towards the ceiling. This will be your starting position. Keeping your upper arm close to your head with elbow in and perpendicular to the floor, lower the resistance in a semicircular motion behind your head until your forearms touch your biceps. The upper arms should remain stationary and only the forearms should move. Go back to the starting position by using the triceps to raise the dumbbell. Repeat for reps, and with the other arm. Perform any of the versions shown.

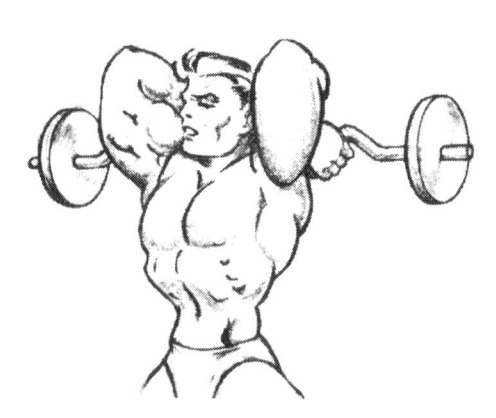

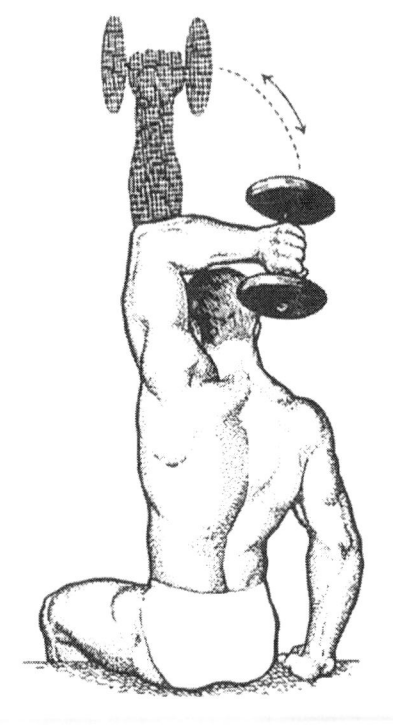

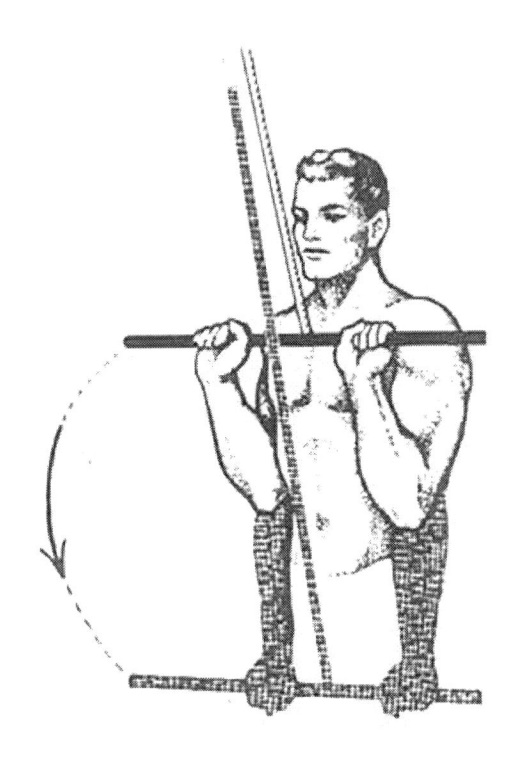

61. Cable Pushdowns

Equipment: cable machine
Effect: Strengthen triceps
Resistance : Light / Medium [Slow]
Hip position: N/A
Spine position: N/A
Scapula position: Neutral / locked
Muscles: Triceps (all heads), anconeus
Typical Poundage: 6-12 kg (women); 12-24 kg (men)
Joints: Elbow, wrist, hand

Face high pulley and grasp cable attachment with overhand narrow grip. Position elbows to side. Extend arms down. Return until forearm is close to upper arm. Repeat. Stay close to cable to provide resistance at top of motion.

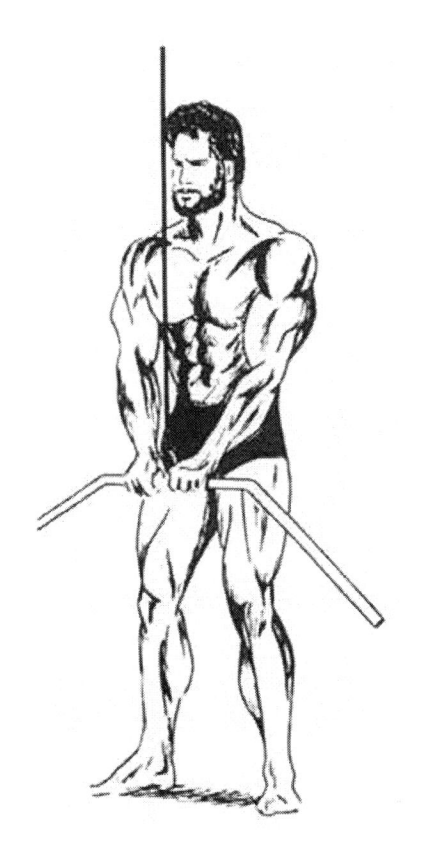

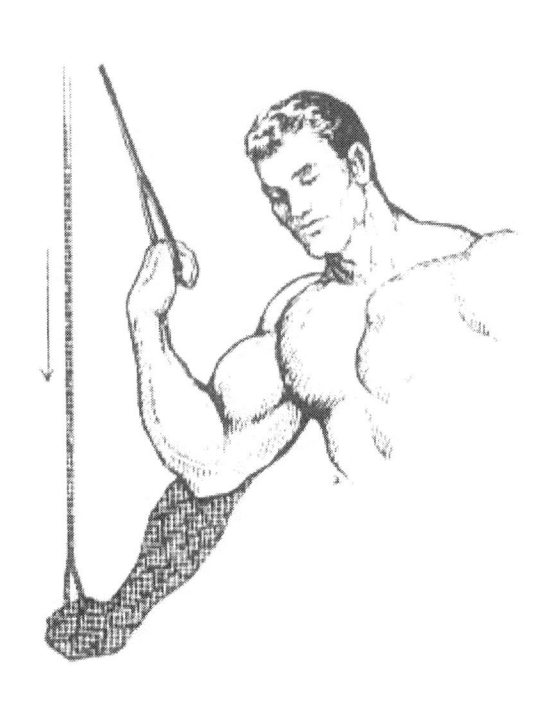

62. Cable Overhead Extensions

Equipment: cable machine
Effect: Strengthen triceps
Resistance : Light / Medium [Slow]
Hip position: N/A
Spine position: Extended / arched
Scapula position: Rotated / locked
Muscles: Triceps (all heads), anconeus, serratus anterior
Typical Poundage: 6-12 kg (women); 12-24 kg (men)
Joints: Elbow, shoulder, wrist, hand

Attach a rope handle to the low pulley of a cable station. Hold at end of the rope in each hand behind your head, with your elbows bent 90 degrees. Stand in a staggered stance, one foot in front of the other, with your back to the weight stack and knees slightly bent. Keeping your back naturally arched, bend at your hips until your torso is nearly parallel to the floor (or stay upright). Without moving your upper arms, push your forearms forward until your elbows are locked, allowing your palms to turn downward as you completely straighten your arms. Pause, then return to the starting position. Repeat for reps. Perform any of the versions shown.

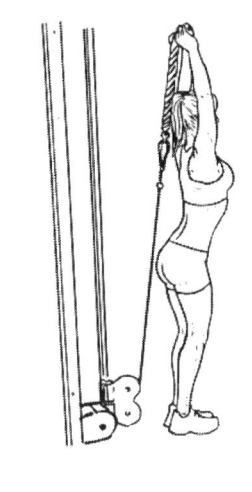

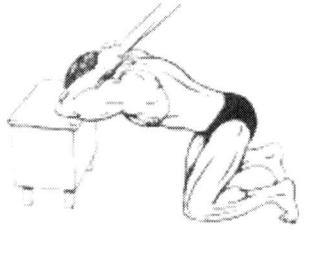

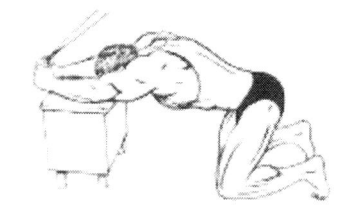

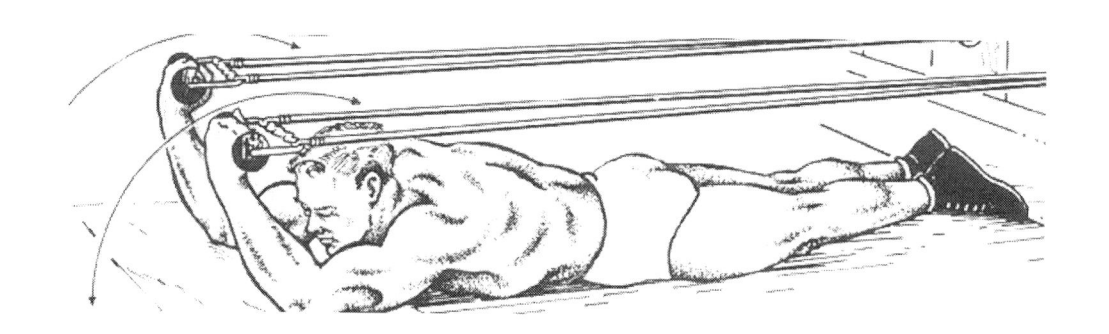

63. Close Grip Bench Press

Equipment: barbell, bench

Effect: Strengthen triceps, chest

Resistance : Light / Medium / Heavy [Slow]

Hip position: N/A

Spine position: N/A

Scapula position: Retracted

Muscles: triceps (all heads), pectoralis major, anterior deltoids

Typical Poundage: 20-50 kg barbell (women); 50-80 kg (men)

Joints: Shoulder, elbow, wrist, hand

This exercise is a superb developer of the triceps muscle. You can use a "reverse grip" as shown below, whereby the hands are reversed on the bar, but remember to wrap the thumbs around the bar as usual for safety. It might be a good idea to do a few partial reps or burns at the end of the movement - whereby you simply perform the top third of the exercise to really pump the triceps. In the old days people used to combine this into a pullover - press exercise for the triceps - where you either do both movements as a single exercise or perform one after the other.

Lie on bench and grasp barbell from rack with shoulder width grip. Lower weight to chest with elbows close to body. Push barbell back up until arms are straight. Repeat. Grip can be slightly narrower than shoulder width but not too close. Too close of a grip can decrease range of motion, plus may tend to hyper-adduct the wrist joint, and unnecessarily decreases the stability of bar. Use overhand or underhand grip.

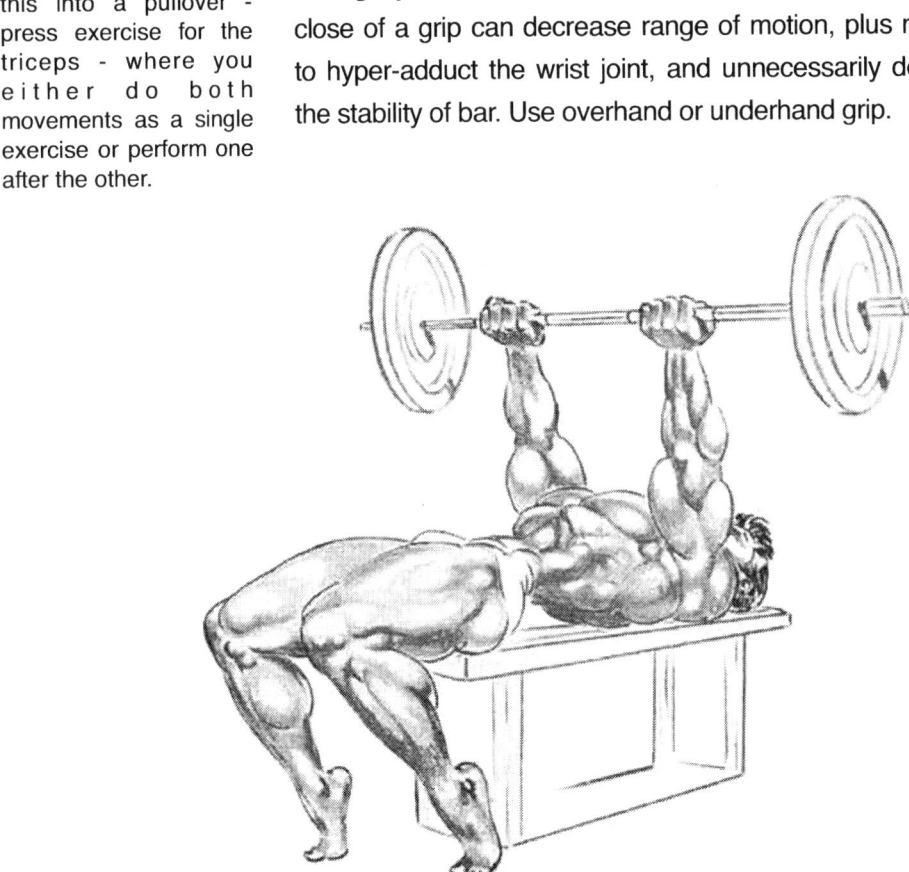

64. Press Up

Equipment: None
Effect: Strengthen chest, shoulders, triceps
Resistance : Light / Medium / Heavy [Slow / Medium]
Hip position: N/A
Spine position: N/A
Scapula position: The scapulae should retract and slightly inwardly rotate (depending on how wide the hands are placed apart) on the down phase of the push-up. As the arms push away from the body, the scapulae should protract and slightly outwardly rotate.
Muscles: triceps (all heads), pectoralis major, anterior deltoids
Typical Poundage: 5-10 kg (women); 10-20 kg (men)
Joints: Shoulder, elbow, wrist, hand

Lie face down on the floor with your palms at shoulder level, fingers pointing forward. Push yourself up until your body weight rests only on your palms and toes. Lower yourself and repeat. To accent the chest, place your hands wider than shoulder-width; to target the back and triceps, bring your hands close together with the thumbs and index fingers touching.

This exercise is great because it requires no equipment and can be performed anywhere. When you place your feet up higher than the body then press-ups become more difficult - also you can try using just one arm if you get really strong. Close/wide grip is another way to vary the resistance and to stave off boredom.

Note that we give no direct exercises for the trapezius muscle in this book (i.e. we do not recommend shrugging motions). This is because we think that the "traps" receive sufficient stimulation from all of the other moves; and furthermore we do not believe in over-developing the trapezius which detracts from a pleasing shoulder shape/ symmetry.

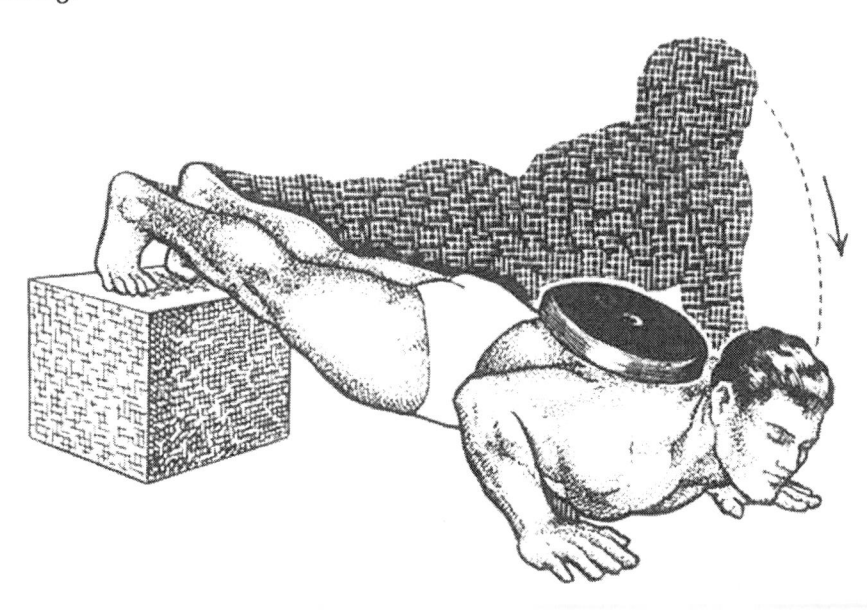

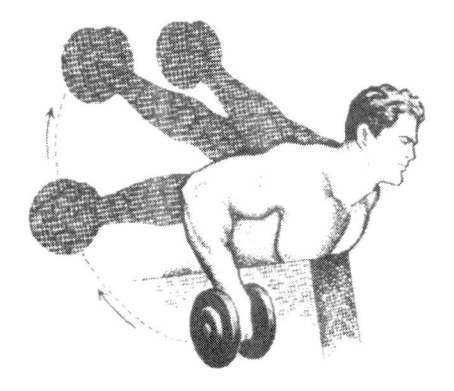

65. Bent Over / Lying Forearm Extension - Triceps Extension

Equipment: dumbbell
Effect: Strengthen triceps (both movements)
Resistance : Light / Medium [Slow]
Hip position: Flexed (fixed)
Spine position: N/A
Scapula position: Neutral / locked
Muscles: Triceps (all heads), anconeus
Typical Poundage: 4-8 kg (women); 8-12 kg (men)
Joints: Elbow, wrist, hand

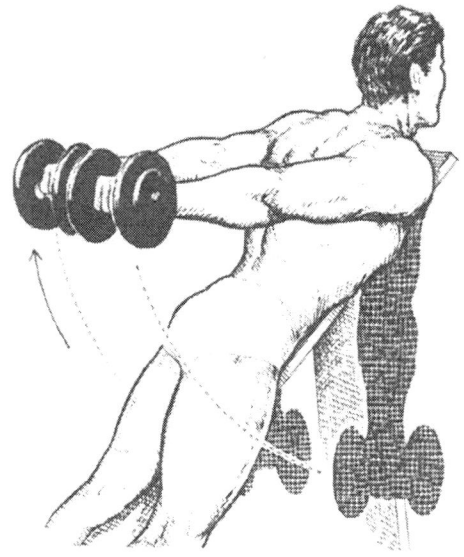

Two different exercises. Firstly the triceps extension. Bend end over at the waist, and lock the elbow into a position next to your hip. Raise and lower the dumbbell (to the rear) by moving only the forearm. Hold at the top for a few seconds to increase the tension on the triceps. In the forearm extension exercise you keep the arm straight and elbow locked and "pulse" the arm backwards and forwards.

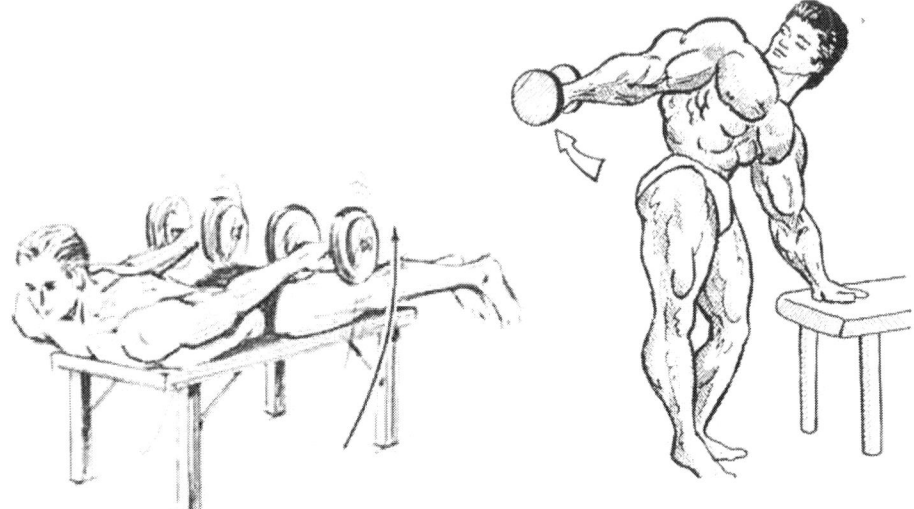

66. Bench Dips

Equipment: bench, weight
Effect: Strengthen triceps
Resistance : Light / Medium [Slow]
Hip position: N/A
Spine position: N/A
Scapula position: Neutral / locked
Muscles: Triceps (all heads), anconeus, pectoralis major
Typical Poundage: 5-10 kg (women); 10-20 kg (men)
Joints: Elbow, shoulder, wrist, hand

Sit on the inside of one of two benches placed parallel, slightly less than leg's length away. Place hands on edge of bench, straighten arms, slide rear end off of bench, and position heels on adjacent bench with legs straight. Lower body by bending arms until slight stretch is felt in chest or shoulder, or rear end touches floor. Raise body and repeat.

Bench dips are another great exercise for the triceps, and normally you want to put extra weight on your thighs or else around the neck to make the movement more effective. Once again you can try performing a few partial reps or burns at the end of the set to really pump the triceps. This movement works well when combined with some form of triceps extension in a superset fashion.

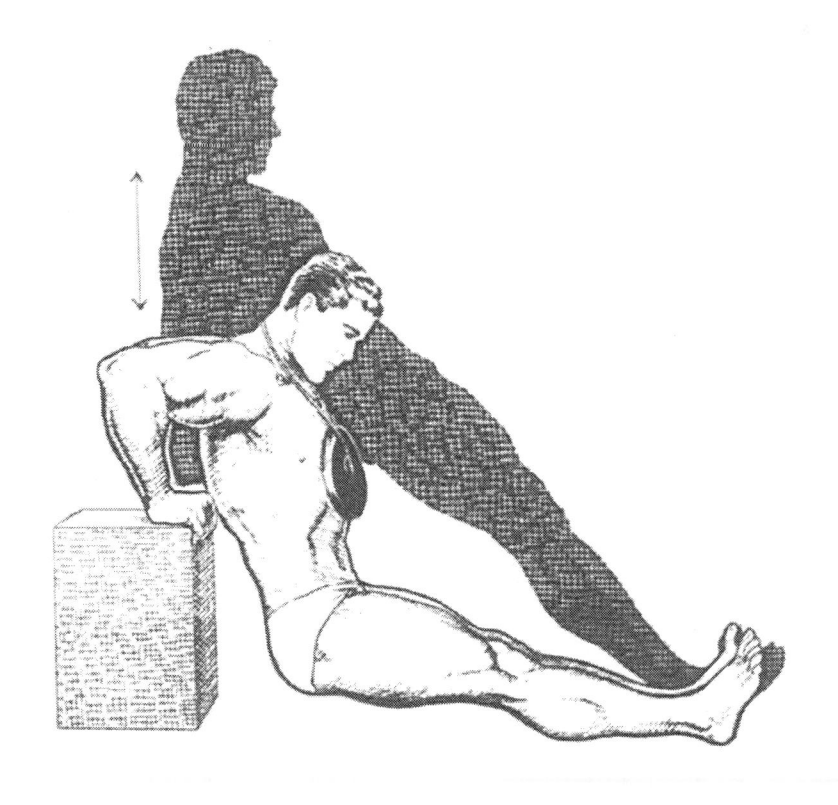

226 ZEN OF DUMBBELL TRAINING

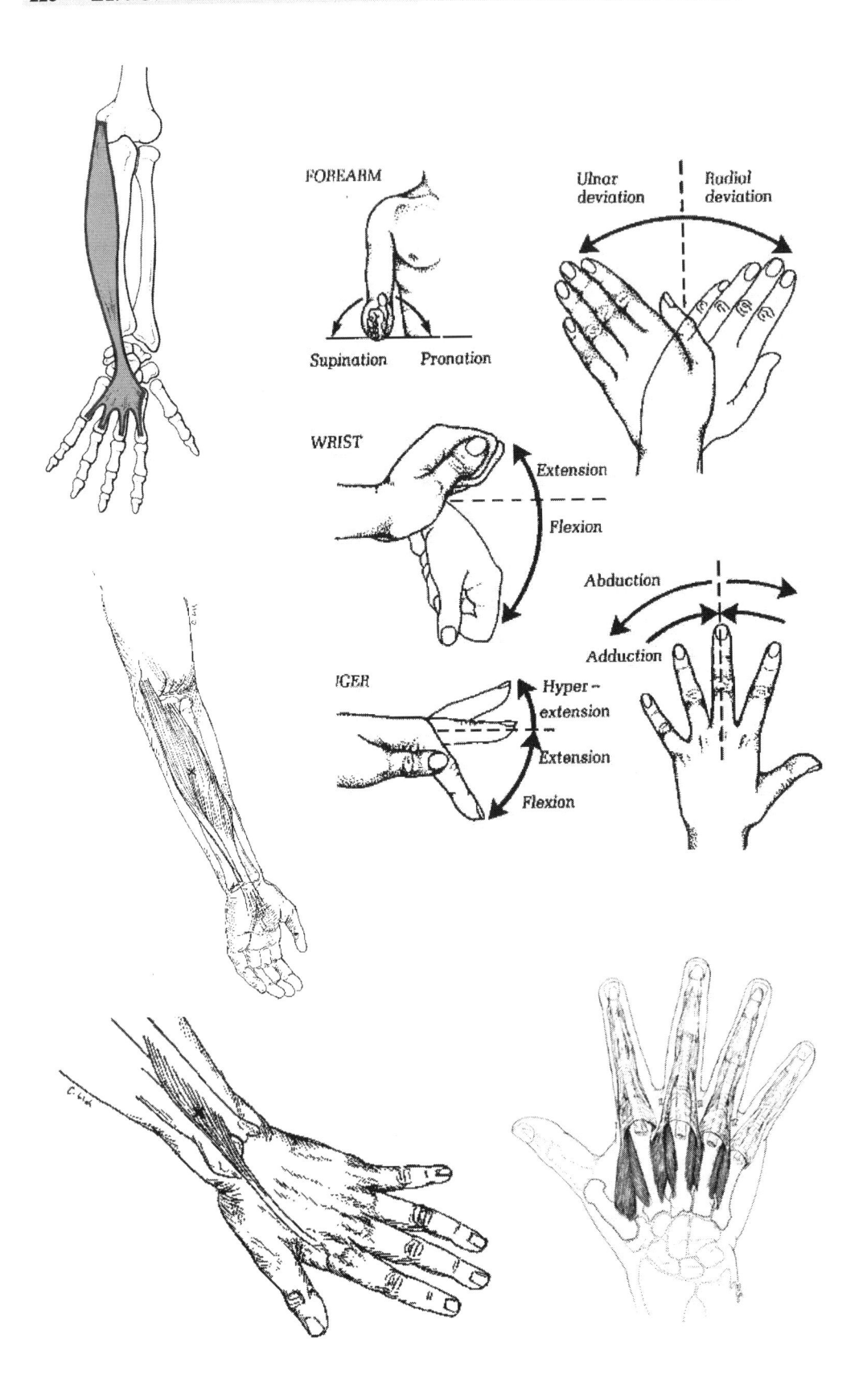

FOREARM

Supination — Pronation

Ulnar deviation — Radial deviation

WRIST

Extension / Flexion

Abduction / Adduction

FINGER

Hyper-extension / Extension / Flexion

CHAPTER TEN

The Wrist and Hand

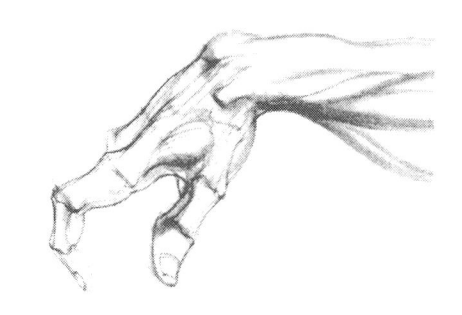

THE HAND, located at the extremity of the upper body, is a versatile tool. This is due to the enormous mobility of the fingers, which are equipped with a complex system of tendons (connecting bone to muscle). The other factor contributing to the hands versatility is the arrangement of the thumb with respect to the fingers. The opposable thumb makes it possible to grasp objects and to accomplish many different tasks.

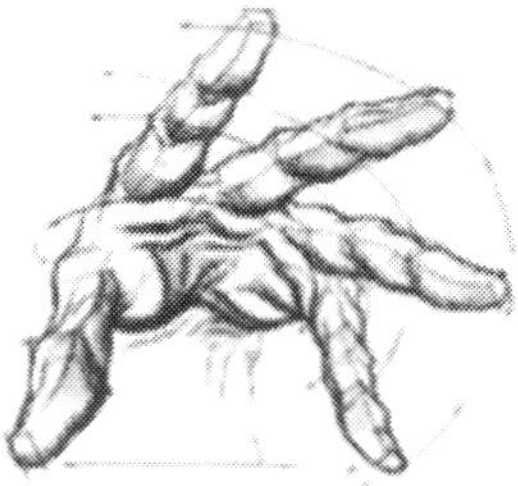

The hand is linked to the forearm via the carpel bones, which form the area of the wrist. Despite the complexity of the wrist and hand, we are able to exercise the region using a relatively small number of movements. And it is important to note that the hand and forearm are naturally exercised every time we pick up and/or grip a heavy object. Therefore just using reasonably heavy weights (i.e. dumbbells) can result in sufficient hand development (and strength) in some individuals. Despite these facts, many want to develop the hands and wrist region to a higher degree of strength, endurance and also flexibility, and to obtain the same often special exercises are required as described in this section.

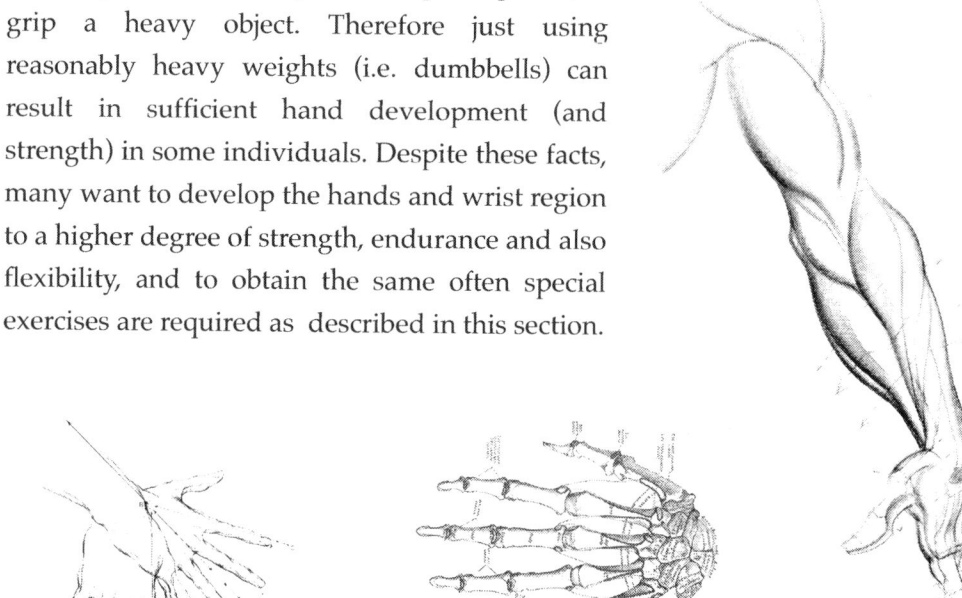

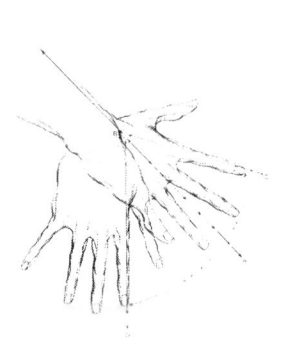

228 ZEN OF DUMBBELL TRAINING

FLEXION and EXTENSION

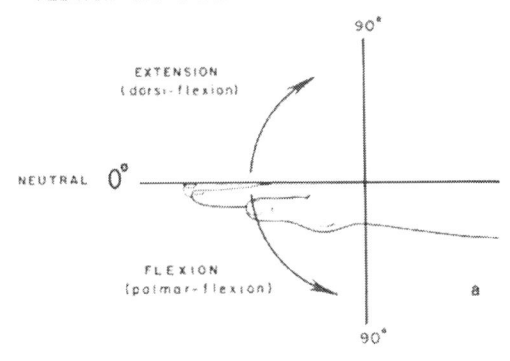

NEUTRAL 0°

EXTENSION (dorsi-flexion)

FLEXION (palmar-flexion)

90°

a

RADIAL and ULNAR DEVIATION

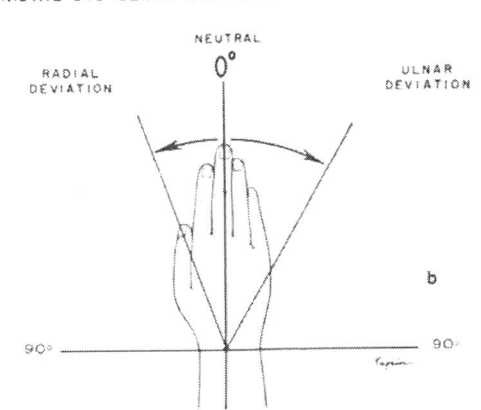

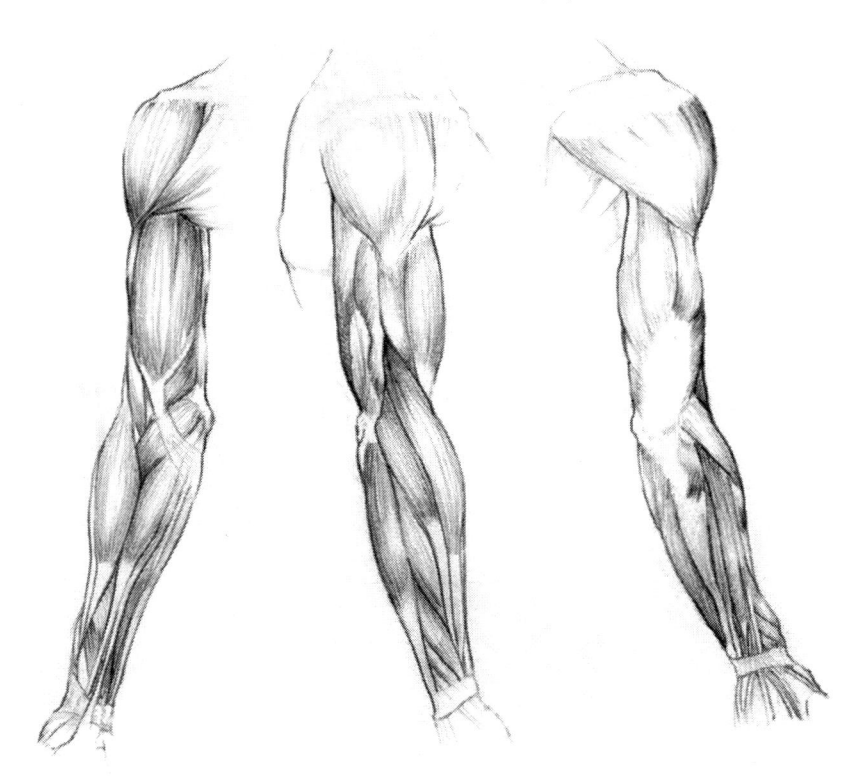

NEUTRAL 0°

RADIAL DEVIATION

ULNAR DEVIATION

90°

b

When we think about ROM of the hand and wrist, we sometimes presume that most people have similar capabilities in this respect. However just as some people have stronger hands and wrists, so people vary in the range of movements possible with their own hands. In particular, arthritis can weaken muscles and degrade ROM in these areas; and in such cases exercises are recommended.

It seems however that few trainees bother to train the forearm muscle(s) to any major degree, and most do not train them at-all. This seems strange when you consider that the forearm and hand muscles are quite easy to develop, and once developed they tend to remain strong throughout life. Plus only a few simple-to-perform exercises are required to develop this area, although these movements are often painful to perform (in a good way).

That said, gaining truly extra-ordinary development of the forearm and hand muscles is difficult and takes significant effort and dedication.

Strong hands are a prerequisite for lifting heavy weights in many movements such as the dead-lift and barbell clean. In fact the simple task of using heavy weights in general will develop stronger hands than average.

But perhaps one of the best ways to develop the hand and forearm muscles is to lift using barbells and dumbbells with very thick handles, and here around 2 inches in diameter seems to be best. Of coarse not everyone has access to such dumbbells, but it may be a good idea to get yourself some think handled adjustable dumbbells if super-strong hands and forearms is a major goal.

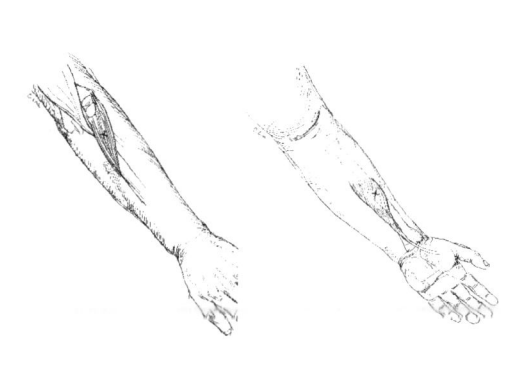

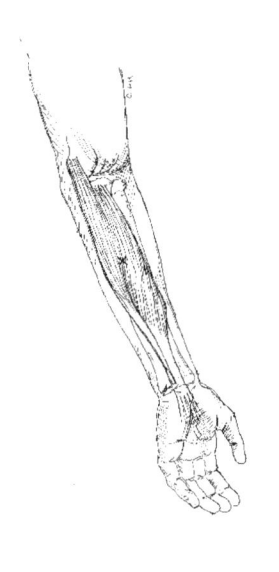

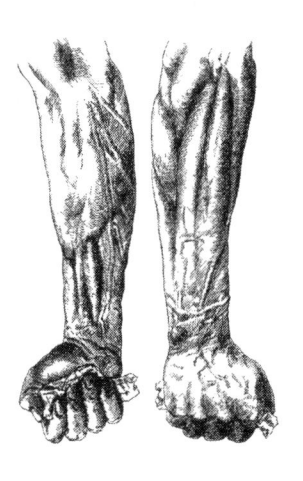

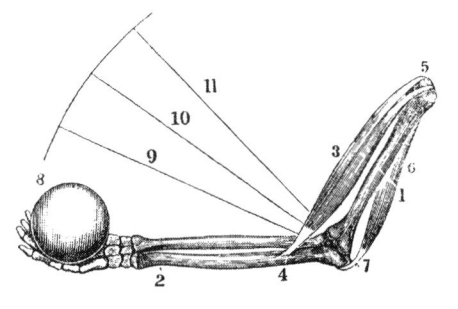

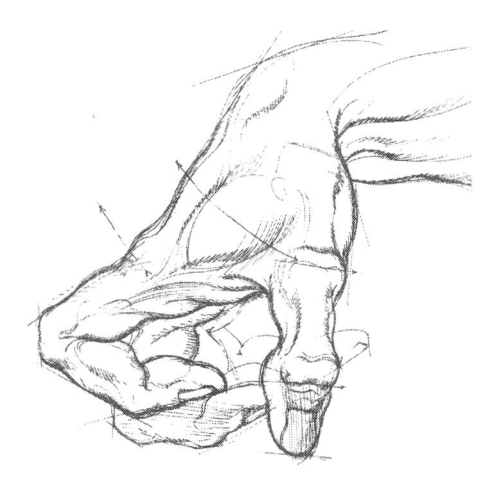

Wrist and Hand Joint(s) - Exercises

67. Seated Wrist Curl
68. Overhand Wrist Extension
69. Thick-Handled Dumbbell Dead-lift (2 inch diameter handle)
70. Thick-Handled Dumbbell Clean / Swing
71. Wrist-Roller
72. Gripper Machine

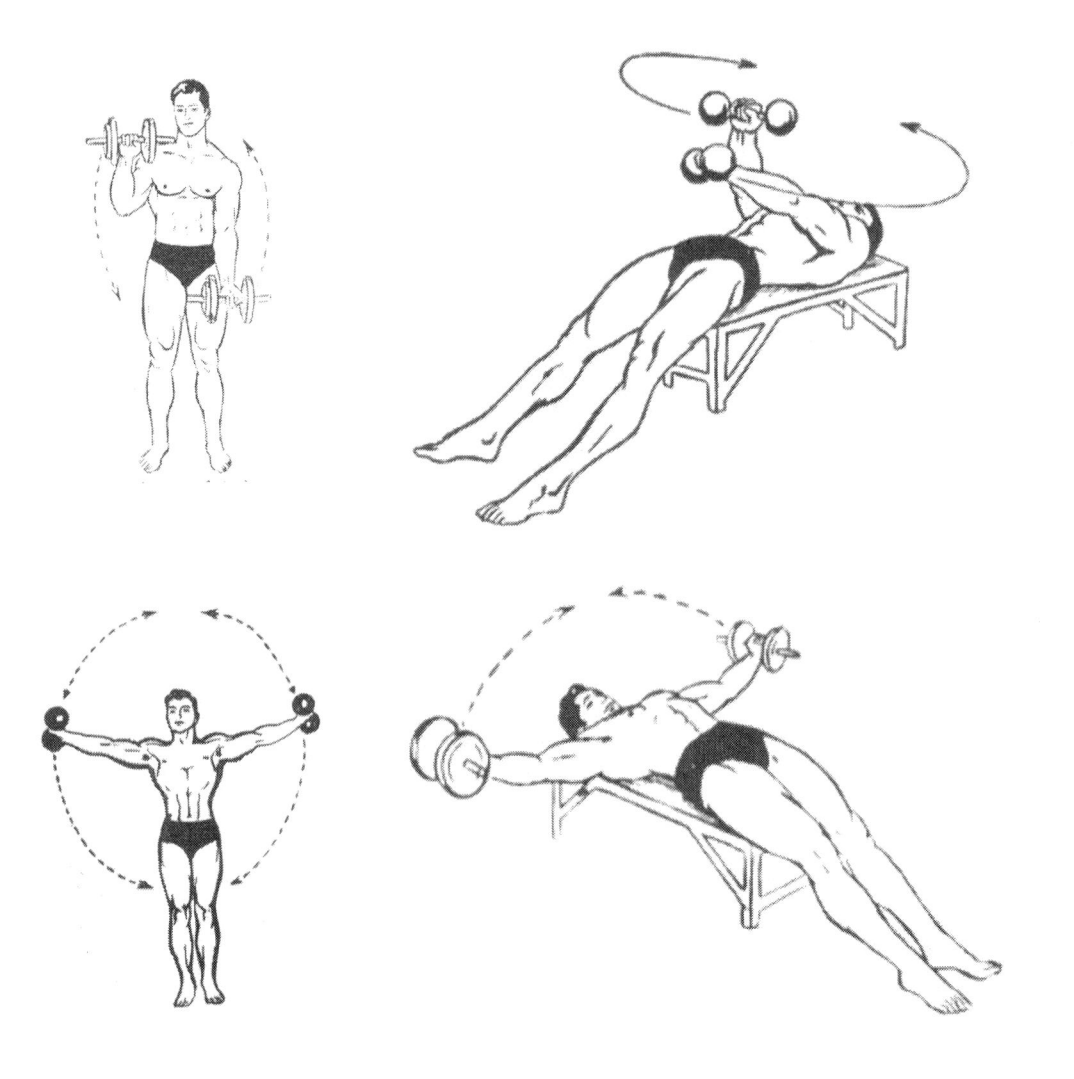

67. Seated Wrist Curl

Equipment: twin dumbbells / barbell
Effect: Strengthen wrist, forearm flexors
Resistance : Light / Medium / Heavy [Slow]
Hip position: N/A
Spine position: N/A
Scapula position: N/A
Muscles: Forearm flexors
Typical Poundage: 10-20 kg barbell (women); 40-60 kg (men) (some strongmen use up to 100 kg to build 15 -16 inch forearms!)
Joints: Wrist, hand

Sit and grasp a dumbbell with an underhand grip. Rest forearm on thigh / bench with wrist just beyond knee. Allow the wrist to "unwrap or extend" the dumbbell downwards, then to roll out of the palm down to finger-tips at bottom. Raise dumbbell back up by rolling bar back up the finger-tips and then flex wrist back up by gripping, flexing wrist and pointing the knuckles up as high as possible. Lower and repeat.

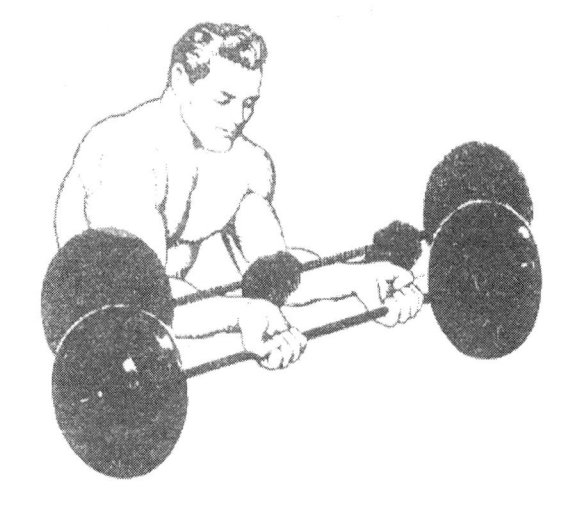

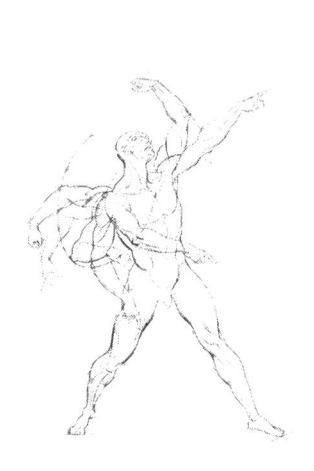

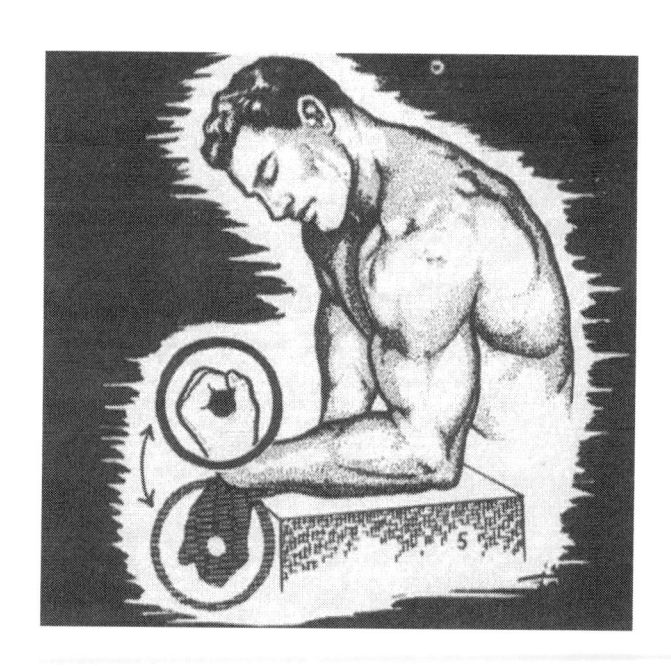

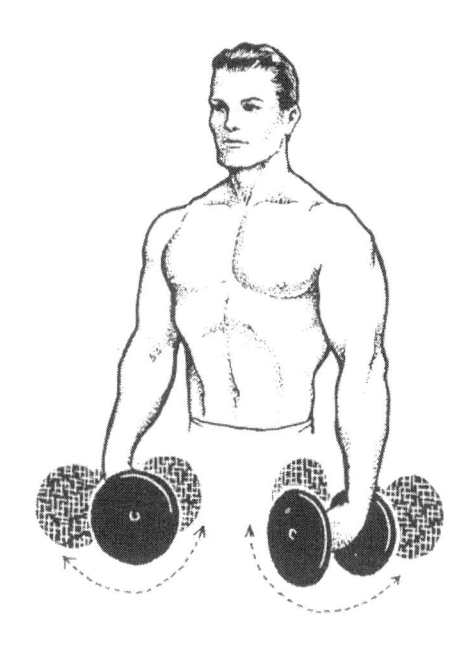

68. Overhand Wrist Extension

Equipment: twin dumbbells / barbell
Effect: Forearm extensors
Resistance : Light / Medium / Heavy [Slow]
Hip position: N/A
Spine position: N/A
Scapula position: N/A
Muscles: Forearm extensors
Typical Poundage: 5-8 kg dumbbells (women); 8-12 kg dumbbells (men)
Joints: Wrist, hand

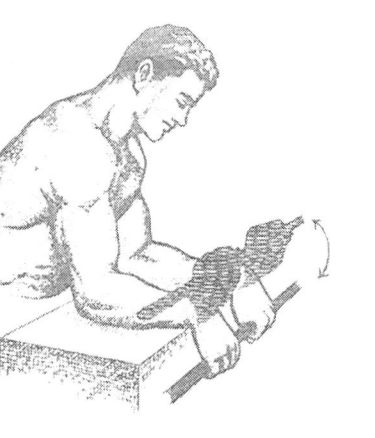

Sit and grip dumbbell with an overhand grip. Rest forearm on thigh with wrist just beyond knee. Raise dumbbell by pointing knuckles upward as high as possible. Return until knuckles are pointing downwards as far as possible. Repeat. This movement can be combined with wrist curls as above.

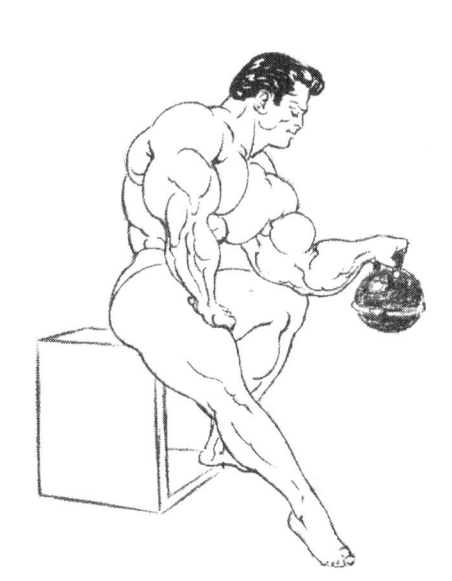

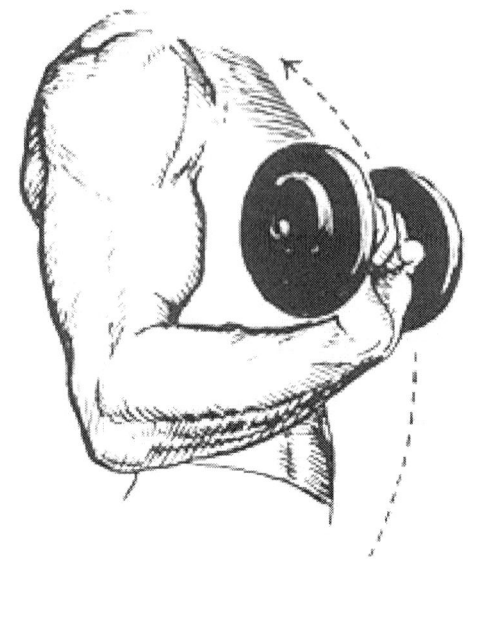

69. Thick-Handled Dead-lift

Equipment: twin dumbbells / barbell
Effect: Strengthen wrist, forearm flexors
Resistance : Light / Medium / Heavy [Slow]
Hip position: Flexion (light)
Spine position: Arched lumbar (extension)
Scapula position: N/A
Muscles: Forearm flexors
Typical Poundage: 8-12 kg dumbbells (women); 20-40 kg dumbbells (men)
Joints: Wrist, hand

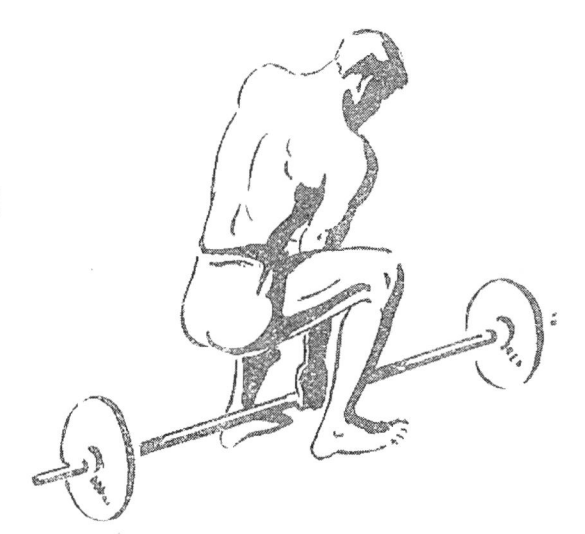

Load up a thick-handled (2 inches diameter or more) dumbbell with weights, and simply dead-lift off the floor and hold for 1-2 minutes or more.

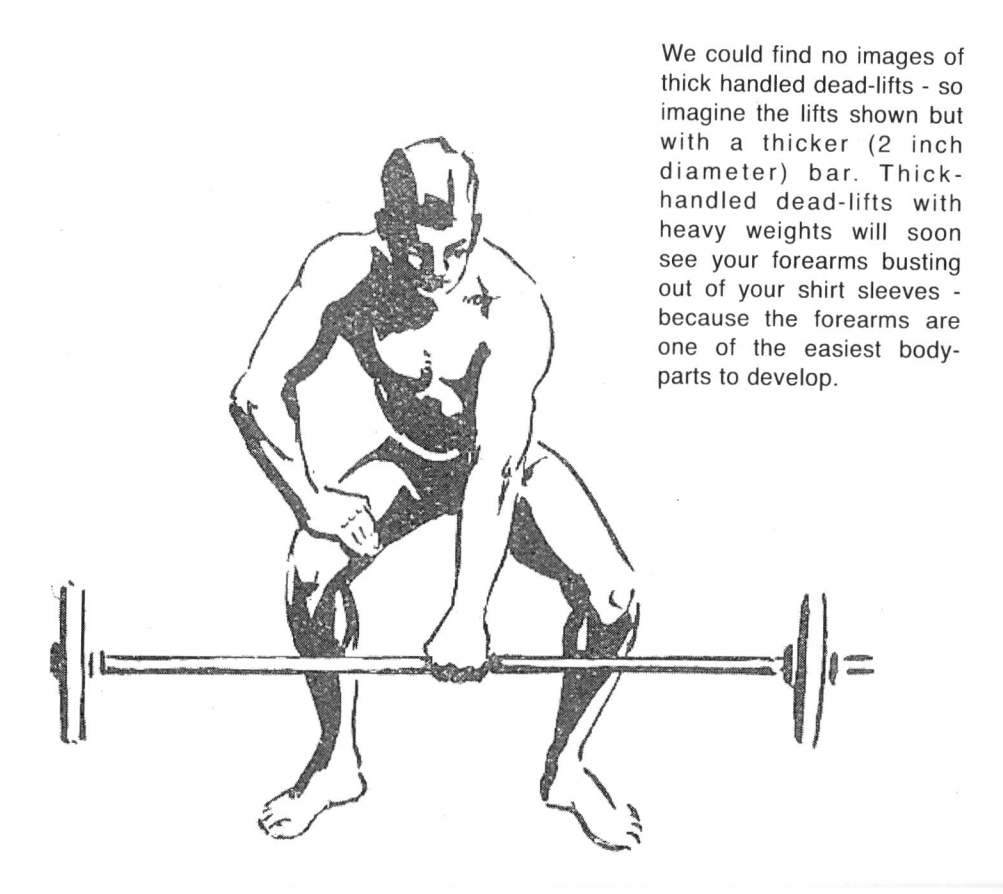

We could find no images of thick handled dead-lifts - so imagine the lifts shown but with a thicker (2 inch diameter) bar. Thick-handled dead-lifts with heavy weights will soon see your forearms busting out of your shirt sleeves - because the forearms are one of the easiest body-parts to develop.

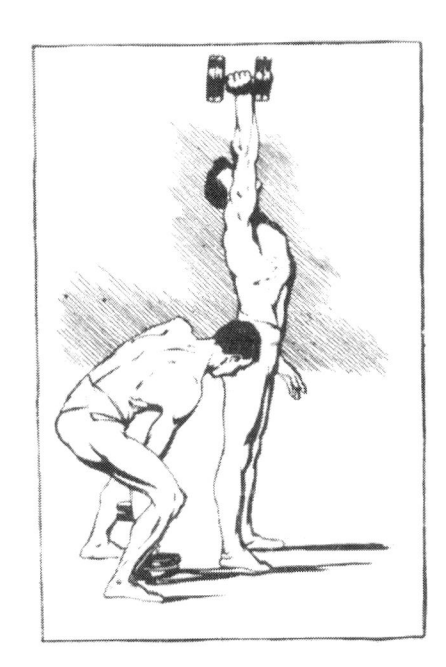

70. Thick-Handled Dumbbell Clean / Swing

Equipment: twin dumbbells / barbell
Effect: Strengthen wrist, forearm flexors
Resistance : Light / Medium / Heavy [Fast]
Hip position: Flexion (light)
Spine position: Arched lumbar (Extension)
Scapula position: N/A
Muscles: Forearm flexors
Typical Poundage: 8-12 kg dumbbells (women); 20-30 kg dumbbells (men)
Joints: Wrist, elbow, hand

Load up a thick-handled (2 inches diameter) dumbbell with weights, and simply quickly clean the weight off the floor (and up to the shoulder). When you "drop" the dumbbell rapidly back to the floor, catch it with a firm grip contraction and do not let it actually touch the floor. This contraction will greatly work the gripping muscles. Can also use a barbell (thick-handle also).

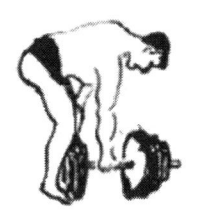

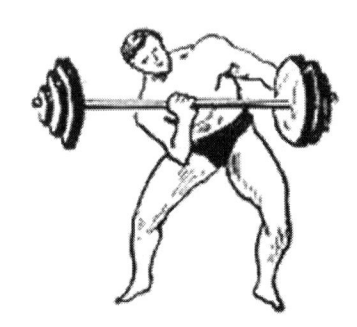

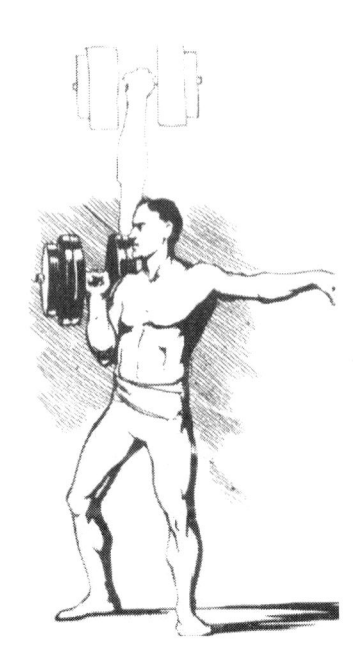

71. Wrist Roller

Equipment: twin dumbbells / barbell
Effect: Strengthen wrist, forearm flexors / extensors
Resistance : Light / Medium / Heavy
[Slow] - best with thick-handled roller
Hip position: N/A
Spine position: N/A
Scapula position: Neutral
Muscles: Forearm flexors + extensors
Typical Poundage: 6-10 kg dumbbells (women); 10-30 kg (men)
Joints: Wrist, hand

Grasp the wrist roller handle with both hands; using an over hand grip. With left hand gripping handle, relax grip of right hand and slide grip behind handle, and re-grip. Relax grip of left hand and flex right wrist. Repeat sequence with opposite hands, alternating back and forth until the weight plate has raised up near hands. Lower weight steadily with opposite movement.

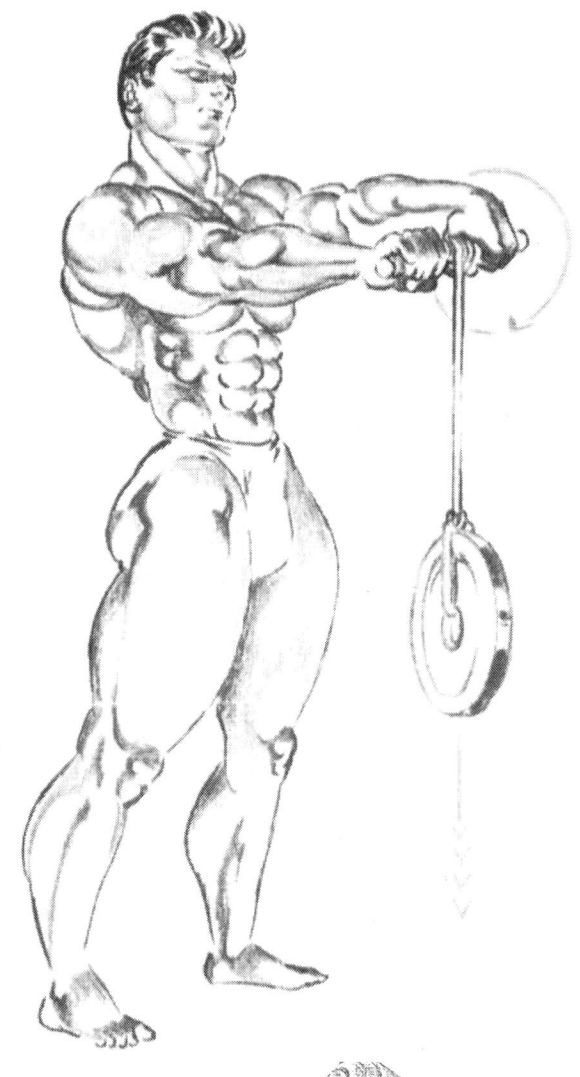

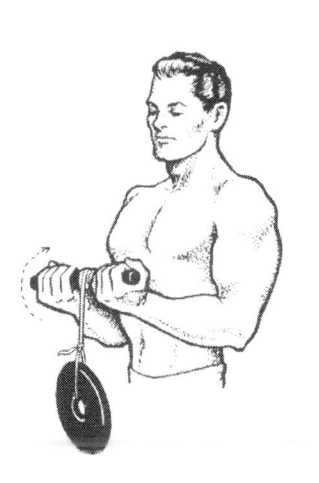

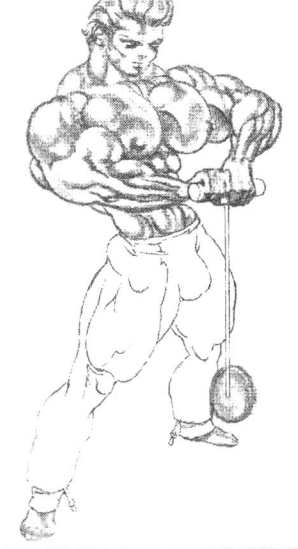

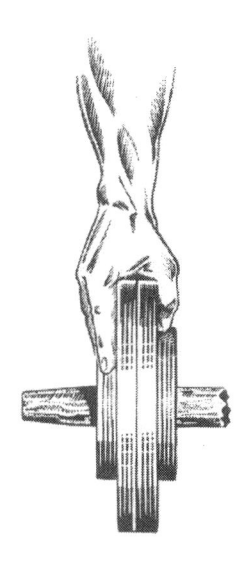

72. Gripper Machine

Equipment: Grip Machine
Effect: Strengthen wrist, forearm flexors
Resistance : Light / Medium / Heavy [Slow]
Hip position: N/A
Spine position: N/A
Scapula position: N/A
Muscles: Forearm flexors
Typical Poundage: 8-12 kg (women); 20-40 kg (men)
Joints: Wrist, hand and fingers

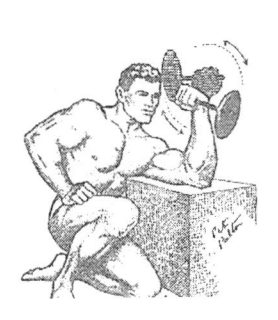

Load up machine with weights, and then work your crushing grip by closing the handles together. By the way I would avoid - and never use wrist straps on any exercise (including dead-lifts). It is far batter to simply grip the heaviest barbells that you can with gripping power alone - your gripping strength will improve naturally as a result. I used to dead-lift 700 lbs without wrist straps - and my hands and forearms were well-muscled as a result of the same. We could find no images of a forearm machine in action - and so instead we show images of hand circles / twists, leverage bars etc.

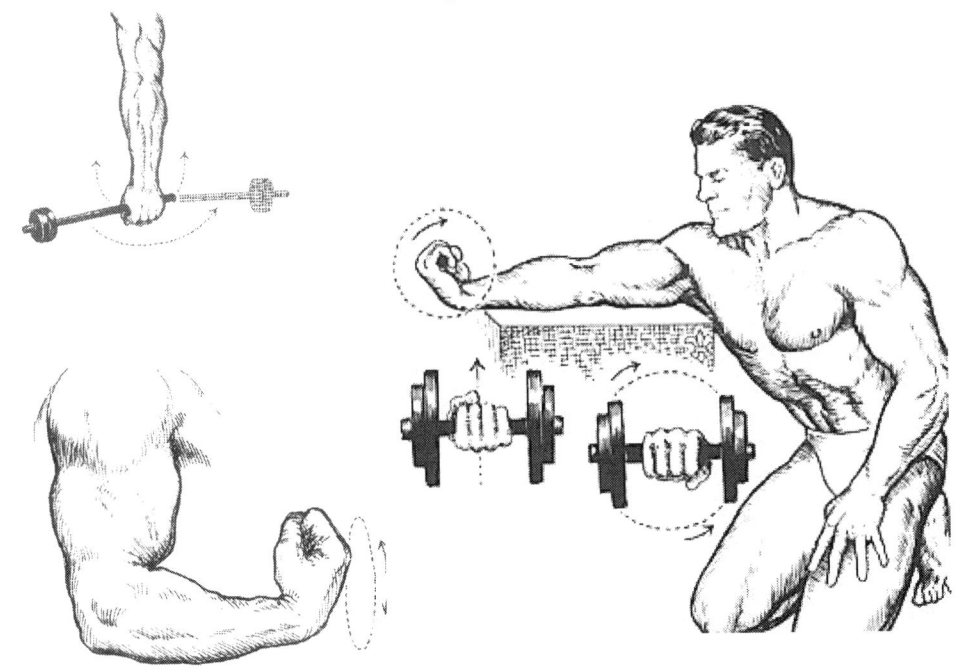

THE WRIST AND HAND 237

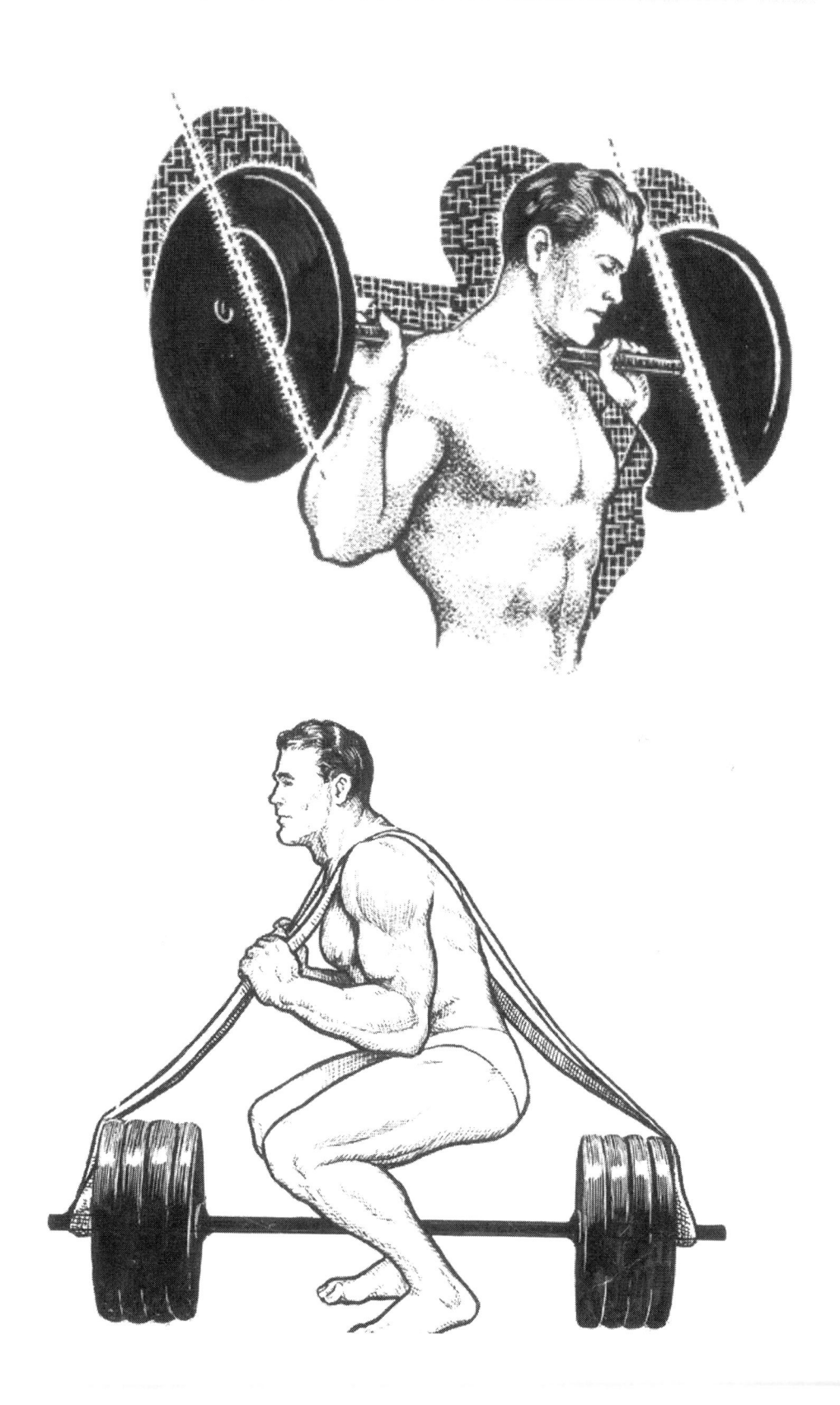

ROM Training

You will notice that we have recommended ROM training (largely) for the shoulder and hip joints - and that we have ignored most of the other joints of the human body (apart from the spine) in this respect. We have done so for a specific reason. The shoulder and hip joints are of the ball-and-socket type - and have a very wide range-of-motions as a result. Both of these joints can move in a variety of ways. Thus ROM training is appropriate because we want to maximise the flexibility potential of these joints. Note that ROM training with weights does of-course improve the strength and stability of these joints; only we label it ROM training to distinguish it from pure strength training. One would not normally want to perform ROM training for pivot/rotating and/or hinge joints such as the elbow, knee or ankle because these joints have limited ROMs. Be careful with ROM training; if performed incorrectly it could damage your joints. Therefore use very light weights and progress in a slow and steady manner.

PREVIOUSLY WE spoke about the dual purpose of weight training; being to produce either range of motion (ROM) improvements and/or strength improvements in terms of the various movements of the human body. Throughout this book we have labelled exercises as being in the ROM and/or strength category; and we have recommended that you treat (and so perform) exercises that are exclusively in one or the other category differently. In particular it is recommended that you use very light weights for ROM exercises, and leave plenty of "freedom" in the movement arc itself for the body to adjust and/or experiment with multiple 3D movement patterns. We recommend that you perform such ROM exercises by experimenting with multiple paths, and to explore very wide ROMs, pauses, static holds, end-of-movement pulses, extreme stretches, circles etc. Also try twisting the dumbbells in various ways, and use your instincts to tell you which weights to use and how to use them. If an exercise is labelled as both strength and ROM, then perform it in two distinct styles, one (strength style) being heavier and in a more fixed movement path and the other in a free movement fashion (ROM style). Strength training relies more on finding a single perfect "groove" that you use every time you lift and in order to maximise skill and strength potential, whereas ROM training is all about exploring movement limitations. I would recommend that you might like to have an entirely separate ROM style workout that you can perform on a daily basis (perhaps on rising first for 15-20 minutes).

The question arises as to how to know (whilst exercising in a ROM fashion) when you are approaching a dangerous over-stretched position at which point the joint may become unstable and be injured? To start with move slowly (always) and stop when you begin to feel a natural movement limitation. For safety perform all movements without bouncing (slow and controlled) - and even end-of-movement pulses should be fairly slow. Put your faith in your own feelings and in bio-feedback - listen to the body at all times.

CHAPTER ELEVEN

The Hip and Knee

THE HIP is the region between the torso and lower limbs, and it connects the femur to the pelvis. The stability and powerful musculature of this joint are essential for standing and walking. Many physical disciplines require good range of motion (ROM) at the hip.

The knee, an intermediate joint on the lower limb, is primarily capable of flexion and extension. Its mobility allows it to vary the distance between the foot and the trunk. Its stability is not due to bone structure, which is rather weak, but rather to the arrangement of ligaments and muscles. The knee receives considerable stress, both from above (body weight) and from below (impact of foot on the ground).

The hip joint can move in many directions. In flexion the angle between the anterior surfaces of the thigh and trunk decreases. ROM for hip flexion is greater when the knee is also flexed. When the knee is extended, hip flexion is restricted by the hamstring muscles, and ROM is reduced.

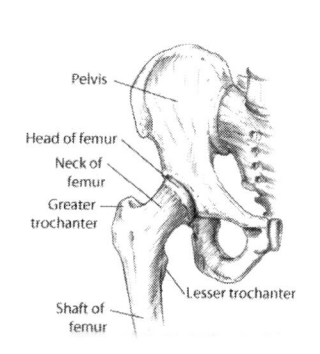

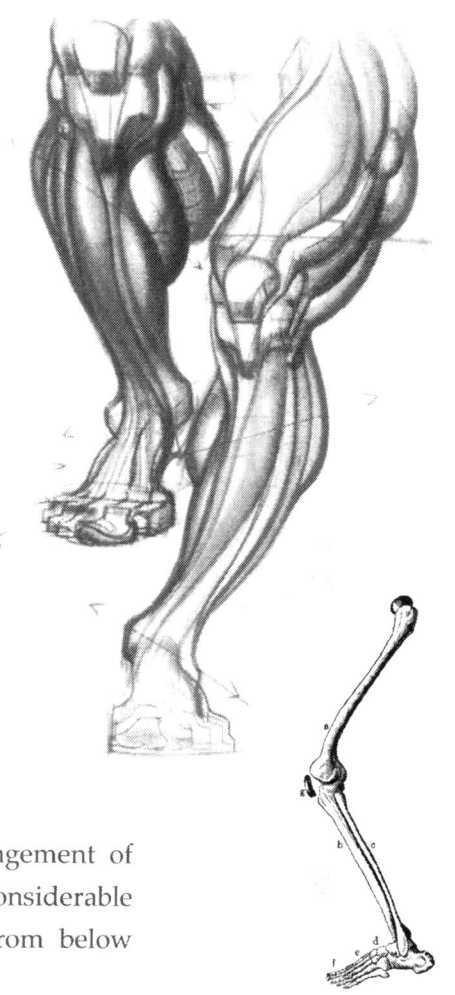

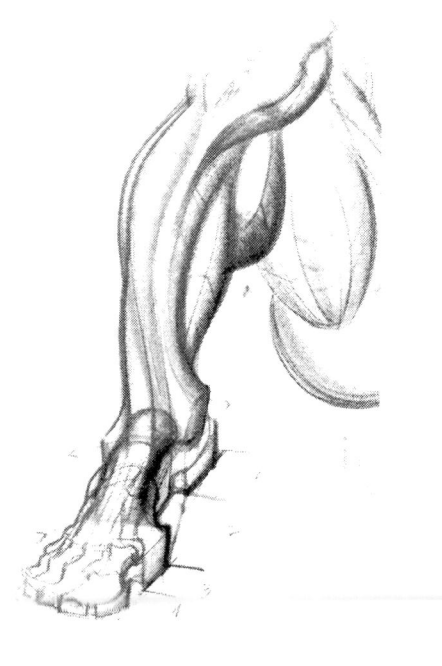

240 ZEN OF DUMBBELL TRAINING

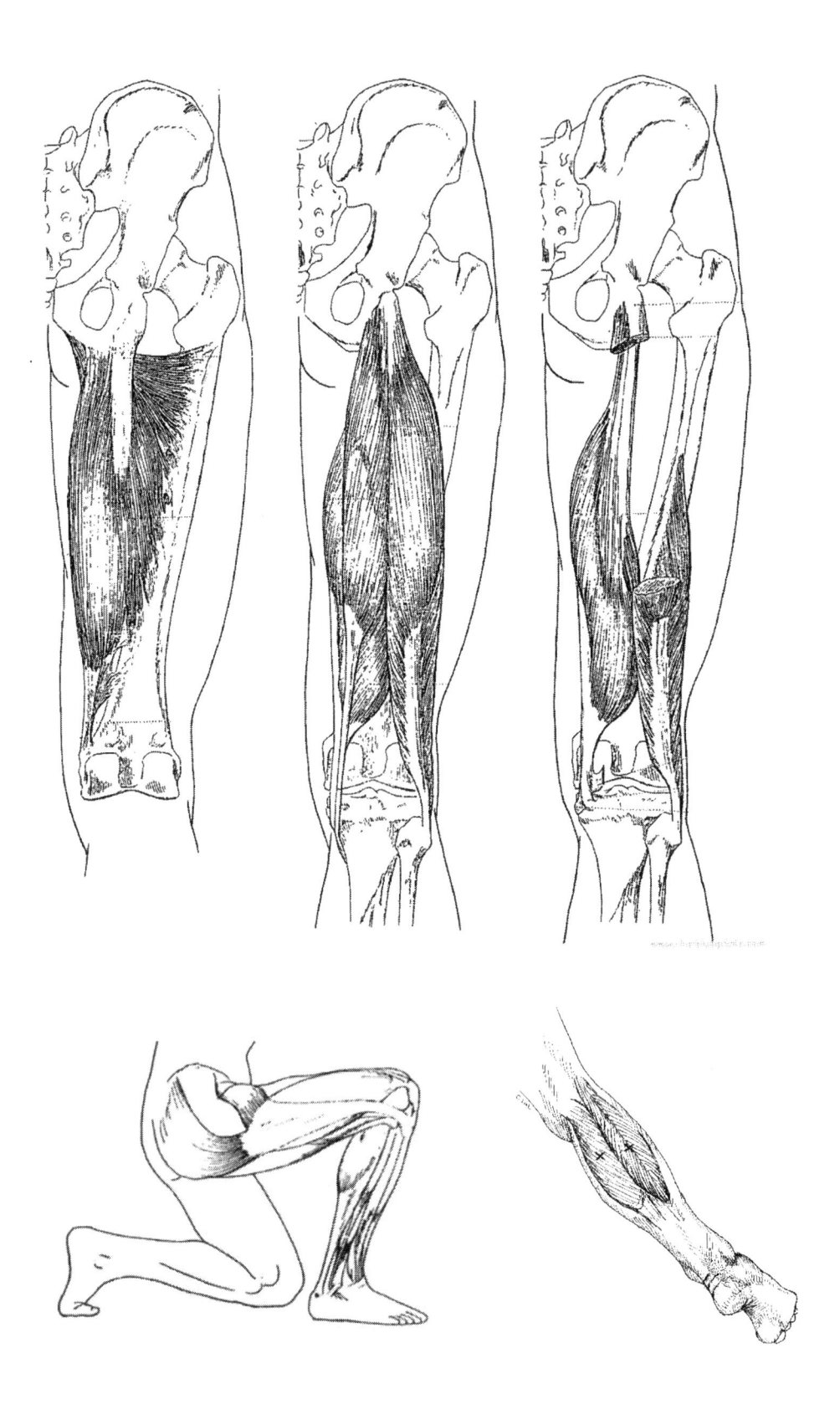

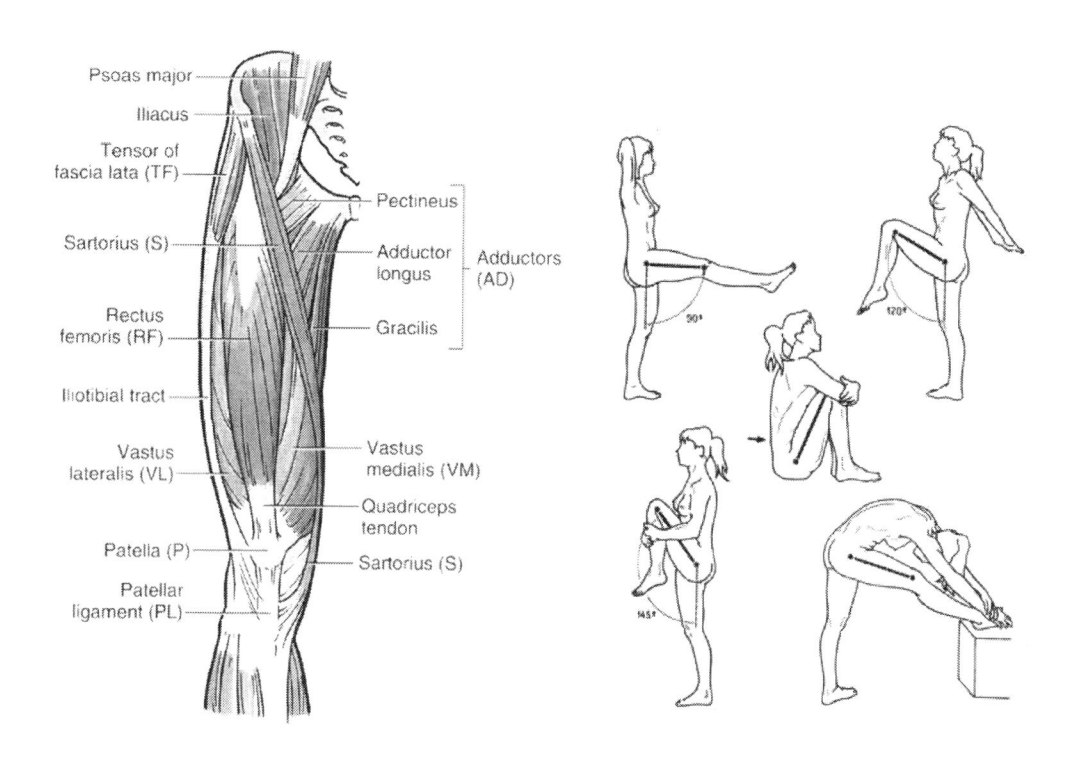

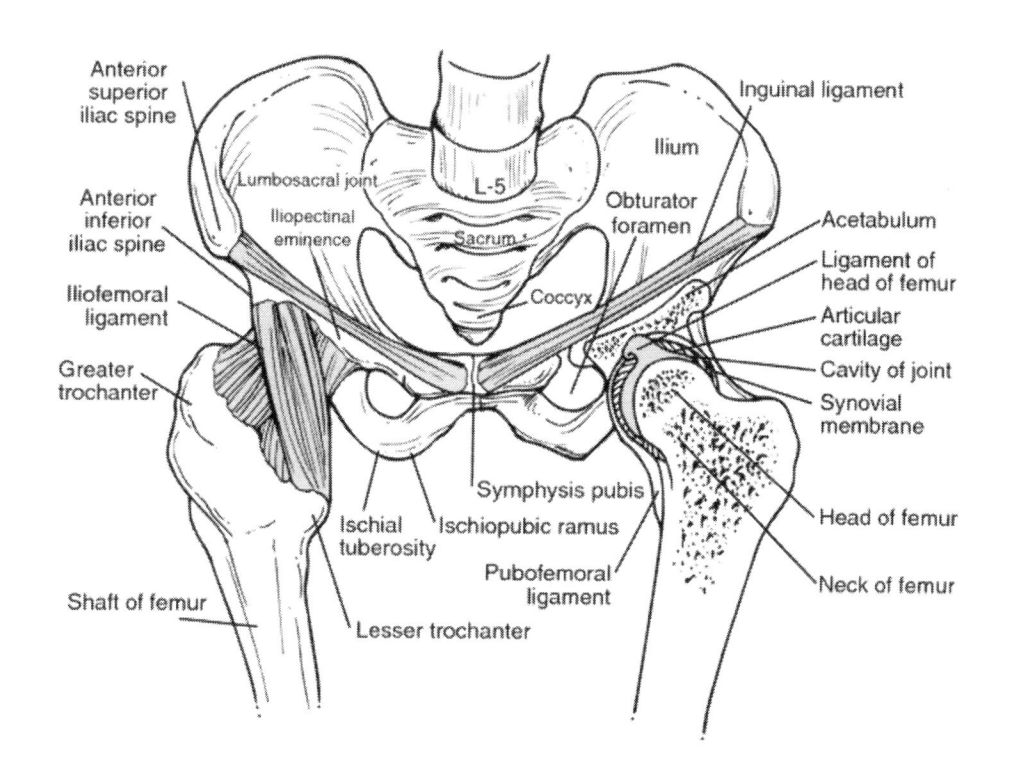

THE HIP AND KNEE 241

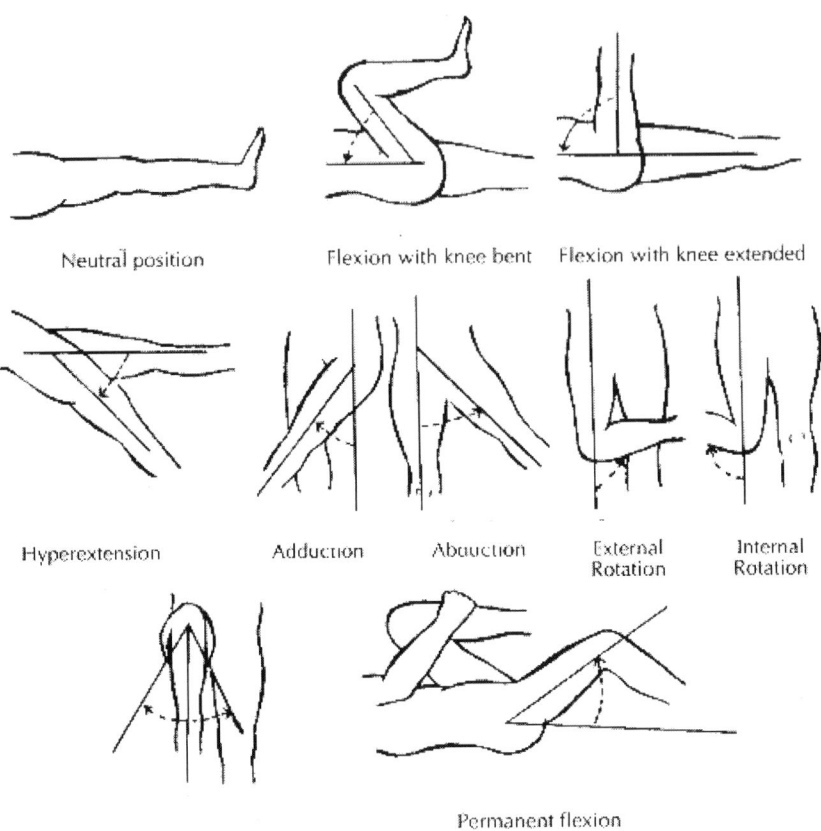

Neutral position   Flexion with knee bent   Flexion with knee extended

Hyperextension   Adduction   Abduction   External Rotation   Internal Rotation

Permanent flexion
(flexor contracture)

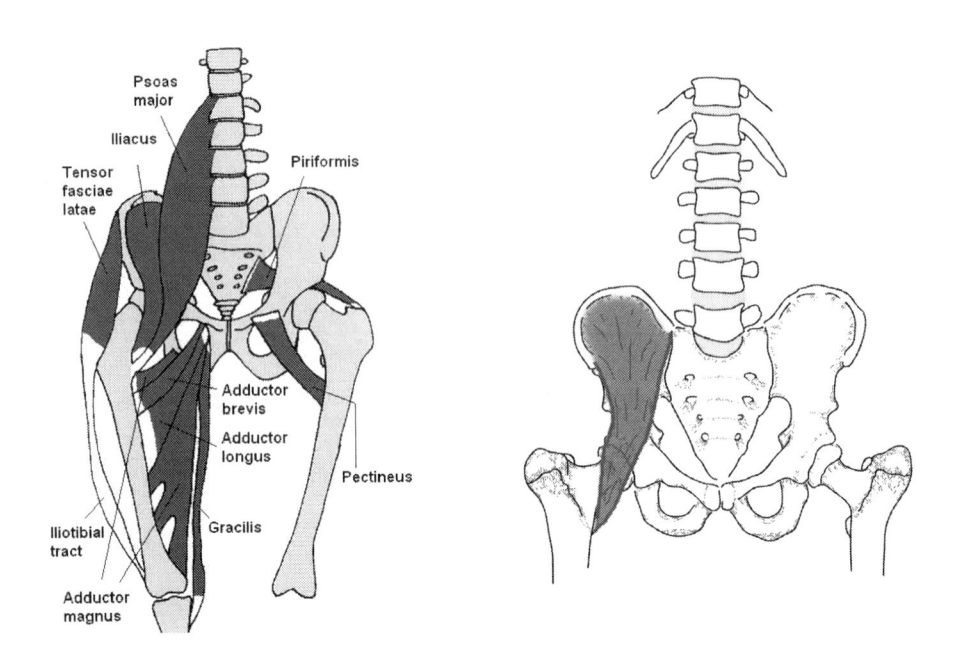

Psoas major
Iliacus
Tensor fasciae latae
Piriformis
Adductor brevis
Adductor longus
Pectineus
Iliotibial tract
Gracilis
Adductor magnus

THE HIP AND KNEE

On these pages, we show diagrams of the internal structures of the hip and leg simply to illustrate that the region is complex. Note that it is not just the bones that hold the hip to the torso and leg (femur), and that a great number of different muscles and tendons are involved (in movement also).

During extension of the hip, the angle between the posterior surfaces of the thigh and trunk decreases. ROM for extension is limited compared to that for flexion. It goes almost without saying that healthy and fit knees and hips are vital if you wish to possess any athletic capability whatsoever. To a great extent the hip structure, including the related muscles and bones etc, is one the strongest areas of the body. It is also one of the most mobile, and is involved in most types of athletic activity. The trained eye can often spot an athlete simply by the development of the buttocks and/or from the strength and/or flexibility of the hip area; because superb development of muscles in this region is a tell-tale sign of a well-trained individual.

The converse is also true, and one can spot illness, arthritis, poor athleticism and/or lameness by the way a person moves in the hip area.

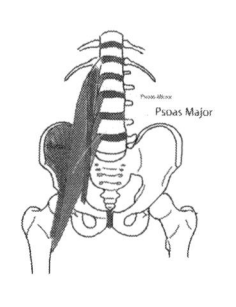

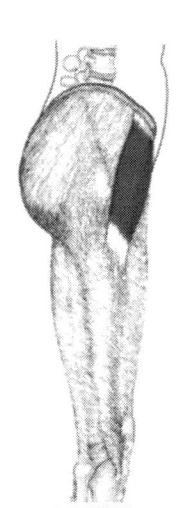

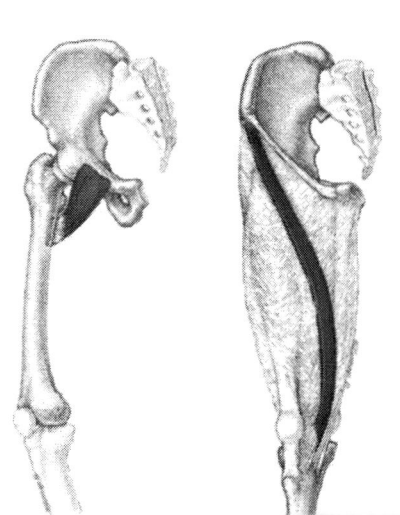

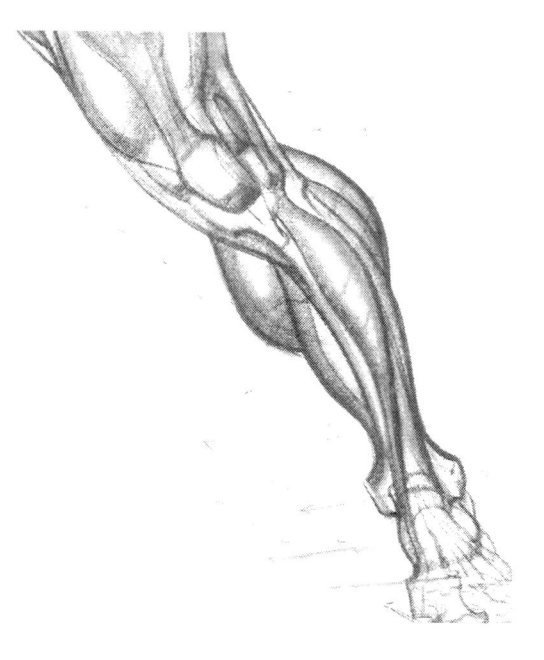

Psoas Major

ZEN OF DUMBBELL TRAINING

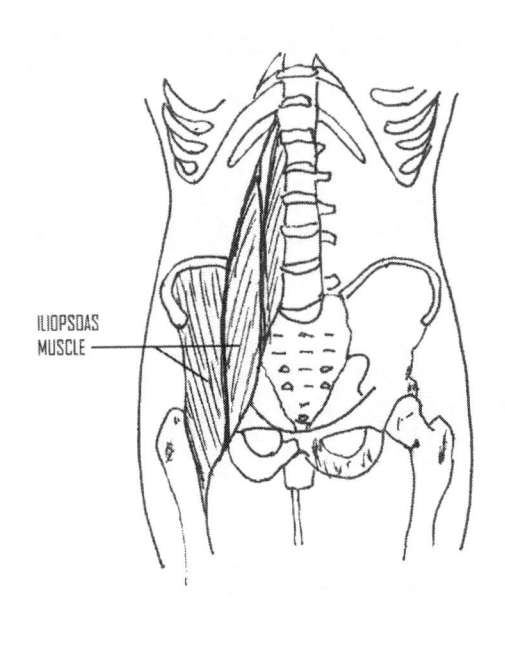

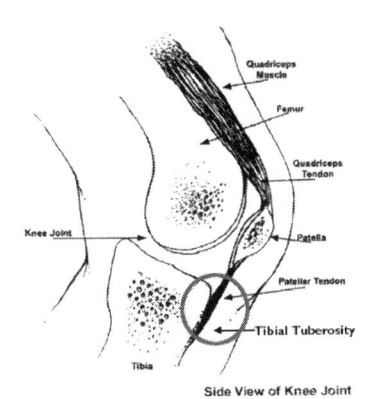

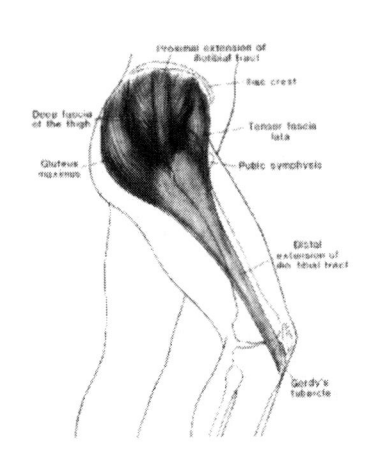

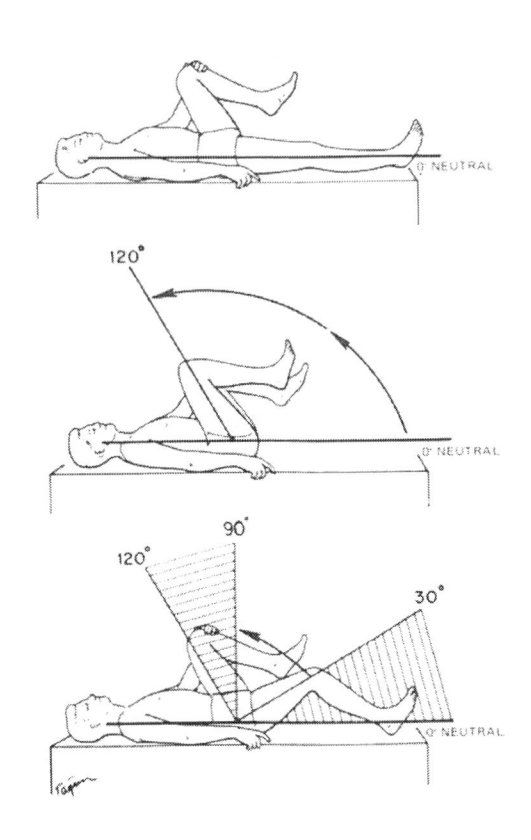

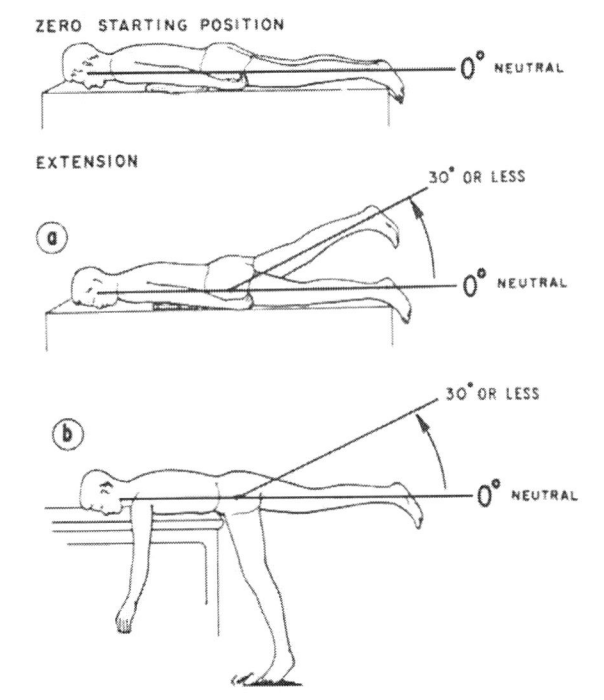

The ball-and-socket hip joint is supposed to have great range of motion, and it is important to exercise the area through as wide a ROM as possible and thus to preserve function as we age. Typical ROM values for hip flexion and extension are shown in these diagrams (on left).

When we turn our attention to the movement of the knee, we find that the knee is primarily a simple hinge joint. Flexion decreases the angle formed by the posterior thigh and leg - and is performed by leg biceps etc. ROM for active flexion is limited by contraction between the bodies of the contacting muscles. ROM for passive flexion is greater since the flexors are relaxed and more easily compressed (sitting with ankles under knees). Knee extension is when you straighten the lower leg, and is performed by the quadriceps muscles etc. Note that the knee is a relatively week joint (compared to the hip), gaining its strength from the structure of ligaments, tendons and muscles.

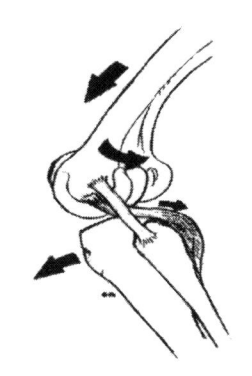

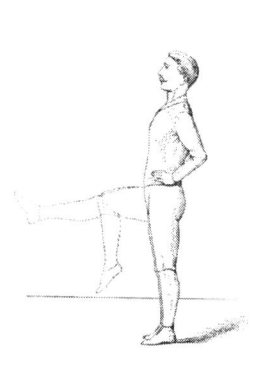

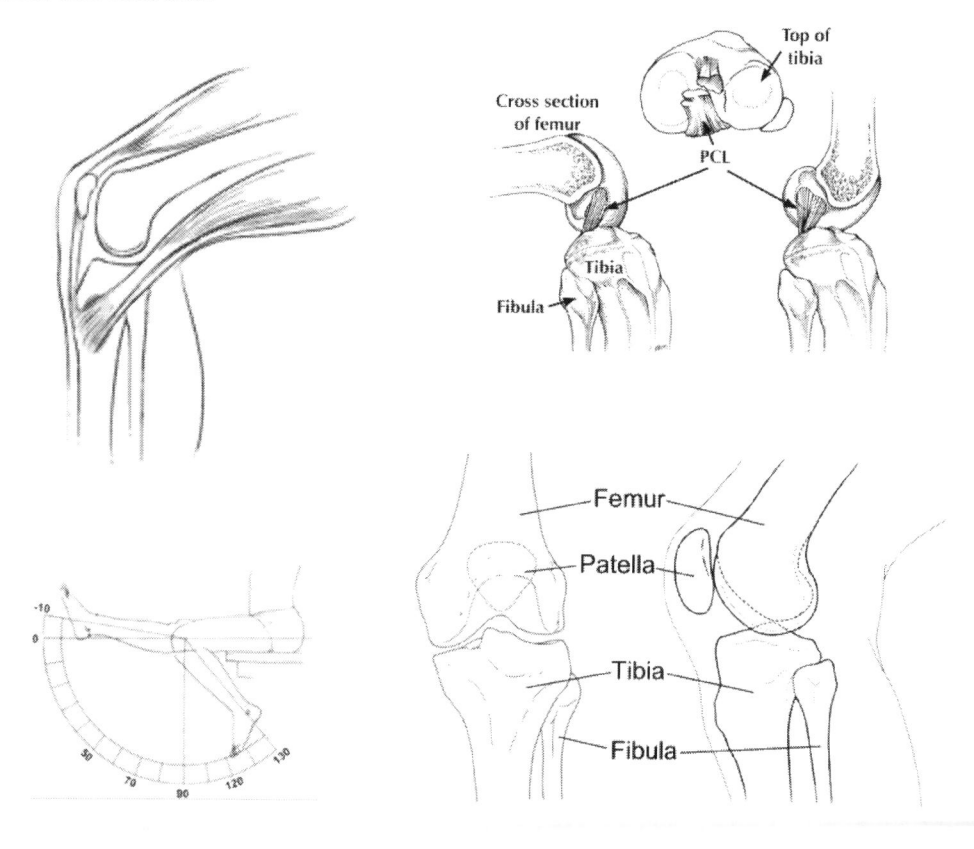

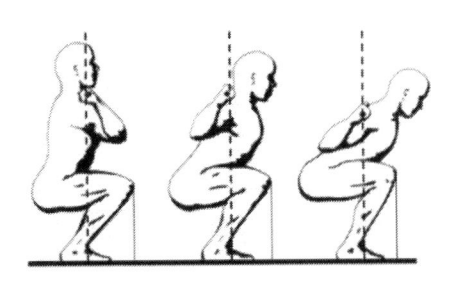

Hip and Knee Joint(s) - Exercises

73. Barbell Squat
74. Overhead Squat
75. Hack Squat
76. One-Leg Squat
77. Leg Curl
78. Bent Leg Raise
79. Front Leg Raise
80. Side Leg Raise
81. Leg Extension
82. Lying Leg Circles
83. Lying Leg Open/Close

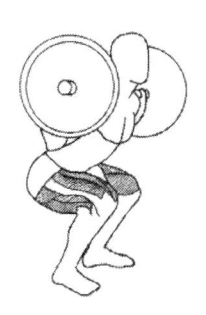

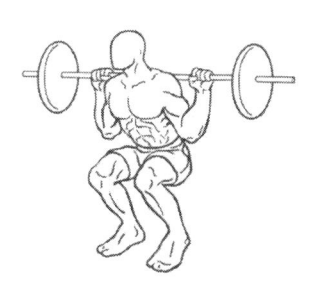

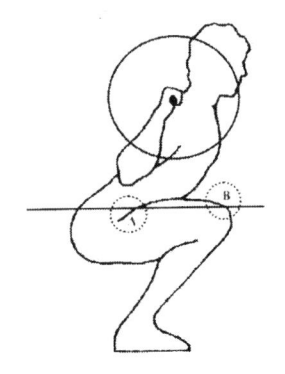

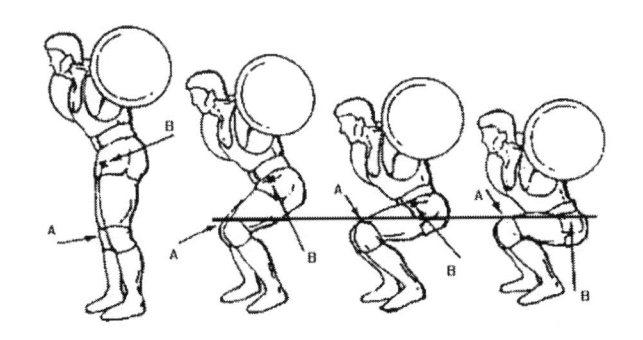

I would now like to briefly go over my earlier comments on simultaneously "creating" rigid and soft body-parts whilst moving. Remember that I said that when lifting it is vital to fix certain parts of the body into "rigid" or "semi-flexed" positions, and in order to allow other parts to move. Here flexed probably refers to the combined flexion of opposing body parts (muscles), as in a combined biceps/triceps flexion to main a fixed and strong arm position which is immovable in either direction. To some extent holding certain areas of the body rigid, whilst allowing other areas to move, is a natural process which is at least partially unconscious. However often when performing (or learning) highly skilled movements, one must consciously flex specific muscles to hold particular parts of the body rigid.

A discussion of the barbell squat is salient at this point. Now the squat is a basic exercise - perhaps the most basic. It is also the most result-producing one that anybody can perform. But it is extremely difficult to learn and to perform correctly. Great skill is required to perform the squat. To start with I would like you to think of each repetition as an athletic event, in and of itself. Before you take the weight off the stands (or clean and place the bar behind the neck), one should already have the lower back arched and stomach muscles fairly tight. You want to maintain a rigid spine position throughout - and under no circumstances should the lower back become de-arched at any point. Keep the torso firm - flex the abs and also flex the lower back. Next step back and set the feet into position, perhaps a little wider than shoulders is best, and with feet pointing slightly outward. Now that everything is in the "set" position - once more check for an arched lower back. Your glutes, hamstrings and quads will also be semi-flexed - if not then you would collapse to the floor. Now slowly begin to "hinge" at the hip joint and also at the knees. It is a slow movement to begin with. Remember no hinging whatsoever at the lower back! Be aware of the knee position in space.

As the movement progresses; the difficulty (in terms of conscious control) becomes how much should the hip hinge (as opposed to the knee bend/hinge) and contribute to the movement of the torso in space. A good rule of thumb is that in a parallel squat (not on toes or deeper than parallel), the knees would not normally extend further forward than the toes.

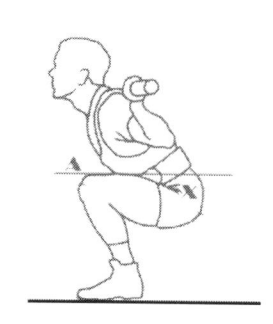

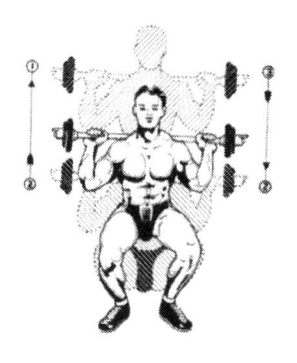

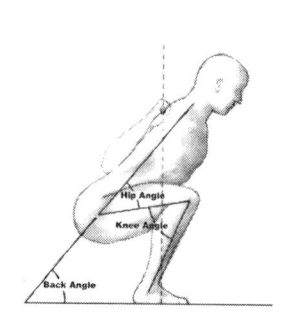

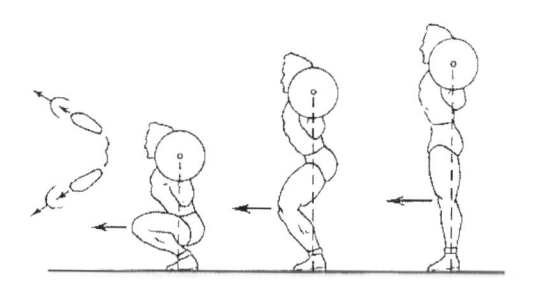

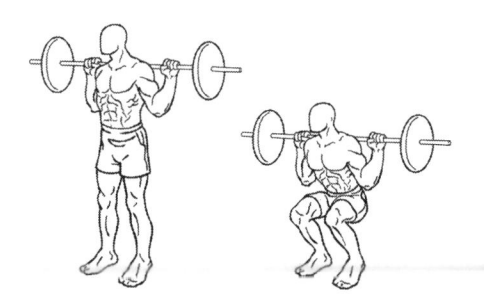

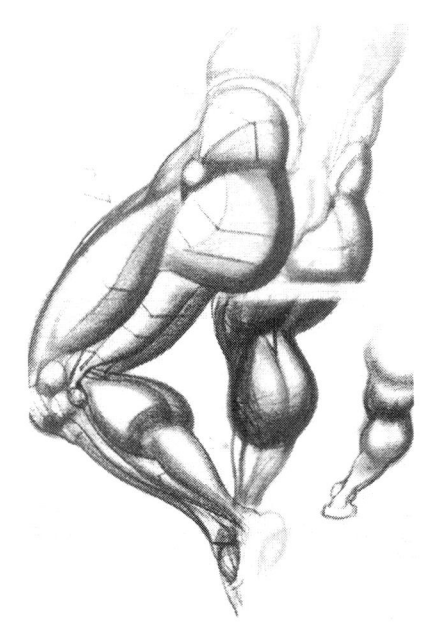

73. Barbell Squat (flat-footed)

Equipment: barbell
Effect: Strengthen hips, quadriceps, biceps femoris
Resistance : Light / Medium / Heavy [Slow]
Hip position: Hip Hinge - Flexion / Extension
Spine position: Extended / arched lumbar
Scapula position: Retracted
Muscles: Erector spinae, gluteus maximus, hamstrings (biceps femoris), quadriceps, rectus abdominis, calves
Typical Poundage: 40-80 kg barbell (women); 60-200 kg barbell (men) [look forward throughout]
Joints: Hip, knee, ankle, spine (arched)

In the old days people often performed the squat exercise on the toes (deep-knee bend) - which is an interesting variation that allows you to squat deeply onto your haunches; and also works your ankles and thighs in a different manner. Also a great variety of different kinds of squats were employed including one-legged and "jumping" versions.

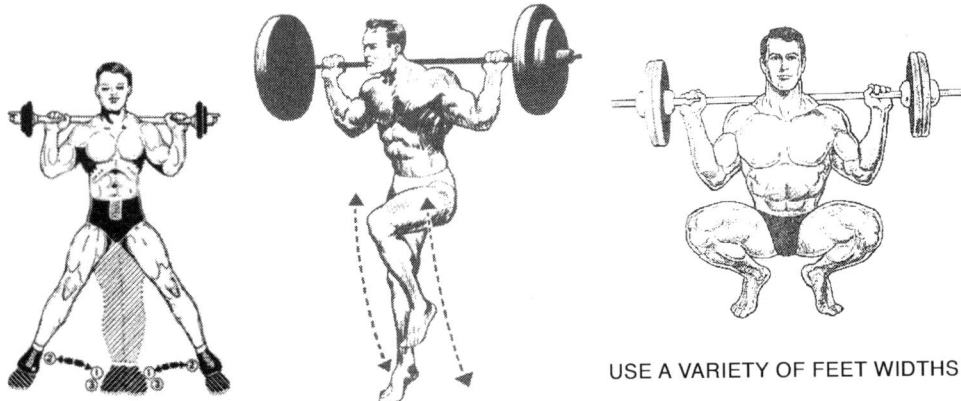

The most result-producing (muscle-growth stimulating) exercise of them all. From a rack with barbell at upper chest height, position the bar high on back of shoulders and grasp barbell to sides. Dismount bar from rack and stand with shoulder width stance. Bend knees forward while allowing hips to bend back behind, keeping back straight and knees pointed in the same direction as the feet. Descend until thighs are just past parallel to floor. Extend knees and hips until legs are straight. Return and repeat. Keep head facing forward, back straight and feet flat on floor; equal distribution of weight throughout forefoot and heel. Knees should point in the same direction as the feet throughout movement.

USE A VARIETY OF FEET WIDTHS

THE HIP AND KNEE 249

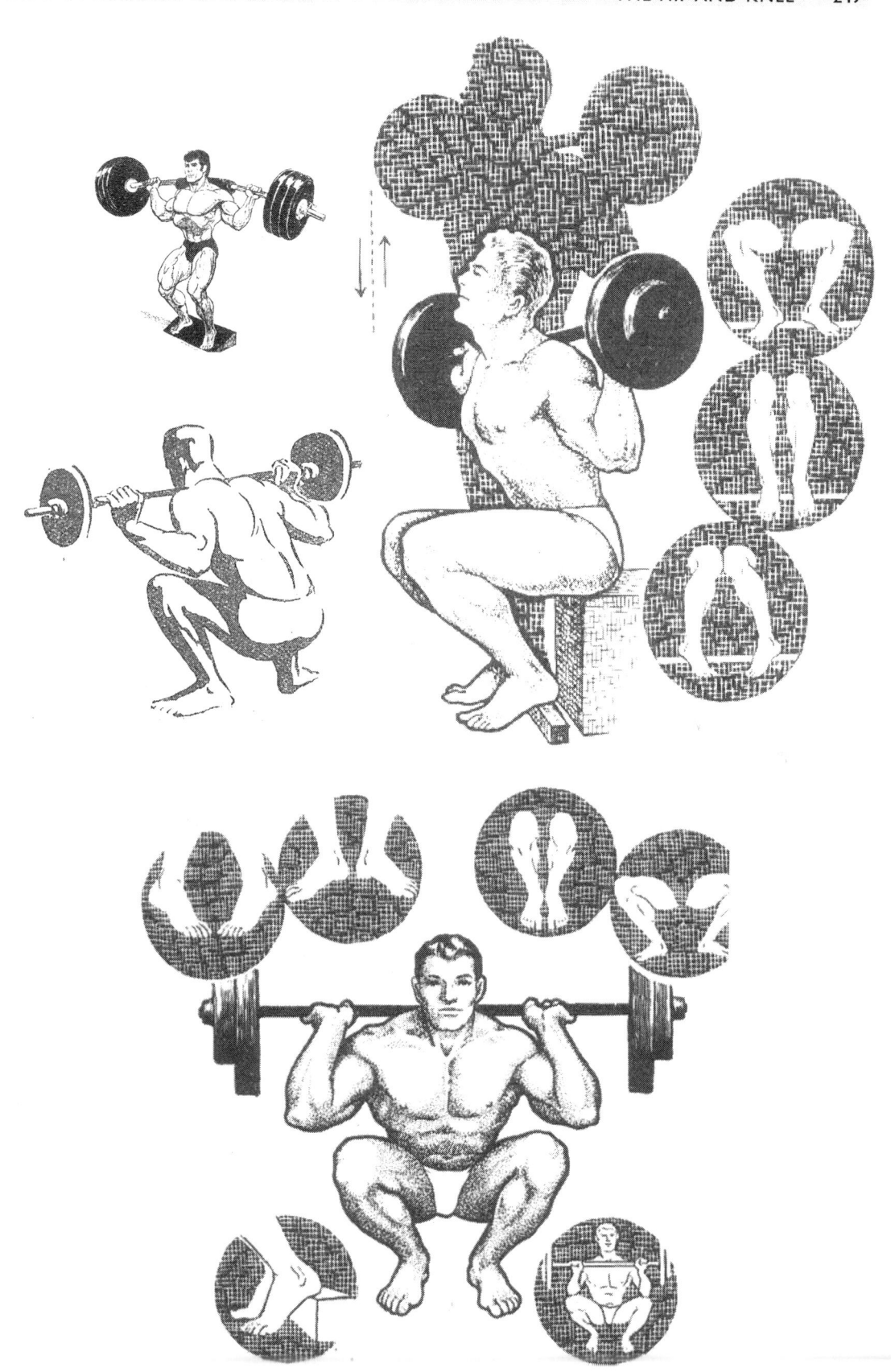

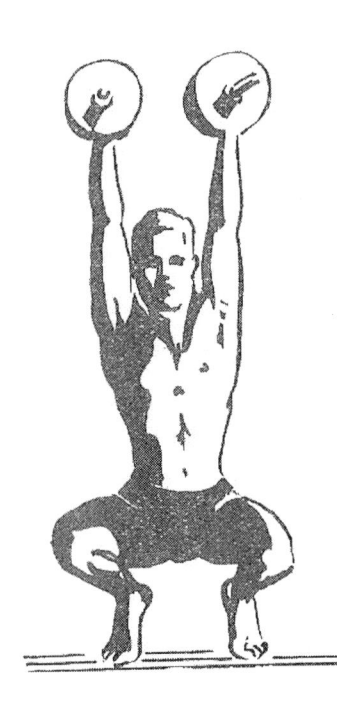

74. Overhead Squat

Equipment: barbell / single or double dumbbells
Effect: Strengthen hips, quadriceps, biceps femoris
Resistance : Light / Medium / Heavy [Slow]
Hip position: Hip Hinge - Flexion / Extension
Spine position: Extended / arched lumbar throughout
Scapula position: Rotated
Muscles: Erector spinae, gluteus maximus, hamstrings, quadriceps, rectus abdominis (supporting), calves
Typical Poundage: 8-15 kg dumbbells (women); 10-24 kg (men) - can use kettle-bells [look forward throughout]
Joints: Hip, knee, shoulder, ankle, spine (arched)

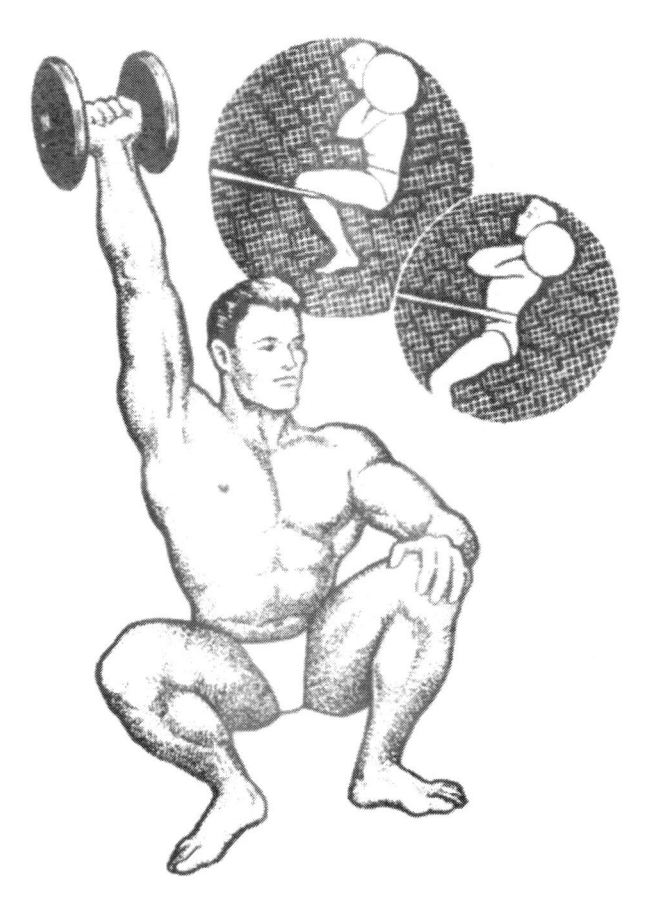

Snatch a light barbell overhead with very wide overhand grip. Position toes slightly outward with wide stance. Maintain bar behind head and with arms extended. Descend until knees and hips are fully bent or until thighs are just past parallel to floor. Knees travel in direction of toes. Extend knees and hips until legs are straight. Return and repeat. Keep head forward, back straight and feet flat on floor; and equal distribution of weight through forefoot and heel.

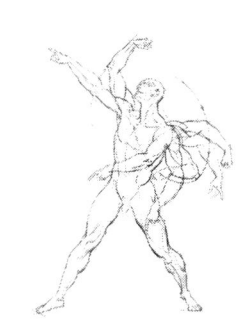

75. Hack Squat

Equipment: twin dumbbells / barbell
Effect: Strengthen hips, quadriceps, biceps femoris
Resistance : Light / Medium / Heavy [Slow]
Hip position: Hip Hinge - Flexion / Extension
Spine position: Extended / arched lumbar throughout
Scapula position: Neutral / locked
Muscles: Erector spinae, gluteus maximus, hamstrings, quadriceps, rectus abdominis
Typical Poundage: 8-15 kg dumbbells (women); 10-30 kg dumbbells (men)
Joints: Hip, knee, ankle, spine (arched lumbar)

With feet flat on floor, squat down and grasp barbell from behind with overhand grip. Lift bar by extending hips and knees to full extension. Bend knees forward slightly while allowing hips to bend back behind, keeping back straight and knees pointed same direction as feet. Descend until thighs are close to parallel to floor and bar is behind lower leg. Repeat. Alternate version is to hold twin dumbbells at sides throughout.

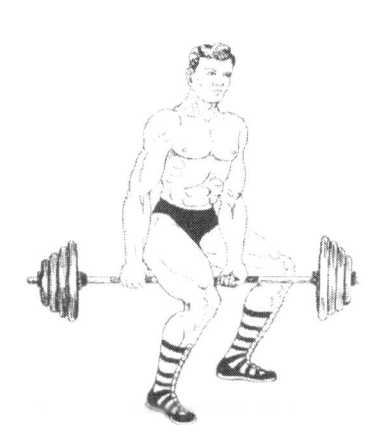

The long and short biceps femoris, semimembranosus and semitendinosus make up your hamstrings. In the squat there is an apparent paradox when examining the contraction of the quadriceps and the hamstrings. In the up phase of a squat, the quadriceps contract to cause extension of the knee joint while the hamstrings are contracting to cause extension of the hip joint. It would seem plausible that both these muscle groups should neutralise the others movements, with no resultant movement. This contradiction has been defined as "Lombards Paradox". On the descent phase of the squat, the leg biceps also eccentrically contract (flex) to slow the bodies decent (bending of the knee) against gravity. On the way down also the quadriceps and gluteus maximus eccentrically contract to slow movement. On the way up the quadriceps contract (concentrically) to extend the knee against gravity and so to straighten the upper leg.

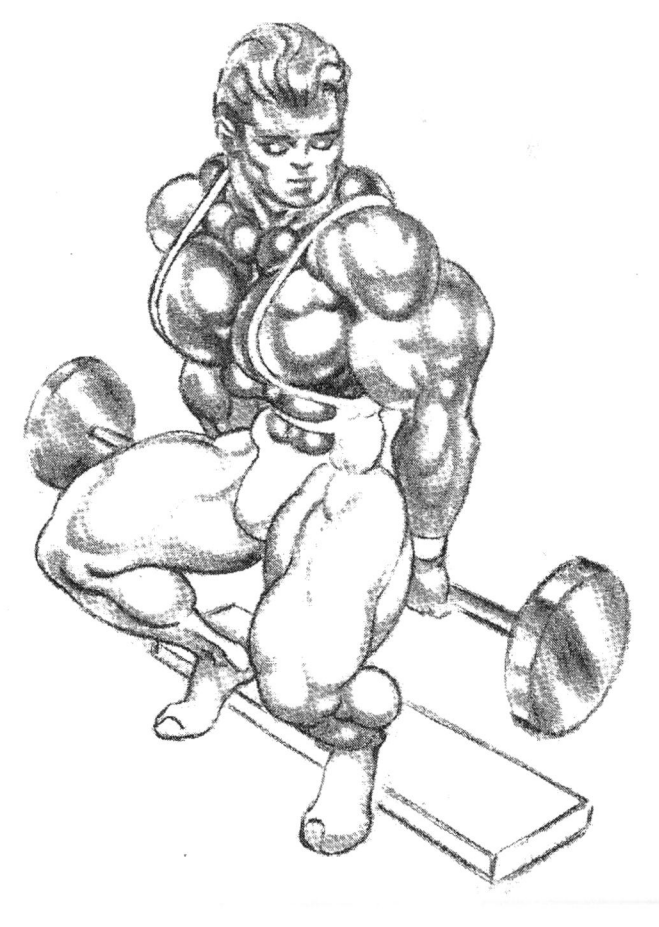

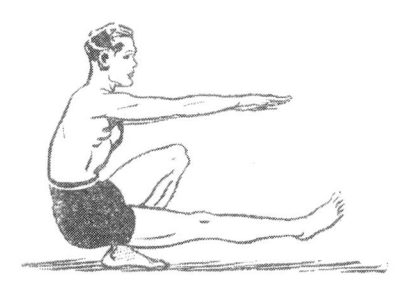

76. One-Leg Squat

Equipment: Nothing / twin dumbbells / barbell
Effect: Strengthen hips, quadriceps, biceps femoris
Resistance : Light / Medium / Heavy [Slow]
Hip position: Hip Hinge - Flexion / Extension
Spine position: Extended / arched lumbar
Scapula position: Neutral / locked
Muscles: Erector spinae, gluteus maximus, hamstrings, quadriceps, rectus abdominis (supporting / conscious flex)
Typical Poundage: None / 8-16 kg dumbbell (women); 12-24 kg (men)
Joints: Hip, knee, ankle

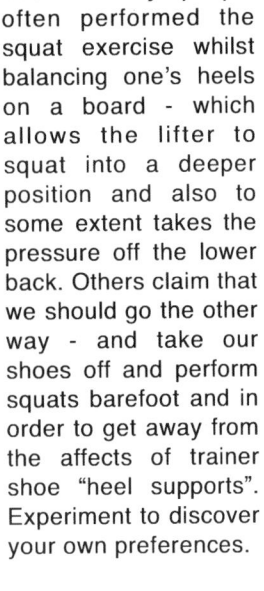

In the old days people often performed the squat exercise whilst balancing one's heels on a board - which allows the lifter to squat into a deeper position and also to some extent takes the pressure off the lower back. Others claim that we should go the other way - and take our shoes off and perform squats barefoot and in order to get away from the affects of trainer shoe "heel supports". Experiment to discover your own preferences.

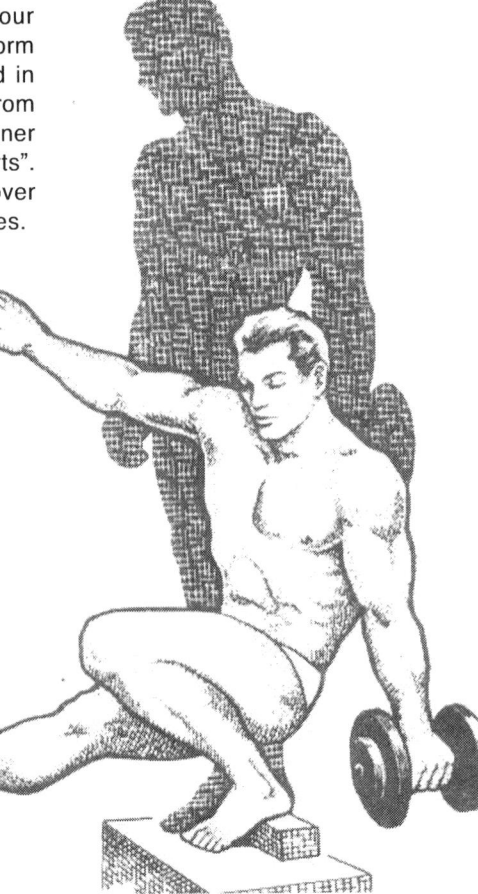

Similar to the standard squat - but use only one leg to move the body. You can either hold a single dumbbell or kettle-bell at the side or on the chest, or hold a barbell behind the head as normal.

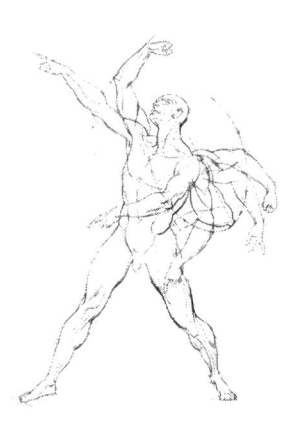

77. Leg Curl

Equipment: barbell / Leg-bell / cable harness + machine
Effect: Strengthen hips, biceps femoris
Resistance : Light / Medium / Heavy [Slow]
Hip position: N/A or Slight Extension
Spine position: Neutral / arched lumbar
Scapula position: Neutral / locked
Muscles: Gluteus maximus, hamstrings, semitendinosus, semimembranosus, gastrocnemius
Typical Poundage: 8-12 kg (women); 12-20 kg (men)
Joints: Knee

Attach foot harness to low pulley (or wear leg-boot or ankle weight). With foot harness on one ankle, grasp support bar with both hands and step back with other foot. Elbows remain straight to support body. Attached foot is slightly off floor. Pull cable attachment back by flexing knee until knee is fully flexed. Return by straightening knee to original position and repeat. Continue with opposite leg.

Alternative is to use a leg-bell and perform the same movement as above. DO NOT USE A LEG CURL MACHINE - SEE DANGEROUS EXERCISES

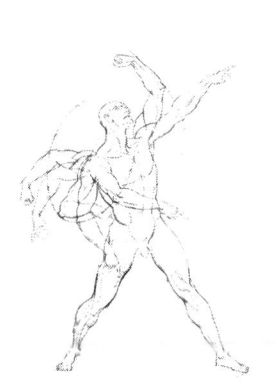

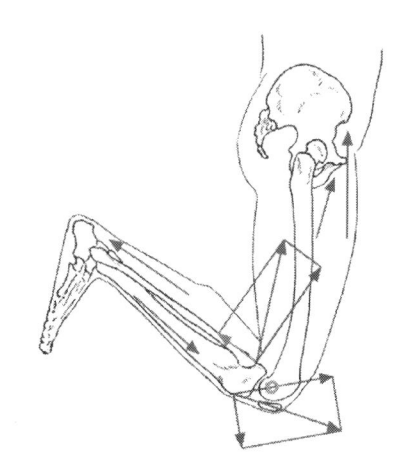

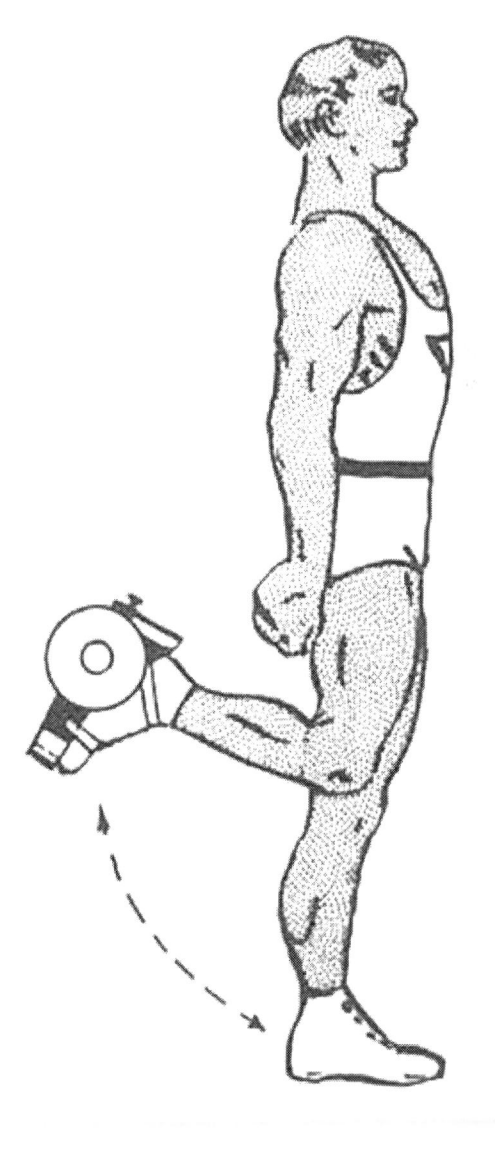

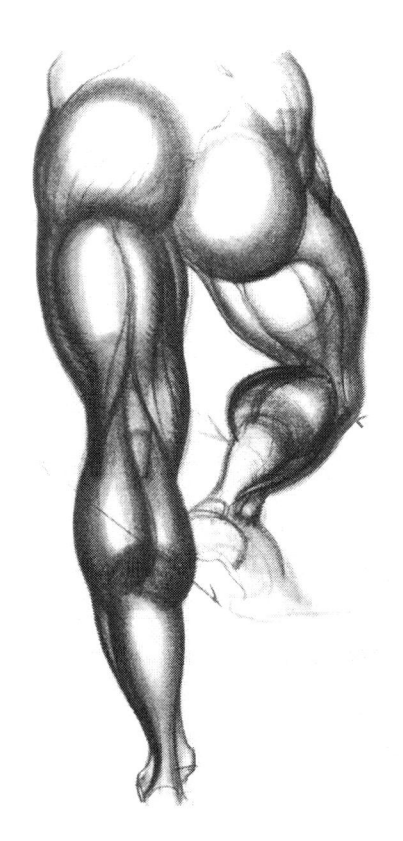

78. Bent Leg Raise (ROM)

Equipment: Nothing / Leg-bell
Effect: Strengthen leg / waist / stomach muscles
Resistance : Light / Medium / Heavy [Slow]
Hip position: Hip Hinge - flexion / extension
Spine position: Neutral
Scapula position: Neutral / locked
Muscles: hamstrings, rectus abdominis, hip region
Typical Poundage: 8-16 kg (women); 12-24 kg (men)
Joints: Hip, knee

Stand upright, bend and raise your leg upwards, keeping the leg bent. Continue with a downward unwinding movement back to straight. Repeat 5-10 times, and then switch legs.

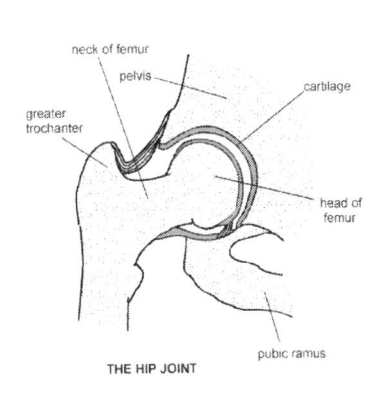

THE HIP JOINT

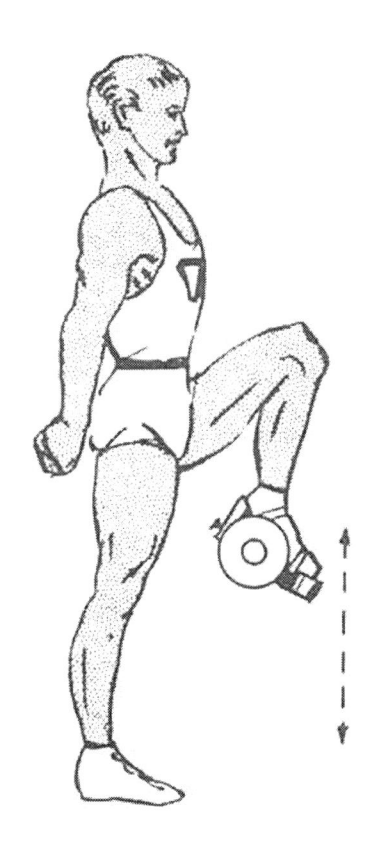

THE HIP AND KNEE 255

79. Front Leg Raise (ROM)

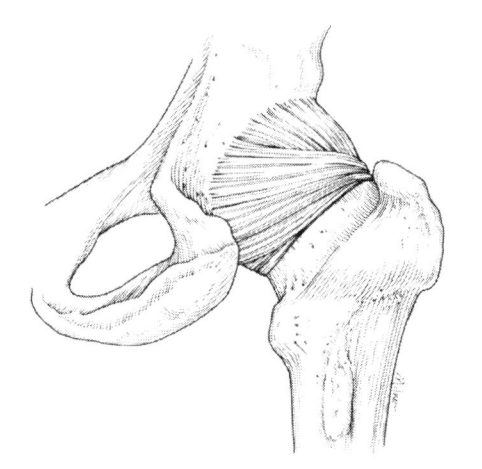

Equipment: Nothing / Leg-bell
Effect: Strengthen leg / waist / stomach muscles
Resistance : Light [Slow]
Hip position: Hip Hinge - flexion / extension
Spine position: Neutral
Scapula position: Neutral / locked
Muscles: hamstrings, quadriceps, rectus abdominis, hip region
Typical Poundage: 8-16 kg (women); 12-24 kg (men)
Joints: Hip

Stand upright, swing your leg forward, keeping the leg straight. Continue with a downward swing, bringing the leg (in either direction) as far as your flexibility allows. Repeat 5-10 times, and then switch legs.

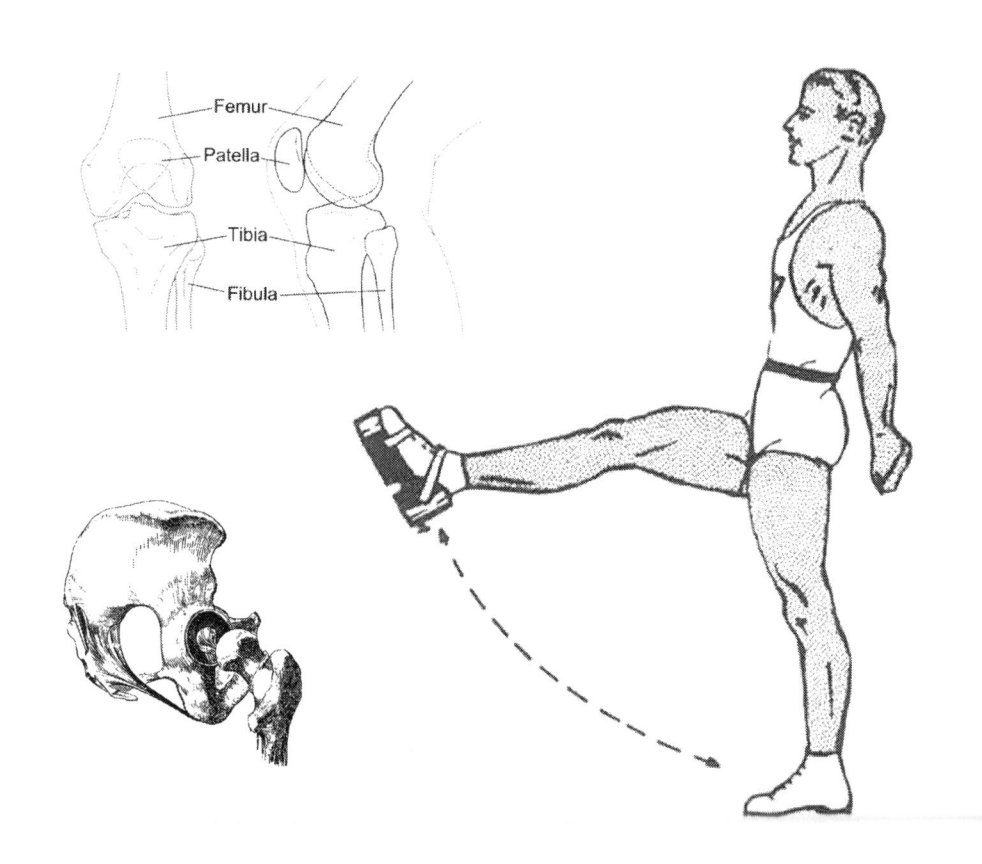

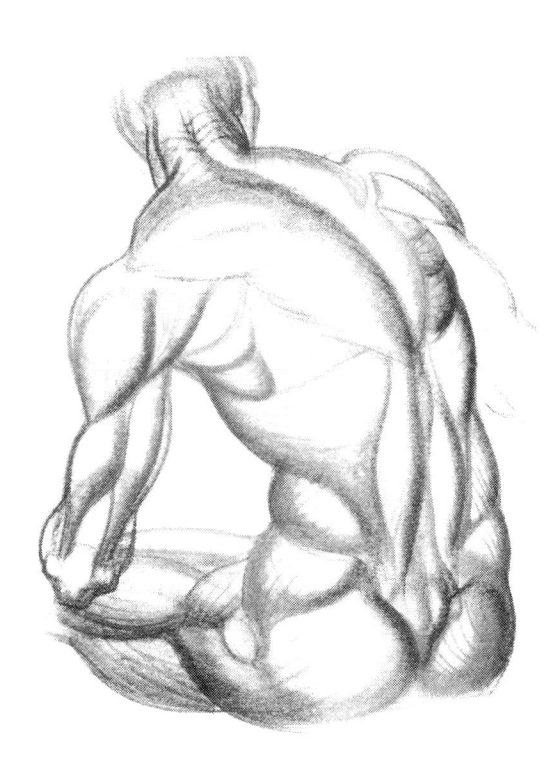

80. Side Leg Raise (ROM)

Equipment: Nothing / Leg-bell
Effect: Strengthen leg / waist / stomach muscles
Resistance : Light [Slow]
Hip position: Neutral
Spine position: Neutral
Scapula position: Neutral / locked
Muscles: Pectineus, adductor brevis / longus, adductor magnus, gluteus medius, hips
Typical Poundage: 8-16 kg (women); 12-24 kg weight (men)
Joints: Hip

Stand upright, swing your leg sideways, keeping the leg straight. Continue with a downward swing, bringing the leg as far as your flexibility allows.

Repeat 5-10 times, and then switch legs.

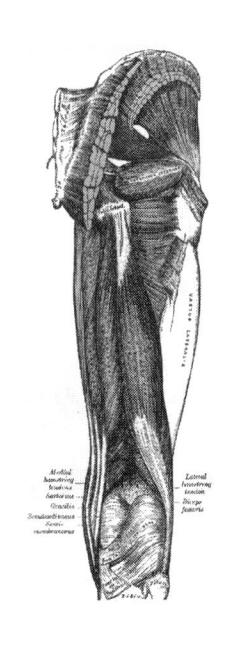

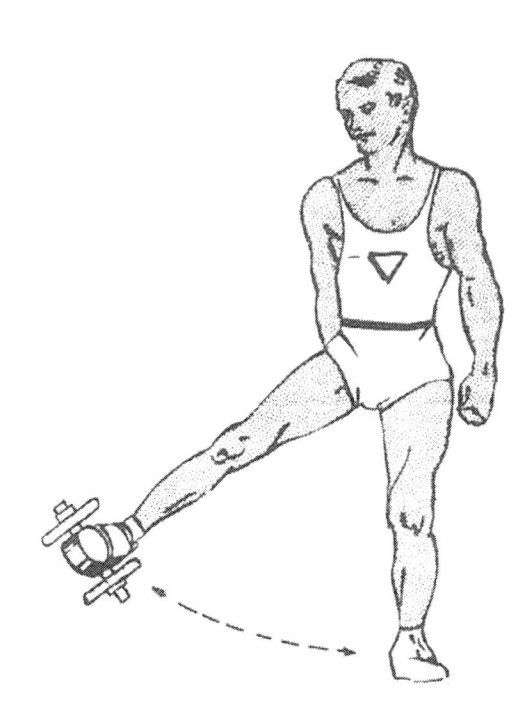

81. Leg Extension (ROM)

Equipment: Nothing / Leg-bell
Effect: Strengthen leg / waist / stomach muscles
Resistance : Light / Medium / Heavy [Slow]
Hip position: Hip Hinge - Flexion
Spine position: Neutral
Scapula position: Neutral / locked
Muscles: Quadriceps (rectus femoris, vastus lateralis, vastus medialis, vastus intermedius)
Typical Poundage: 8-16 kg (women); 12-24 kg (men)
Joints: Knee, hip

Stand upright, bend and raise your leg out and hold the knee in place. Now extend and de-extend the knee. Repeat 5-10 times, and then switch legs.

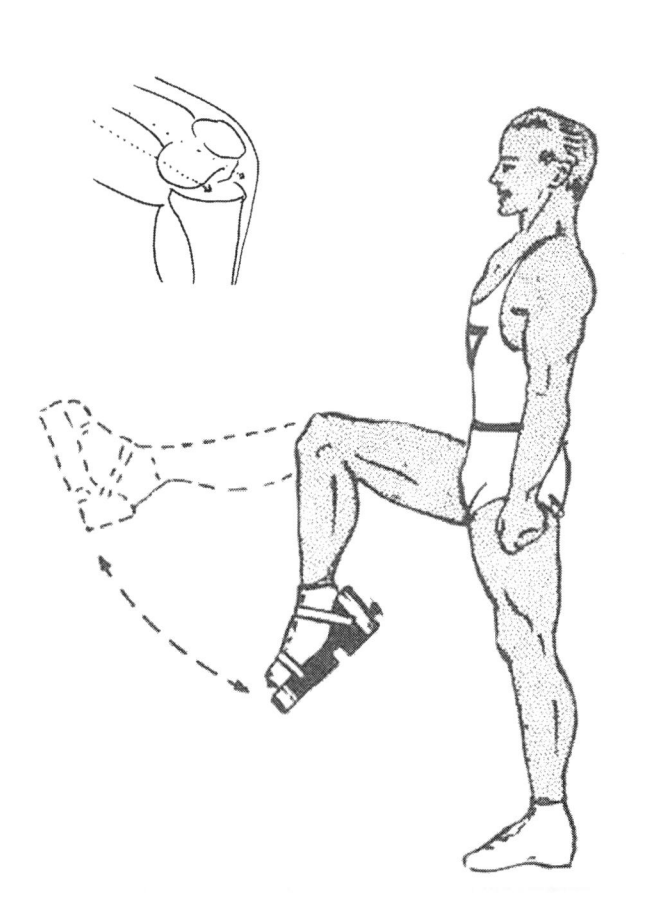

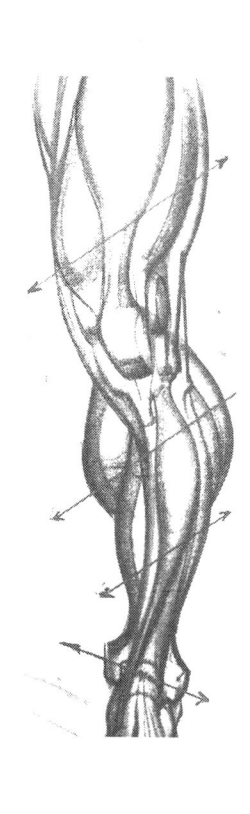

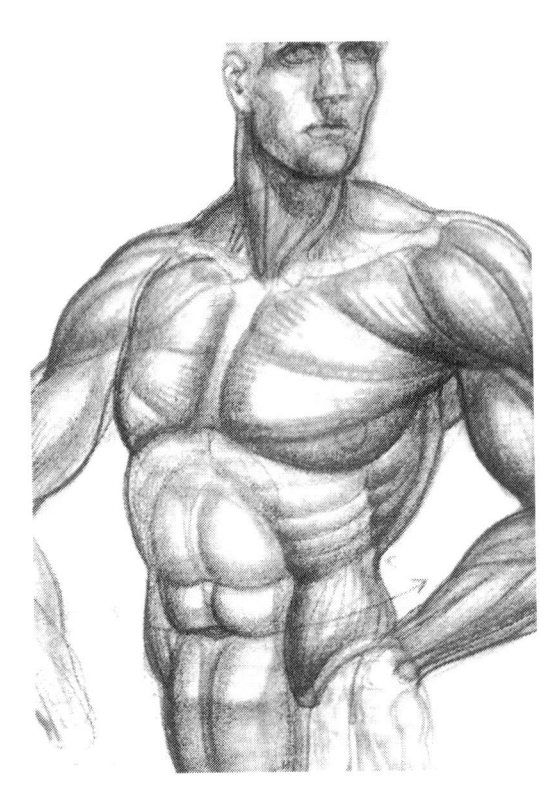

82. Lying Leg Circles (ROM)

Equipment: Nothing / Leg-bell / Iron Boots
Effect: Strengthen leg / waist / stomach muscles
Resistance : Light / Medium / Heavy
[Slow speed]
Hip position: Flexion / Slight Extension
Spine position: Neutral
Scapula position: Neutral / locked
Muscles: Gluteus maximums, hamstrings, rectus abdominis, entire hip structure / musculature
Typical Poundage: 8-16 kg (women); 12-24 kg (men)
Joints: Hip, knee, spine (supporting)

Lie down and bend at the hip, raising legs up and keeping holding straight at the waist level.

Now perform a cycling movement whilst keeping the hips flexed and the knees high.

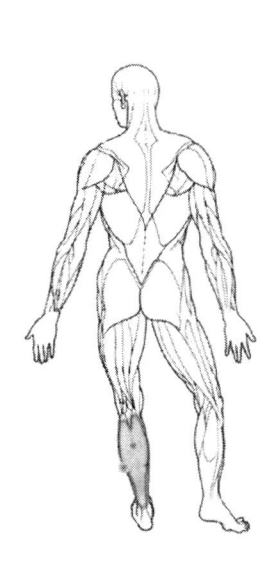

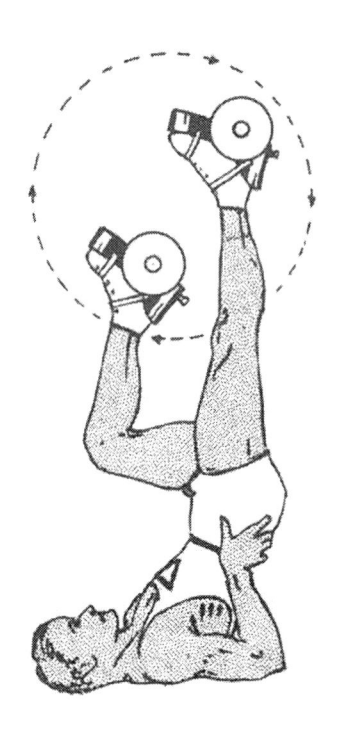

83. Lying Leg Open/Close (ROM)

Equipment: Nothing / Leg-bell / Iron Boots
Effect: Strengthen leg / waist / stomach muscles
Resistance : Light / Medium / Heavy [Slow]
Hip position: Hip Hinge - Flexion
Spine position: Neutral
Scapula position: Neutral / locked
Muscles: Hamstrings, hips, rectus abdominis
Typical Poundage: 8-16 kg (women); 12-24 kg (men)
Joints: Hip

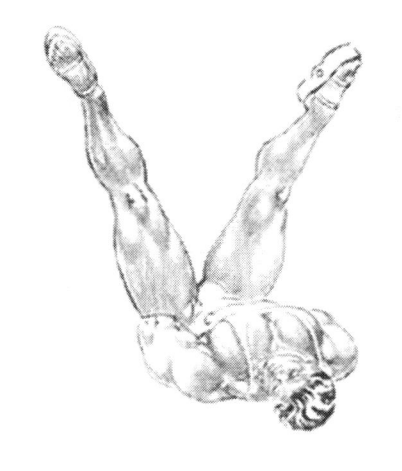

Lie down and bend at the hip, raising legs up and keeping them straight at the waist level. Now open and close legs whilst keeping the hips flexed and the knees locked.

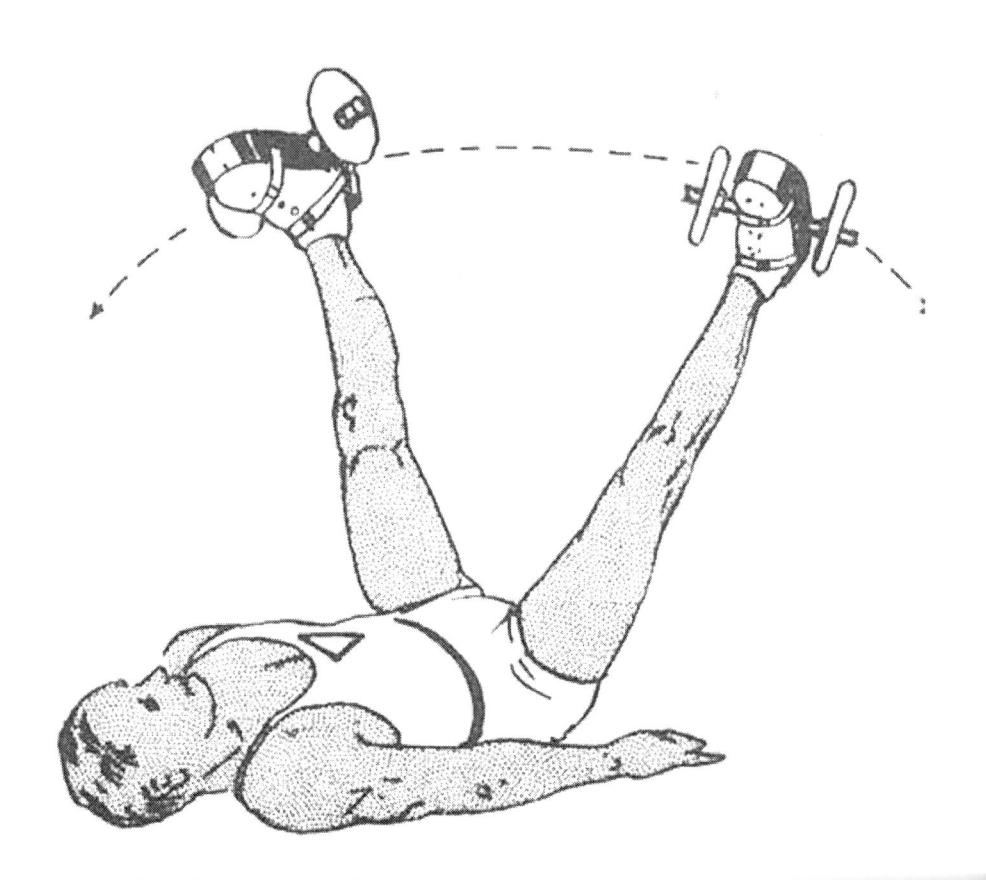

"THE WISE FOR CURE ON EXERCISE DEPEND."—Dryden.

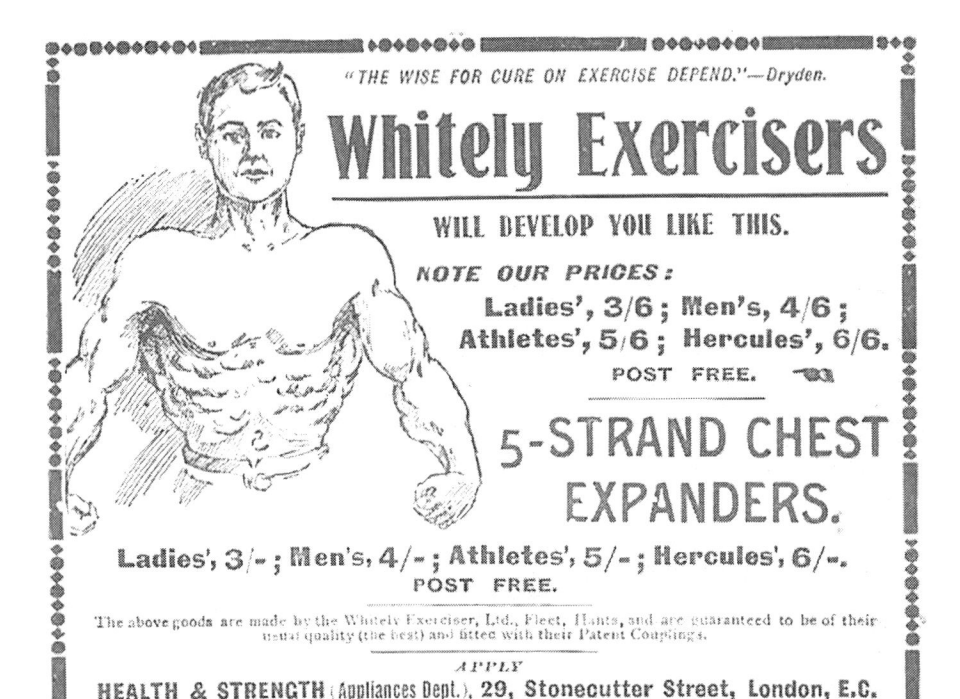

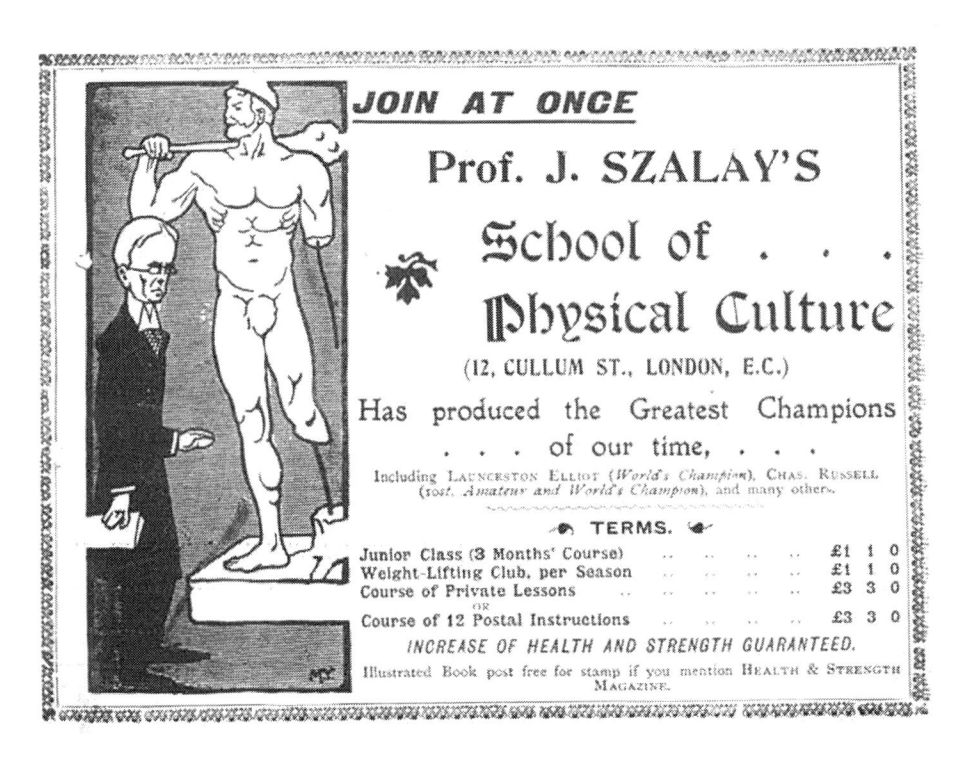

Whitely Exercisers

WILL DEVELOP YOU LIKE THIS.

NOTE OUR PRICES:
Ladies', 3/6; Men's, 4/6;
Athletes', 5/6; Hercules', 6/6.
POST FREE.

5-STRAND CHEST EXPANDERS.

Ladies', 3/-; Men's, 4/-; Athletes', 5/-; Hercules', 6/-.
POST FREE.

The above goods are made by the Whitely Exerciser, Ltd., Fleet, Hants, and are guaranteed to be of their usual quality (the best) and fitted with their Patent Couplings.

APPLY
HEALTH & STRENGTH (Appliances Dept.), 29, Stonecutter Street, London, E.C.

JOIN AT ONCE

Prof. J. SZALAY'S School of Physical Culture

(12, CULLUM ST., LONDON, E.C.)

Has produced the Greatest Champions of our time,

Including LAUNCESTON ELLIOT (*World's Champion*), CHAS. RUSSELL (101st. *Amateur and World's Champion*), and many others.

TERMS.

Junior Class (3 Months' Course)	£1 1 0
Weight-Lifting Club, per Season	£1 1 0
Course of Private Lessons	£3 3 0
OR	
Course of 12 Postal Instructions	£3 3 0

INCREASE OF HEALTH AND STRENGTH GUARANTEED.

Illustrated Book post free for stamp if you mention HEALTH & STRENGTH MAGAZINE.

THE ANKLE AND FOOT

CHAPTER TWELVE

The Ankle and Foot

THE FOOT serves a double function, bearing the weight of the entire body, and helping to perform the dynamic movements necessary for walking/running. This requires both strength and flexibility. The foot contains 26 bones, 31 joints and 20 muscles.

The ankle joint combines the malleability of the foot with the strength of the leg bones. Now the ankle can twist left and right, and perform circular movements etc. However here we are largely concerned with flexion and extension of the ankle, and with associated movements. You often see that ballet dancers and track athletes have excellent calf, ankle and foot muscles which obviously helps to propel them about in a variety of ways.

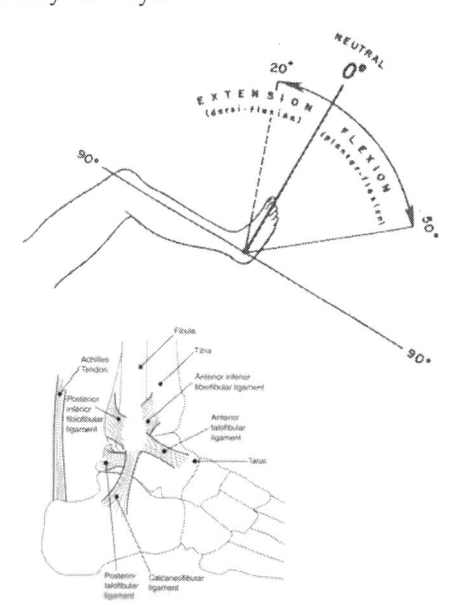

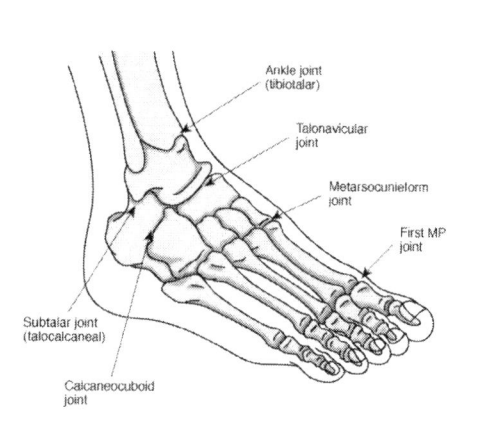

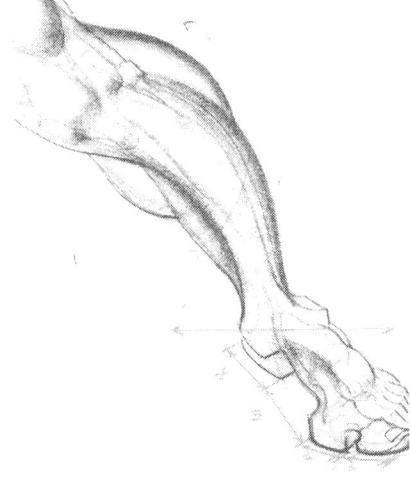

Ankle and Foot Joint(s) - Exercises

84. Standing Calf Raise
85. Seated Calf Raise
86. Donkey Calf Raises

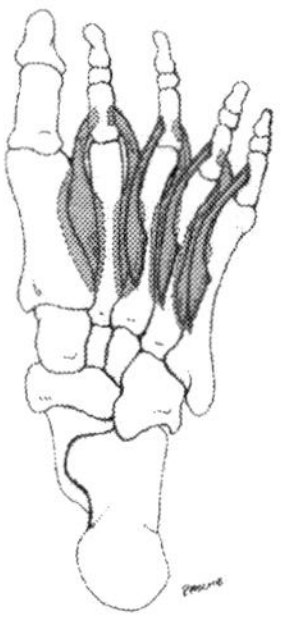

Largely in terms of power movements, the foot can either extend or flex with resistance. Normally flexion causes the muscles of the calf - including gastrocnemius and soleus to develop or grow stronger. Now in some people these muscles naturally develop very quickly, whereas in other people no matter what they do the muscles of the lower leg fail to develop to any great degree. Genetics is to blame!

Thus when it comes to lower leg muscles, it seems that genetics takes an even bigger role than in most other muscles in the body which can normally be developed through careful and prolonged training. A few tips might perhaps help - and set you on the road to progress. In my experience standing calf raises with heavy weights - plus a full range of movement - will develop the calves to the maximum extent. But remember that each time you take a step (when walking about) you raise up on your full bodyweight, so this is like lifting 400 lbs on a calf machine with 2 legs. Therefore even heavier weights are required to develop the calves fully.

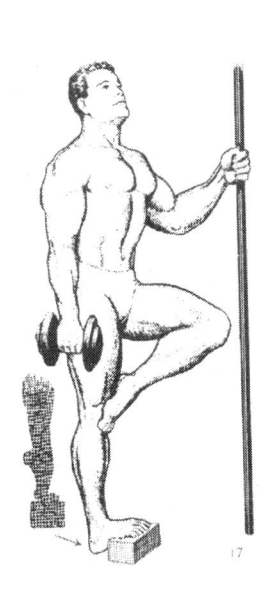

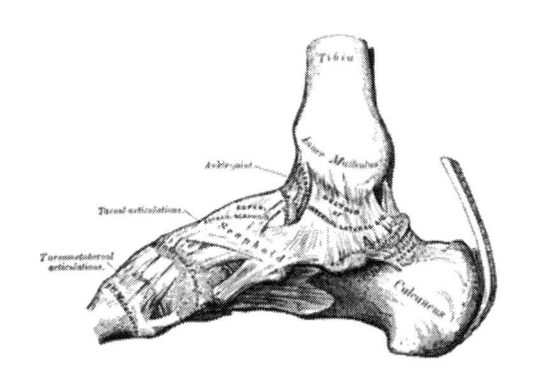

84. Standing Calf Raise

Equipment: barbell, calf raise machine
Effect: Strengthen calves
Resistance : Light / Medium / Heavy [Slow]
Hip position: N/A
Spine position: Extended / arched lumbar
Scapula position: Neutral / locked
Muscles: Plantaris, Gastrocnemius (all heads), soleus
Typical Poundage: 40-200 kg (women); 80-300 kg (men)
Joints: Ankle

Set barbell on power rack at upper chest height with calf block under barbell. Position back of shoulders under barbell with both hands to sides. Position toes and balls of feet on calf block with arches and heels extending off. Lean barbell against rack and raise from supports by extending knees and hips. Support barbell against verticals with both hands to sides. Raise heels by extending ankles as high as possible. Lower heels by bending ankles until calves are stretched. Repeat.

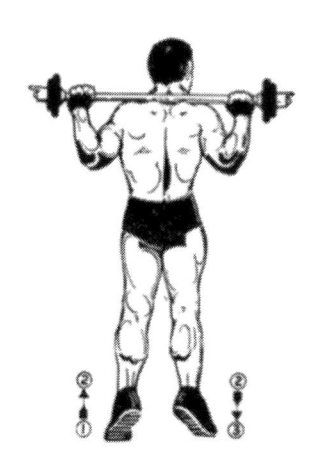

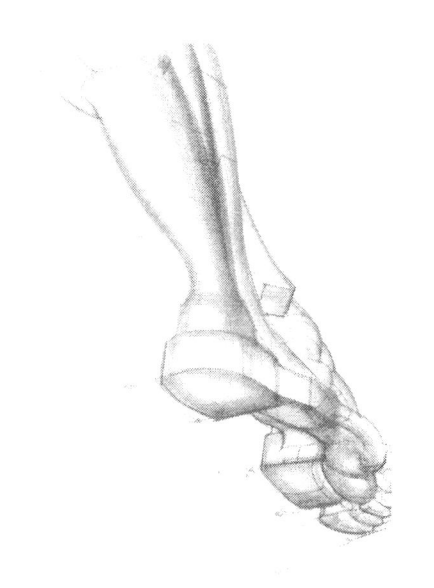

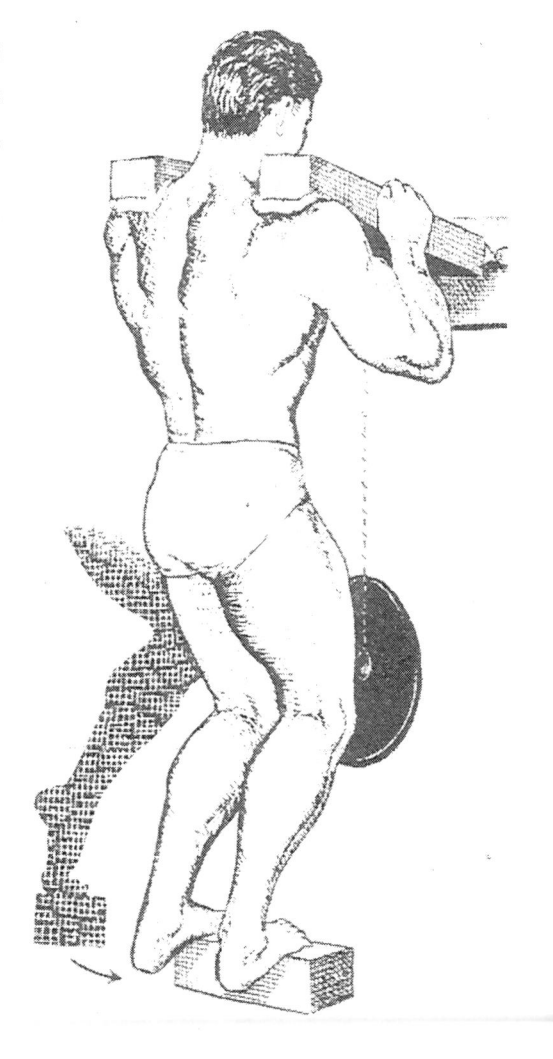

85. Seated Calf Raise

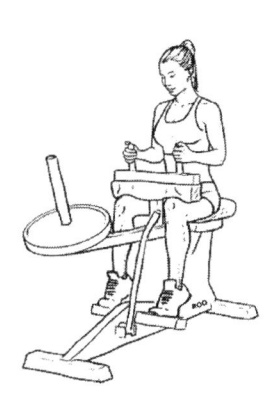

Equipment: Calf raise machine / barbell
Effect: Strengthen calves
Resistance : Light / Medium / Heavy [Slow]
Hip position: Hip Hinge - Fixed position
Spine position: Extended / arched lumbar throughout
Scapula position: Neutral / locked
Muscles: Soleus
Typical Poundage: 15-30 kg (women); 25-40 kg (men)
Joints: Ankle

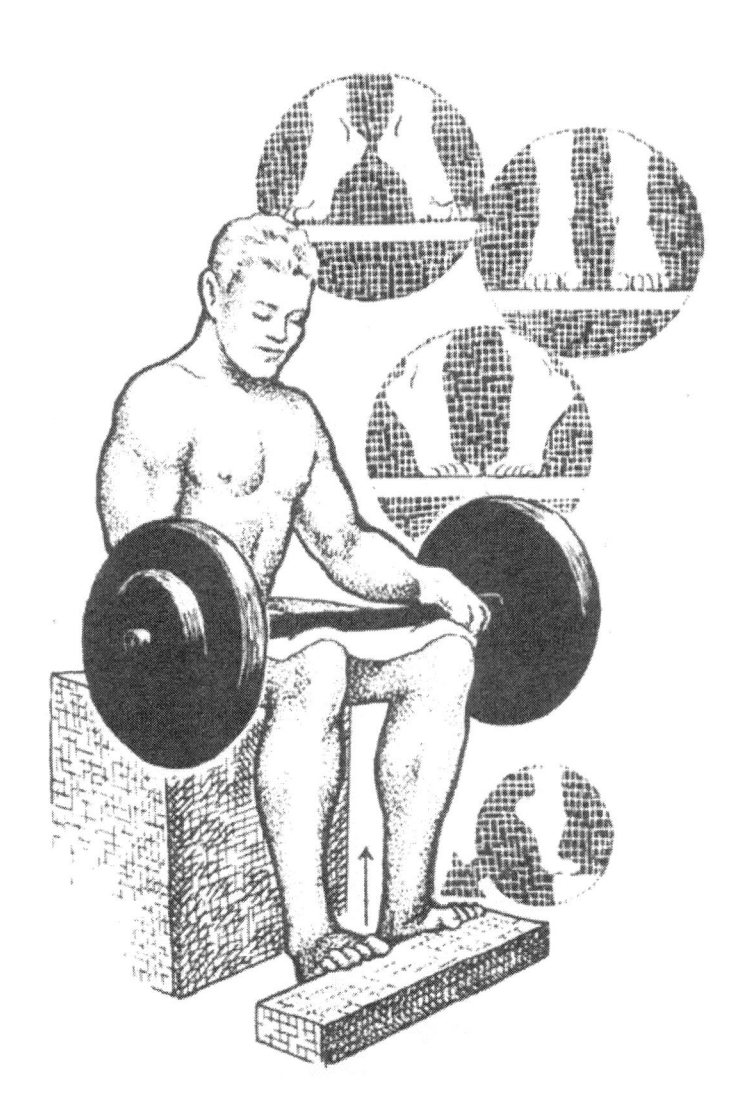

Sit on seat facing lever. Reach forward and pull hand lever toward body. Place forefeet on platform with heels extending off. Position lower thighs under lever pads. Release hand lever by pushing away from body. Place hands on top of thigh pads. Raise heels by extending ankles as high as possible. Lower heels by bending ankles until calves are stretched. Repeat.

THE ANKLE AND FOOT

86. Donkey Calf Raise

Equipment: support, blocks, training partner
Effect: Strengthen calves
Resistance : Light / Medium / Heavy [Slow]
Hip position: Hip Hinge - Fixed position
Spine position: Extended / arched lumbar throughout
Scapula position: Neutral / locked
Muscles: Gastrocnemius (all heads), soleus
Typical Poundage: 50-100 kg (women); 50-100 kg (men)
Joints: Ankle

Stand on edge of platform, toes and balls of feet on calf block with arches and heels extending off. Bend over and grasp knee high bar or place forearms on thigh high surface. Allow training partner to mount hips or lower back from bench. Raise heels by extending ankles as high as possible. Lower heels by bending ankles until calves are stretched. Repeat.

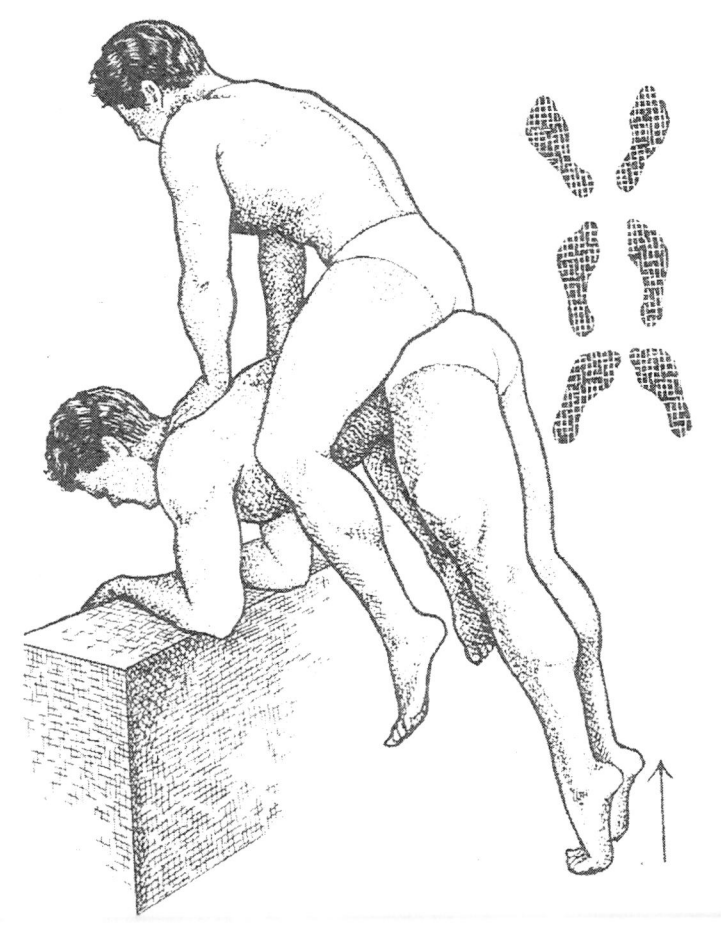

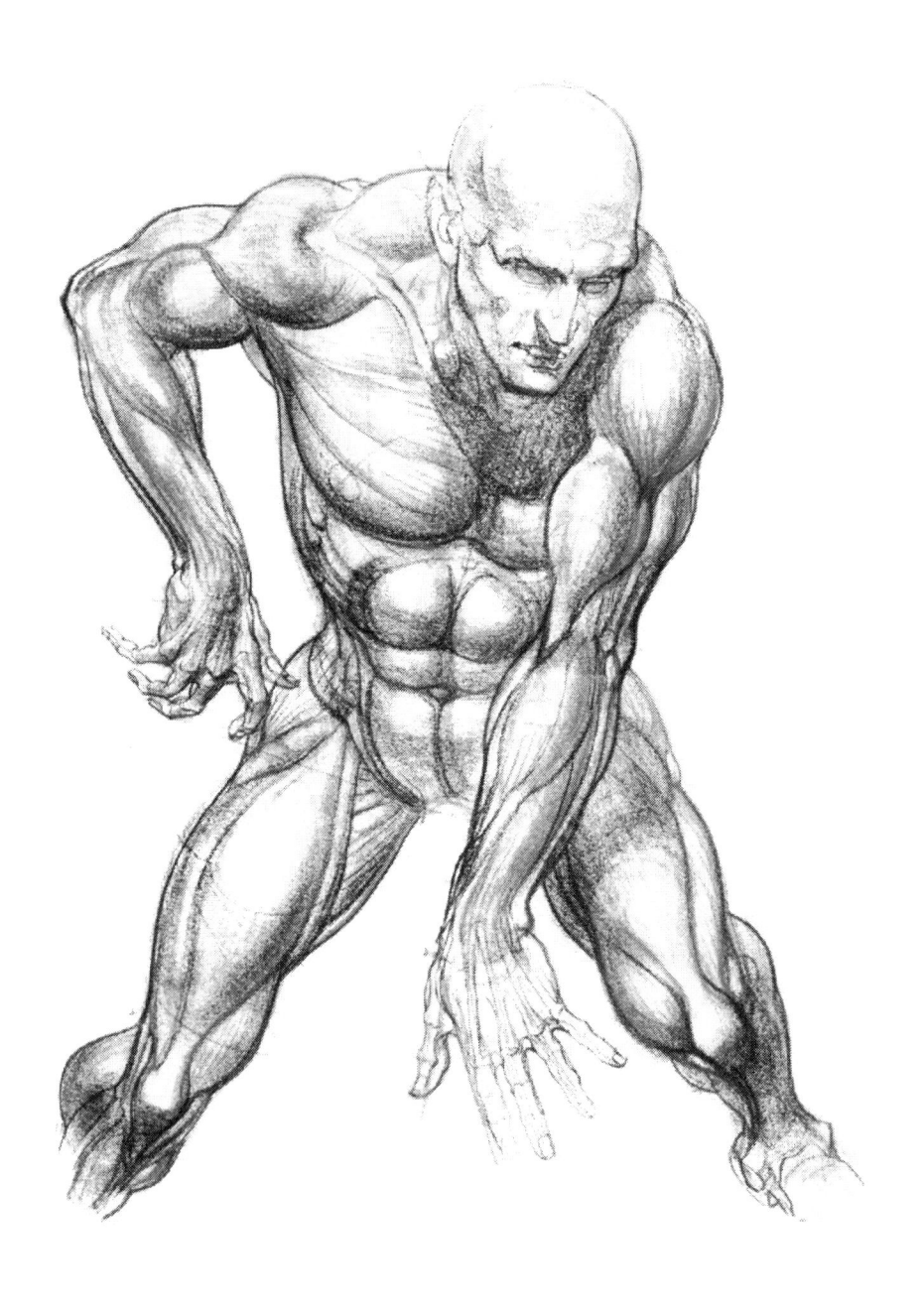

CHAPTER THIRTEEN

Gravity

IN THE early 1970s Arthur Jones, of Nautilus fame, spoke about the "resistance profile" of weight-training exercises. In particular, he noted the descending resistance profile of certain exercises, such as the standing curl. Here the resistance experienced on the biceps varies from zero (1A arms hanging), to a maximum when the forearm is at right angles to the body (1C), and then it goes back to zero (1E at the top) again.

Arthur correctly observed that this resistance profile was in direct opposition to the actual strength profile of the muscle (the biceps), which are strongest at the end (top), and weakest at the beginning. He surmised that if we could find a way to reverse this resistance profile, effectively making the resistance greatest at the finish, then this would maximise the work on the muscle and hence increase the growth potential of the exercise (the biceps curl).

Arthur's solution was the Nautilus cam - shaped like a nautilus shell - that altered the strength profile of the movement. The cam effectively maximised resistance at the end point where the muscle is

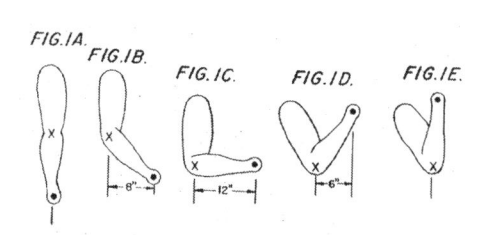

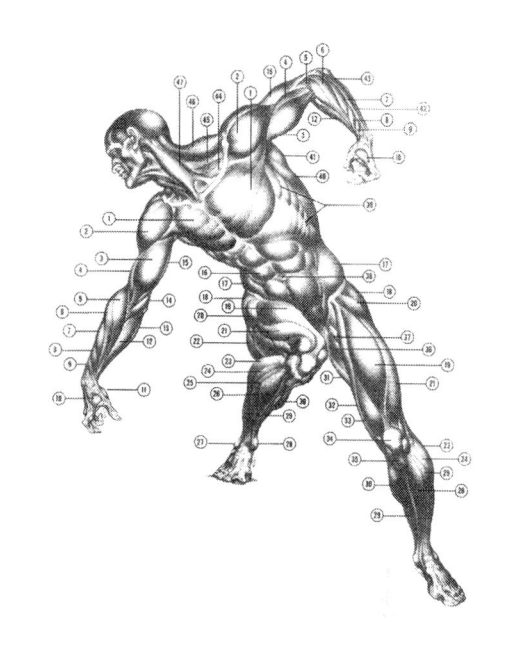

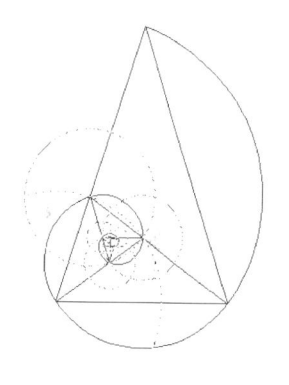

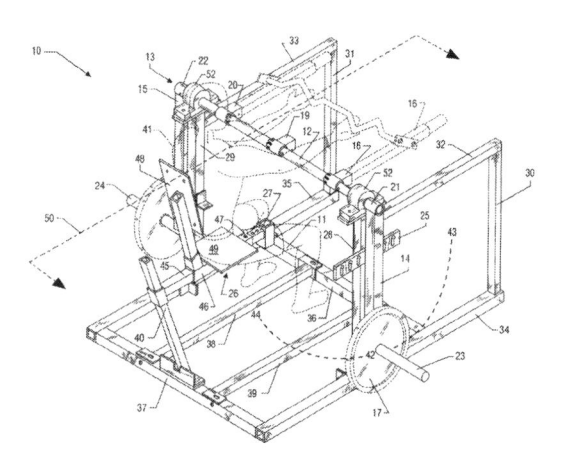

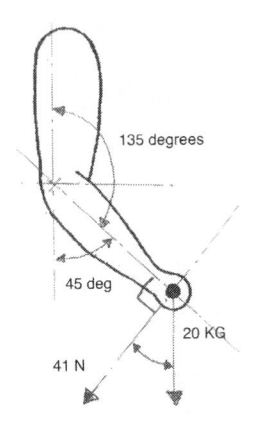

An analysis of the torque force on the bicep when standing upright and curling a 20 KG dumbbell at a point when the lower arm (forearm) is bent to an angle of 135 degrees with respect to the upper arm. The bicep "feels" a force of 41 Newton Metres (Nm). This force goes to zero as the arm is fully straightened. Below we see an analysis of the force on the bicep when curling a 20 KG dumbbell on a preacher bench. We use the same 135 degree angle between upper and lower arm. Here we find the bicep "feels" a force of 56 Newton metres (Nm) at this point in the curl. Therefore the preacher bench increases resistance on the bicep at this point.

strongest. And if you have ever used a Nautilus machine; (I have an original Nautilus arm curl machine in my house), then you will find that you do get a very intense contraction of the muscle at the top position. Your biceps will become sore almost immediately, and definitely you will notice soreness the next day after a few sets on such a machine. Perhaps at the very least such a machine gives variety, and allows the trainee to progress if he has reached a sticking point in his training.

I do believe that such machines can be useful, being ones that alter the resistance profile, but only so long as they are not detrimental in other ways (see Chapter 23). But I do not believe that one should perform all exercises on these types of machines, and for many different reasons. In particular such machines do not (in general) allow for the trainee to choose his/her own 3D movement pattern in space. Plus they fail to tailor the movement to the trainee's own unique characteristics in terms of arm length, joint positions etc. I think that Arthur simplified reality to some extent. And he forgot that the biceps are called upon (in everyday life) to match resistance profiles of all different kinds. For example when chopping wood, or swinging weights to the shoulder ballistically, the biceps will experience varying resistance profiles. Rarely do we move in such a constrained and robotic fashion as in a biceps curl.

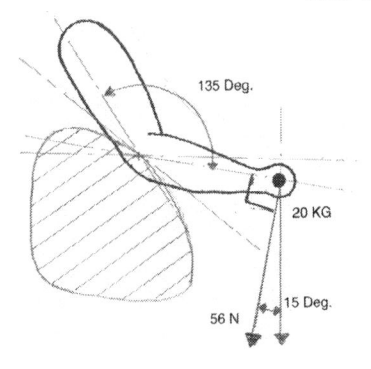

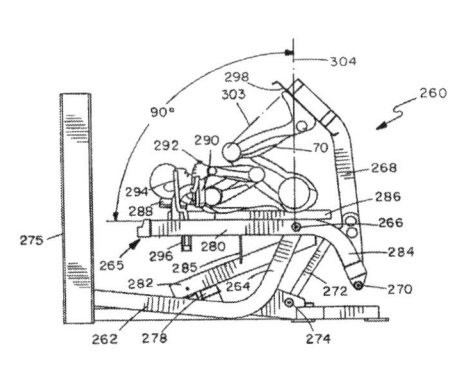

Nevertheless by drawing attention to the resistance profile, Arthur moved the field of exercise science forward. Today we should consider the "gravity" vector (or direction) of resistance, and its profile when lifting weights of any kind. Performing (for example) the incline press can more effectively target the upper pectorals. Also lying down and performing side laterals and/or side crunches can allow us to use the direction of gravity (relative to the body) in unique ways. Also cable machines allow us to obtain resistance in unusual positions, relative to our bodies. In effect a cable side bend or cross-over brings gravity through a 90-degree rotation!

Another important example relates to the preacher bench curl. Here due to the 45 degree angle of the bench, we get greater resistance in the bottom half of the curl (resistance direction is moved relative to the biceps), really stretching the biceps under load as a result. Normally we get very little resistance in the bottom half of the curl, and none when the bar is held at arms length (see analysis on left). Stretching the biceps under load is very important, and preacher bench curls will really make your biceps grow in this manner, if done with a full range of motion. Combining preachers (stretching position resistance) with a Nautilus biceps machine curls (contraction position resistance) in one workout; will really work your biceps harder than when using only the standing (upright) version - that much is certain!

I suggest that you experiment with how to use the direction of gravity (or unusual resistance profiles) in your own training. Another example (in a standing curl) is to keep the elbows well back, which will also keep the biceps under tension at the top. Another interesting point relates to biceps function, which (as everyone knows) is to bend the elbow as well as to supinate the hand. But the biceps have another third function; and are also active when you raise your arm in front and to the side of your torso. The upshot is that bicep curls can be very effective (you get a tighter contraction) when you curl with a raised elbow position (fixed elbow better here).

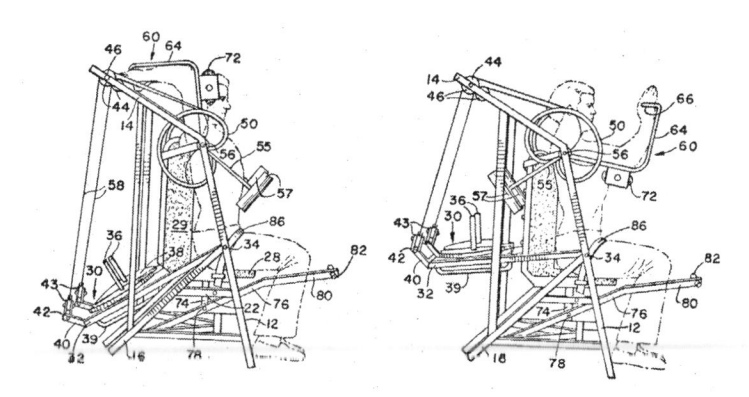

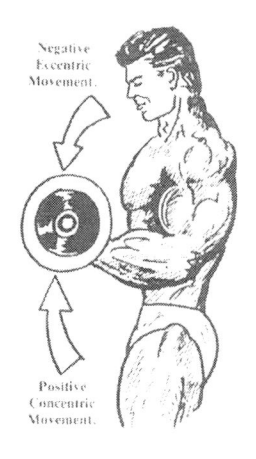

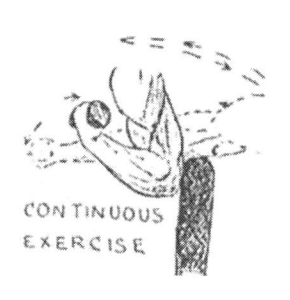

A nice technique to alter the resistance profile of a barbell on certain exercises is to use chains and/or bands on the bar; and in order to make the exercise more difficult in the strongest part of the movement. Chains work well on exercises like squats, the bench-press and on the standing press. They also work for exercises like dips and even flys if you can find a way to attach a chain or band to the bar/body. To learn about such (advanced) resistance training techniques; you might want to study the training methods of elite powerlifters such as the Westside Barbell Club and IronMind in the USA.

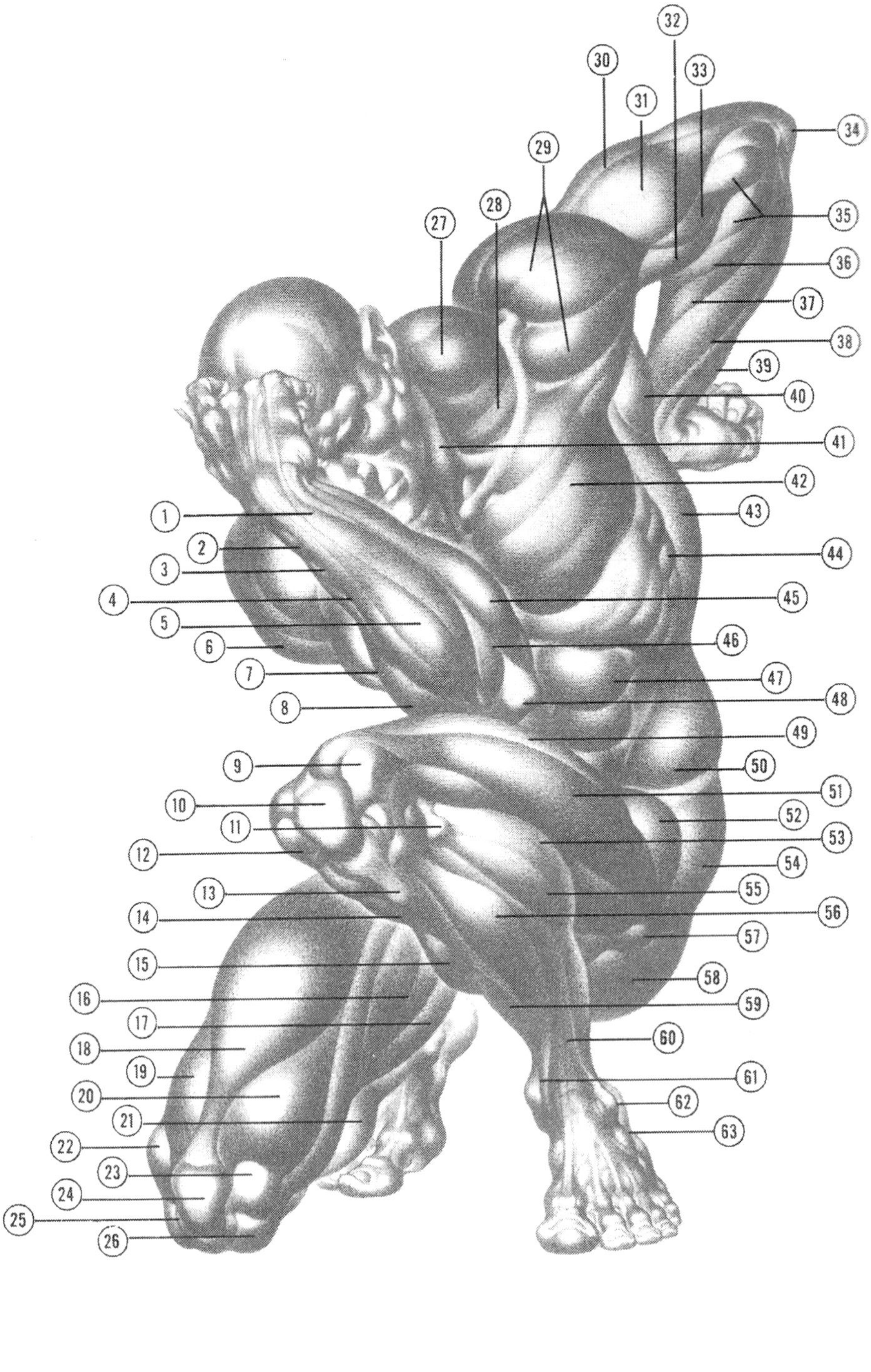
1
2
3
4
5
6
7
8
9
10
11
12
13
14
15
16
17
18
19
20
21
22
23
24
25
26
27
28
29
30
31
32
33
34
35
36
37
38
39
40
41
42
43
44
45
46
47
48
49
50
51
52
53
54
55
56
57
58
59
60
61
62
63

CHAPTER FOURTEEN
Training Techniques

RESISTANCE TRAINING has a long history going right back to the ancient Greeks and Romans. Aristotle commented on the tendency of some athletes to train for beauty alone, whilst others trained for strength. Even today, one can (theoretically) split strength training techniques into two kinds, being those methods that produce structural changes and the others that produce purely functional changes.

However in practice often one type of training effects both types of changes to one degree or another. The present book is a general purpose text, and it is not concerned with specific training techniques which are beyond the scope of our analyses (we ignore specific strength training for olympic lifting etc).

Rather here we shall attempt to set the trainee on the path to efficient and effective general-purpose training methods; in the hope that if and when more specialised techniques are required that he could find that information in the form of a coach and/or specialised texts.

Perhaps the best book ever produced on strength training is *"Super Training"* by Yuri Verkhoshansky. We heartily recommend that book when you wish to learn more about training techniques both generally and specifically; whereas here we shall briefly overview the

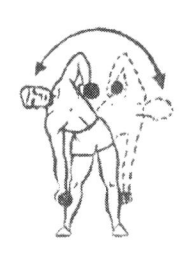

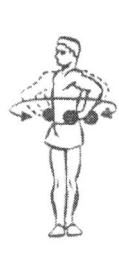

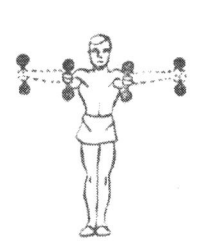

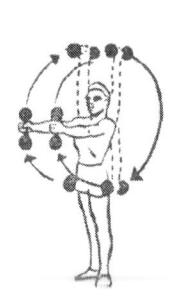

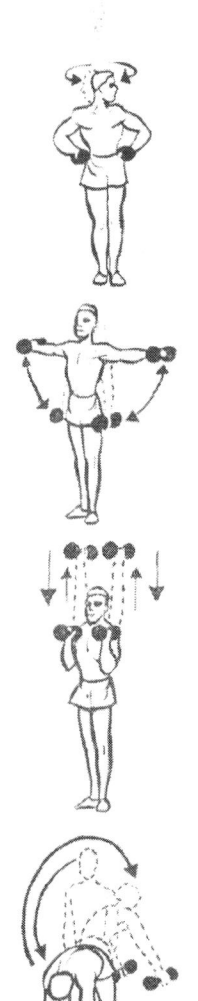

Sometimes a period of exercise specialisation is called for. For example as a youth (19-20 years old) I would regularly complete two weekly 1 hour workouts (along with my normal routine) whereby I just performed countless sets of heavy full squats pyramiding up to 500 lbs for 4-5 reps. After 2 years on such a routine I easily gained 20 lbs of solid muscle; and I believe that the heavy squats stimulated my metabolism to make such gains.

Other techniques can prove useful. For example, heavy dead-lift specialisation and/or specialisation on the clean and press with a barbell and/or twin dumbbells can stimulate muscular gains. The strongest I ever had my deltoids was when performing just standing presses (countless sets) for 1 hour twice weekly. At the end of this period; I was standing pressing a 225 lb barbell for 10 reps and cleaning and pressing (standing up) a pair of 120 lb dumbbells for 2-3 reps (twice weekly).

different training methods in the hope that the reader can find more detailed information elsewhere.

It is useful at this point to mention the difference between training to produce muscle hypertrophy, as opposed to training for improved skill/capability (or nervous system training). A stronger athlete may be one with bigger muscles; or he may in fact not be. Often skill, leverage issues, and overall capacity to apply strength are important, as in the sport of weightlifting for example.

Now anyone who has spent any period of time on a weight-training program will have noticed that progress comes fast at first, when the muscles grow bigger and stronger quickly; but that after a while, progress slows or stops altogether and new (more demanding) techniques must be used to cause progress to continue. In terms of lifting weights; one can distinguish between concentric contraction (positive) movements - where the weight is moved in the direction of flexion; and static contraction where the weight does not move but the muscle is contracting to maintain its position. Also there is eccentric contraction where the weight moves in the opposite direction to flexion - but the weight is "slowed down" relative to gravity. In passing it is worth noting that eccentric and static contractions (that is strength) are stronger than the concentric type.

One can hold a weight or let it slowly drop, being a weight that is heavier than one can concentrically (positively) lift. Different techniques have been developed to work these various and specific aspects of strength.

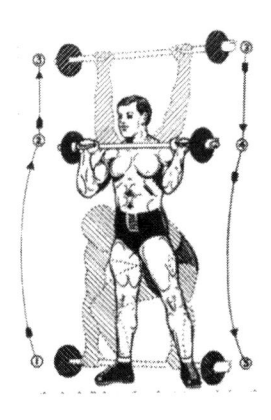

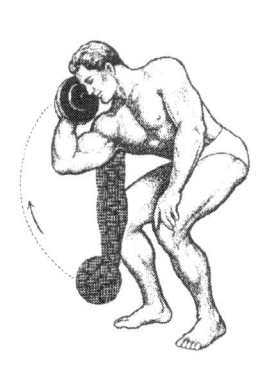

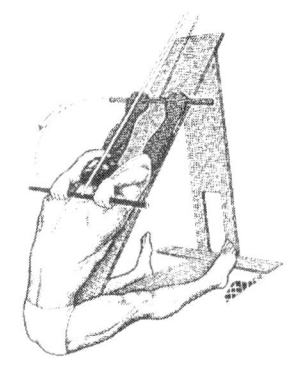

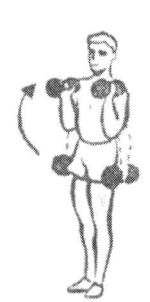

Supra-maximal Methods

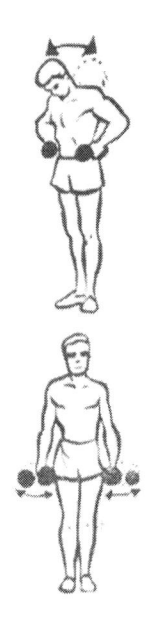

These are methods which allow the continuation of training movement beyond that which is normally possible after the concentric (positive) movement fails.

Forced repetitions are one such method. You work to failure with a given load, and you then execute a few more repetitions with the aid of a training partner. The partner helps on the concentric phase, whilst the eccentric phase is performed without help.

Cheating is the use of momentum, by swaying the body, or bouncing the bar against the body, or using "loose" form, and in order to complete more repetitions than one normally could perform.

Ballistics is another technique, and involves lowering or dropping a weight rapidly to recruit the stretch reflex or to exploit elastic energy in the tendons and other connective tissues (not recommended).

Restricted Range Repetitions are an excellent method to increase the intensity of exercise. The athlete chooses a load which is heavier than the maximum that he can use for a complete cycle of the exercise, he then performs a few small range concentric-eccentric repetitions near the strongest region of that particular exercise. If these are performed after the end of a completed normal set of repetitions - then the technique is called "burning".

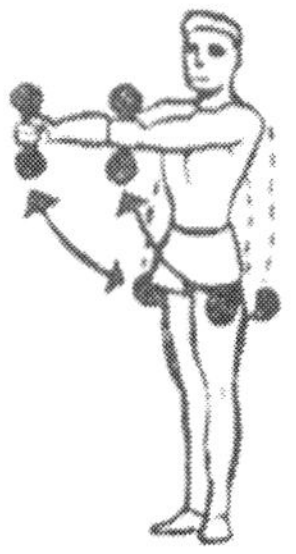

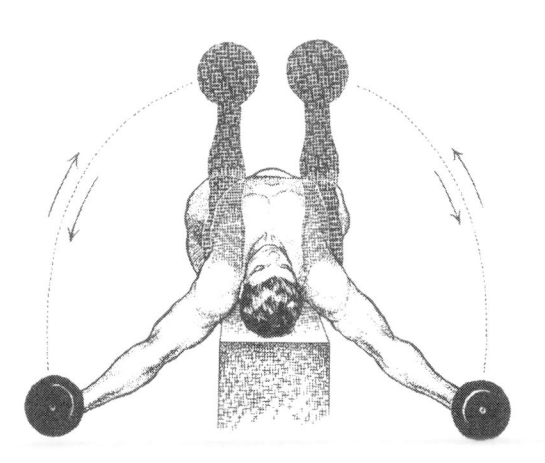

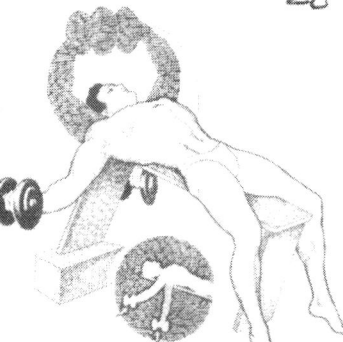

Circa-maximal Methods

These methods imply training with loads that are close to the 1 rep-maximum. All the preceding methods may be used with such training.

Sub-maximal Methods

Sub-maximal or repetition methods characteristically involved training with loads of about 60-80 percent of one's 1 rep maximum. These methods are normally performed for muscle hypertrophy and/or for bodybuilding and/or for increasing muscular definition.

Methods include a classical bodybuilding regime, consisting of 3 to 5 sets of 8-10 repetitions with each movement. Here often the load (or weight) is increased from one set to another (plus decreasing reps) in the so-called pyramid system (allows warm up and gradually increasing resistance over time). At other times (and on other programs) the weight remains constant between sets.

Use of super-sets is a well-known method; whereby two separate exercises are performed one immediately after another. Sometimes the super-set is performed for the same muscle, and at other times for different muscles (i.e. bench press plus chin-ups). Sometimes a giant set is performed with several exercises completed one after another without any rest in-between. Pre-exhaustion is a method whereby a single-joint exercise is used to preferentially exhaust one muscle prior to performing a multi-joint exercise; and in order to work one muscle group intensely.

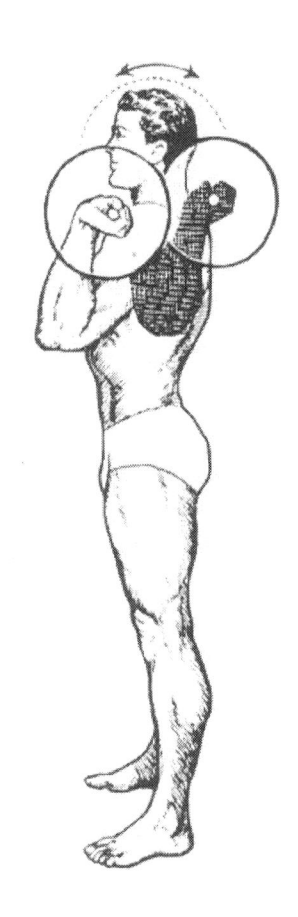

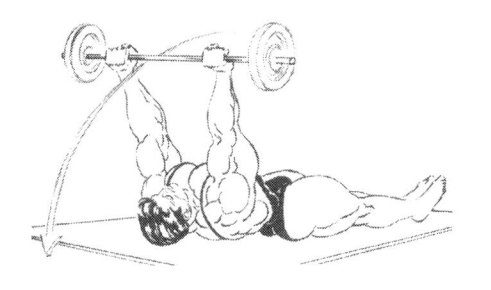

Use of a split routine is common in weight-training; whereby you divide a routine into distinct components and then perform one part on one day and the rest on another day (for example - upper body day 1, lower body day 2). Stripping or drop-sets is yet another method; whereby you work the same exercise with progressively lighter weights - and without any rest.

Many other methods have been, and/or are currently used in the field and sport of weight-training; and all are employed normally to increase the stress on the various muscles of the body. For many people the hope (and constant wish) is to increase the size and strength of the muscles of the body. Of-coarse this should not be the only reason to train, as discussed previously.

A few words on drugs are salient at this point. Right away I shall state that I don't believe in using performance enhancing drugs under any circumstances. I have never taken them myself, for example. Yet it is undoubtedly true that if you use drugs, then you may obtain more strength and muscular development than you ever could with natural training. This is not certain, but it is likely. I know this because studies have shown that beginners can gain more solid muscle (12 pounds in 3 months) simply by taking drugs alone (and not training) than you can by training without them (8 lbs in 3 months).

But the drugs have many down-sides. Two drug-taking "acquaintances" died of drug-related complications before they reached the age of 40. And I was always stronger then either one of these chaps in the gym (plus I am still alive).

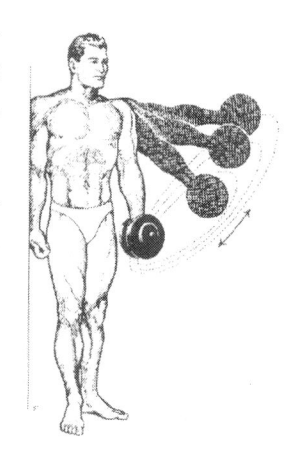

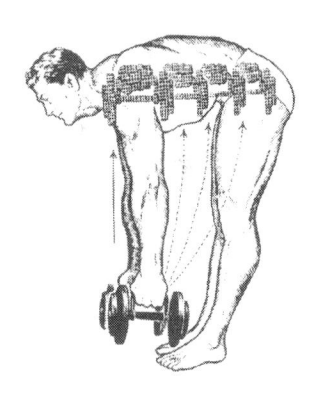

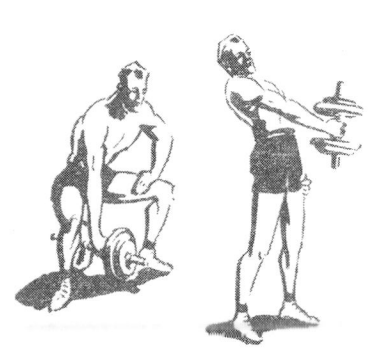

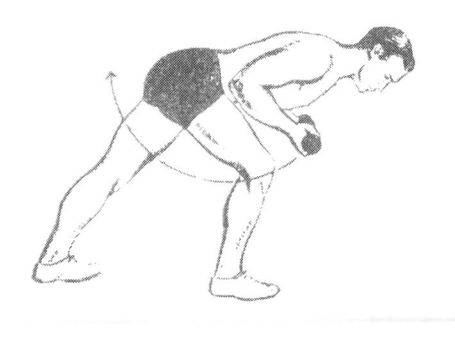

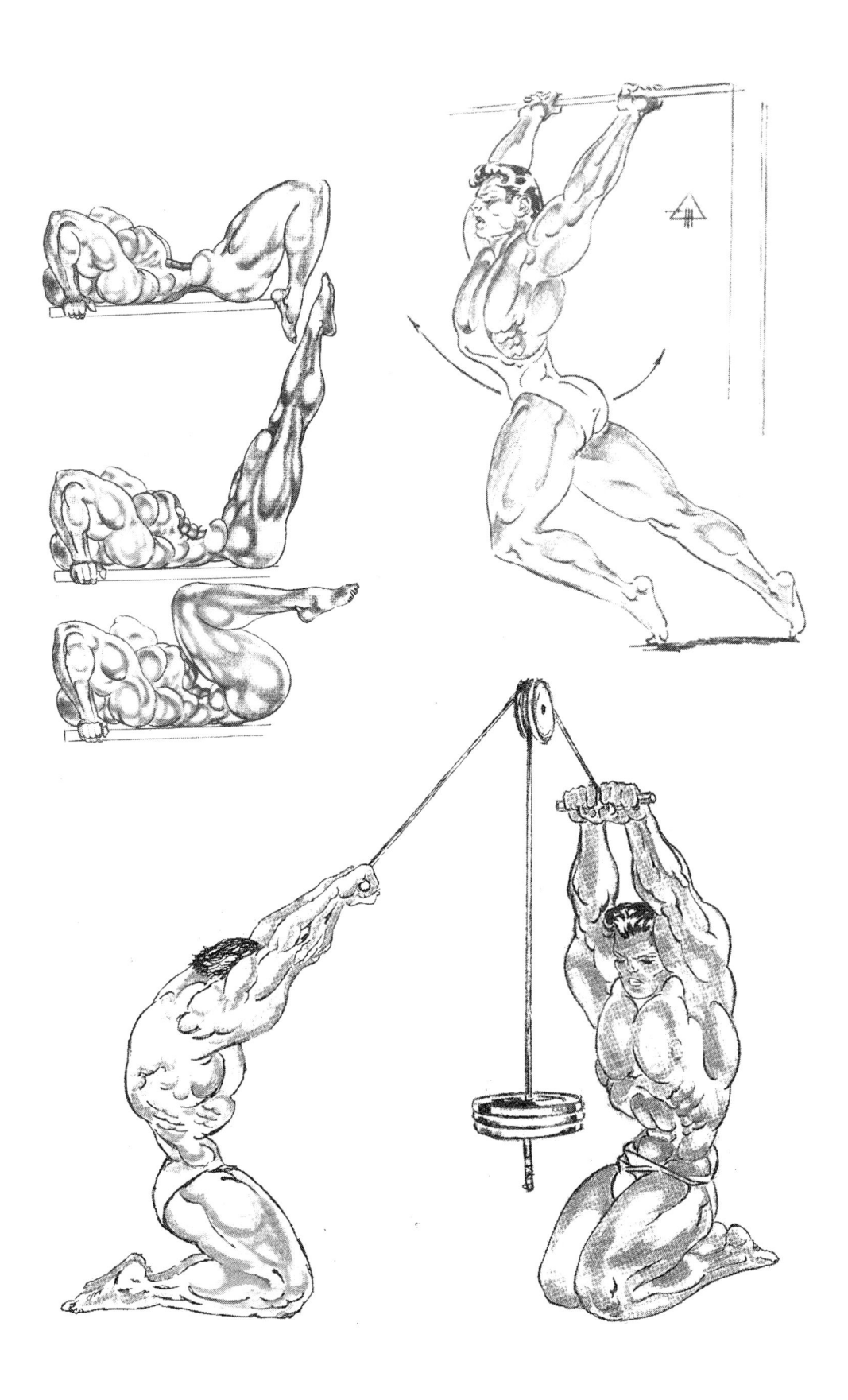

CHAPTER FIFTEEN

Training for Health

IN EARLY chapters we spoke about the definition of fitness, but we failed to discuss health. Of course what each of us means when we speak of a "healthy" person will be different, and especially when we apply the term to ourselves. Myself when I think of health, I do not imagine how I shall be on any particular day of the week; but rather visualise how I shall look (and be) in the far future - perhaps years from the present time.

This is how I have always felt, that fitness training is the ideal route or path to a good/better life physically, and as an aid to the creation and preservation of my long term health. I shall not recite examples of people who think differently than I do, or the occasions that others have felt compelled to instruct me in the apparent dangers and supposed pointlessness of strength training.

My aim here is not to convince you of the positive benefits of the fitness lifestyle. Rather I shall recite best-practice in terms of health promotion; and from the perspective (largely) of personal experience.

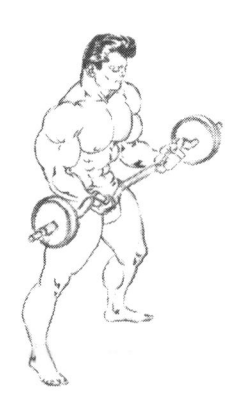

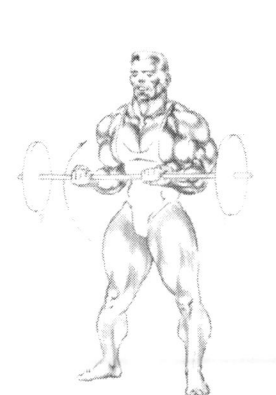

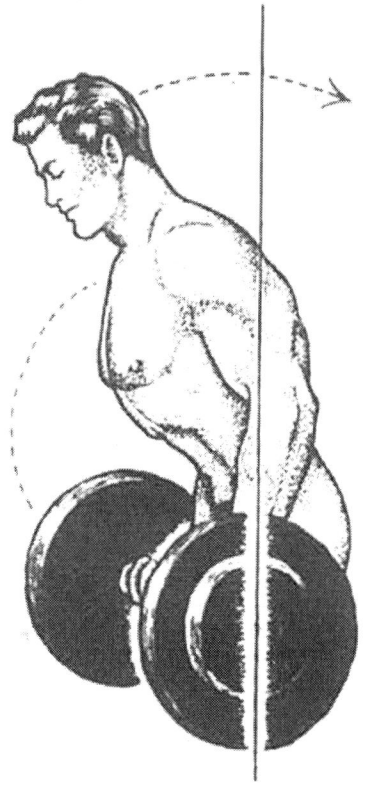

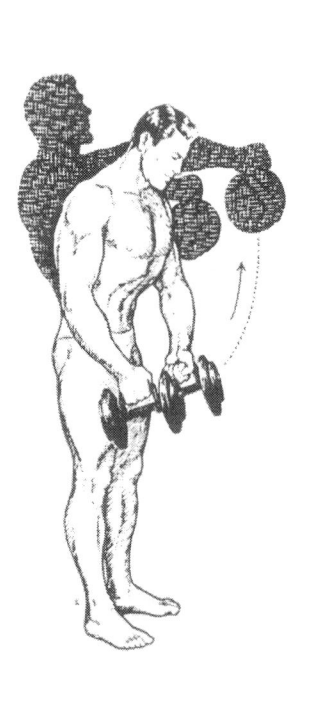

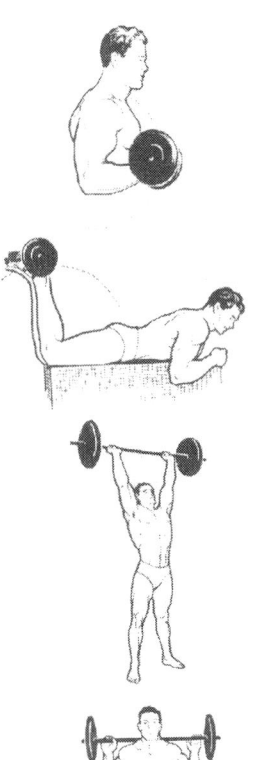

Right away I shall state that I have always felt better training around 5 days per week with weights (1 hour sessions); and running 3-4 times a week (at least 45 minutes per run). Sometimes I notice that when I need to loose fat, daily running is even better, in terms of overall health and the way that I feel in myself. Normally I would include walking sessions of around 1 hour daily as well, and in order to feel at the absolute peak of physical fitness.

Myself I do not seem to need any more than this, so far as physical exercise is concerned. It also seems that the routines performed (in terms of resistance training) do not really seem to matter; as long as I work everything (each muscle group) around 2-3 times weekly. Therefore I believe in combining equal amounts of weight-training and running (aerobics), and in order to achieve balanced physical fitness. I have noticed that it is nice also to include some stretching (yoga etc) in my routine; but on the whole I have noticed that the weight-training itself does provide sufficient flexibility in my various joint ROMs.

In terms of diet (dealt with previously), I have found that I don't need much food to maintain an ideal bodyweight. As stated earlier, I believe in limiting sugar, white flour and junk foods (although I love all of these and greedily consume them on occasion). I do notice that I feel and look better when I supplement my diet with 50-100 grams of whey protein, although I do not eat anywhere near 1g of protein per lb of bodyweight, but more like 0.75 g per lb. I also like fruit and vegetable juices, and eat oatmeal daily, and I like fish, plus fruits of all kinds etc.

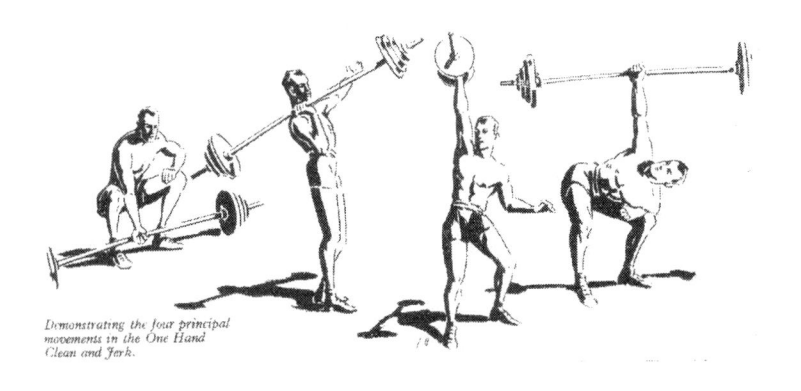

Demonstrating the four principal movements in the One Hand Clean and Jerk.

TRAINING FOR HEALTH   279

I believe in one day of complete inactivity per week also (at least). A good example health routine is as follows:

Health Routine

Day 1 - Full-body workout

Day 2 - Run/Walk

Day 3 - Full-body workout

Day 4 - Run /Walk

Day 5 - Full-body workout

Day 6 - Bike / Walk / Swim

Day 7 - Complete Rest

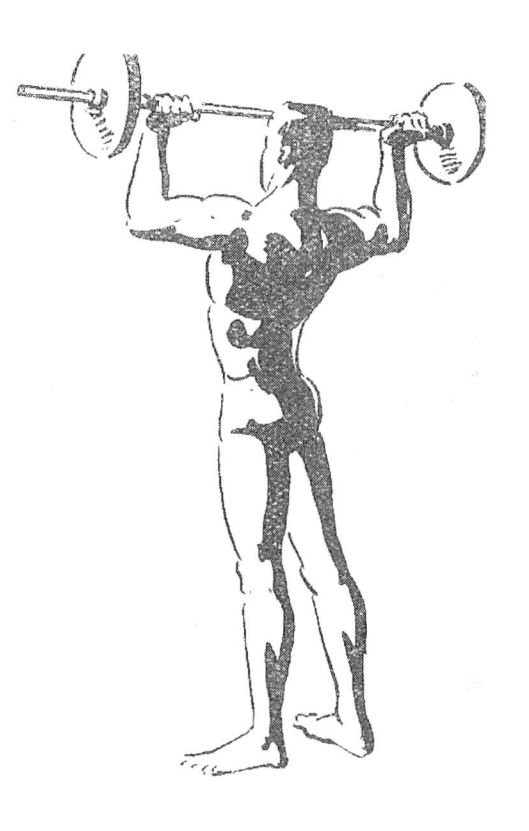

Overall one should aim for an every-other day walk/run of 1-1.5 hours; because moving about using the legs is the fundamental human activity. I do not recommend that you train on the same routine (i.e. use all of the same exercises) for more than 1-2 months, but rather constantly swap-in, and swap-out, different movements as desired.

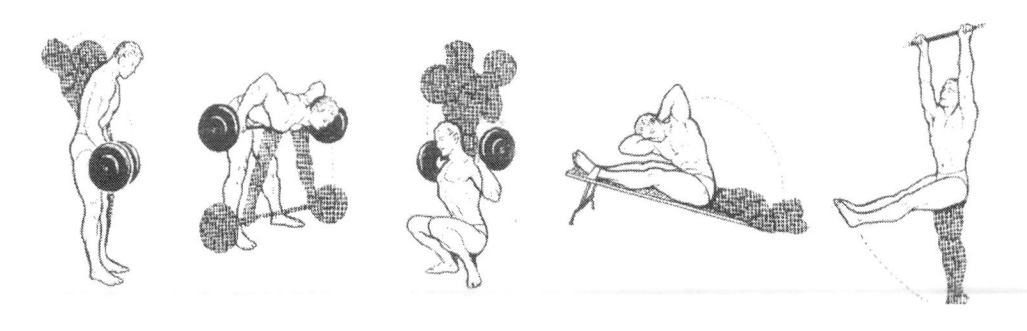

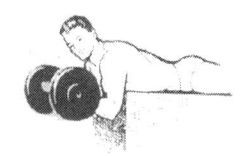

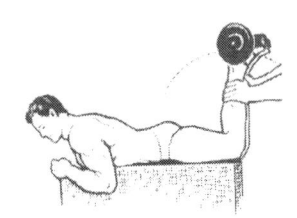

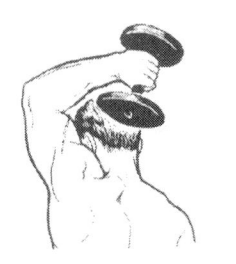

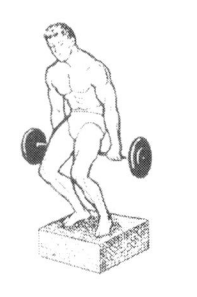

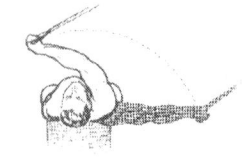

Exercises

You will be performing a full body workout 3 times a week. Many people think - and have found - that this is the ideal routine allowing 4 days of complete rest for muscles to recover and grow from the exercises (Steve Reeves belief).

Perform the following exercises (order not important):

Barbell Squats (+ dumbbell hack squats): 6 sets of 8-10 reps
Barbell Dead-lifts (once per week if heavy): 6 sets of 8- 10 reps
Dumbbell Stiff-Legged Dead-lifts: 3 sets of 8-10 reps
Chin-ups: 3 sets of as many as possible
Dumbbell Bent over rows: 3 sets of 8-10 reps
Barbell Bench Press (or dumbbell): 3 sets of 8-10 reps
Lying Round the World: 3 sets
Lying Fly (bent + straight arm) + Hang: 3 sets
Lying Dumbbell Pullovers: 3 sets
Standing dumbbell press: 3 sets of 8-10 reps
Standing Overhead Lateral: 3 sets of 8-10 reps
Standing Front Lateral: 3 sets of 8-10 reps
Standing Dumbbell Curls (or preacher curls): 3 sets of 8-10 reps
Cable Triceps Pushdown: 3 sets of 8-10 reps
Seated knee-ins for abdominals: 3 sets
Abdominal crunches: 3 sets / Calf Raise: 3 sets

Total sets = 57 - complete in 1 hour to 1.5 hours
[N.B all are suggested exercises only]

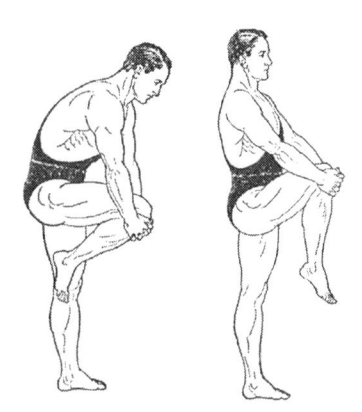

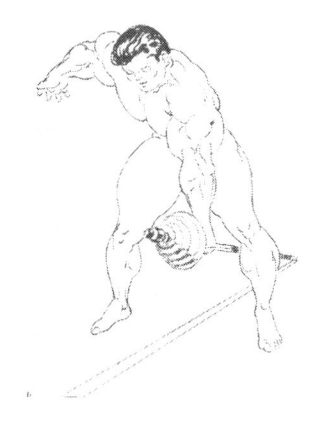

Notes

For most people, it is probably ideal (in terms of health) to train 3 times a week with free-weights on a routine similar to the one laid out here. Note that you should change the exercises around often. It is best to train alone (to prevent waisted time talking) and to perform the routine at quite a fast pace. On the 3 days when you do not train you will be walking and/or running for 1 hour - or else substituting some other form of cardiovascular training for the same. If you are over-weight, then you may need to perform aerobics on your weight-training days as well. The exercise routines given here are quite strenuous and will result in allot of calories burned.

Body-part training frequency is a very important consideration; and depends upon personal preference, muscle recovery, goals, weights used and the intensity of training effort etc. The basic rule is that you should have recovered (in a body-part sense) from the last workout before you once again work the same region of the body. Recovery ability depends on many factors, including the body-part(s) worked, weights used, rest and activity between workouts and nutrition. Steroids can greatly increase recovery ability and reduce the time between workouts (not recommended). A heavy dead-lift workout with maximum weights may take a week or more to recover from fully, and before you are ready to perform at such a level again.

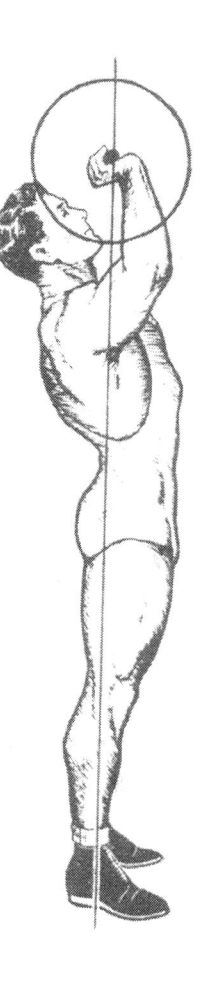

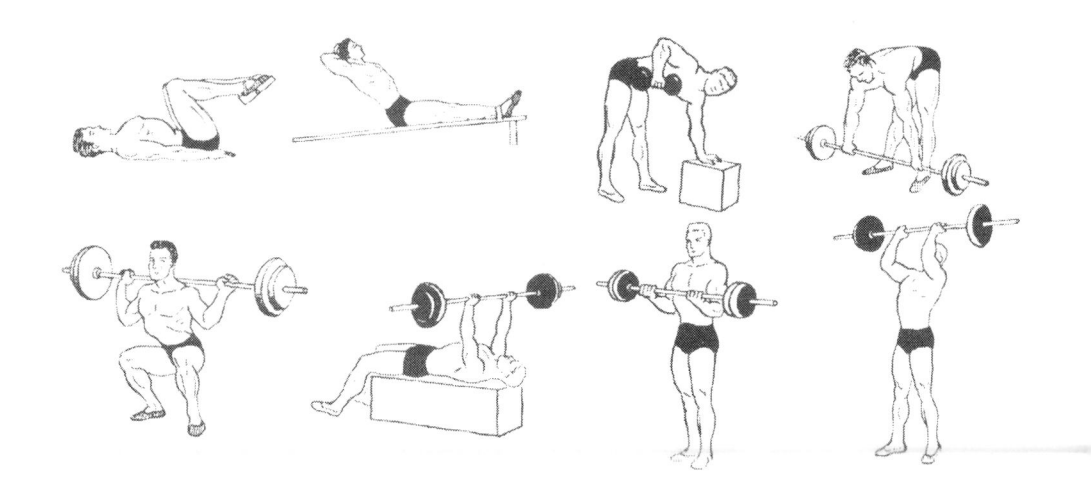

SANDOW'S MAGAZINE

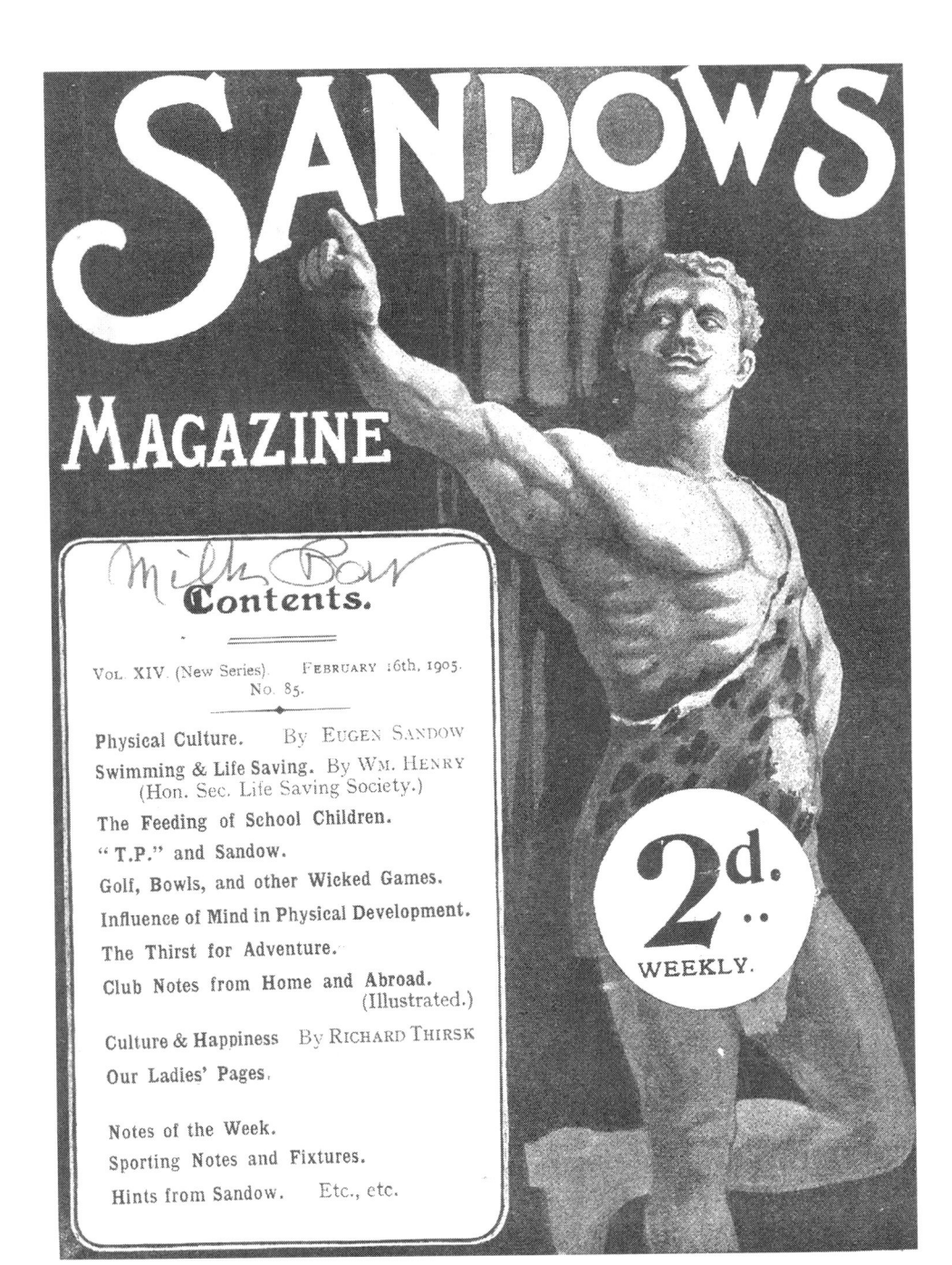

Contents.

Vol. XIV. (New Series).   February 16th, 1905.
No. 85.

Physical Culture.   By Eugen Sandow

Swimming & Life Saving. By Wm. Henry
(Hon. Sec. Life Saving Society.)

The Feeding of School Children.

"T.P." and Sandow.

Golf, Bowls, and other Wicked Games.

Influence of Mind in Physical Development.

The Thirst for Adventure.

Club Notes from Home and Abroad.
(Illustrated.)

Culture & Happiness   By Richard Thirsk

Our Ladies' Pages.

Notes of the Week.

Sporting Notes and Fixtures.

Hints from Sandow.   Etc., etc.

2d. WEEKLY.

CHAPTER SIXTEEN

Training for Strength

OUR OWN age has seen *Bodybuilding*, or developing shapely muscles for an improved appearance, steadily rise in prominence to the point where in the 21st Century most people now go to the gym *to get some muscles.* It was not always so - and even 20 years ago (pure) muscle builders were thought to be oddballs. Now trends do come and go, for example *Physical Culture*: the building of health, strength and beauty in the human body, was trendy around 100 years ago when Eugene Sandow first popularised the body-beautiful. But it seems that we are now placing too much emphasis on the actual look of the body.

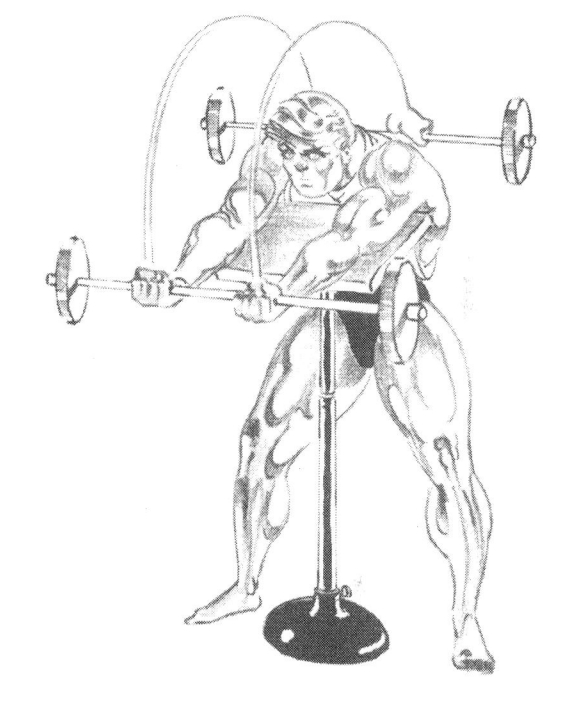

Rather in this book I have stressed the need to perform exercises according to functional movement patterns. I have emphasised good movement techniques; as opposed to focussing on the muscles being exercised. It is my belief that function is more important than

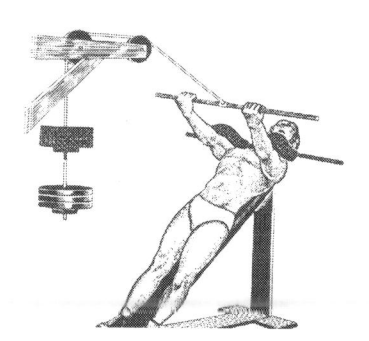

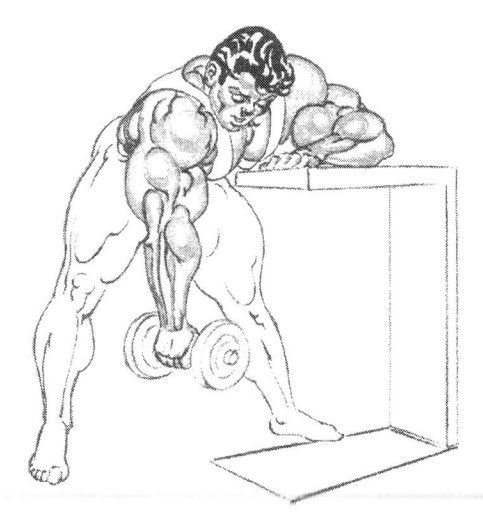

In the old days a great exercise for stimulating overall muscular strength improvement was the clean and press with a barbell (or twin dumbbells); performed as a single exercise. So you clean the weight(s) from the floor and press them overhead (1 repetition), before lowering the same to the floor and beginning again (for multiple repetitions). Lifters might perform say 5-6 sets of 5-1 reps; pyramiding the weight up on each successive set. You end with a limit attempt to see what you can do for a single repetition. Progress is measured by higher weights lifted over time. Another technique is to do the same, but this time using just a single dumbbell, and possibly a thick-handled dumbbell.

form in this respect, and that muscular development will take care of itself if we emphasise natural training in accordance with the normal capacities of the human body. Therefore, our focus here is on capability, and on finding ways to enhance basic ROM functionality (plus strength).

A key movement related capability of the human body is strength. Unfortunately many let their bodies become weakened due to inactivity, poor diet and/or illness. Strength training can restore the body to its natural state in this respect; and if performed correctly, a kind of super-strength can be developed which sees capability go far beyond the norm in terms of the physical powers.

Perhaps a few words to define strength are useful at this point. According to Wikipedia *Physical Strength is the ability of a person to exert force on physical objects using muscles*. The online encyclopaedia also states that strength is determined by several factors, including muscle size/type, tendon strength, joint angles, limb lengths etc. Obviously these factors differ from one individual to another, and an individual's strength varies according to genetics, sex, age, diet, rest, mood etc.

Strength has always held a somewhat mysterious aspect, perhaps because we all admire the physically powerful who can bend others to their will. Some people link possession of physical strength to the brutish aspects of the human soul, however in so doing they err significantly. Many great and intelligent men and women were also fitness buffs, and those known to possess unusually large and powerful muscles include Plato, and Leonardo da Vinci.

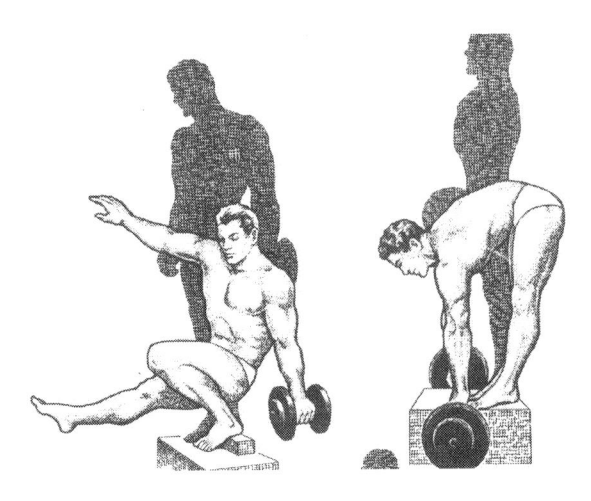

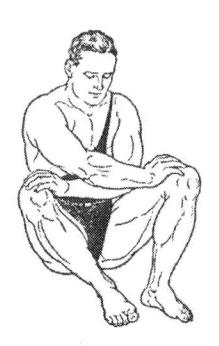

TRAINING FOR STRENGTH

Physical Culture links mind and body with spiritual health, and the Ancient Greeks believed that all 3 must be equally developed in the ideal person. They named this quality of superiority Arete, and young men would train daily in the gymnasia to attain the same, which were also libraries and centres of learning for the mind.

Today scientists are finally realising that being physically fit can improve one's health and well being, plus studies show that fitness may be linked to superior intellectual capabilities as well. So strength is an enviable quality to possess - or obtain - then. What concerns us here is change; how you can become a better, stronger and fitter version of yourself and perhaps, in fact, the ideal version. And to do so naturally. A common saying is that *many paths lead to the same goal*, and we do not claim that the path(s) described here are the only ones leading to super-fitness - nor do we recommend that anyone slavishly follow any other person's advice in this respect.

There are often many routes to the same end, and when it comes to training for strength, we find that possible are many types of routines and exercises which will bring about significant improvements. Strength is very much a specific factor in an individual. It is not just about big muscles. Speed, skill and discipline all play a big part in any demonstration of physical strength; as evidenced by light-weight women weight-lifters who can lift 300 lbs or more overhead in the olympics.

So specific strength must be specifically trained. Here I am assuming that you want to improve your strength in a more general aspect, and the following routine gives one example of how to achieve the same.

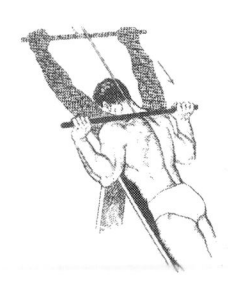

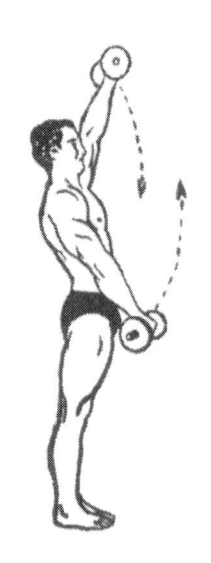

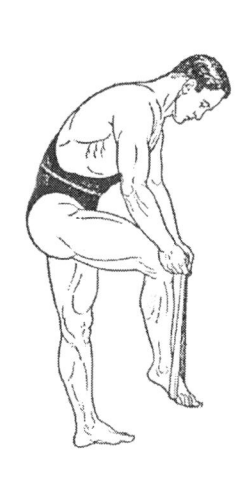

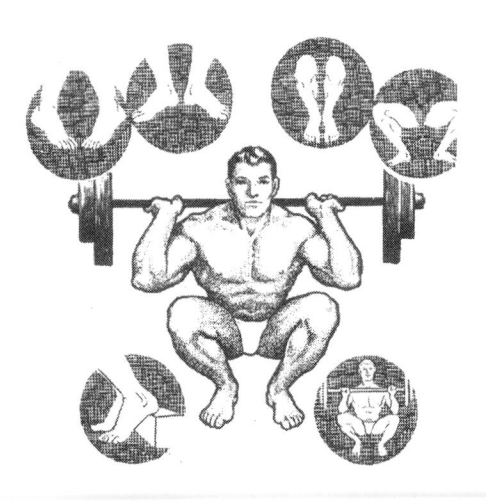

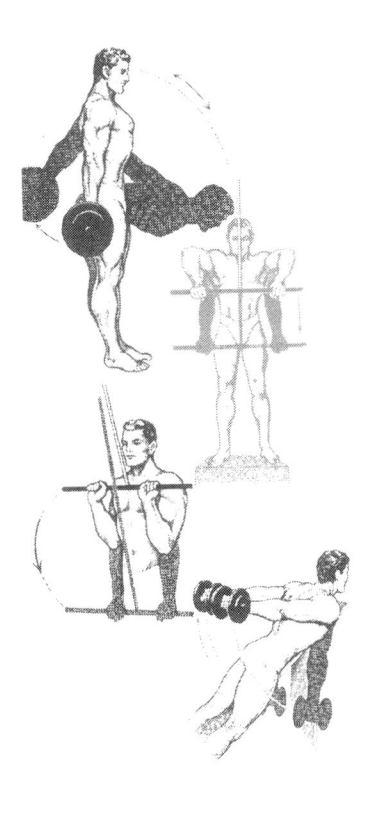

Strength Routine

Day 1 - Chest, Shoulders, Arms + Walk/Run

Day 2 - Legs, Back, Abs, Calves

Day 3 - Complete Rest

Day 4 - Chest, Shoulders, Arms + Run /Walk

Day 5 - Legs, Back, Abs, Calves

Day 6 - Bike Ride / Walk / Swim

Day 7 - Complete Rest

Pavel Tsatsouline says:

"*until one becomes 'entry level strong', a strict bodyweight military press for men or strict pull-ups for women, no priority other than strength can be justified for a healthy athlete*".

I also recommend that all (younger) athletes concentrate on gaining the strength to perform a bodyweight standing press (1 rep with a barbell), and perhaps a double bodyweight squat and dead-lift as well. In order to achieve the same, you will need to go on a strength specialisation routine.

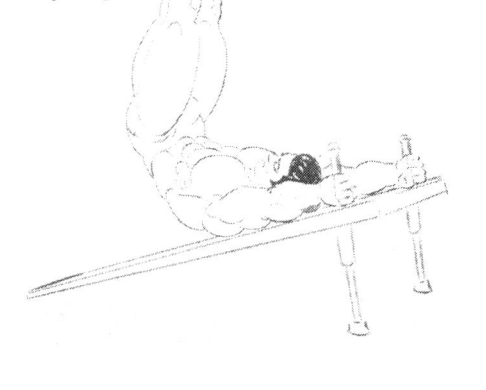

To improve strength you would want to exercise the biggest muscles in the body with heavy weights, because in so doing you stimulate your system to grow. It is best to train each muscle approximately twice each a week. Concentrate on lifting heavier weights on the barbell and/or dumbbell squat and dead-lift. Also practice the bench press and standing dumbbell press. Aim to increase the weights used over time - which may require an increase in bodyweight.

Exercises

You will be performing a half body workout four times weekly. Many people think - and have found - that this is the ideal routine allowing 3 days of complete rest for muscles to recover and grow from the exercises. We have cut down aerobics to 3 days to allow for growth of muscles. Perform the following exercises (order of performance is not so important): Total sets = 20 sets, completed in 1 hour.

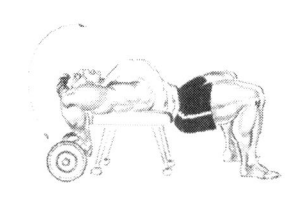

Day 1: [use heavy weights on all exercises / pyramid]
Standing dumbbell press: 5 sets of 8-3 reps
Barbell Bench Press (+ Dips): 5 sets of 8-3 reps
Lying Round the World + Pullover - 3 sets
Lying Fly + Hang (straight and bent arm): 3 sets
Standing Overhead Lateral: 3 sets of 8-10 reps
Standing Front Lateral: 3 sets of 8-10 reps
Standing Dumbbell Curls (+ dumbbell preacher curls): 3 sets of 8-3 reps
Cable Triceps Pushdown (or one-arm extension): 3 sets of 8-3 reps
Seated knee-ins for abdominals: 3 sets

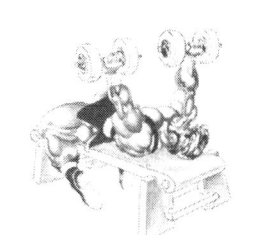

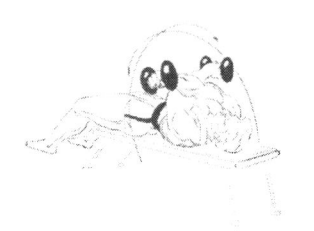

Day 2: [use heavy weights on all exercises / pyramid]
Barbell Squats (+ dumbbell hack squats): 10 sets of 8-3 reps
Barbell Dead-lifts (once per week if heavy): 6 sets of 8- 3reps
Dumbbell Stiff-Legged Dead-lifts: 3 sets of 8-10 reps.
Chin-ups: 3 sets of as many as possible
Dumbbell Bent over rows: 3 sets of 8-3 reps
Seated knee-ins for abdominals: 3 sets
Abdominal crunches: 3 sets
Calf Raise: 3 sets > [N.B all are suggested exercises only]

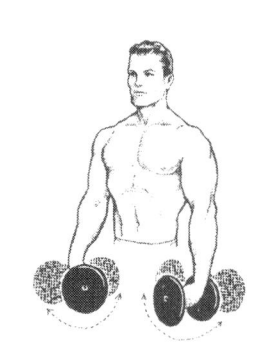

An important factor is the order in which you perform the exercises; and especially when training for strength. On squat day I always do squats first, then dead-lifts, followed by lighter moves. On chest / shoulders day, I normally like to begin with standing shoulder presses before going onto flat/ incline bench presses and then my ROM moves. Note that to some extent the order of exercises is a personal preference, although it can speed-up progress on a specific exercise if you specialise on a lift by doing it first.

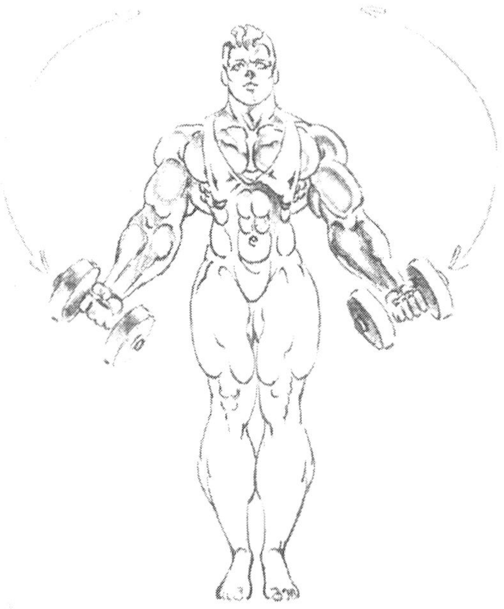

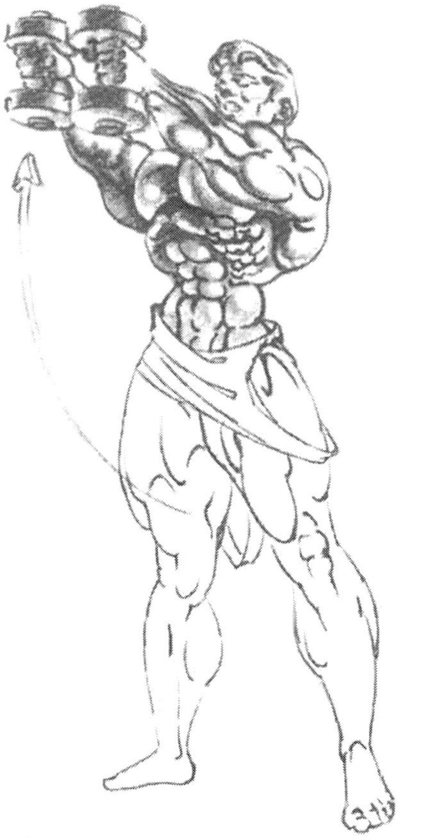

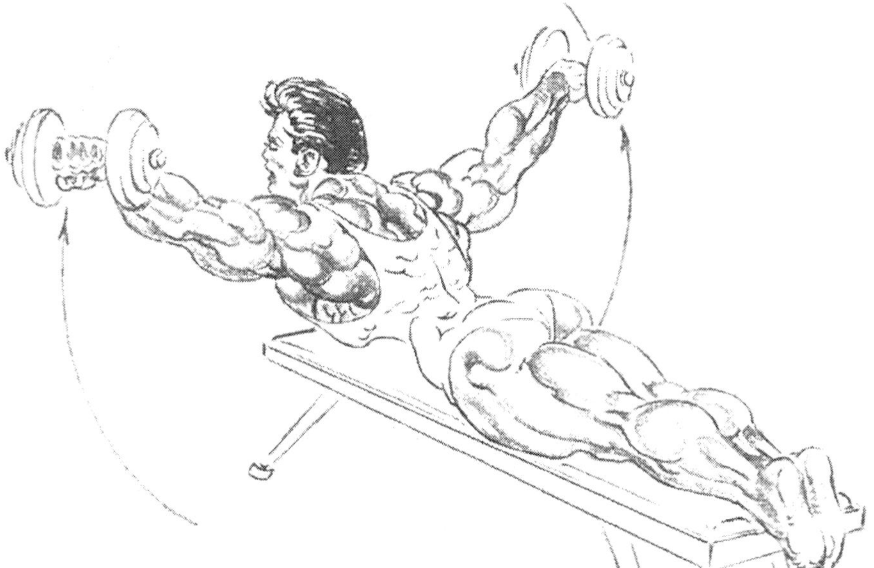

CHAPTER SEVENTEEN

Training for Figure

TRAINING FOR an improved figure or body-shape is often called bodybuilding or body-sculpting. One may assume that men and women, since they have such differently shaped bodies, would require entirely different routines in terms of bodybuilding. And whilst that may be partially true, at least in the beginning year or two of training, both men and women will benefit from the same type of routine.

My reasons for recommending the same routine for both men and women, relate to the fact that both sexes have the same muscle groups and basic physiology. Although men may have an easier time of it in terms of making more rapid progress in response to training, largely because they have higher levels of the muscle-building substance testosterone in their systems.

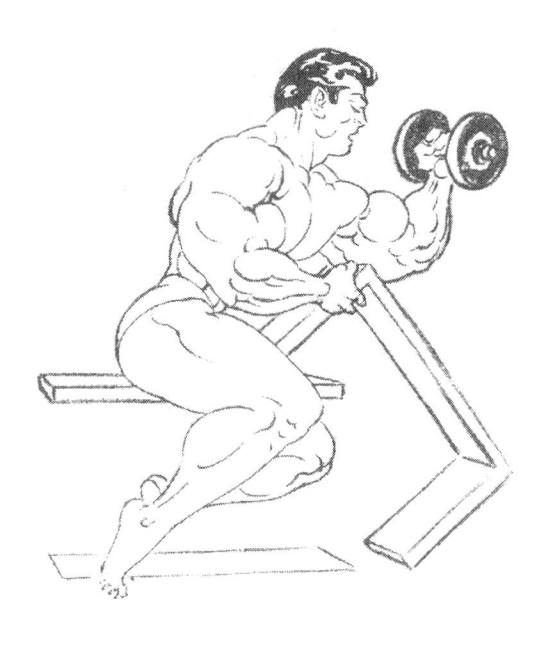

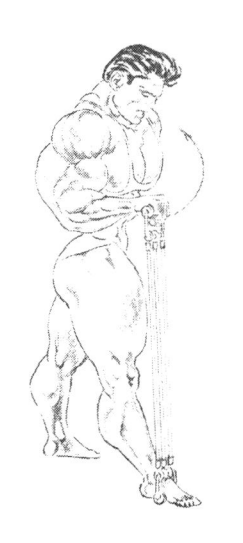

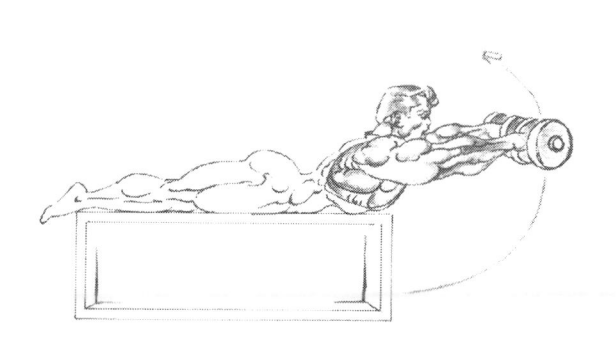

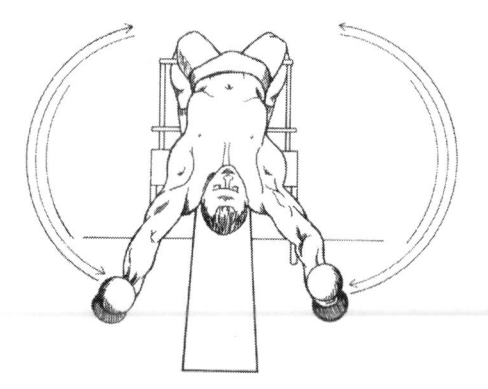

Many train to obtain a more pleasing and/or sexy body image. And men and women alike can quickly alter their body-shape using free-weight-raining. This is because it is the muscles of the body that give it a shapely outline, and particularly important in this respect are muscles such as the quadriceps, buttocks, calves, shoulders, back and abdominals etc. So long as you are not carrying large amounts of body-fat, it will be your muscles that bring shape to your overall physical form.

Training for shape may seem to be more complex than simply training for health and/or strength. This is so because each has his or her own unique body shape, and specific areas that they would like to improve and/or work on. But in actuality, improving body-shape can be quite a simple process once you get a few basic principles in your head. Right away I am going to state that I don't believe that there is any such thing as spot-reducing. It is not really possible to remove fat from one area alone for example, as fat loss happens everywhere on the body at once. However apparent spot reducing may be in fact possible by building up the major muscles of the body, and so altering ones physical profile or form. How exactly can one attain a better shaped physique?

The principles of so doing are quite simple. Firstly one identifies an ideal bodyweight (difficult I know), but using tables and looking at others of a similar (desirable) build can help. Once you decide on an ideal - identify if you need to loose or gain weight. If you need to loose more than about 15 pounds, then go on the health routine given previously for as long as necessary, combined with a healthy diet which reduces calories by the required amount. If you need to gain weight, then I suggest that you go on the strength program outlined previously, combined with high-protein drinks 1-2 times daily, with 30-50 grams of whey protein each time. On such a program you are attempting to gain high quality muscular bodyweight.

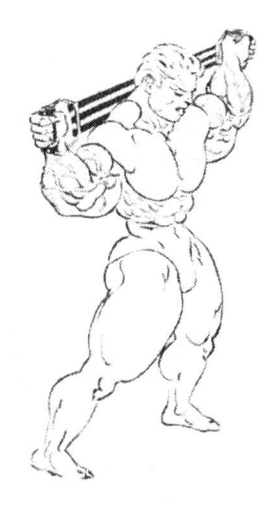

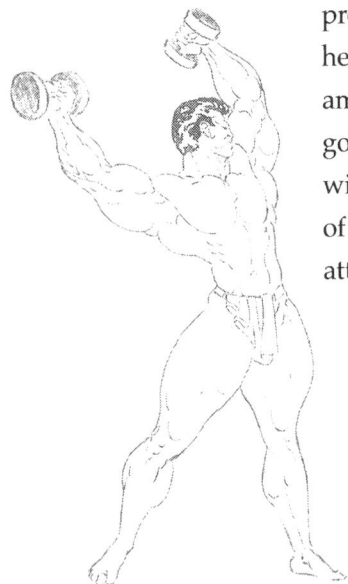

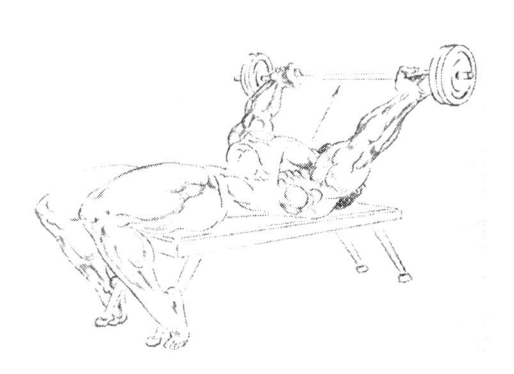

It may take you up to 1 year or so, in order to see real progress in terms of either gaining, or loosing significant bodyweight, and in order to approach your ideal bodyweight.

Once you are within about 15 pounds (higher or lower) than your ideal bodyweight, I suggest that you can then go on a specialised program of weight-training (if necessary) and in order to work on those areas that you would like to improve (you can build up muscles, one relative to another, and so influence body shape). What I am recommending is to engage in a bodybuilding program, whereby you now split your routine into different types of workouts and attack specific muscle groups directly.

Day 1 - Chest, Shoulders + Walk/Run
Day 2 - Legs, Abs, Calves
Day 3 - Upper Back, Arms + Walk Run
Day 4 - Complete Rest

An example schedule is shown above. You will find that you can concentrate on specific muscle groups, and that you will be able to train them with more intensity and make faster progress. I leave exercise selections up to yourself. After perhaps 6 months on such a program you should notice significant improvements in terms of shapelier muscles and a more pleasing overall physical form.

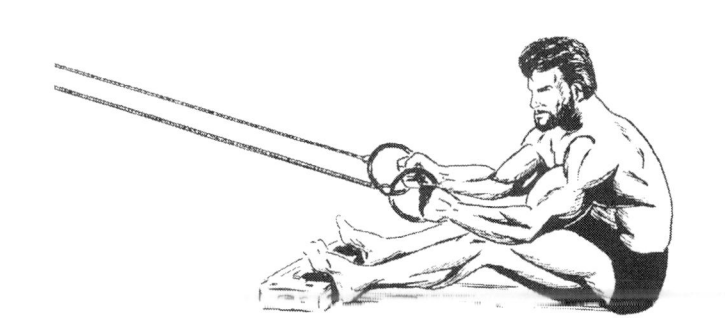

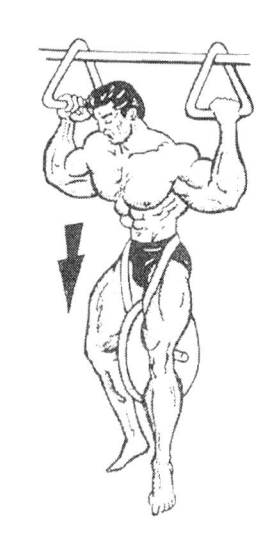

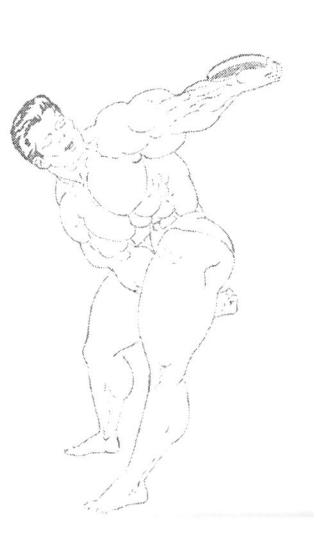

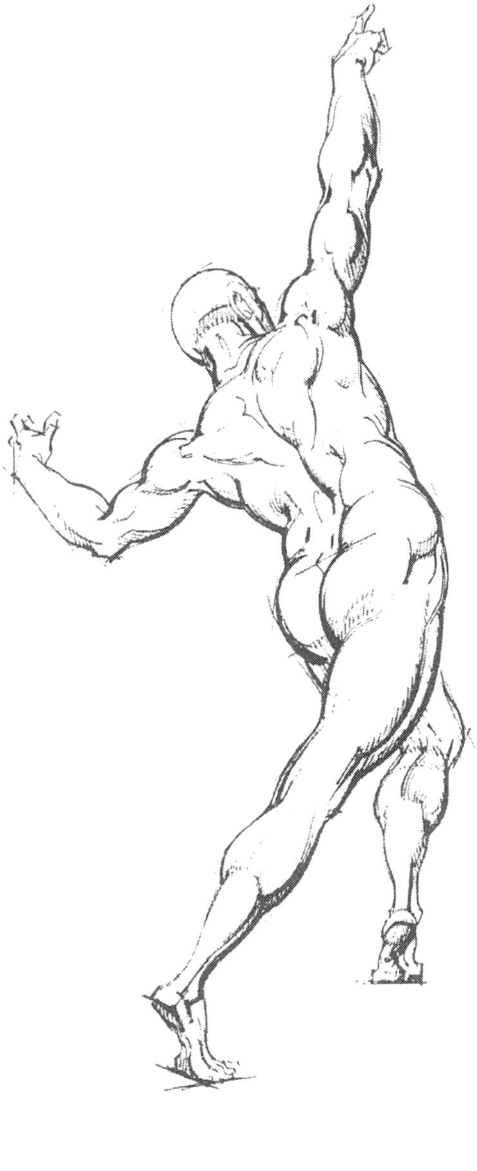

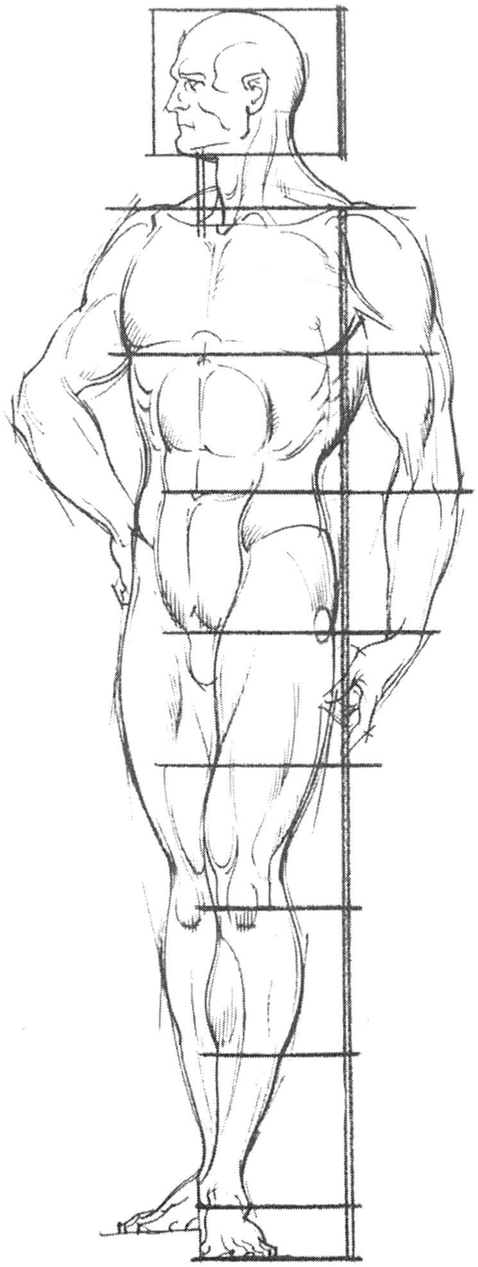

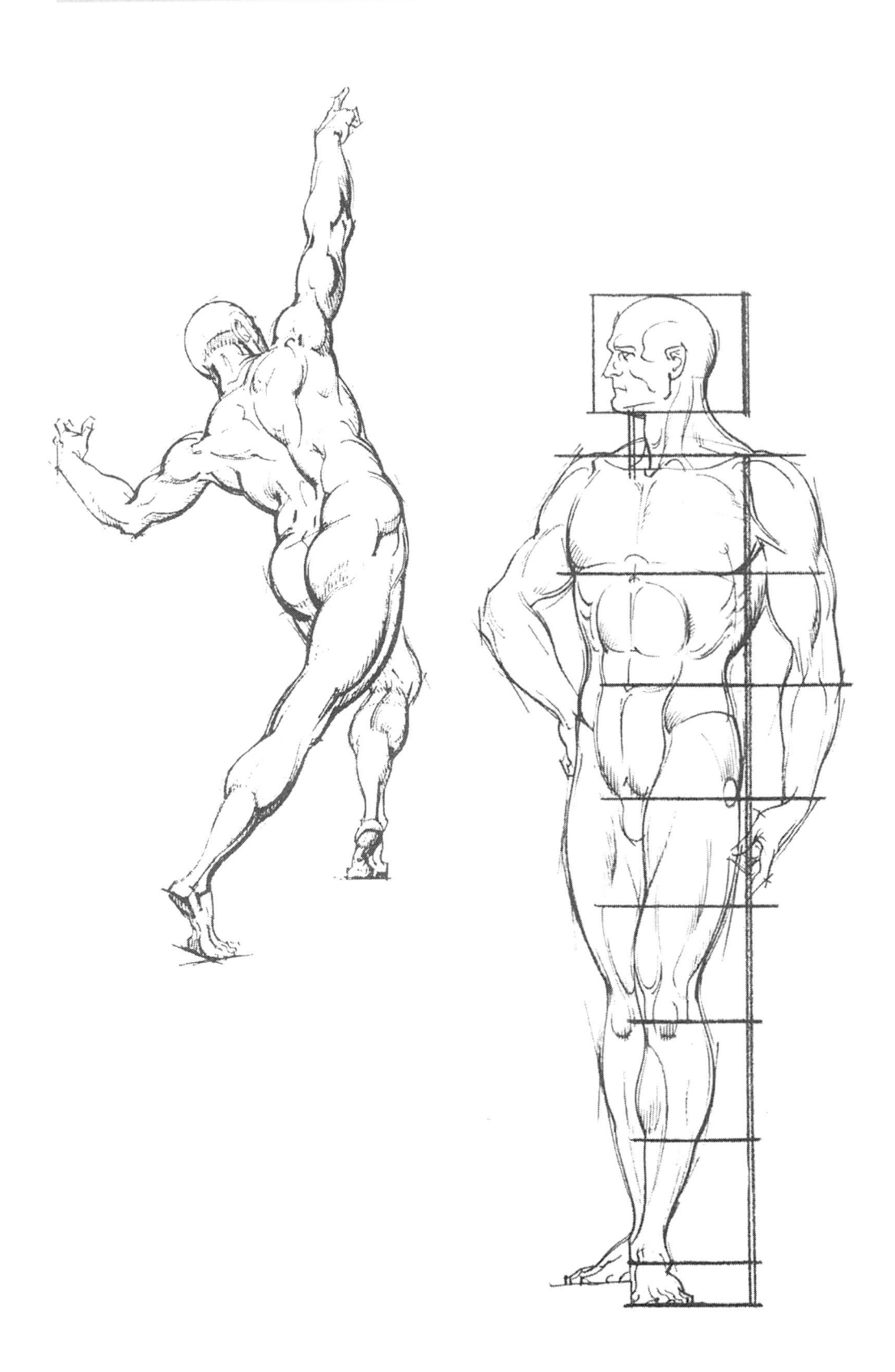

CHAPTER EIGHTEEN

Training for Therapy

MANY PEOPLE have physical deficiencies and/or injuries and/or they simply cannot move as other people do, or else they experience problems moving about as they get older. It is in the area of physical transformation, injury correction/prevention and rehabilitation; that weight-training finds its most important application.

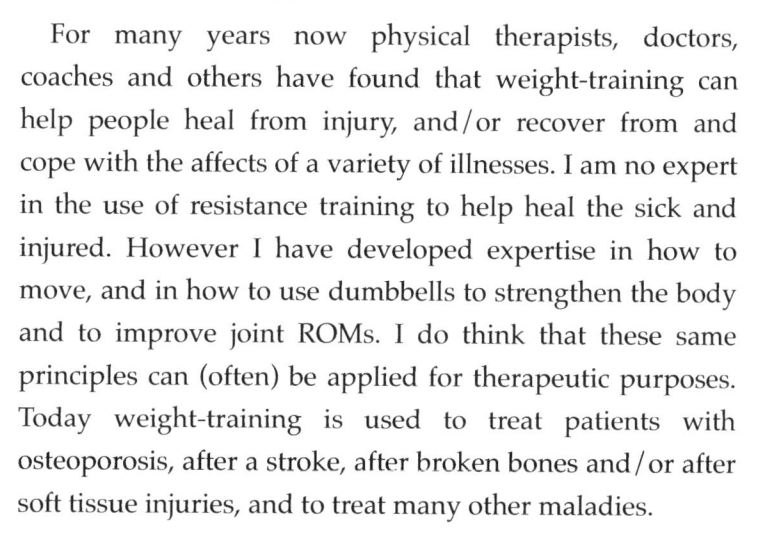

For many years now physical therapists, doctors, coaches and others have found that weight-training can help people heal from injury, and/or recover from and cope with the affects of a variety of illnesses. I am no expert in the use of resistance training to help heal the sick and injured. However I have developed expertise in how to move, and in how to use dumbbells to strengthen the body and to improve joint ROMs. I do think that these same principles can (often) be applied for therapeutic purposes. Today weight-training is used to treat patients with osteoporosis, after a stroke, after broken bones and/or after soft tissue injuries, and to treat many other maladies.

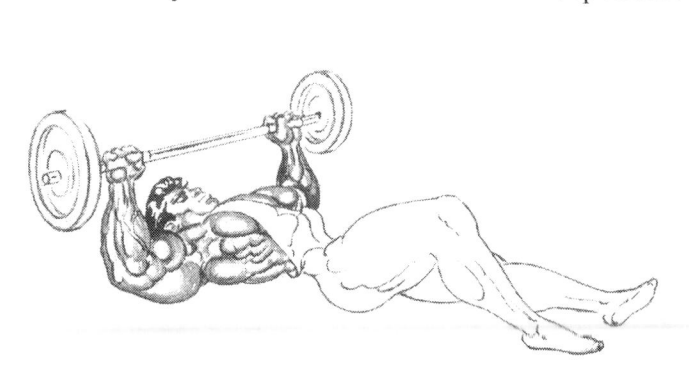

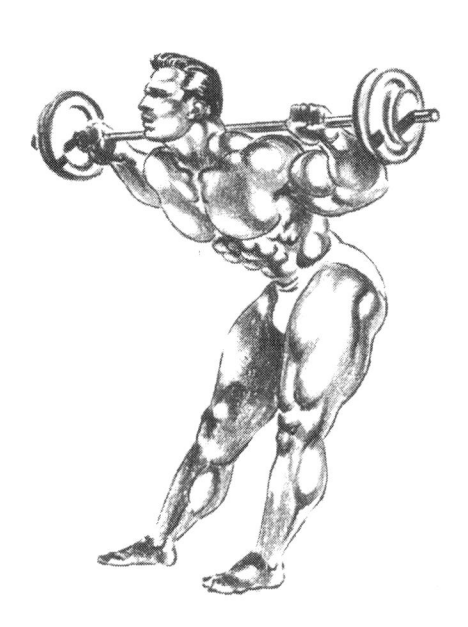

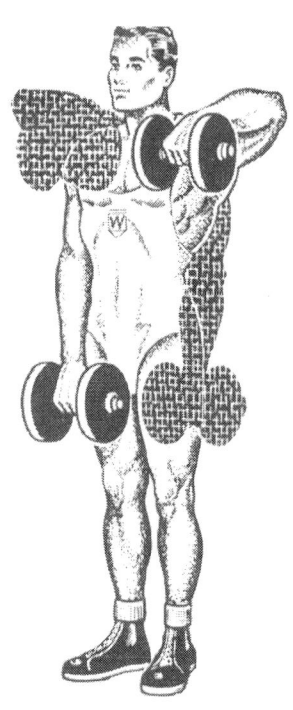

Resistance training for therapeutic use may be different to it's application in normal fitness training. I do recommend that you take the advise of a doctor/specialist in relation to your specific injury and/or personal circumstances and in relation to the type of weight-training routines to use, and also in relation to the likelihood of positive or negative results from the same.

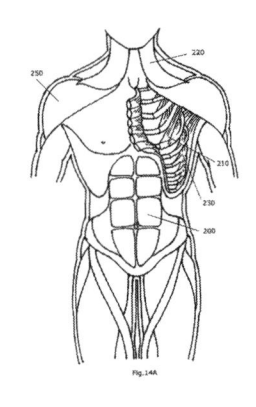

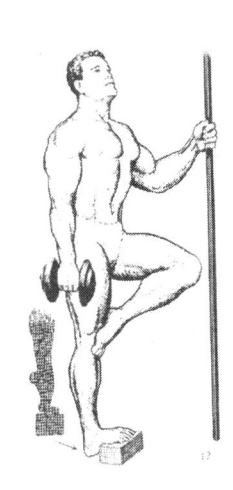

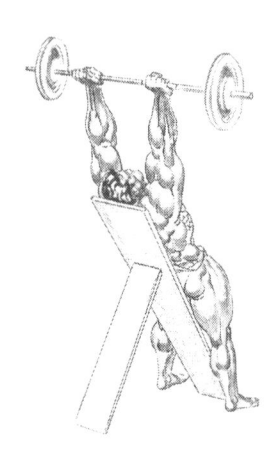

Today resistance training is part of the core set of treatments for certain diseases. For example, did you know that weight training for osteoporosis can help protect your bones and prevent osteoporosis-related fractures? Studies show that strength training over a period of time can help prevent bone loss, and may even build new bone.

In one study, postmenopausal women who participated in a strength training program for a year saw significant increases in their bone density in the spine and hips, areas affected most by osteoporosis in older women. Maintaining strong muscles through weight training helps to keep up your balance and coordination; a critical element in preventing falls, which can lead to osteoporosis-related fractures. There is also evidence that weight-training can help treat asthma, and possibly enable people to become medication free. So all-in-all the evidence is now clear that weight-training can help in the treatment of a wide-range of diseases.

Weight training isn't just for bodybuilders and professional athletes. In physical therapy, it can be an important component of a treatment plan that can help to rebuild lost muscle mass, balance the body as it recovers from injury, and increase physical endurance – all things which can help speed your return to total wellness.

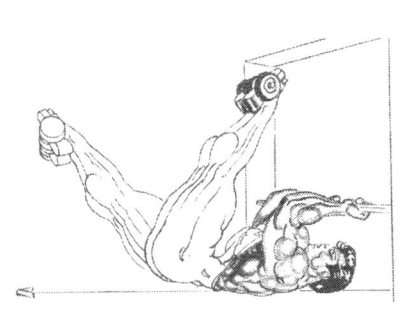

Just as physical therapy exercises are designed to recover proper function of a specific area of injury or stress, weight training is utilised to prepare your muscles and joints for a return to the demands of everyday living. Weight training is one of the best ways to restore damaged muscles, develop muscle size and strength, and give you the endurance to avoid re-injury – whether at work, rest or play. Resistance training has many benefits including restoring damaged muscles, the rebuilding of size and strength, and it develops stronger joints and increased joint ROMs. Properly performed, weight-training is a comprehensive physical therapy system that is difficult to better in terms of both speed and degree of recovery in a great many circumstances. In fact I do not have the space here to discuss all of the many different studies that provide incontrovertible evidence that weight-training is truly the supreme health promoting activity.

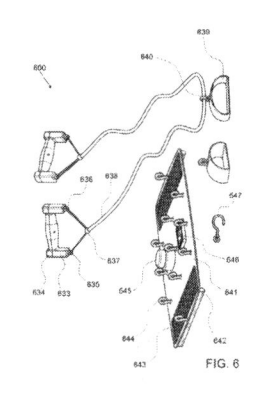

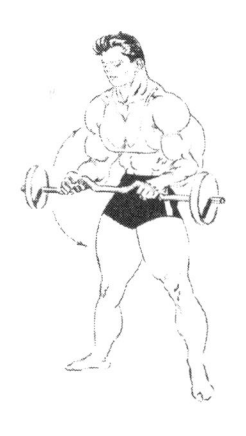

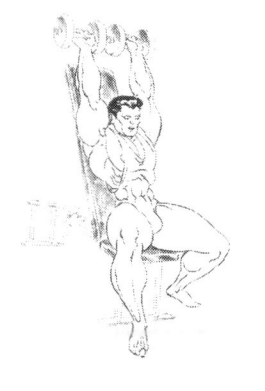

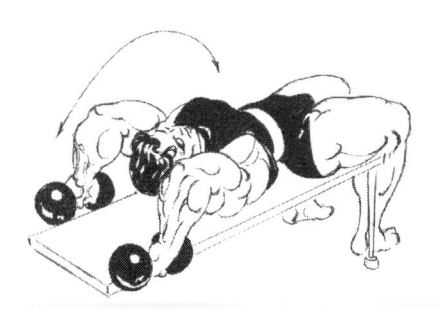

But the facts may be even more unbelievable in terms of the wider benefits to be obtained from resistance training. It appears that weight-training may keep a person young, in terms of so-called *biological age* - and could even prolong life! Several studies have been made to discover if there is a relationship between lifespan and weight-training. A growing body of research shows that working out with weights has health benefits beyond simply bulking up one's muscles and strengthening bones. Studies are finding that having more lean muscle mass may allow kidney dialysis patients to live longer, give older people better cognitive function, reduce depression, boost good cholesterol, lessen the swelling and discomfort of lymphedema after breast cancer and help lower the risk of diabetes etc.

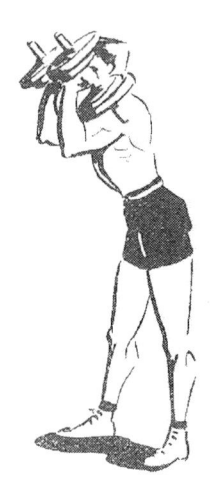

A new study that involved more than half a million participants over age 40 found that modest exercise increases life expectancy regardless of weight. That's right, it doesn't matter whether you are morbidly obese or have a normal body mass index (BMI), exercise helps you to live longer regardless. In fact, participants who were active but with class I obesity lived an average of 3.1 years longer than those who were at a normal weight but didn't engage in physical activity.

But let us get back to my primary aim, being to instruct you in the proper use of dumbbells, in this case for therapy. What I would say first, is that you will have to design the exact nature of the specific program that you can/will follow for yourself, and/or in consultation with your physician. There may be certain exercises that are simply not suitable for you, or that you cannot currently perform, or in fact that you could never perform due to physical limitations. It may be that dumbbells are not usable by yourself due to "gripping" problems, and in such cases machines may be a good substitute.

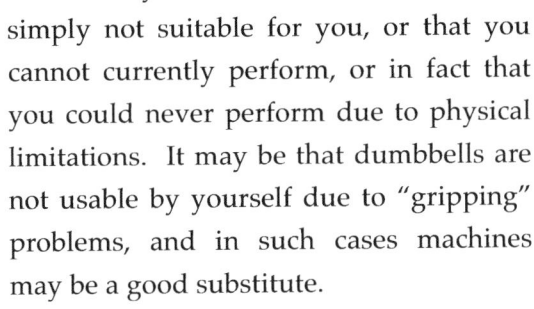

Certain general principles can be adopted when using dumbbells for physical therapy. Firstly it would be normal to use much lighter weights, and to (perhaps) aim at improving joint flexibility and ROMs over strength, at least initially until you become stronger.

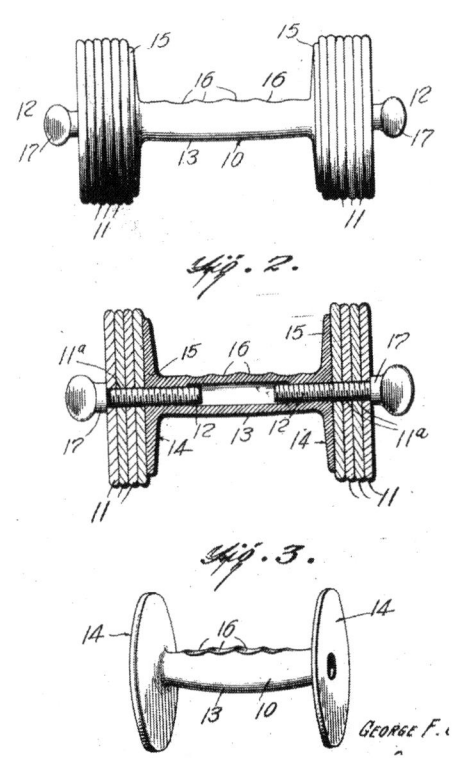

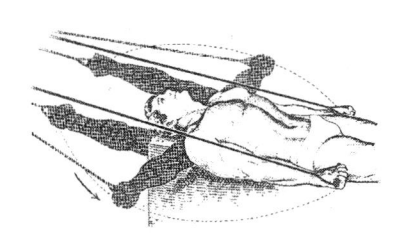

Having said this, back injury/performance expert Stuart McGill speaks about the need to work on back stability first, and before attempting to stretch back structures (in any way) in training. His reasoning is that if the back is not at least stable to a certain degree - then flexibility training will only make matters far worse, and may actually cause new injury. In such cases it may be that compound exercises such as (light) squats and/or overhead circles etc can work the inner muscles around the spine and so develop sufficient stability of the spine and in order to allow for greater improvements in strength and flexibility. McGill gives a series of special exercises for the lower back, and places emphasis (as we do here) on proper exercise form and on functional (strength + ROM) training methods.

I am not going to recommend any specific exercises for physical therapy, because each person needs a particular set of exercises according to his/her personal circumstances. Selecting movements from those presented here in this book may allow you to proceed in safe manner. The mechanism of healing is interesting. When you lift a weight, in fact you create micro-damage in the muscle and ligaments, and in terms of many tiny injuries etc. The body "spots" these injuries, and proceeds to heal itself.; and thus a natural "therapy" process is stimulated!

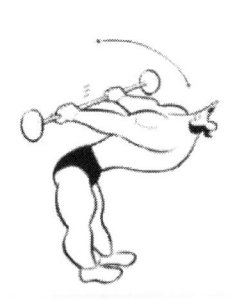

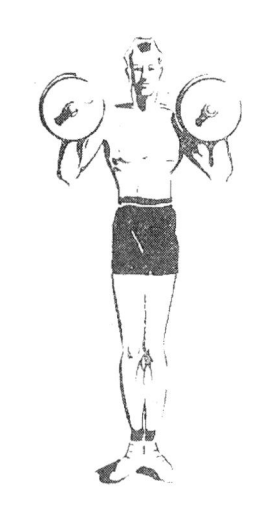

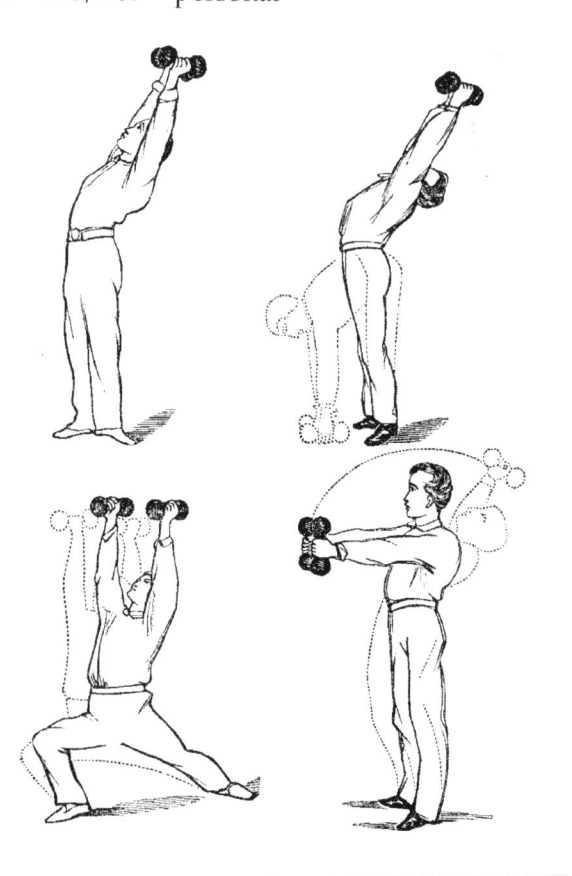

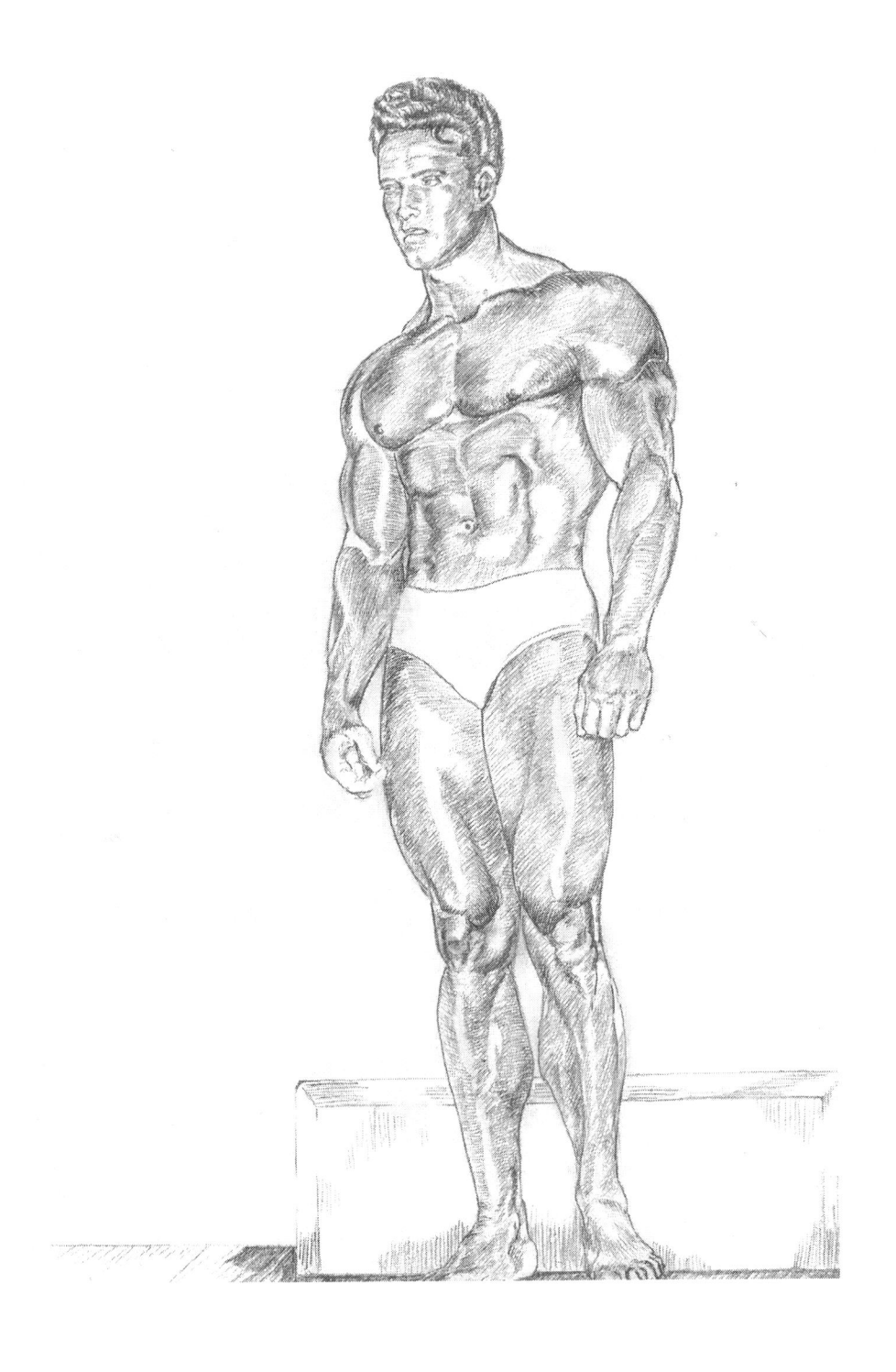

CHAPTER NINETEEN

Conclusions

WE HAVE come to the end of the Zen of Dumbbell Training. And looking back over the range and content of material covered, it is my hope that will be able to find various nuggets of information that allow you to progress in your fitness goals.

You may not actually agree with everything that I have said. That is OK, and is to be expected. In the preface I warned you to take what others say with a pinch of salt. But I would urge you to consider - and definitely to test - my opinions. Because this book is nothing less than the end result of some 10,000 hours of barbell/dumbbell training and countless hours spent reading books, magazines and periodicals about strength training. To say nothing of many hours spent discussing weight-training with friends, coaches and some champion athletes.

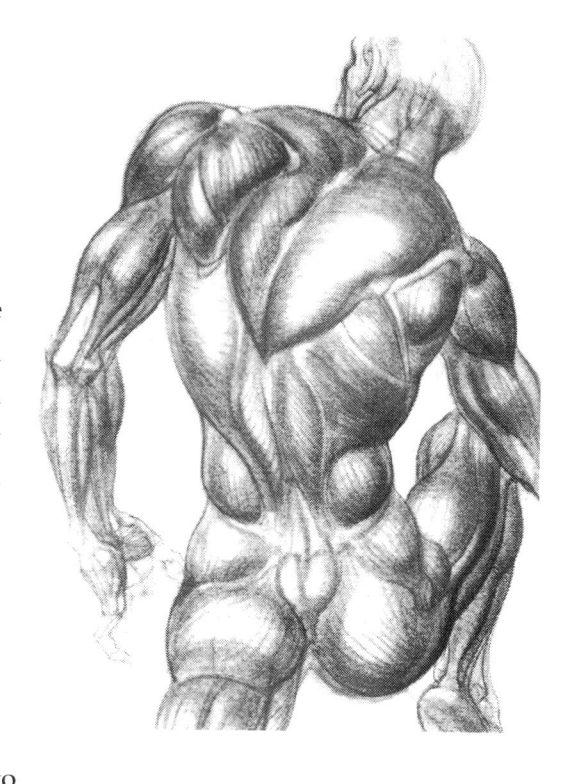

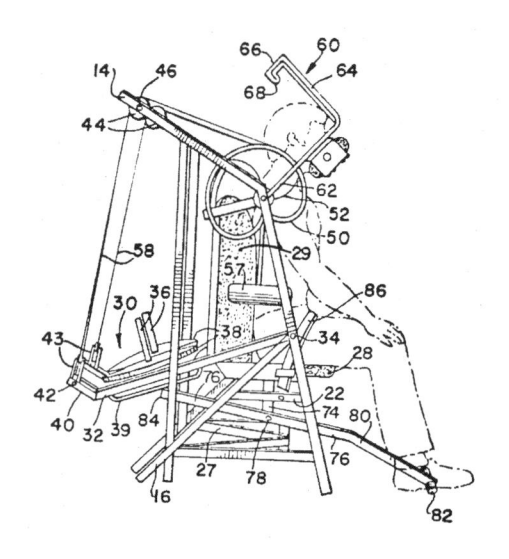

It would be incredible if I had not learned something useful and/or correct along the way. Yet it is sometimes not actually the correct pieces of information which have the most affect on other people. At times it is the incorrect opinions. These can be damaging. Sometimes information is given with the best intentions, but turns out to be useless for the intended recipient. This is because each of us has unique responses to our environment. So be wary of everything you read and are told.

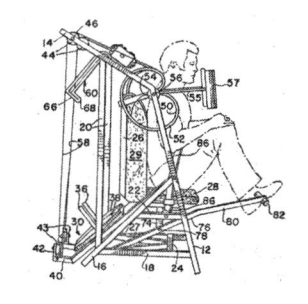

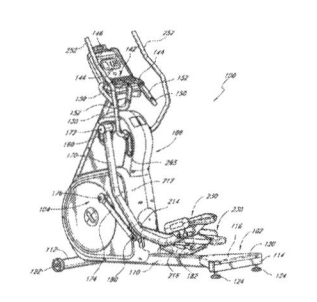

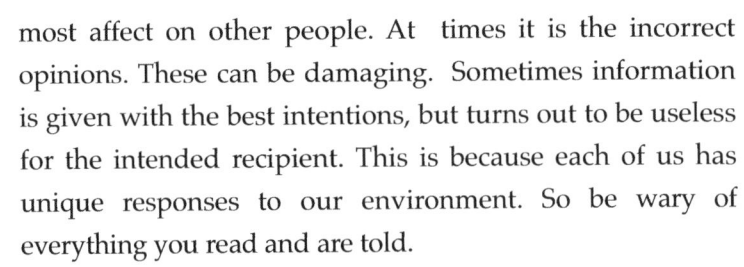

And be especially wary of well-built and obviously fit people who instruct you about the best way to train. What works for them might be genetic superiority, youth, diet, or some other factor that they themselves might not even be aware of. And people do succeed despite doing many things incorrectly. Even great athletes sometimes have the belief that one exercise has a particular effect, whilst in actual fact it is something else altogether which is producing the same.

And beware of listening to drug-taking individuals who can often grow muscles despite the fact that they are doing almost everything wrong in terms of correct training practices. You can get fantastically strong naturally in any case. But you have to train correctly to progress naturally. Myself I have bench pressed 400 lbs and dead-lifted just under 700 lbs - and I am a natural-for-life lifter. These achievements took 10 years of daily training, 5-6 days a week, and never missing a workout.

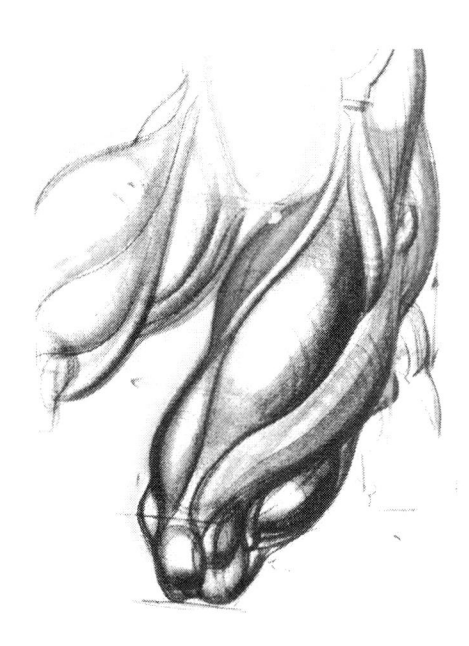

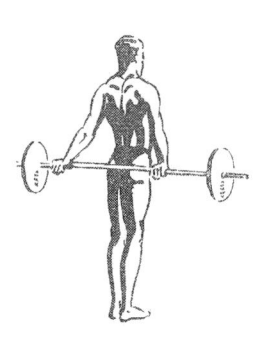

But bodyweight and muscle size are not the primary aim of Zen Training, rather you should shoot for an athletic look and high levels of general fitness from both muscular and aerobic exercises. You MUST include such activities as running, walking and swimming in your routine in order to attain an overall athletic capability.

In my experience natural training will give you a better build than the steroid men. Natural training builds a symmetrical body. You get larger legs, back, chest and shoulders etc; in good proportions, one muscle relative to another muscle. And natural training will not, and cannot, give you muscles that are too large for your frame (normally - although there are exceptions).

It really does not matter how strong someone is relative to another person, truly. Rather you should focus on yourself, and on becoming the best version of you.

Back to the title of this book. You can get anything you like (in terms of health and strength) from dumbbell training. This I truly believe. You just have to go about the process of training with the correct attitude, and using the right techniques. And you must apply knowledge appropriately. Take your time, the results will be far superior to rushing.

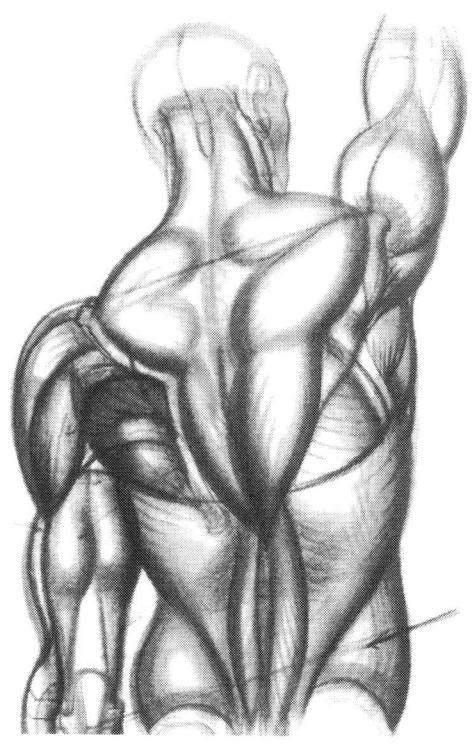

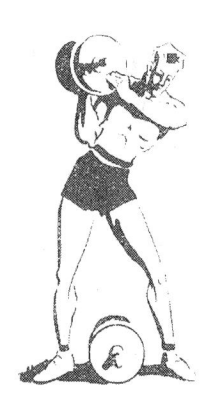

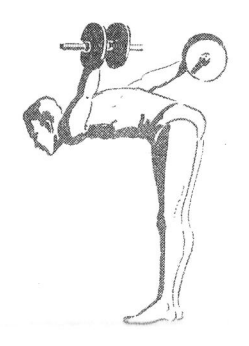

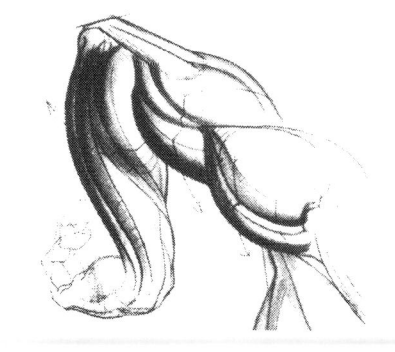

An important point also, is that not everyone can, or should, perform all exercises. Naturally as we age and/or become weaker or injured, we must adjust our aims and train according to our limitations. Plus we must choose appropriate exercises according to our stage of training and the degree of training adaption (level of fitness). Switching movements regularly can avoid over-training and "staleness".

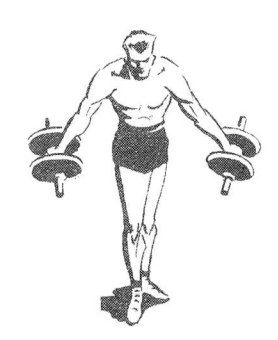

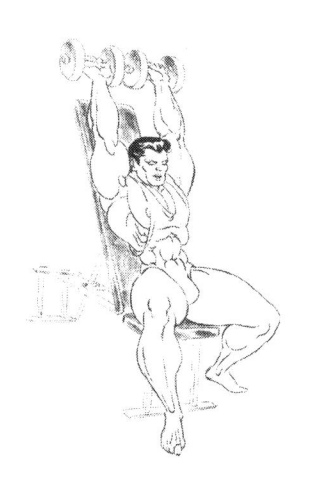

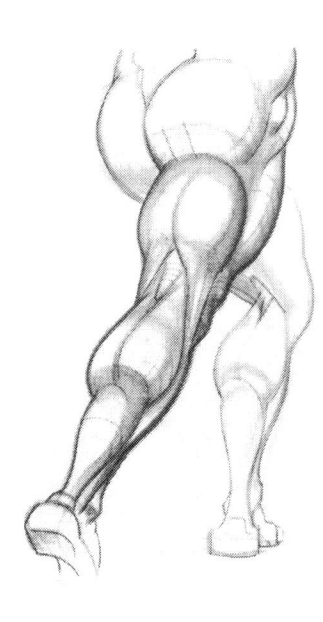

I would now like to bring attention to a *major problem* that exists in the fitness industry.

The vast majority of fitness programs and exercises performed in gyms right across the world *are completely worthless*! That is, people everywhere are performing exercises and routines that are without any merit whatsoever, and they are a total waste of time! I would estimate that we are easily talking about 90 percent of all the exercises performed, period (in terms of the actual number of movements performed by people everywhere).

I refer here to weight-training exercises, and to machine, dumbbell and barbell movements. A great many of the exercises performed are dangerous, and actually can do more harm to the trainee's physique, strength, fitness capabilities, and flexibility than if he/she had stayed at home and done nothing whatsoever. In fact, that is what I recommend, to stay at home, if you are going to train like everyone else, and simply don't bother.

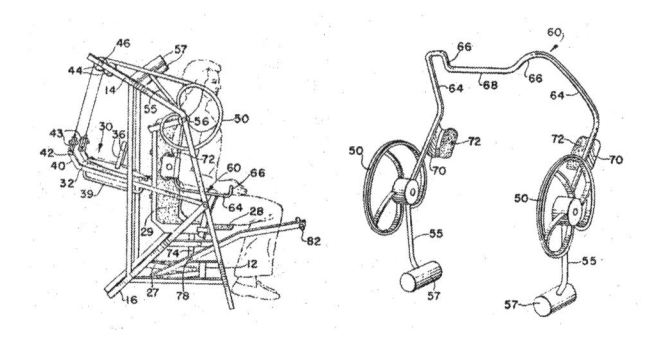

How did I come to the conclusion that most exercises are useless? Put simply, by observing the complete lack of results achieved by the average trainee. NO STRENGTH IMPROVEMENTS; NO ROM IMPROVEMENTS; AND A PHYSIQUE THAT NEVER CHANGES. It seems that everyone is getting everything wrong in relation to resistance training. And I am referring here not only to exercise selections, and the associated performance techniques, but also to the applicability (or usefulness) of the same to the actual needs of the trainee himself.

Arthur Jones, of Nautilus fame, spoke about 10 basic principles behind effective weight-training; as follows:

1. Indirect Effect

When you exercise, any muscle growth produced as a result will also effect, to a lesser extent, all of the other muscles of the body. It has also been noticed that the effect is proximity related. The closer a muscle is to the exercised muscle, the more it is effected. Also, the larger the muscle, the greater its affect on overall growth.

2. Limit Exercise Number

Best results will almost always be produced by selecting from a number of the best exercises which involve the major muscle masses. The human body very rarely utilises a movement in which a muscle is isolated. Therefore why would we attempt to cause muscle growth by using a large number of isolation exercises.

3. High Intensity

According to Jones, you should carry each set to a point where you force against the weight on a rep even after the weight has stopped moving upward. When the weight stops mid-rep and will not move another inch, you are done.

4. Secondary Growth Factors

Regardless of how hard you work in the gym there are certain factors that must be provided if growth is to occur. These factors are: nutrition, adequate rest, avoidance of overwork (i.e. overtraining) and psychological factors.

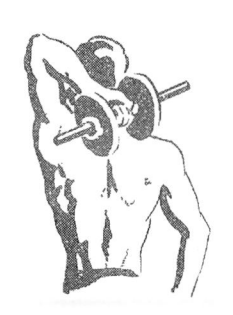

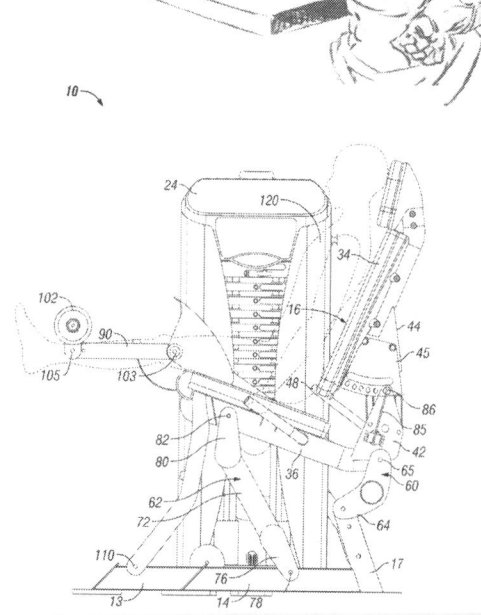

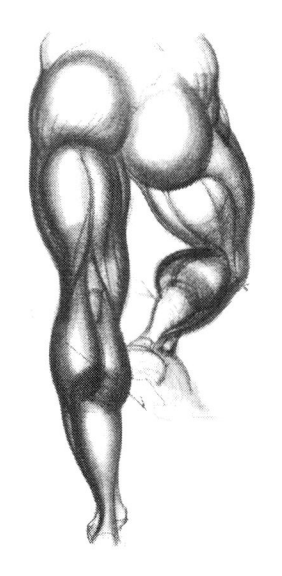

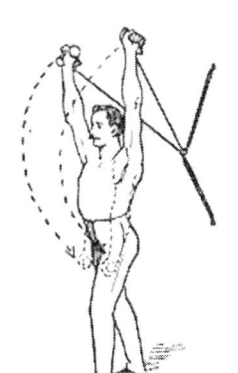

5. Reciprocity Failure

If bodybuilding training were a simple mathematical calculation it would stand to reason that if one set gave results, then 10 sets would give ten times the measured result. Unfortunately, this is not the case. There is an intermediate point, somewhere between these two extremes, where optimal results will be achieved. Experiment with volume, but do so carefully.

6. Strength and Endurance

Muscular endurance, as opposed to cardiovascular endurance, is directly correlated with the strength of the muscle. That is to say that if you can complete 12 reps with x pounds of resistance you should be able to predict, with some accuracy, the amount of weight that you could move for 3, 9, 20 reps, etc. For this reason training for muscular strength and endurance yield the same results; stronger, more powerful, larger muscles.

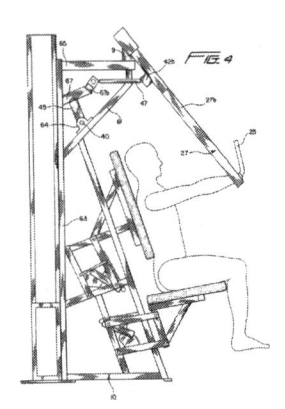

7. The Time Factor

In order to accurately assess muscle gains and to maximise training efficiency, time must be considered in every training routine. At its very basic level it means recording the time, in minutes, that each entire workout takes. This works well for comparing whole workouts to one another.

Time keeping can also be applied to individual exercises. Jones' solution was to carefully control the time between the beginning of one set to the beginning of the next set.

Another control measure that Jones introduced was rep speed. He suggested a rep tempo of about a 4 second negative, and a 2 second positive. He recommended that there be no more than five hours of training weekly and preferably 4 hours or less.

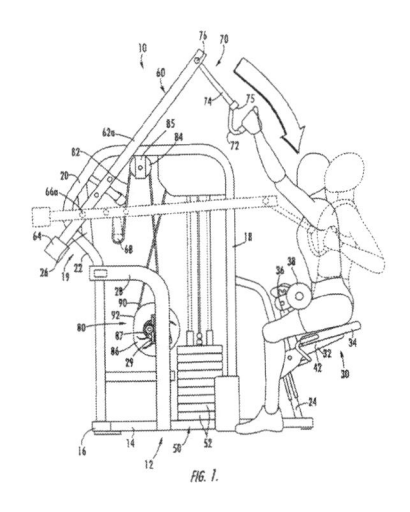

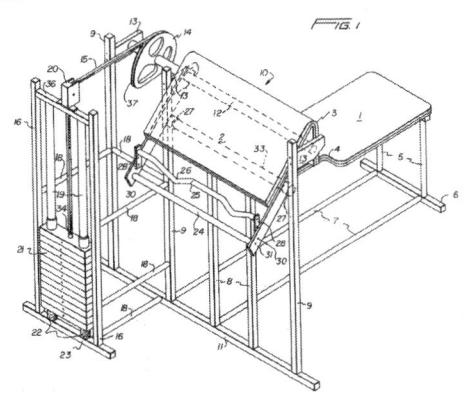

8. Instinctive Training

"For anything even approaching the best possible results from training, it is absolutely essential to work in direct opposition to your instincts" - *Arthur Jones.* He is referring here to the need to train hard, in contrast to natural desires.

9. Low Volume

One set, two, never more than three sets. Jones was a firm believer that any more than three sets of an exercise was wasted effort and unnecessary. In general he stated the "best rep scheme" was the 10, 8, 6 format. The first set of an exercise would use a sufficient amount of resistance to cause failure at 10 reps. The weight is increased on the second set to permit only 8 reps and again on the third set to allow for only 6 reps. Squats would be one of a few exceptions to this rule. More sets and/or reps can be performed here to stimulate the body into growth.

10. Layoff

For the best possible results a trainee needs to take some time off every once in awhile.

Conclusion (Jones)

Jones used the above principles in order to produce an example "ideal" training routine; being one designed to produce the maximum degree of muscle growth. He recommended that people do the following in each session:

1. Squats
2. Stiff-legged dead-lifts
3. Close supinated grip chins/pull down
4. Standing press
5. Parallel bar dips
6. Barbell curls
7. Barbell wrist curls
8. One-legged calf raise

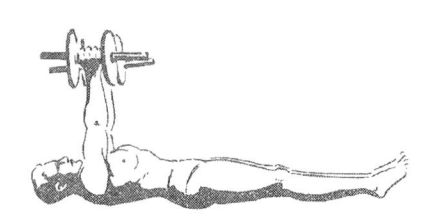

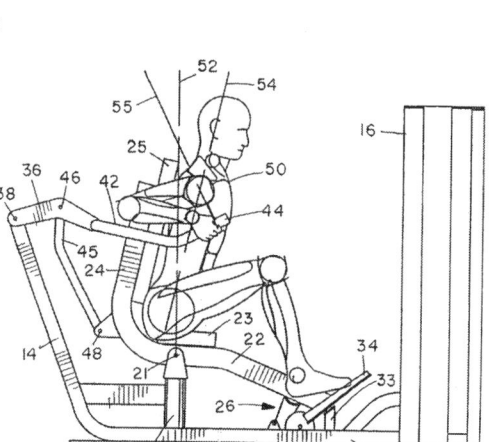

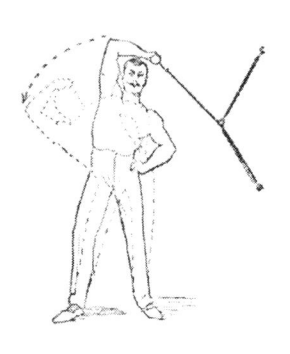

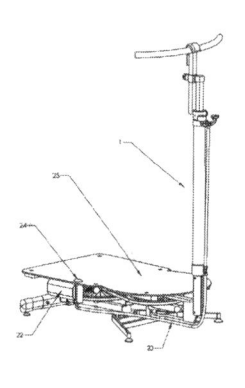

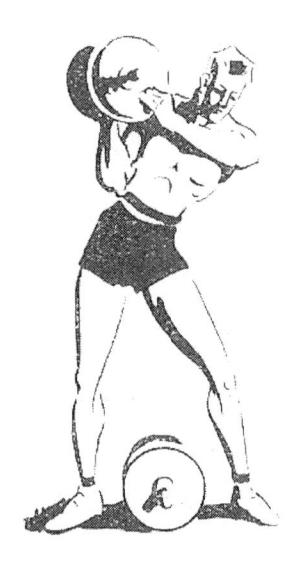

Jones stated that just these eight exercises done twice weekly is all that is needed, provided that you take each set to absolute failure (failure is not recommended by myself). If the desired results are not achieved then the volume/frequency can further be reduced by dividing the program into two sessions per week of only four exercises each.

The above principles (and the program itself) do make allot of sense, both intellectually, and in terms of my own experience of what works in practice. Jones placed most emphasis on avoidance of over-training, and upon consideration of the systematic effects of exercise on the human organism as a whole. Without a shadow of a doubt this is the correct approach, both to maximise the results obtained from training, whilst simultaneously avoiding the danger of injury and the negative effects of over-training. The lesson is to do a few basic exercises, and to work briefly, but intensely.

At the same time we should be aware that Jones was focussed on muscle growth alone, and he worked almost exclusively with bodybuilders for much of his career. I believe, conversely, that it is vital for the trainee to perform additional lighter weight-training exercises aimed not at muscle growth - but rather at joint ROM. As a result (and unlike Jones) I do not believe in machines, but prefer to use dumbbells for the vast majority of the exercises contained in any training program.

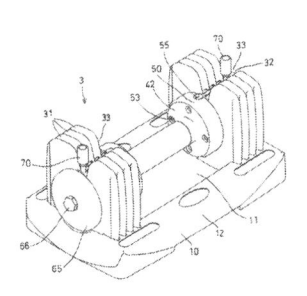

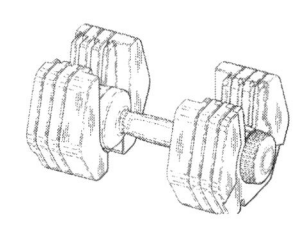

That said, I do believe in applying Jone's principles, only here instead of using machines and barbells, by performing the vast majority of work with dumbbells. That is, performing exercises 2,4, & 6 on his list with dumbbells. I do also believe in widening the routine by including very light dumbbell (ROM) stretching moves such as lean-backs, overhead circles, twists, overhead laterals, front laterals, pullovers, round-the-world, and dumbbell hangs etc. These are performed for joint ROM, are easy and light, and do not deplete energy or encroach on recovery capability.

Jones believed (incorrectly I think) that weight-training, properly performed, would produce all of the cardiovascular benefits required by the individual. I cannot agree with such an approach, because I am a believer in taking a balanced approach to fitness. I think that cardiovascular training is required to produce optimal fitness. Even walking may be enough.

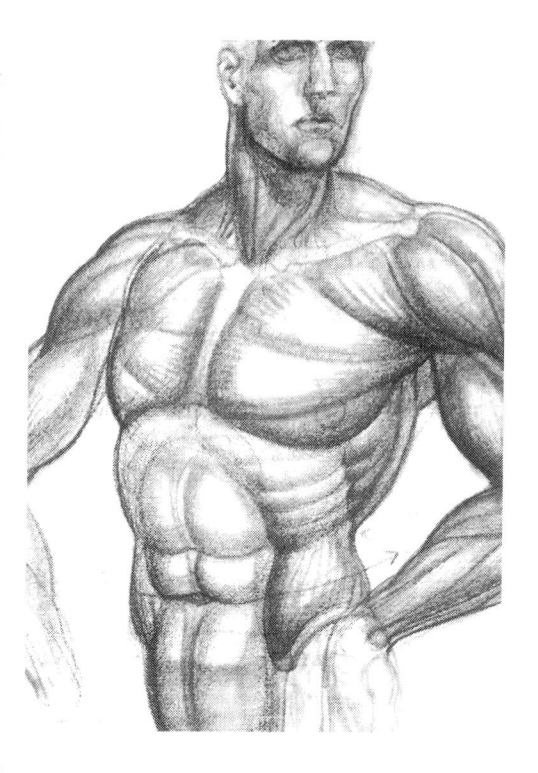

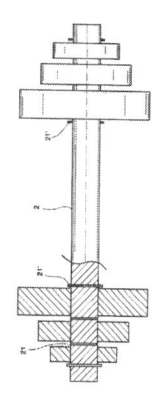

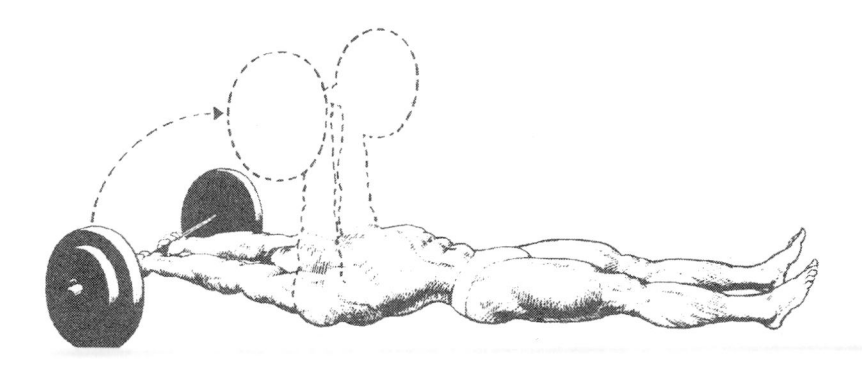

Back to my statement about people wasting time in gyms. I believe that weight-training is performed solely for two purposes; to improve *movement efficiency,* and to improve *strength*. Any health and/or appearance benefits are purely secondary (perhaps pleasant) effects of achieving improvements in these two areas. That said, I believe it is important to measure strength based exercise routines in relation to Jone's 10 principles of effective exercise. The lesson here is: fairly intense (but brief) work using compound (not isolation) movements.

Put simply, it is clear that most people do all of the wrong exercises for strength building, at too low an intensity, plus they do no ROM exercises whatsoever.

As stated, it is true that most trainees make very little progress, in terms of either strength or ROM, and/or in terms of any kind of movement efficiency gains. I am not expecting "drug-like" effects here, only some progress, basically any progress in terms of any improvement whatsoever. In fact (due to lack of progress) the vast majority of people either give up training or else cannot really see the point - and simply go through the motions.

And it's no wonder because they do everything wrong, and do not have a systematic approach as recommended by Jones. I often use my own principle in order define a safe and effective exercise program for any human being.

That evaluation principle is as follows:

A safe and effective fitness program forms part of a planned lifestyle; with appropriate exercise choices and performance styles that effect beneficially (improve) the fitness capabilities of the individual; including factors such as aerobic capacity, strength, natural movement patterns and/or movement ROMs.

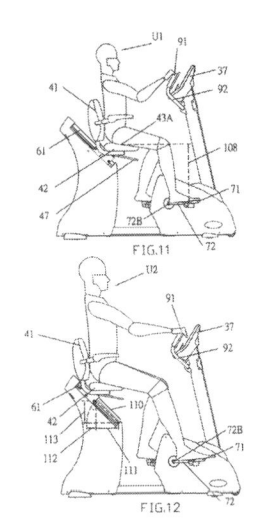

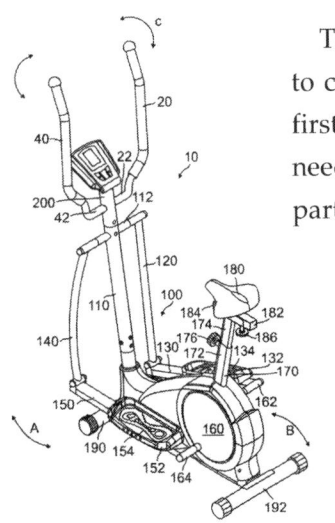

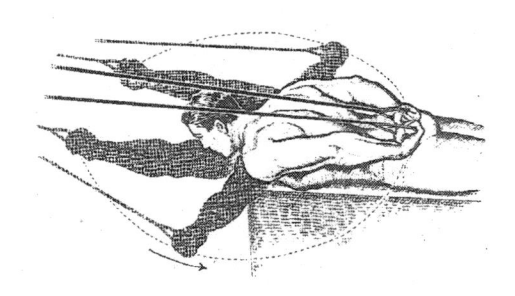

The first concern in any resistance training program is to consider why you are engaging in such training in the first place. What are your goals? What does your body need. Do you need more strength and/or greater ROM in particular joints? There are basically two goals in this respect, to either increase these same factors in your body; or else to maintain the same.

Nobody (normally) wants to actually reduce strength, or else to attain lower levels of joint ROM. You might tell me that muscle shaping is your goal, but truthfully that is nearly impossible to achieve in and of itself, because muscle shapes are largely determined by genetics. You may very well obtain a more shapely physique from training, but this is gained from larger muscles overall, and/or lower levels of body fat across your entire physique.

So weight-training is all about improving and/or maintaining overall body strength and joint ROMs. Sorry to repeat myself here, but there simply is no other reason to engage in such exercise. Of-coarse you may be training primarily for reasons of health, shape or therapy; and (correct) weight-training will provide incredible benefits in these respects. However any benefits in these areas are dependent upon making progress in strength and movement ROMs. Improvements in flexibility, balance, stability and coordination will follow any properly gained (and measured) strength and ROM improvements.

Once you get these twin goals of weight-training in your brain, most of the poor training techniques and useless methods will fall-away, and are recognised as a pointless waist of time.

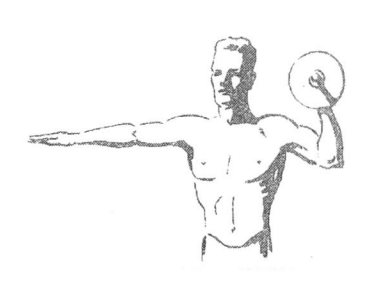

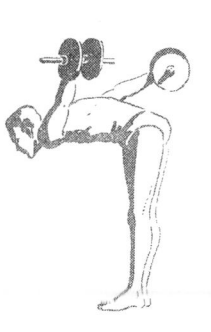

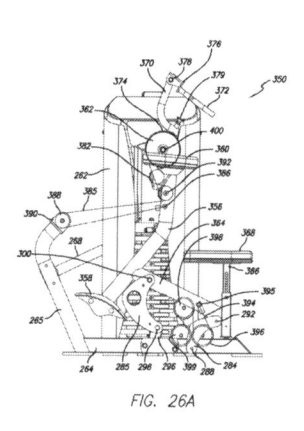

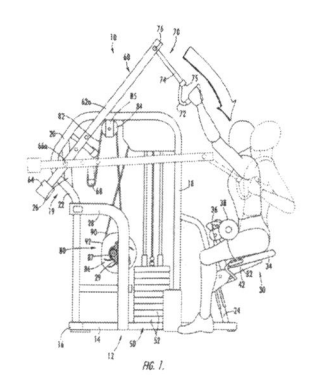

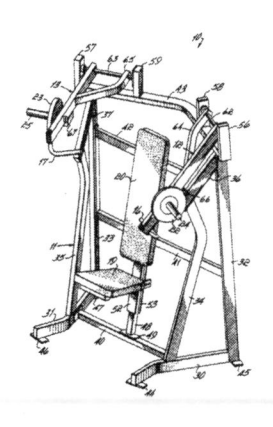

I refer here to overall body strength, and not stronger biceps or pecs. Arthur Jones said that there is a specific and a general effect from weight training. And along with this basic fact is another unassailable truism; that it is not possible (generally) to improve strength in one muscle alone, or at least by a significant factor. Rather you must improve the strength of your entire physique all at once.

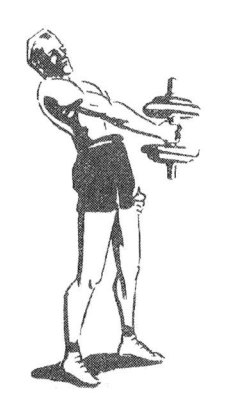

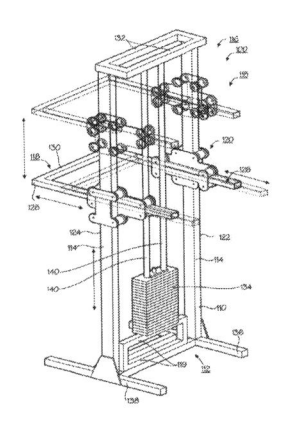

Thus performing lots of biceps curls will improve the strength of your biceps to some (usually small) degree. But you would (often) get a far larger and stronger biceps by doing less curls and concentrating on squatting with heavier weights to obtain a generalised growth spurt across your entire physique. In fact sometimes your biceps will grow just by performing heavier and heavier squats over a period of a couple of months or so, and without even doing any direct work for the biceps whatsoever. This is the indirect effect in action.

Most people are performing all of the wrong exercises to achieve either one of these two primary goals of weight training. They waste time with low-intensity machine exercises, or do lots of short little isolation moves. They often perform exercises in the wrong style; either too strict or too sloppy. They use an incorrect number of repetitions and very low levels of intensity. In actuality you need to employ a range of repetitions, using low reps (1-3 for strength) and higher ranges (8-12) to hit the different types of muscle fibres. It is best to use a pyramid method on strength movements, gradually increasing the weight and lowering reps, so start with 8 reps, go to 6 then 3.

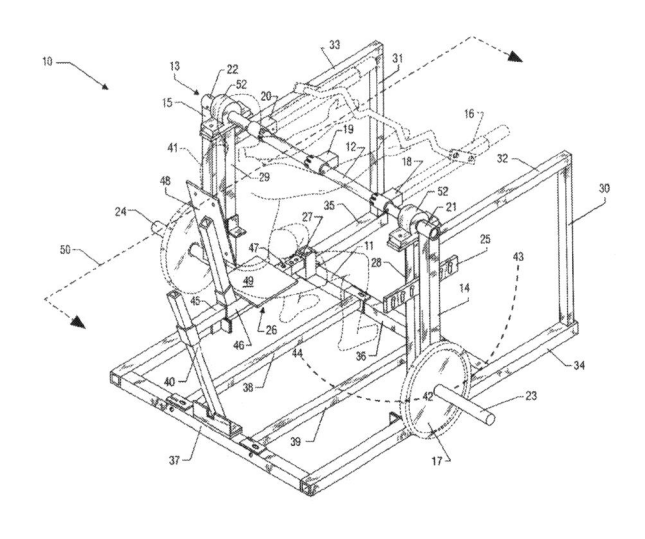

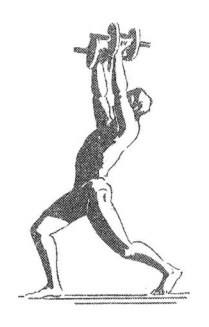

I think Arthur was right in that 3 sets of any exercise is normally enough (for squats you may need more sets). And decide if the exercise is being used for ROM or strength building, and vary the intensity accordingly. ROM training is no where near failure and can be performed with high reps (10+), plus a faster and/or a much slower rep speed may be desired. Do not confuse ROM training with typical isolation moves (not recommended) such as heavy (partial) side-laterals and/or heavy (partial) flys. ROM training is often performed over a far wider movement arc (round-the-worlds), and/or with narrow end-of-movement "pulses" etc, and with much lighter weights (1-5 lbs). ROM training uses methods such as static holds and circular movement patterns.

A note on repetitions and weight selection is vital at this point. Here I refer to strength building (not ROM training). I notice that low reps (1-3) are somewhat out of fashion in the modern gym. But it is low reps that give you the most strength gains. Think about it this way, a 1 rep set (with close to the maximum weight that you can handle) is performed at 90-100 percent intensity. That is, you must recruit almost 100 percent of your muscle fibres in order to complete the repetition successfully. Such a set will build more muscle, because it involves **all of the muscle**, and your body gets the message (instantly) that you don't have enough muscle at present - and sets up the muscle growth process in response.

I don't know why low reps have gone out of fashion. Perhaps low rep training is too much like hard work, or people are afraid of using heavier weights? Possibly the current "perceived wisdom" comes from the drug-taking bodybuilders who use high reps to build muscles, and would (in any case) build larger muscles no matter how they trained, due to the significant help of the drugs.

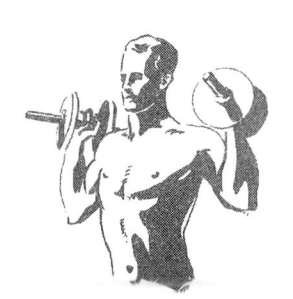

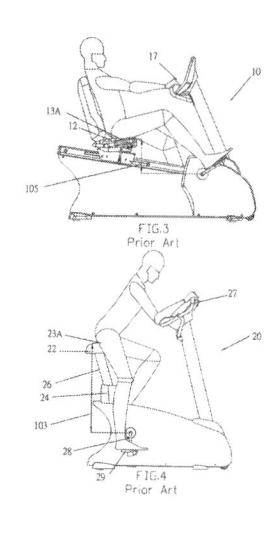

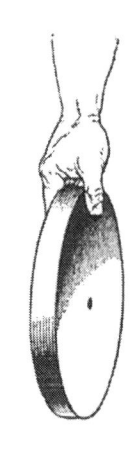

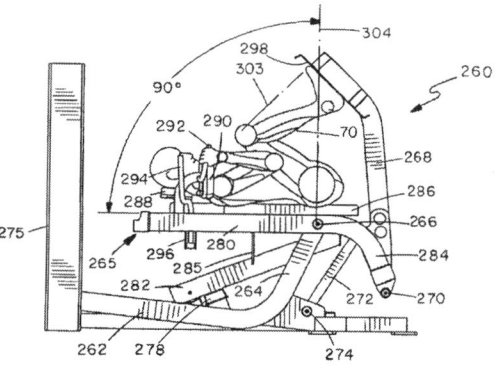

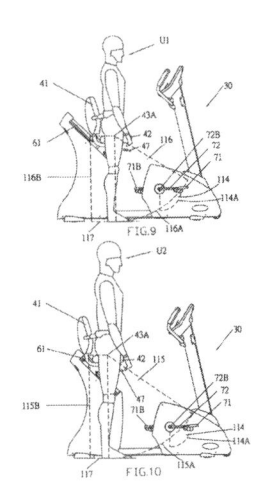

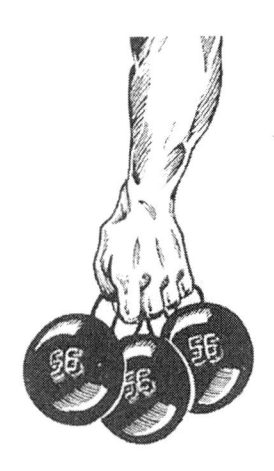

With low reps you do not wear out the joints with constant repetitions, and you build stronger tendons and joints very quickly indeed. Plus training is more intensive and is much faster to perform, and it's not boring. You leave the gym sooner.

But do not take my word for it, try low rep training for yourself. I am not talking here about struggling with limit weights in a poor/cheating style; but rather performing nice and controlled single-rep (or 3 rep) sets with a strict, intense and slow style. Choose a fairly heavy weight, but one that you can handle safely, and do not go near failure. Rather than going near to failure, perform lots of sets, say 5-6 singles quickly and rest only 15-20 seconds between sets. This type of training is different (in tempo) from higher-rep training, because you will need to perform more sets in a relatively fast succession. Once again, go no-where near failure, and perform a couple of higher rep sets before and (perhaps) after the lower rep sets.

Safety is an issue with low reps because you are handling heavier weights, so use spotter and/or stay well-within your limits. I do not recommend low rep training for all exercises. For squats and dead-lifts maybe use slightly higher reps (4-6), because very low reps (1-2) can sometimes be dangerous here. Some exercises are better for ROM (round-the-world, pullovers, straight-arm flys, laterals, arm, shoulder and body circles, etc) and others for strength. Do not use low reps for lighter ROM movements. Low reps are best used for chest and shoulder presses, curls, chins, rows, and dips.

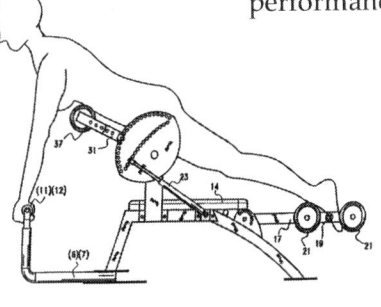

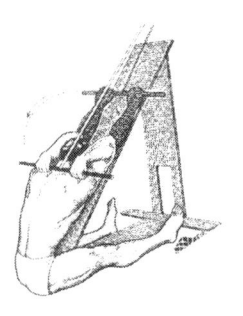

People also commonly use the wrong speed for exercise performance. Some perform reps too fast, almost being ballistic moves. Ballistic exercises are sometimes OK, and normally for ballistic-type moves such as cleans or swings. Once more, sometimes you need faster reps and sometimes quite a slow performance speed depending on movement feeling. Employ both where prudent.

Another key point relates to style and form of training. Despite the fact that I have given some recommended routines in terms of sets and reps, I do not believe that such an approach is always best, that is the most effective and efficient way to train. Sets and reps are a useful way to describe and measure a routine, but there are other "tricks" that you should use to improve your training technique.

The great natural bodybuilding champion John Grimek used to train in a very "free", or un-regimented style, performing moves outside of the normal sets and reps regime. He would (perhaps) start off doing normal full reps for a few cycles, but then perform only half reps at the top, before holding the weight for as long as possible at different (varying) points in the movement arc. In fact he might perform a "static-hold" or do mini-circles (shoulder or lying lateral circles) for even several minutes in the full stretch position whereby the weight is held in that position without moving any part of the body. This technique is especially useful for end point holds in movements such as flys and round-the-worlds or on dumbbell pullovers and off-bench dumbbell "hangs."

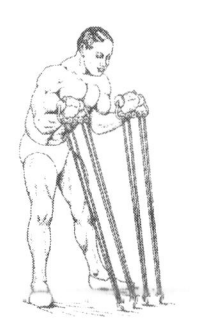

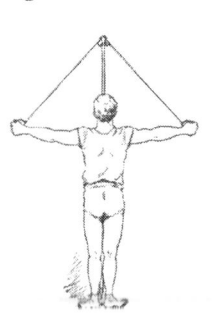

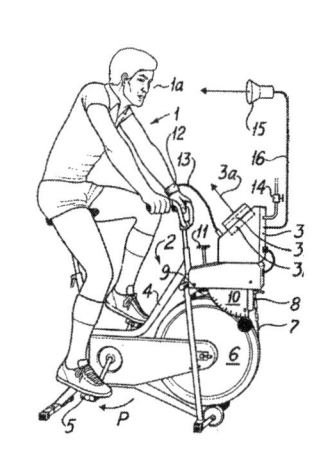

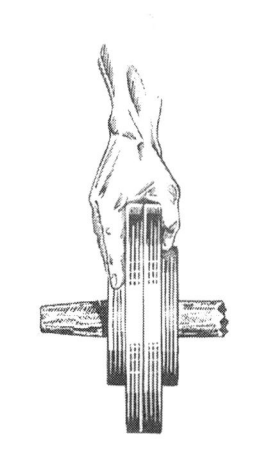

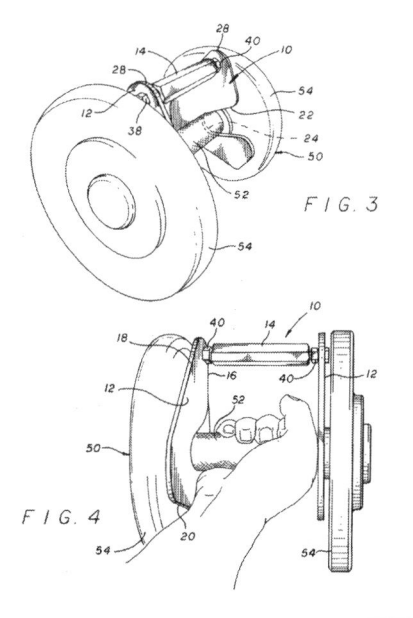

When you try these static holds and circles don't be surprised if you are not very sore the next day, and in a place right "inside" of the joint. And don't be surprised as well if you find that such training gives you a new freedom of motion in the joint, and with a corresponding greater joint ROM. The aim of such training (in one form) is to hold the weight at an extreme stretch position, and wait for the joint to give a little and increase the stretch to attain a new level of flexibility not accessed before. Be warned - use only very light weights here (perhaps 1-2 lbs).

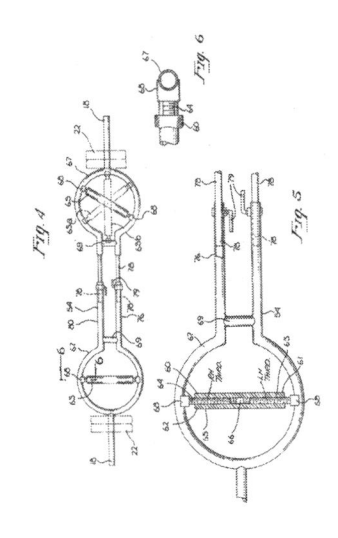

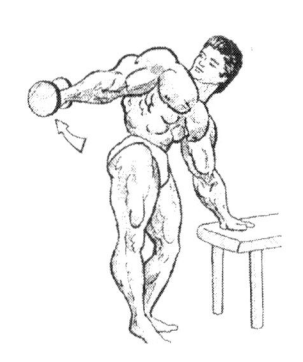

One could call this "stretch" or "joint-flexibility" weight-training? Plus there are other related techniques that you can use to further work the joint from odd angles. Get into an outstretched (end of movement) dumbbell lying "hang" position (or an extended straight arm fly or pullover position); and then perform tiny circular motions with the weight whilst the joint is held under full or partial stretch. Such movements may be very difficult at first, and you may find that they hurt (in a good way) quite a bit. There is a certain good "stretch" feeling that you are after here, and the aim is to stretch right into the joint in new ways and with VERY light weights, perhaps only 1-2 lbs.

Such full "joint-stretching" movements will give you much greater mobility in your shoulders, and it can work for other joints including the calves (slight bouncing moves at the bottom and top position of the calf raise). Note that some less mobile (single plane) joints should not be "circled" or "bounced" in this way - including the knees and elbows.

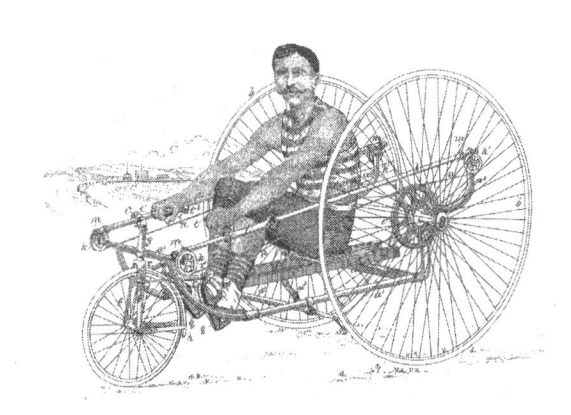

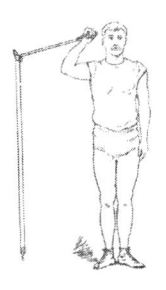

You can still focus on getting a complete stretch and full contraction on any movement. Slowing down moves helps allot also, and so to be able to "feel" what is going on to the fullest possible degree. Try 4 seconds on the concentric phase and 5-6 seconds on the eccentric phase of each rep! Constant tension is key.

As far as performing "static holds", this is a good technique on almost any exercise, because it not only increases training intensity, but seems to drive blood into the muscles and joints, in addition to helping the trainee to control the movement pattern to the optimum degree. Try pressing a weight up, and then on the way down performing 5-6 separate 10 second holds at different points in the movement. Talk about difficult!

Another mistake people make relates to choice of exercises and in terms of the design of an overall program with balanced exercise choices that work all of the regions of the body equally. Take a look at Arthur's abbreviated 8 exercise routine, and notice how it contains exercise combinations that hit every area of the body. This routine also includes lots of multi-joint, and major muscle mass movements. Plus 4 of the movements are performed in a standing position, thus meeting a primary goal of Zen Training, and so exercising the many supporting muscles, tendons, ligaments and structural factors.

We are upright creatures and we should perform the majority of our physical exercises from a standing position. Our body is supposed to work as an integrated unit, and with many muscles/joints working together at once.

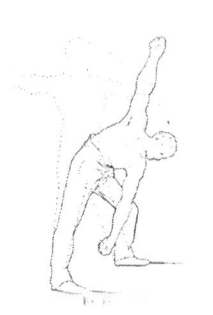

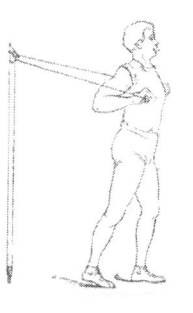

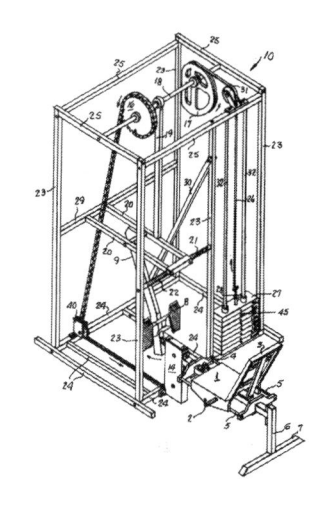

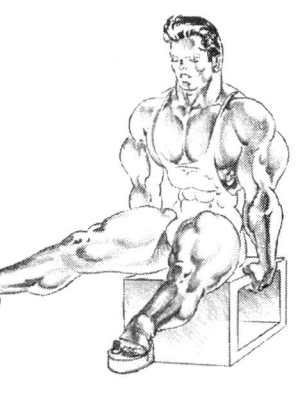

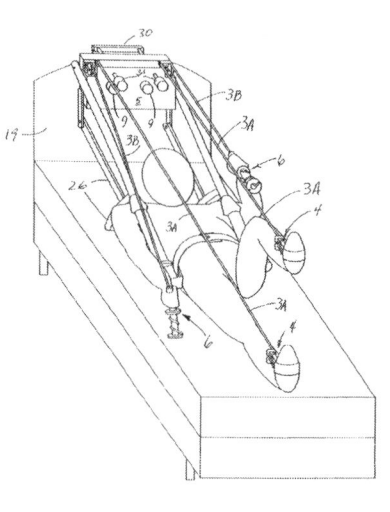

Body-part favouritism is another mistake. Many people spend too much time exercising their strong points. So chaps with great chests spend all the time bench pressing, men with good arms all day curling, and women with nice legs lots of time squatting etc. By all means work your strong points, but take an objective look at what your physique needs, and it might actually be a smaller chest or biceps and more calf development, or improved joint ROMs.

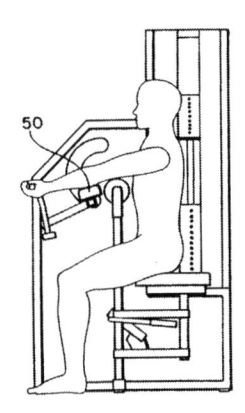

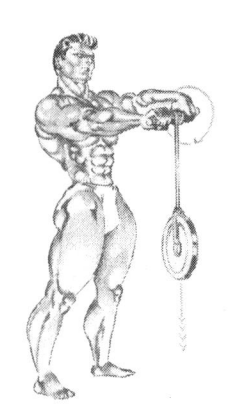

When I see a person who "knows what they are doing" with respect to fitness, I see them strength training intensely for at best 30-40 minutes, on prime-mover exercises like squats, chins, rows or the overhead press (preferably with dumbbells). But even knowledgeable people often spend little time on joint ROM training. I would encourage everyone to spend time getting to know 1-5 lbs dumbbells, and on fantastic ROM exercises like round-the-worlds, dumbbell hangs, dumbbell pullovers, front raises, overhead laterals, plus dumbbell circles of various types. Do not be embarrassed by using light weights, remember they are heavy anyway in terms of stretching movements. Later you can revel in, or show-off, superior joint ROMs, with respect to the bench press "addicts".

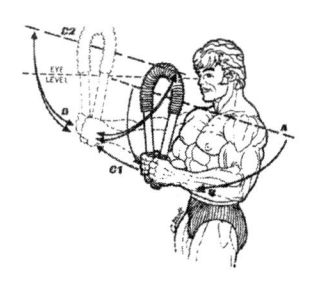

Now I would like to make another important point that relates to fitness training. We are social creatures, and we like to copy one another when it comes to behaviours and attitudes. Next time you are in the gym look around carefully, and watch how people train. Do they seem to be copying everyone else, simply doing a few bench presses and curls. Sometimes it is hard to take your own path, and especially when it is an unusual one. The difficulty comes from going against the "perceived wisdom", and in forcing yourself into unfamiliar territory. Going against the grain is difficult psychologically. Nobody really wants to be different - at least not too much - and in (possibly) the wrong way. Another point relates to "trendy" and complex theories of fitness training.

On the whole I do not believe in any of the latest theories, or else in very involved scientific explanations of the best way to train. I believe in the basics. Therefore stick mostly to the exercises listed here; because they are the very best ones that you could ever perform. But do try experimenting with using multiple movement paths also, and on individual exercises. But use only natural type moves.

I also think that the human body - despite it's complexity - is supposed to move about in a relatively simple fashion. All talk of "core" training, front and back movement "chains" and/or "cross" training leaves me cold. And when I watch a so-called cross-training workout, often performed at speed and including fast ballistic moves with weights - and usually in poor form - I shake my head. Such "leaping about" type workouts are not what the human body is supposed to do.

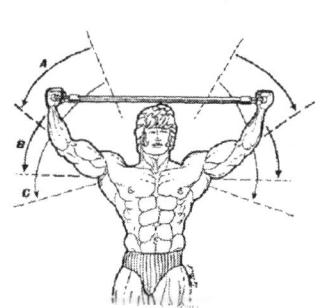

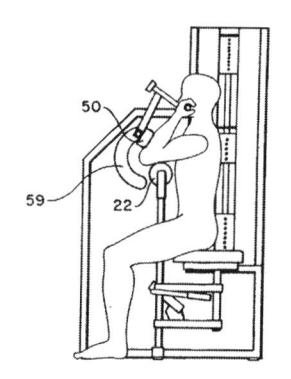

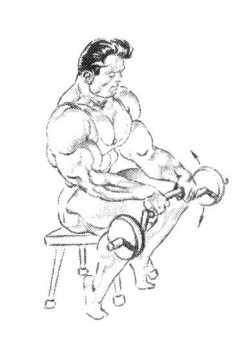

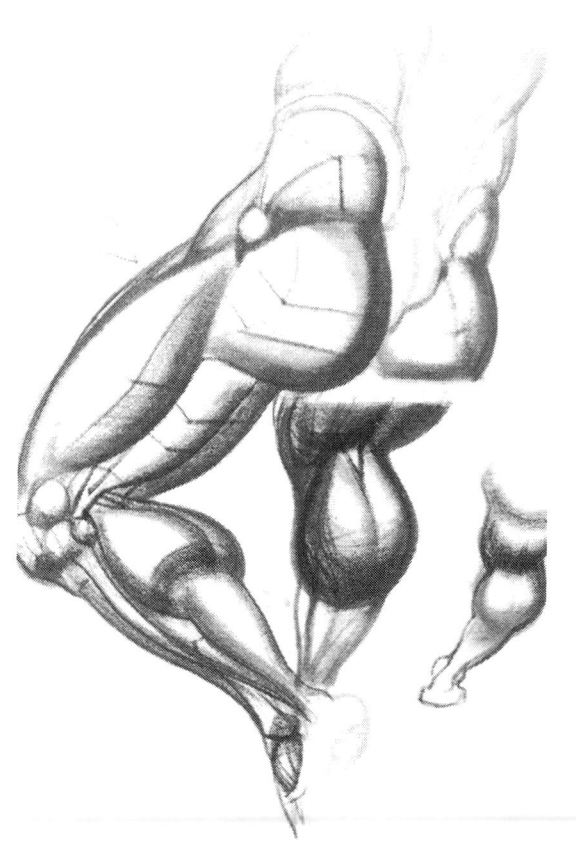

Once again Arthur Jones comes to the rescue here, because in his opinion weight training moves should be performed in a slow, deliberate and controlled manner (in terms of rep speed). And so no fast or ballistic moves with weights! He thought that the chances of injury are vastly increased when you move quickly holding a heavy weight, because the forces involved are effectively doubled.

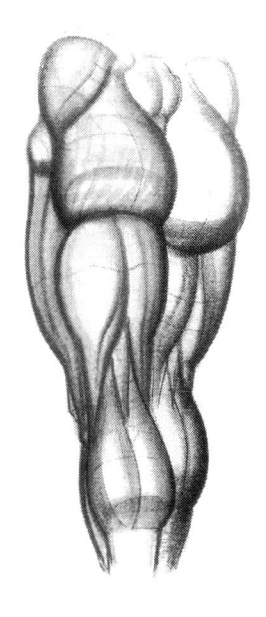

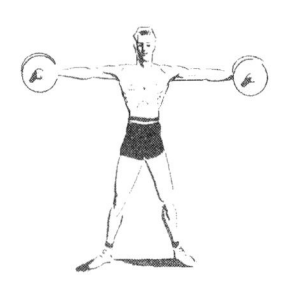

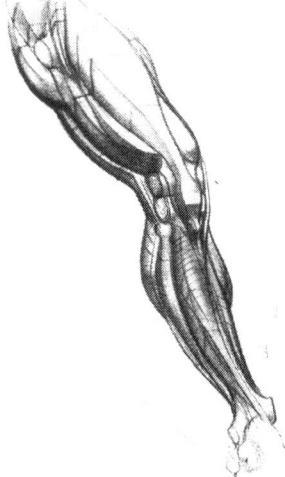

I agree with Arthur here, and I think that resistance moves should be performed in a slow and deliberate manner (generally). There are exceptions, and movements such as the barbell clean, overhead jerk, snatch and the swing can be performed quickly. However these "quick' lifts require significant skill to perform correctly, and one (normally) needs to be taught how to correctly move the body (as a whole) for such fast lifts , and in order to avoid becoming injured. Yet another point relates to integrated use of the body. Athletes, dancers and gymnasts learn to use every part of the body in order to excel at feats of amazing athleticism. Likewise I think that whenever we exercise, we should make maximum use of as many different parts of the body as possible (prime-movers, stabilisers etc). Performance of a compound movement such as a squat, or clean and press with twin dumbbells, exercises a majority of the moving levers (and core plus non-moving stabilisers) in the body.

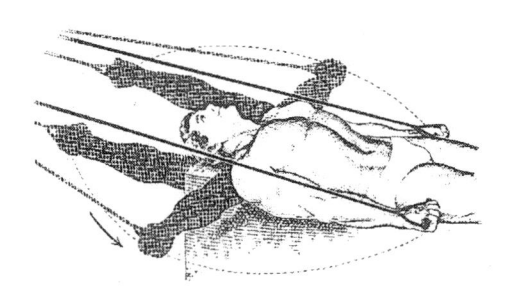

Especially useful is low rep (close to limit) training with the recommended (strength) movements, say 1-3 reps with heavy weights because this forces you to use all of the bodies capacities in order to succeed. In a way this is the opposite of isolation movements, where one tries to avoid using any joints/muscles apart from a specific one. I believe that the vast majority of training (in terms of strength) should be performed with compound movements, which provide the greatest benefits to the overall system and teach you to move the body in an integrated fashion. Also in terms of so-called "core training", lifting dumbbells using the suggested routine(s) will do more for your core muscles and inner structures than anything else you could possibly do - of that I am certain. You don't need silly "made-up" exercises like the plank etc; when you lift dumbbells! In this respect old-school style training is best. How strong do you think your core (and entire body, for that matter) will be when regularly performing dead-lifts, twisting lean-overs, trunk circles, stiff-legged dead-lifts to the feet, and overhead squats etc. Extremely strong, almost "indestructibly" strong, to be sure. On the whole, I believe that great results can be obtained by training according to the principles described herein.

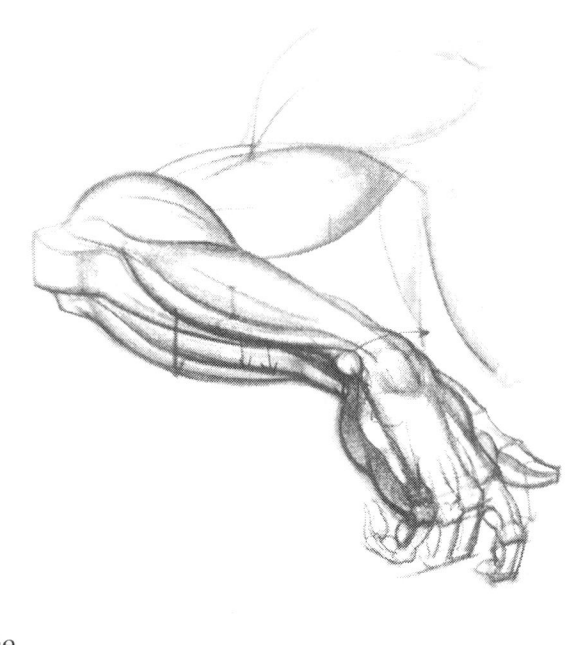

I know I told you not to listen to others, me included. But I really meant to suggest that you should look for general principles that might (possibly) work for yourself, then try them out, and either adopt them or discard them as necessary. Seek your own path. Hence this book.

Listening to your body is the key to successful Zen Training. For optimal health, exercise on a daily basis, using a wide variety of movements, including (where possible) walking, running, swimming, cycling and weight-training with dumbbells. AND AVOID MACHINES!

Finally, I wish you an abundance of love, health and strength throughout your life. Good luck.

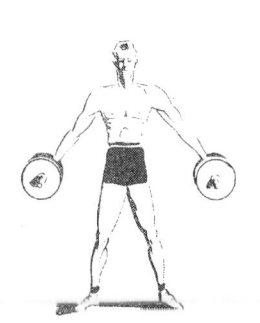

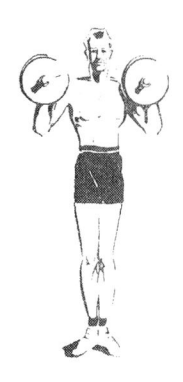

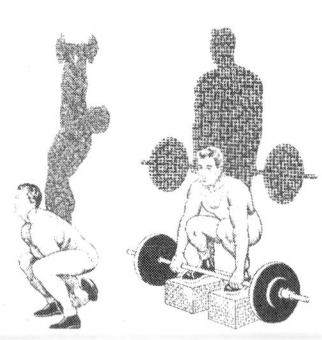

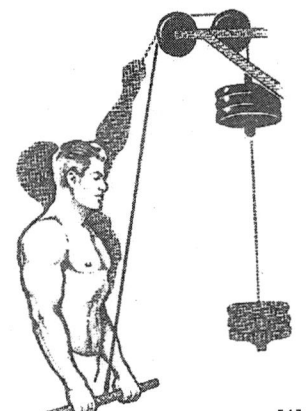

CHAPTER TWENTY

Bibliography

Recommended Books

[1] Chapman, David, Sandow The Magnificent, Eugene, 1994, University Illinois Press.

[2] Pearl, Bill, Keys to The Inner Universe, 1978, Bill Pearl Enterprises.

[3] Scott, Larry, Loaded Guns, Larry Scott and Associates.

[4] Willoughby, David, The Super Athletes, 1970, A.S.Barnes and Co.

[5] Reeves, Steve, Classic Physique, 1999.

[6] Zane, Frank, Fabulously Fit Forever, Zananda Inc.

[7] Fair, John.D., Muscletown USA, 1999, Pensiveness University Press.

[8] Little, John, Bruce Lee, The Art of Expressing the Human body, 1999.

[9] Tsatsouline, Pavel, Enter The Kettle-bell, 2006.

[10] Bass, Clarence, Ripped, 1981, Ripped Enterprises.

[11] Gaines, Charles, Butler, George, Pumping Iron, The Art and Sport of Bodybuilding.

[12] Paris, Bob, Gorilla Suit.

[13] Sandow, Eugene Sandow's System of Physical Training, 1888.

[14] Zinkin, Harold, Remembering Muscle Beach.

[15] SuperTraining, Yuri Verkhoshansky, Mel Smith, 2009.

[16] Strength Training Anatomy, Frederic Delavier, 2010.

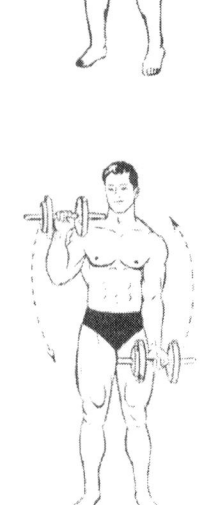

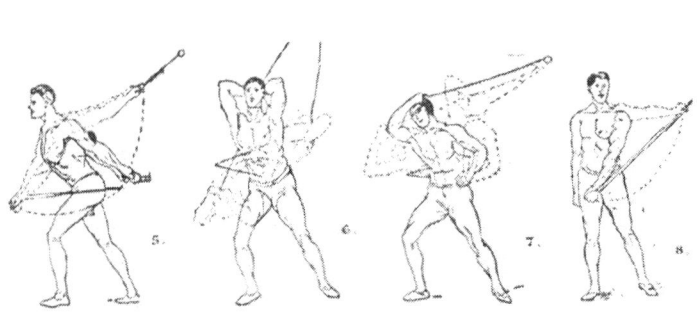

Periodicals

[1] Health and Strength magazine. 1900 - 1984, 1998 onwards.

[2] Classic Physique, 1994 onwards. Steve Reeves International Society.

[3] Iron Man, 1960 onwards.

[4] La Culture Physique, 1904 to 1950.

[5] Muscle and Fitness, Muscle Power, Muscle Builder, Your Physique,1950s - 2000s.

[6] Apollo's Magazine. 1903 - 1911.

[7] Health and Vim. 1914.

[8] Muscle Mag International, Late 1970s to present.

[9] Sandow's Magazine, 1900-1901.

[10] Strength and Health, 1950's to 1970s.

[11] The Gymnasium, 1886 onwards.

[12] The Health Magazine, 1880.

[13] The Strand Magazine, 1900 to 1901.

[14] Vim Magazine, 1914.

[15] The Cross Training Journal, 1999 - present.

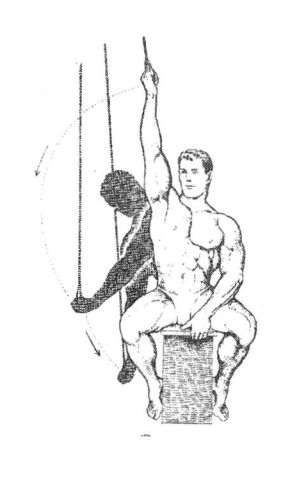

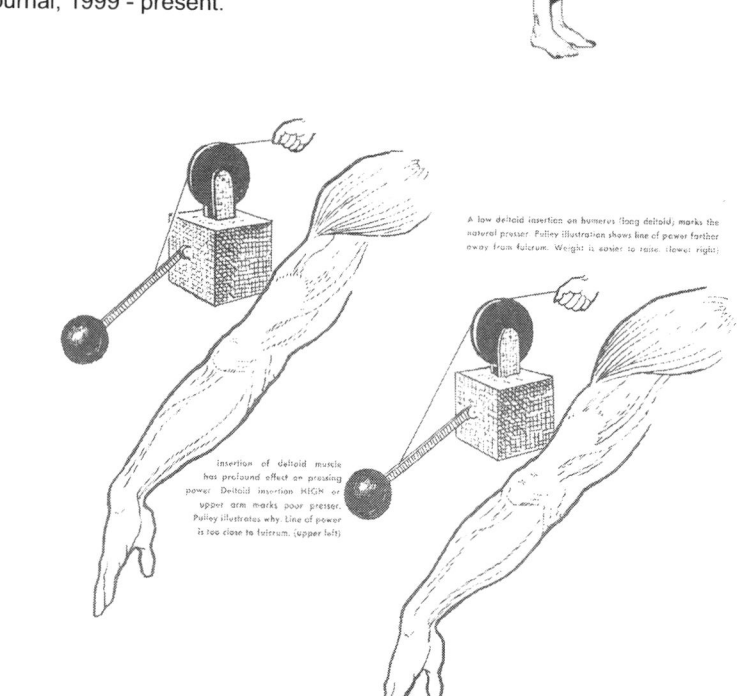

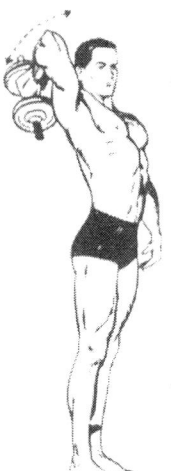

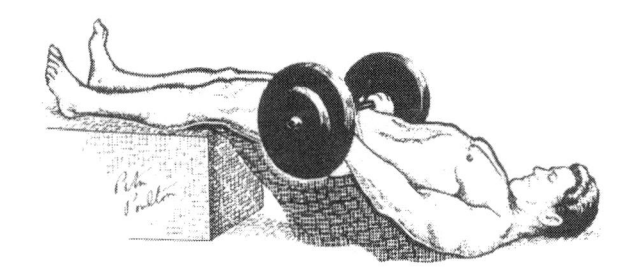

General

[1] Radley, Alan. The Illustrated History of Physical Culture: The Muscular Ideal. 2001.

[2] Brunei, Philippe et al. Sculpture From Antiquity to the Middle Ages.

[3] Shakespeare, William. The Complete Works, Oxford, 2005.

[4] Chapman, David. Sandow the Magnificent, 1998.

[5] The Sandow Museum (http://www.sandowplus.co.uk/)

[6] Sandow, Eugene. Sandow's Magazine of Physical Culture, 1901.

[7] Sandow, Eugene. Strength and How to Obtain It, Gale and Polden, 1901.

[8] Sandow, Eugene. Sandow's System of Physical Training, 1894.

[9] Reeves, Steve. Classic Physique with John Little, 1995.

[10] Maxick. Muscle Control, Ewart Seymour and Co.

[11] Fair, John D. Muscletown USA, 1999, Pennsylvania University Press.

[12] Pullum, W.A. How to Use a Barbell, Pullum and Sons, 1925.

[13] Hackenschmidt, George. "The Way to Live" 1915.

[14] Willoughby, David P. The Super Athletes, 1970, A.S.Barnes and Co.

[15] Webster, David. Barbells and Beefcake, 1979.

[16] Trevor, Chas, T. Sandow the Magnificent, The Mitre Press.

[17] Stewart Andrew. Greek Sculpture, 1990, Yale University.

[18] Roberts K.B. The Fabric of the Body, 1992, Oxford University Press.

[19] Miller, Stephen G. Arete, Greek Sports From Ancient Sources, 1991, California Press.

[20] Macfadden, Bernard. Enc. of Health and Physical Development, 1940.

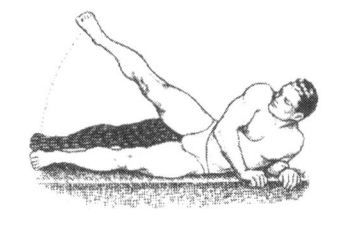

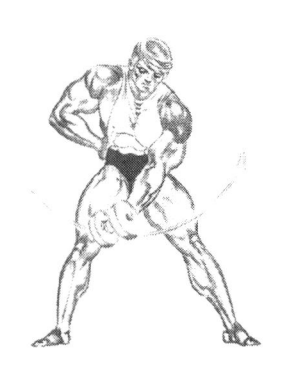

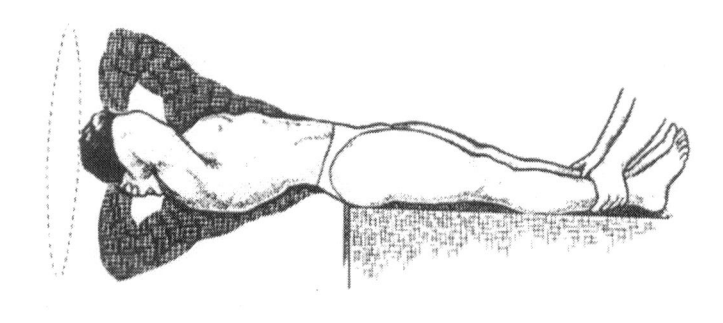

[21] Klein, Sig. Super Physique, Bodybuilding Barbell Course.

[22] Inch, Thomas. Developing the Grip and Forearm.

[23] Gupta, P.K. My System of Physical Training, 1928.

[24] Gentle, David. John Grimek, Monarch of Muscledom, 1999.

[25] Frost, Thomas. The Old Showmen, 1875.

[26] Alcott, William A. Lecturers on Health, 1853, Phillips.

[27] Anton, M. Sculpture Machine, Physical & Body Politics in the Age of Empire, 1997.

[28] Blunder, John F. The Muscles and their History From the Earliest Times, 1864.

[29] Butts, E.C. Manual of Drill for US Army, 1897.

[30] Rice, Emmet. A Brief History of Physical Education, A.S Barnes Company.

[31] Saxon, Arthur. The Development Of Physical Power, 1906.

[32] Touny, A.D. Sport in Ancient Egypt, 1969, Leipzig.

[33] Sweet, Waldo. Sport and Recreation in Ancient Greece, 1987, Oxford.

[34] Samsaye, Terry. A History of the Motion Picture, 1926.

[35] Onions, Richard. The Origins of European Thought, 1951.

[36] Kyle, Donald G. Athletics in Ancient Athens, 1987, Leiden.

[37] Sandow, Eugene. Chest Expander Booklet, 1920.

[38] Inch, Thomas. Free Exercise Courses. 1910's.

[39] McGill, Stuart. Low Back Disorders. 2007

[40] Lutz, E.G., Practical Art Anatomy, 1918.

[41] Radley, Alan. Gentle, David., 1001 Dumbbell Exercises, 2013.

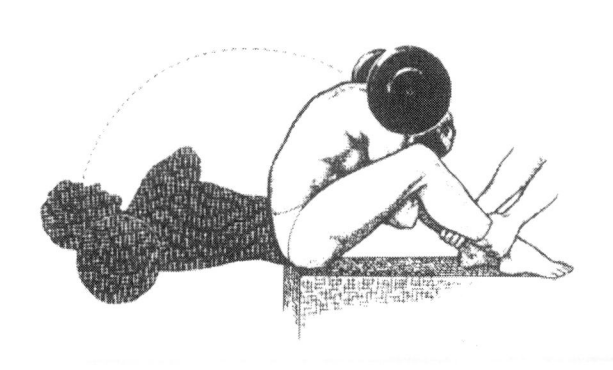

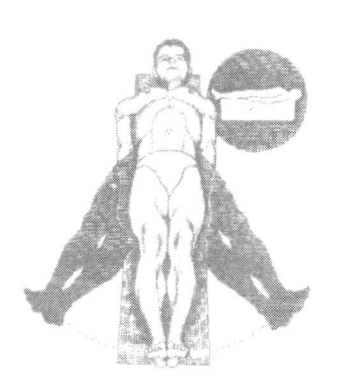

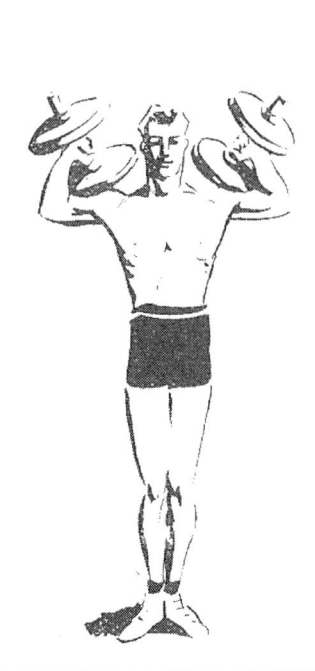

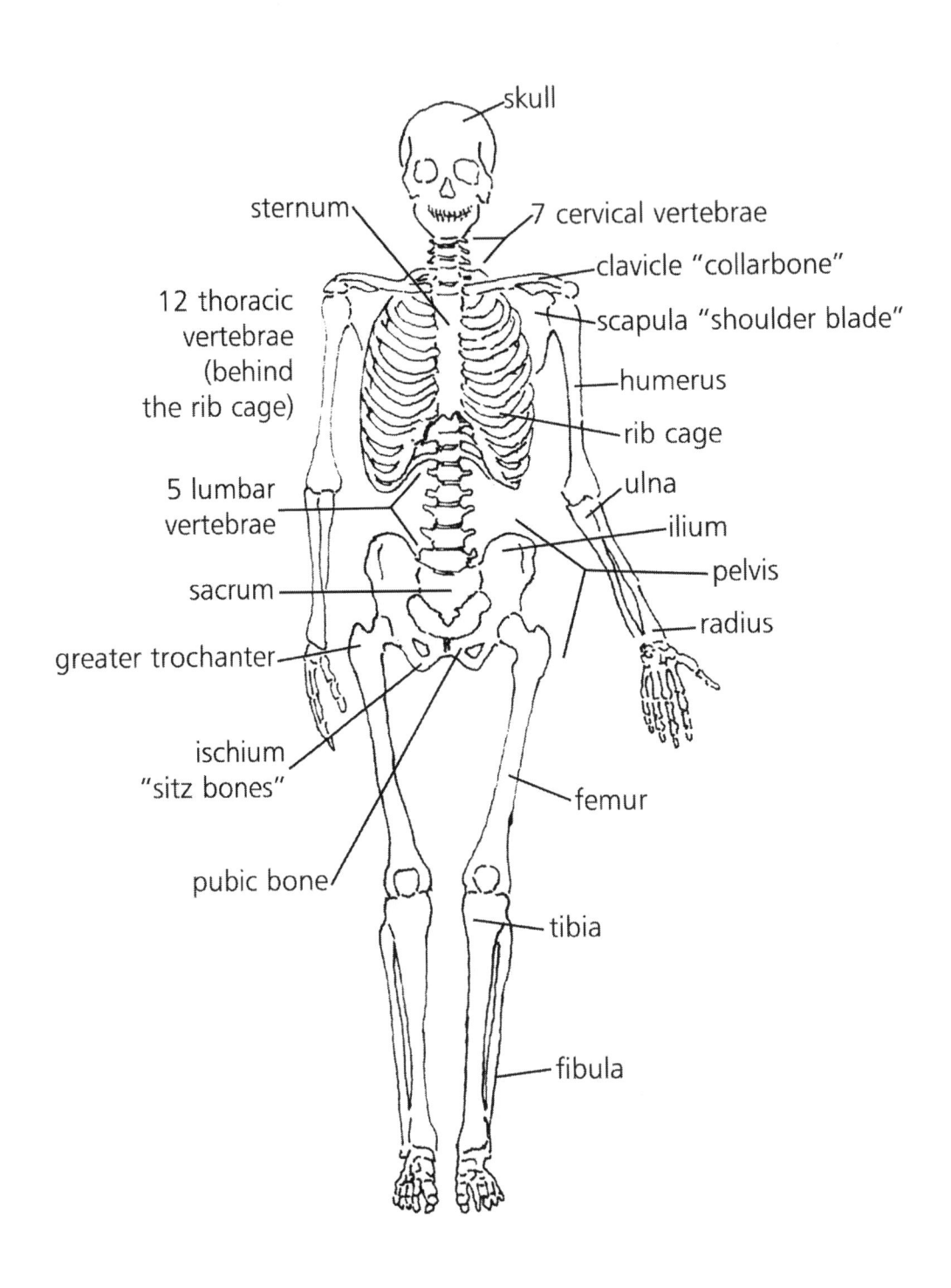

- skull
- sternum
- 7 cervical vertebrae
- clavicle "collarbone"
- 12 thoracic vertebrae (behind the rib cage)
- scapula "shoulder blade"
- humerus
- rib cage
- 5 lumbar vertebrae
- ulna
- ilium
- pelvis
- sacrum
- radius
- greater trochanter
- ischium "sitz bones"
- femur
- pubic bone
- tibia
- fibula

ANATOMY CHARTS 325

PIVOTAL
Between the atlas and axis

BALL-AND-SOCKET
Shoulder

HINGE
Elbow – between the humerus and ulna

ROTATING
The head of the radius turning in the lesser sigmoid cavity of the ulna

BALL-AND-SOCKET
Hip

HINGE-LIKE
Movements in the knee

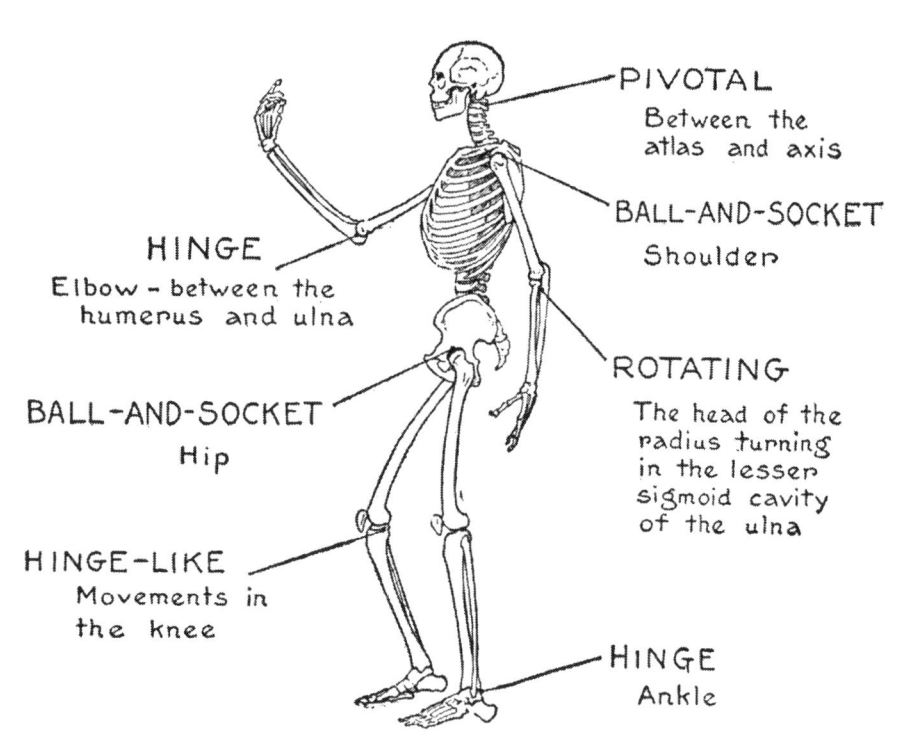

HINGE
Ankle

ARTICULATIONS OF THE SKELETON ILLUSTRATING VARIOUS KINDS OF MECHANICAL JOINTS AND MOVEMENTS.

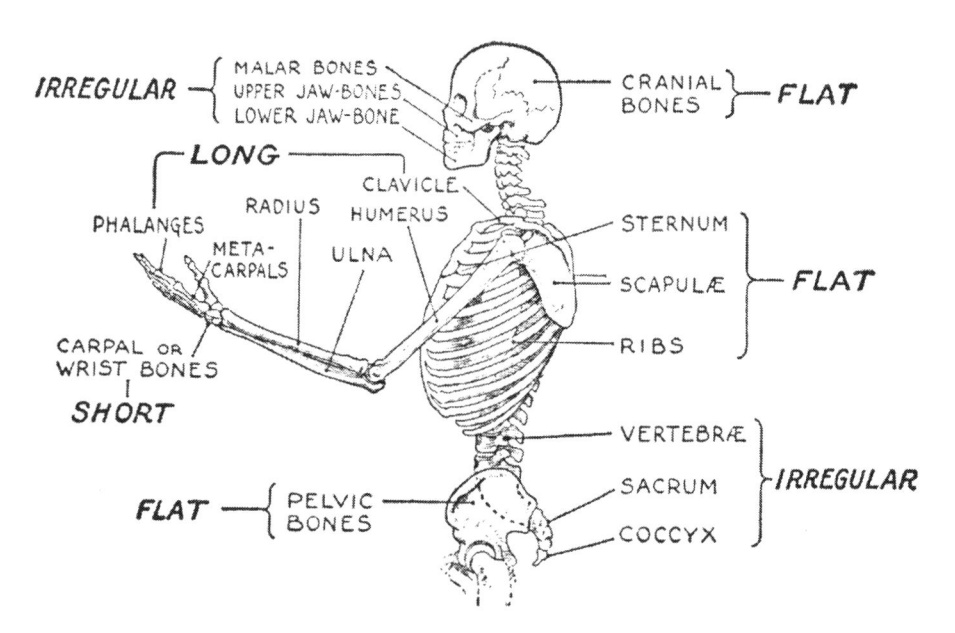

IRREGULAR { MALAR BONES, UPPER JAW-BONES, LOWER JAW-BONE

CRANIAL BONES } FLAT

LONG
PHALANGES, RADIUS, CLAVICLE, HUMERUS, META-CARPALS, ULNA

STERNUM
SCAPULÆ } FLAT
RIBS

CARPAL OR WRIST BONES
SHORT

VERTEBRÆ
SACRUM } IRREGULAR
COCCYX

FLAT { PELVIC BONES

DIAGRAM TO ILLUSTRATE THE FOUR CLASSES OF BONES.

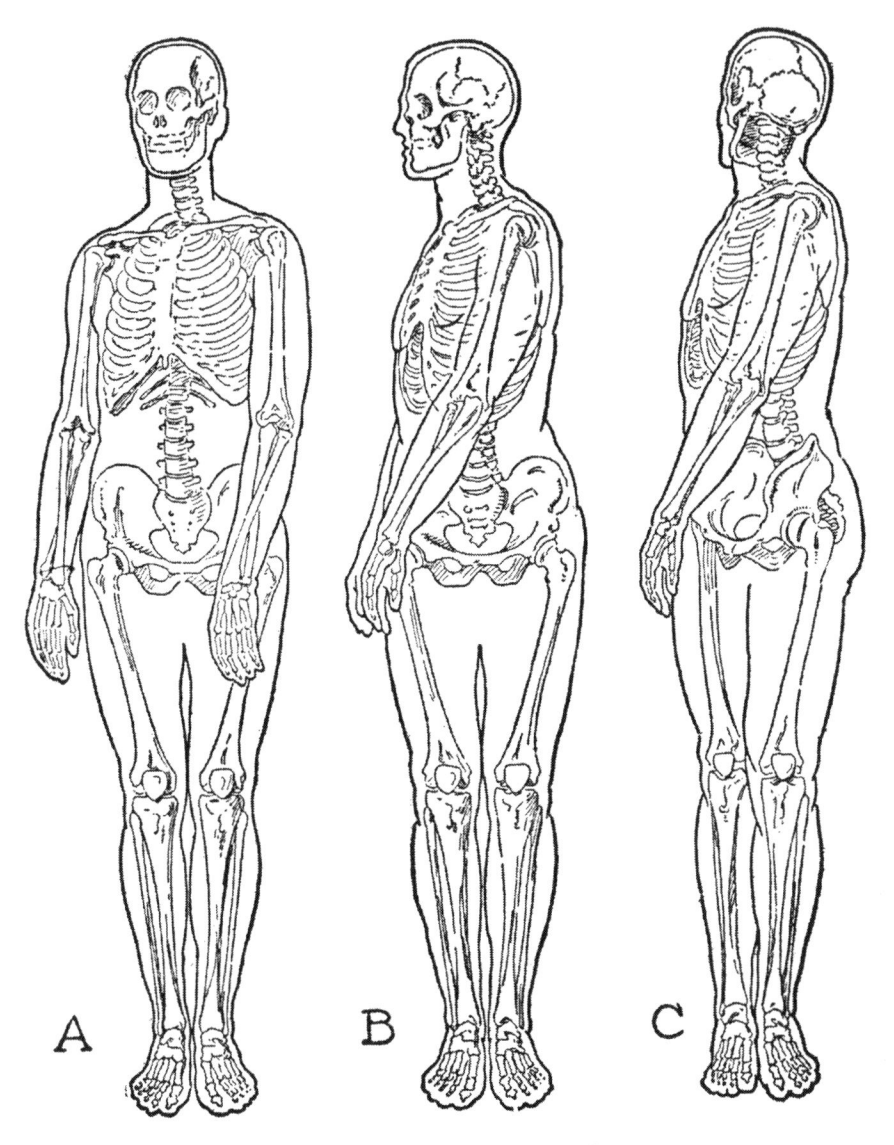

A and *B*. Rotation of the trunk.
C. The action is continued by movement in the bones of the pelvic region.

ANATOMY CHARTS 327

- FRONTAL BONE
- MALAR BONE
- LOWER JAW BONE
- SCAPULA
- HUMERUS
- RADIUS
- ULNA
- 5 METACARPAL BONES
- 14 PHALANGES OF THE THUMB AND FINGERS
- FEMUR OR THIGH BONE
- PATELLA OR KNEEPAN
- 7 TARSAL BONES
- 5 METATARSAL BONES
- 14 PHALANGES OF THE TOES
- SKULL OR CRANIUM
- CLAVICLE OR COLLAR-BONE
- ACROMION PROCESS OF THE SCAPULA
- STERNUM OR BREAST-BONE
- THORAX
- 7 TRUE RIBS
- 5 FALSE RIBS
- CARPUS OR WRIST OF 8 BONES
- BONES OF THE HIPS OR HAUNCH BONES
- TIBIA - THE LARGER OF THE TWO LEG BONES
- FIBULA THE SMALLER AND OUTER LEG BONE

ANTERIOR VIEW

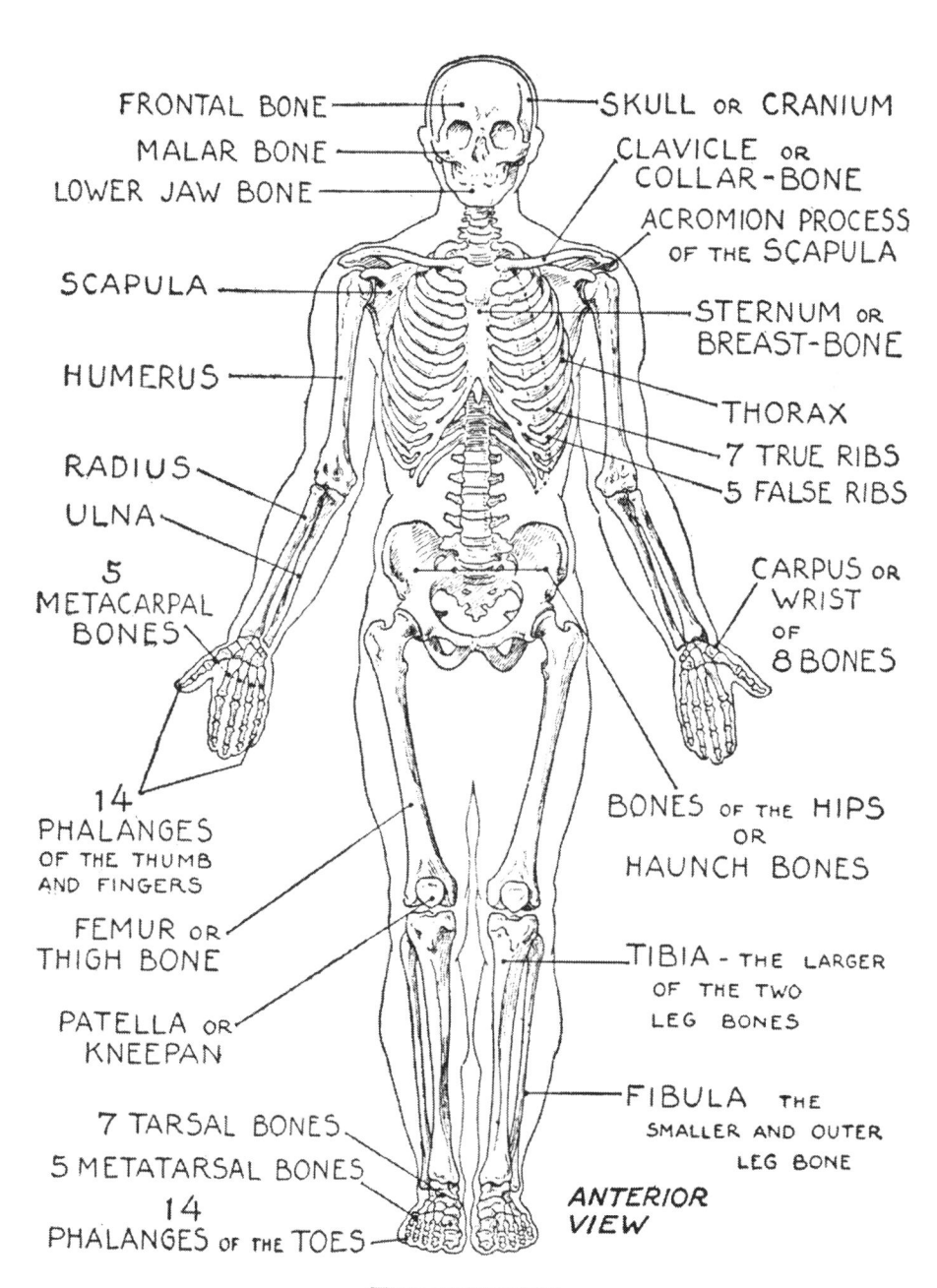

THE SKELETON.

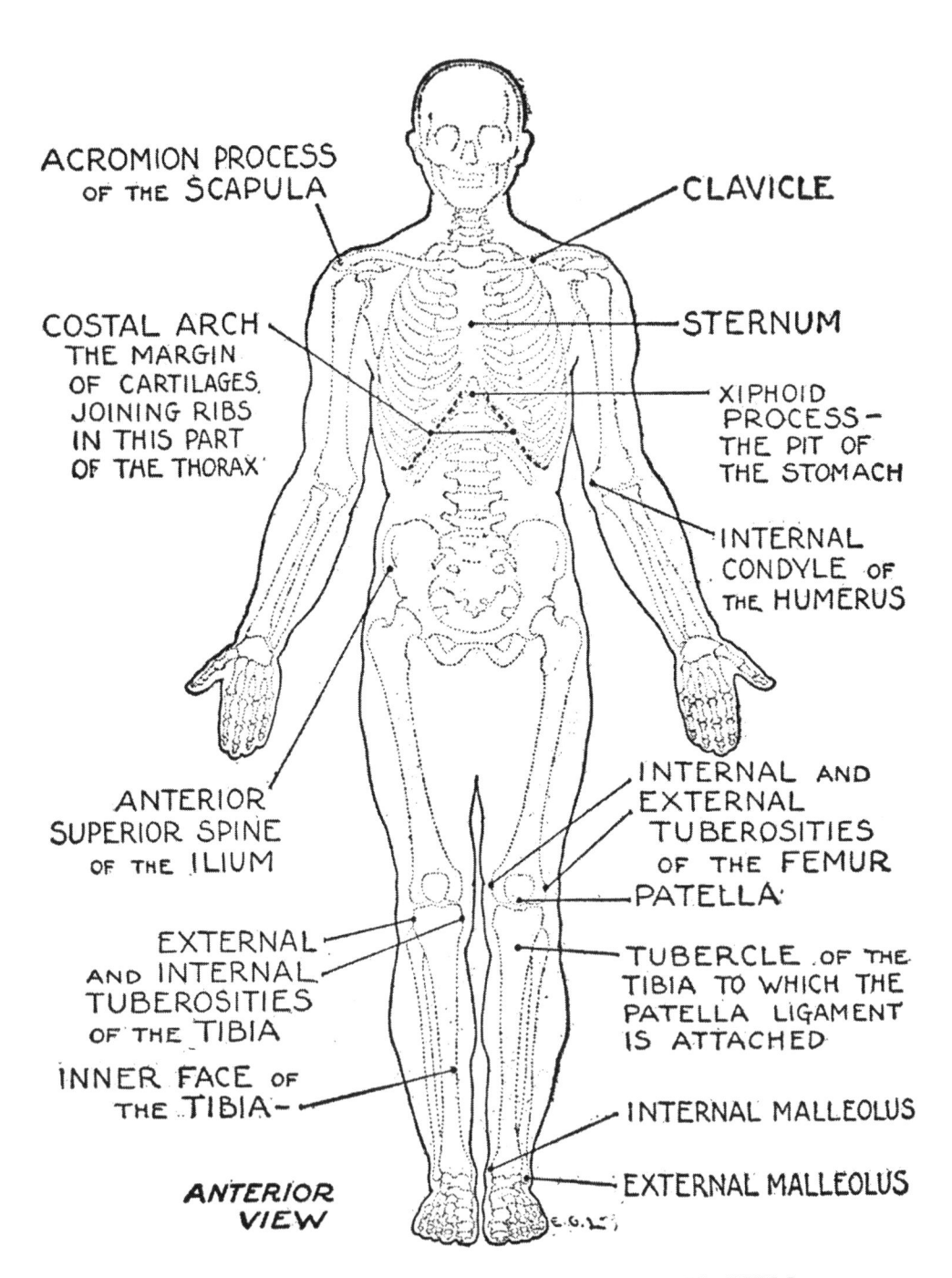

WHERE THE BONES INFLUENCE THE OUTER FORM.

ANATOMY CHARTS 329

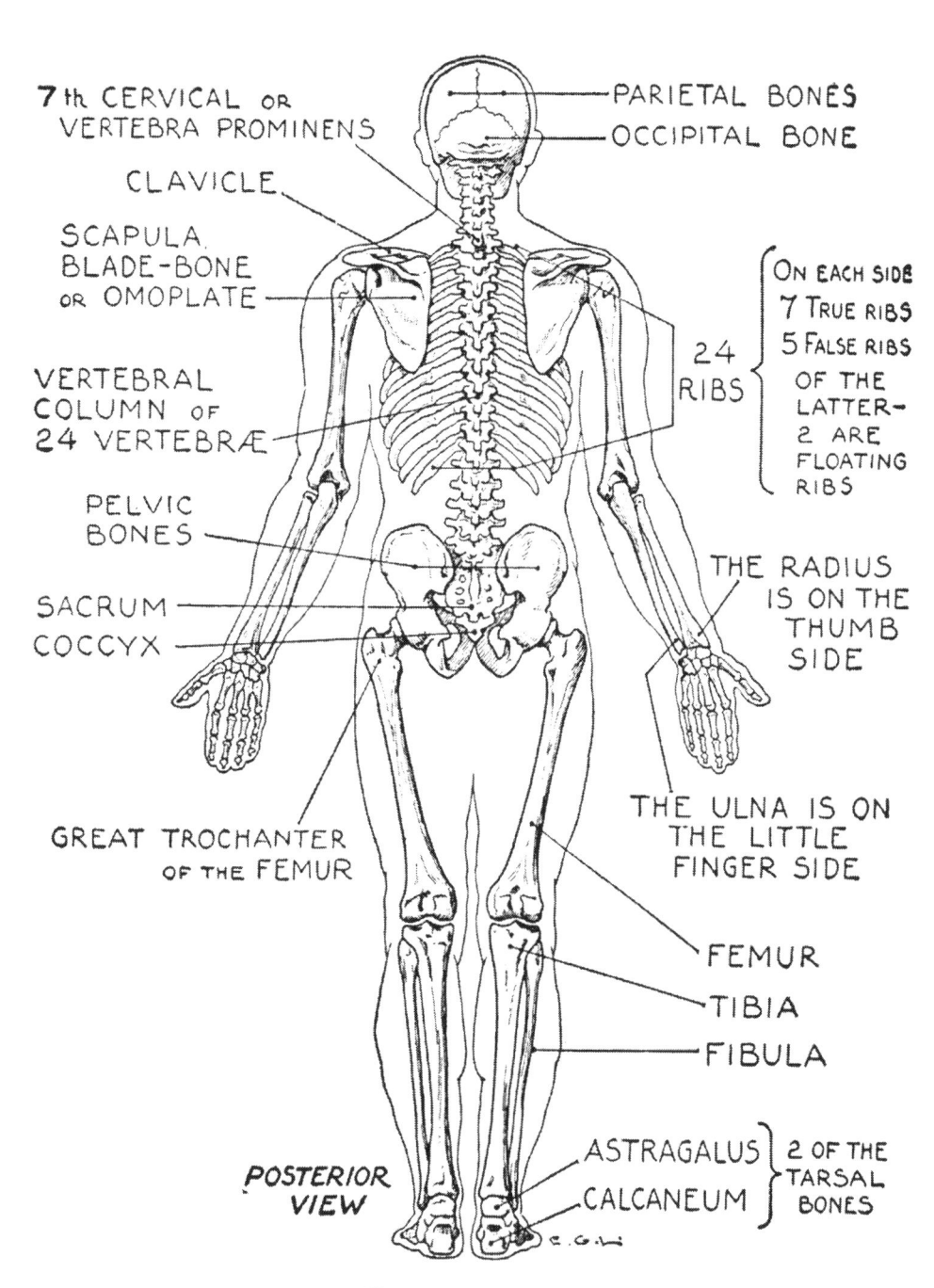

THE SKELETON.

VERTEBRA PROMINENS

ROOT OF THE SPINE OF THE SCAPULA – A DEPRESSION

EXTERNAL CONDYLE OF THE HUMERUS

LOWER END OF THE RADIUS

LOWER END OF THE ULNA

GREAT TROCHANTER OF THE FEMUR

INTERNAL MALLEOLUS

EXTERNAL MALLEOLUS

SPINE OF THE SCAPULA

INNER BORDER OF THE SCAPULA

OLECRANON THE TIP OF THE ELBOW

ULNA ALONG THE ULNAR FURROW

POSTERIOR SUPERIOR ILIAC SPINE MARKED BY A DEPRESSION

HEAD OF THE FIBULA

CALCANEUM

POSTERIOR VIEW

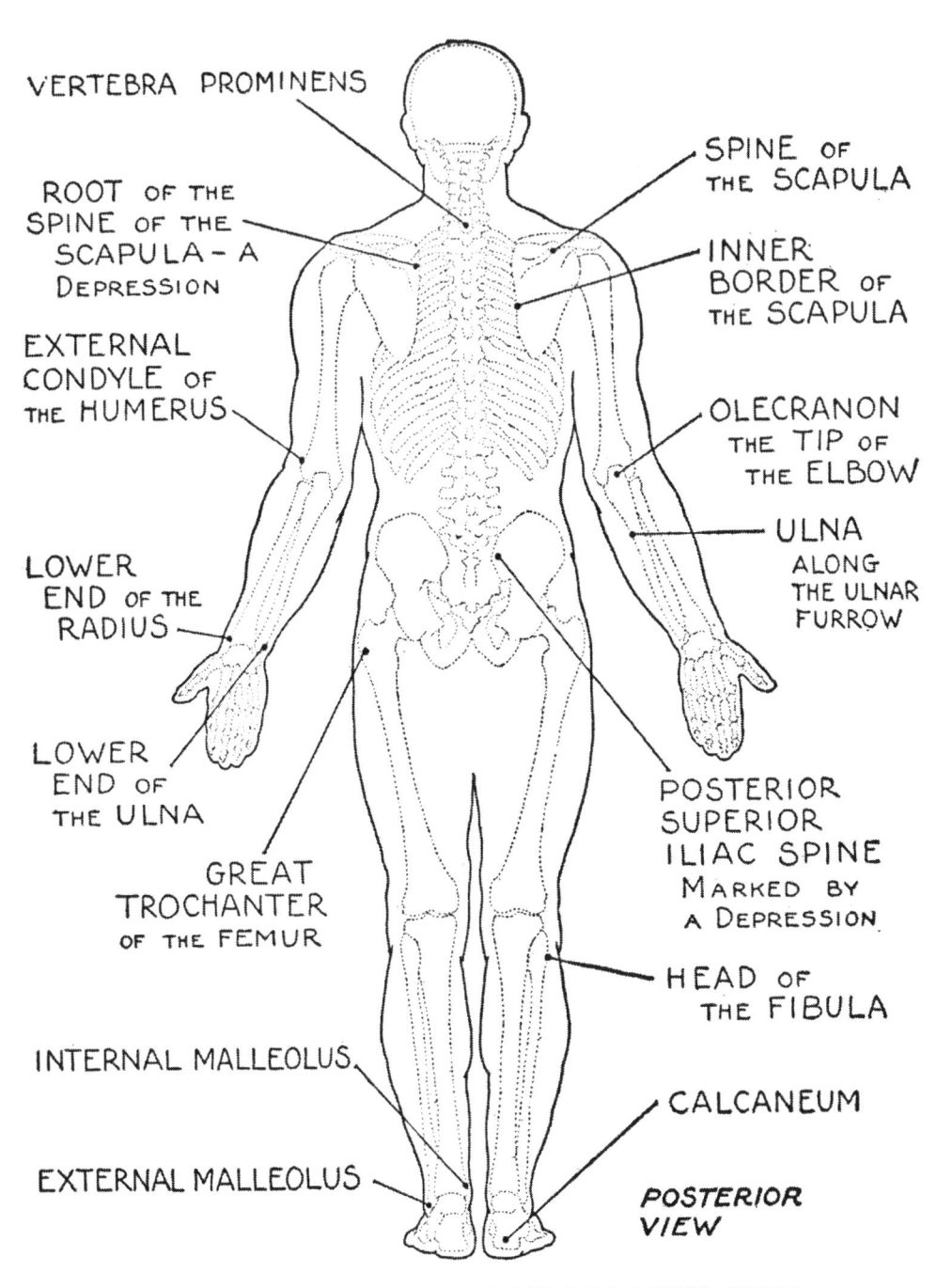

WHERE THE BONES INFLUENCE THE OUTER FORM.

ANATOMY CHARTS 331

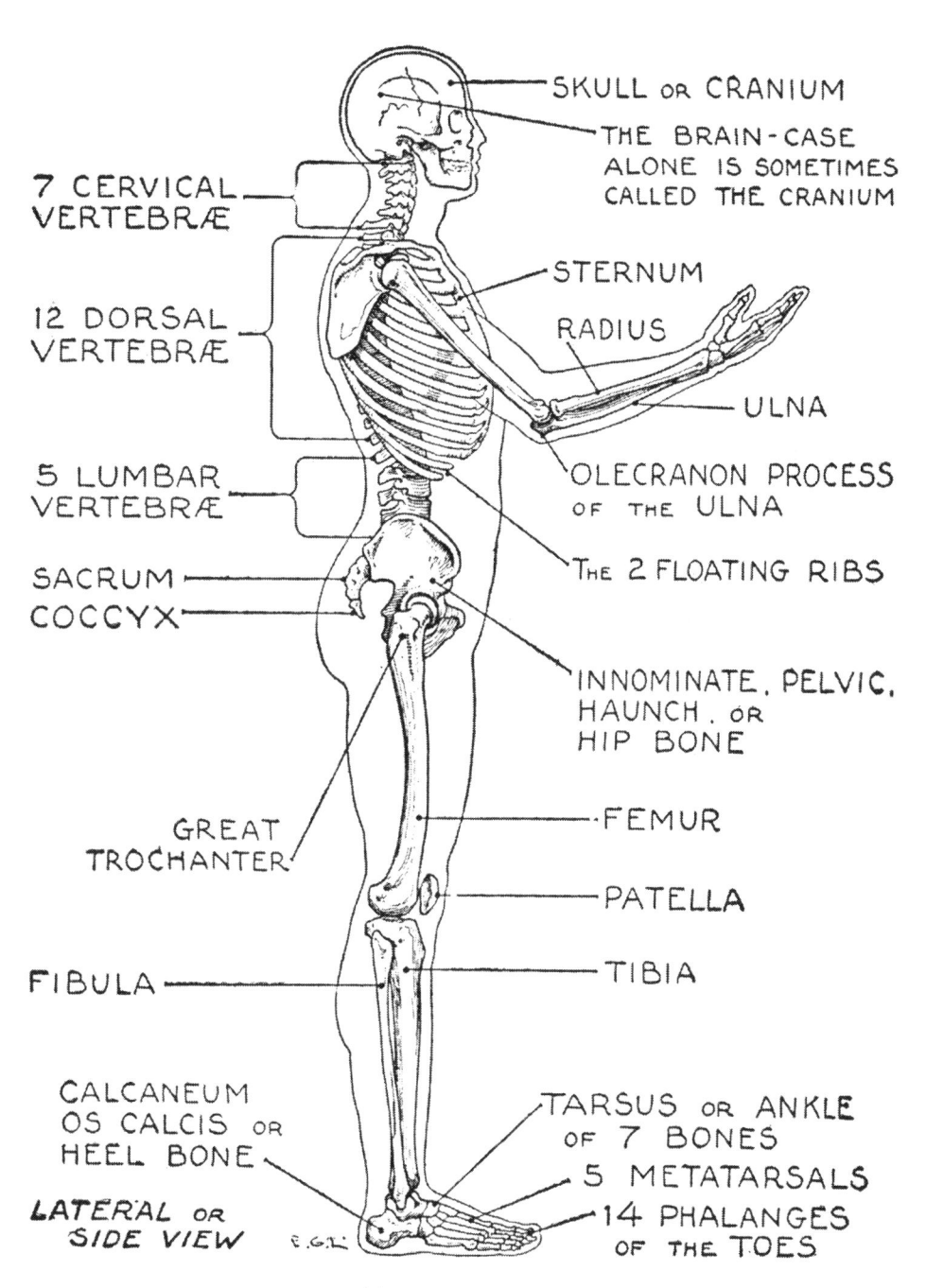

- SKULL or CRANIUM
- THE BRAIN-CASE ALONE IS SOMETIMES CALLED THE CRANIUM
- 7 CERVICAL VERTEBRÆ
- STERNUM
- RADIUS
- 12 DORSAL VERTEBRÆ
- ULNA
- OLECRANON PROCESS OF THE ULNA
- 5 LUMBAR VERTEBRÆ
- THE 2 FLOATING RIBS
- SACRUM
- COCCYX
- INNOMINATE, PELVIC, HAUNCH, OR HIP BONE
- FEMUR
- GREAT TROCHANTER
- PATELLA
- TIBIA
- FIBULA
- CALCANEUM OS CALCIS OR HEEL BONE
- TARSUS OR ANKLE OF 7 BONES
- 5 METATARSALS
- 14 PHALANGES OF THE TOES

LATERAL OR SIDE VIEW

THE SKELETON.

ZEN OF DUMBBELL TRAINING

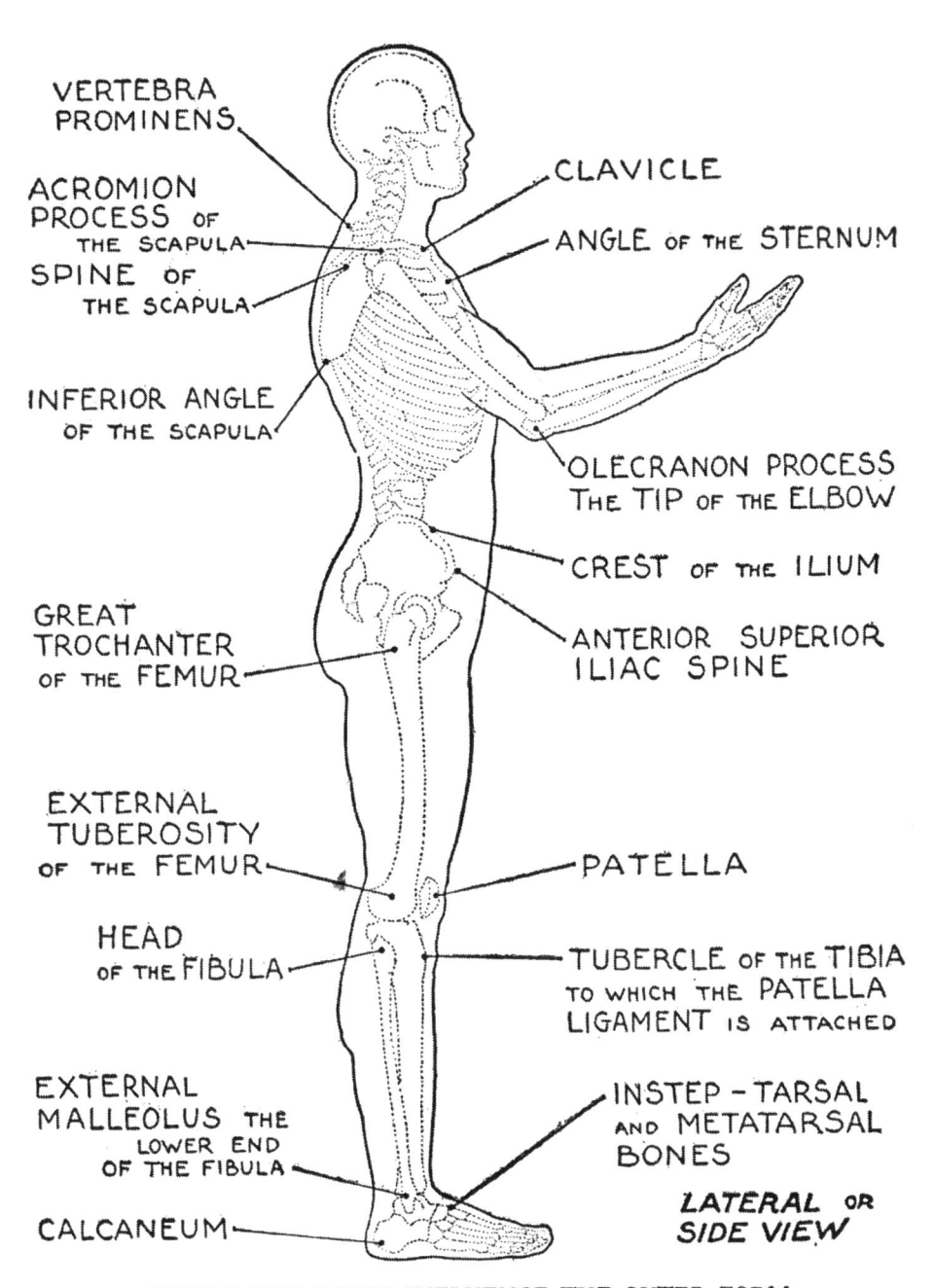

- VERTEBRA PROMINENS
- ACROMION PROCESS OF THE SCAPULA
- SPINE OF THE SCAPULA
- INFERIOR ANGLE OF THE SCAPULA
- GREAT TROCHANTER OF THE FEMUR
- EXTERNAL TUBEROSITY OF THE FEMUR
- HEAD OF THE FIBULA
- EXTERNAL MALLEOLUS THE LOWER END OF THE FIBULA
- CALCANEUM
- CLAVICLE
- ANGLE OF THE STERNUM
- OLECRANON PROCESS THE TIP OF THE ELBOW
- CREST OF THE ILIUM
- ANTERIOR SUPERIOR ILIAC SPINE
- PATELLA
- TUBERCLE OF THE TIBIA TO WHICH THE PATELLA LIGAMENT IS ATTACHED
- INSTEP — TARSAL AND METATARSAL BONES

LATERAL OR SIDE VIEW

WHERE THE BONES INFLUENCE THE OUTER FORM.

ANATOMY CHARTS 333

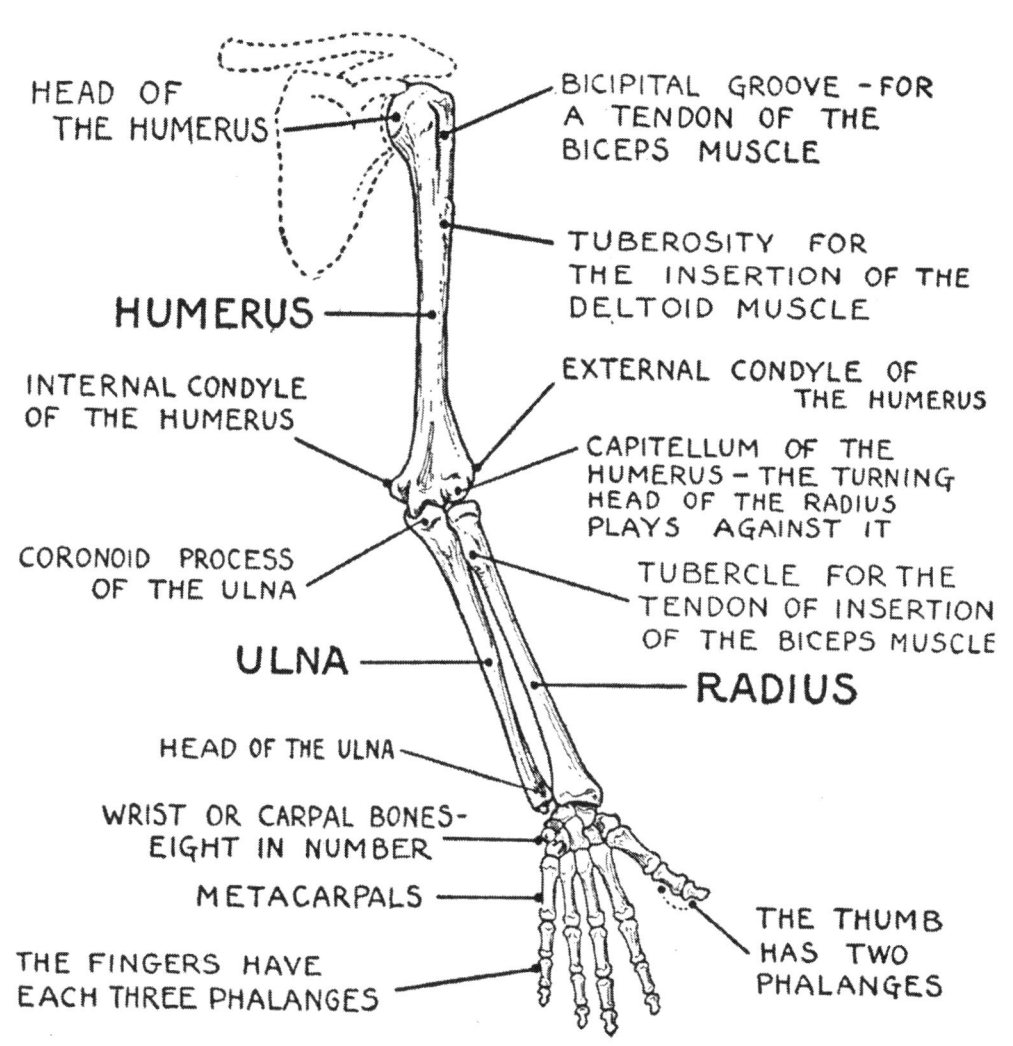

- HEAD OF THE HUMERUS
- BICIPITAL GROOVE – FOR A TENDON OF THE BICEPS MUSCLE
- TUBEROSITY FOR THE INSERTION OF THE DELTOID MUSCLE

HUMERUS

- INTERNAL CONDYLE OF THE HUMERUS
- EXTERNAL CONDYLE OF THE HUMERUS
- CAPITELLUM OF THE HUMERUS – THE TURNING HEAD OF THE RADIUS PLAYS AGAINST IT
- CORONOID PROCESS OF THE ULNA
- TUBERCLE FOR THE TENDON OF INSERTION OF THE BICEPS MUSCLE

ULNA — RADIUS

- HEAD OF THE ULNA
- WRIST OR CARPAL BONES – EIGHT IN NUMBER
- METACARPALS
- THE THUMB HAS TWO PHALANGES
- THE FINGERS HAVE EACH THREE PHALANGES

LEFT ARM ANTERIOR VIEW

THE BONES OF THE UPPER LIMB.

Frontalis
Temporal
Orbicularis palpebrarum
Zygomatic major
      "   minor*
Masseter
Depressor anguli oris
Orbicularis oris
Sterno-mastoid

Deltoid

Pectoral major
Serratus magnus
Brachialis anticus
Serratus magnus
External oblique

Rectus abdominus
Supinator longus
Extensor carpi radialis longus

Muscles of forearm

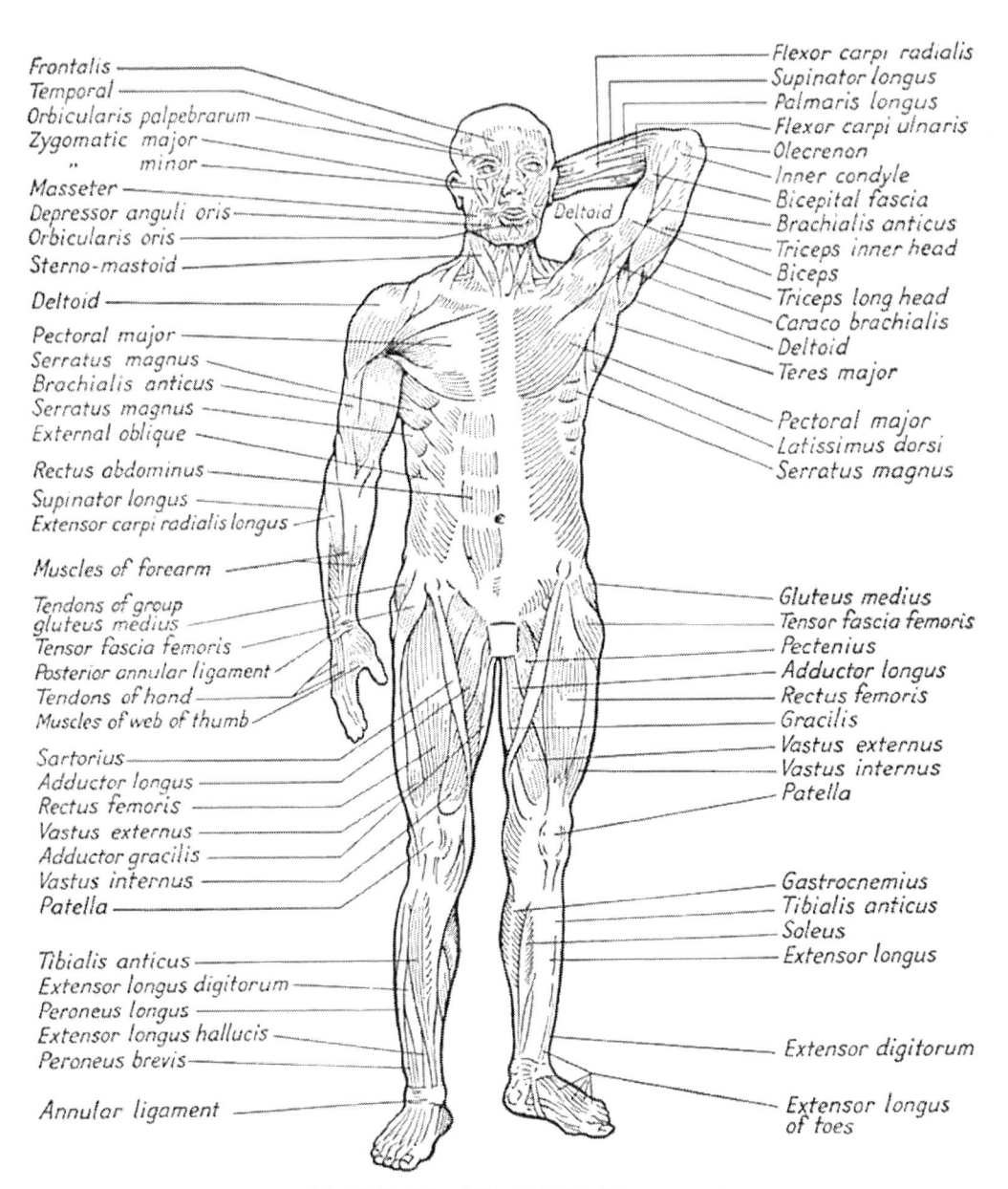

Tendons of group
gluteus medius
Tensor fascia femoris
Posterior annular ligament
Tendons of hand
Muscles of web of thumb

Sartorius
Adductor longus
Rectus femoris
Vastus externus
Adductor gracilis
Vastus internus
Patella

Tibialis anticus
Extensor longus digitorum
Peroneus longus
Extensor longus hallucis
Peroneus brevis

Annular ligament

Flexor carpi radialis
Supinator longus
Palmaris longus
Flexor carpi ulnaris
Olecrenon
Inner condyle
Bicepital fascia
Brachialis anticus
Triceps inner head
Biceps
Triceps long head
Caraco brachialis
Deltoid
Teres major

Pectoral major
Latissimus dorsi
Serratus magnus

Gluteus medius
Tensor fascia femoris
Pectenius
Adductor longus
Rectus femoris
Gracilis
Vastus externus
Vastus internus
Patella

Gastrocnemius
Tibialis anticus
Soleus
Extensor longus

Extensor digitorum

Extensor longus
of toes

Deltoid

MUSCLES OF BODY (front view)

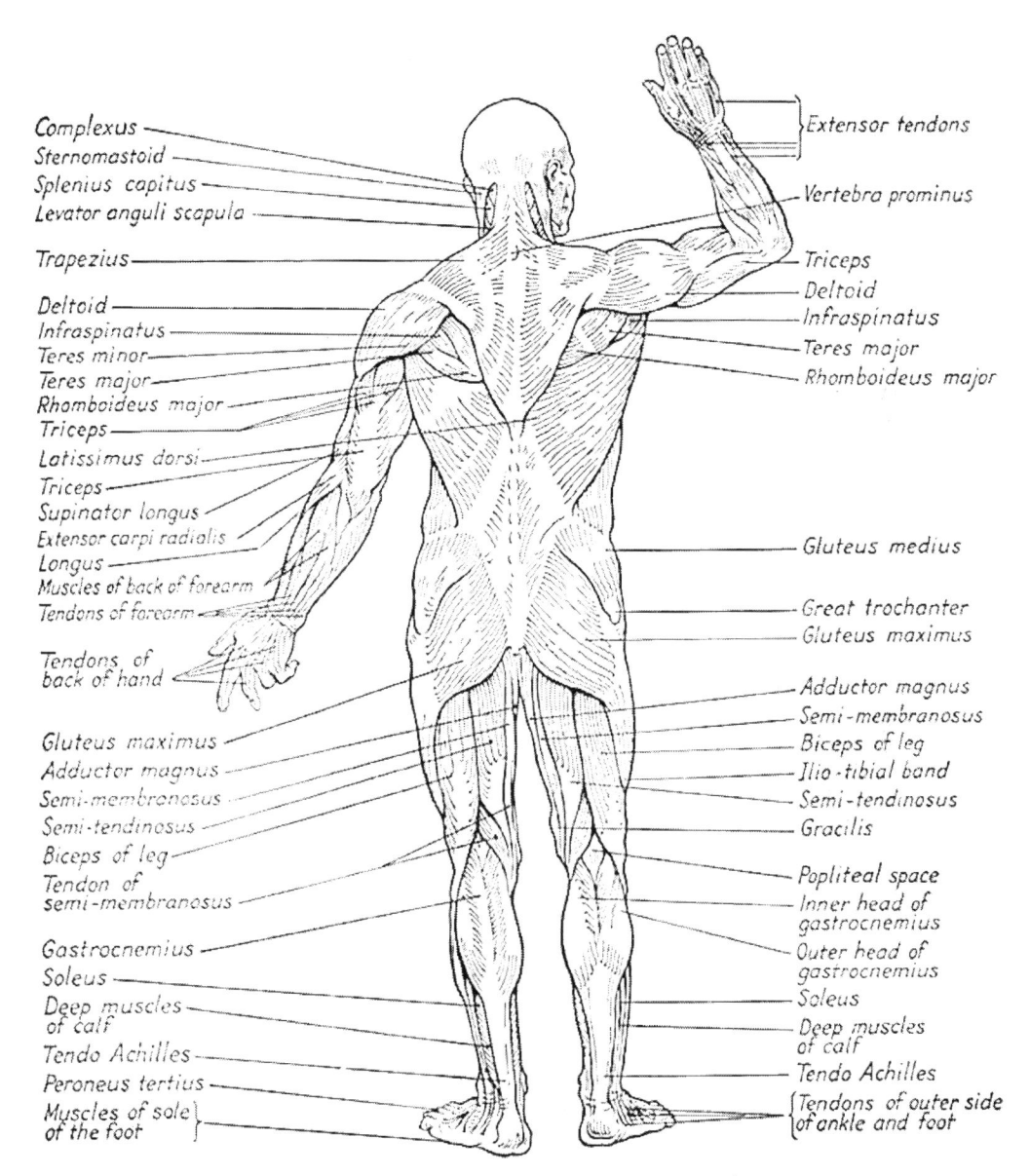

ANATOMY CHARTS 335

Complexus
Sternomastoid
Splenius capitus
Levator anguli scapula
Trapezius
Deltoid
Infraspinatus
Teres minor
Teres major
Rhomboideus major
Triceps
Latissimus dorsi
Triceps
Supinator longus
Extensor carpi radialis
Longus
Muscles of back of forearm
Tendons of forearm

Tendons of back of hand

Gluteus maximus
Adductor magnus
Semi-membranosus
Semi-tendinosus
Biceps of leg
Tendon of semi-membranosus

Gastrocnemius
Soleus
Deep muscles of calf
Tendo Achilles
Peroneus tertius
Muscles of sole of the foot

Extensor tendons
Vertebra prominus
Triceps
Deltoid
Infraspinatus
Teres major
Rhomboideus major

Gluteus medius

Great trochanter
Gluteus maximus
Adductor magnus
Semi-membranosus
Biceps of leg
Ilio-tibial band
Semi-tendinosus
Gracilis

Popliteal space
Inner head of gastrocnemius
Outer head of gastrocnemius
Soleus
Deep muscles of calf
Tendo Achilles
Tendons of outer side of ankle and foot

MUSCLES OF BODY (back view)

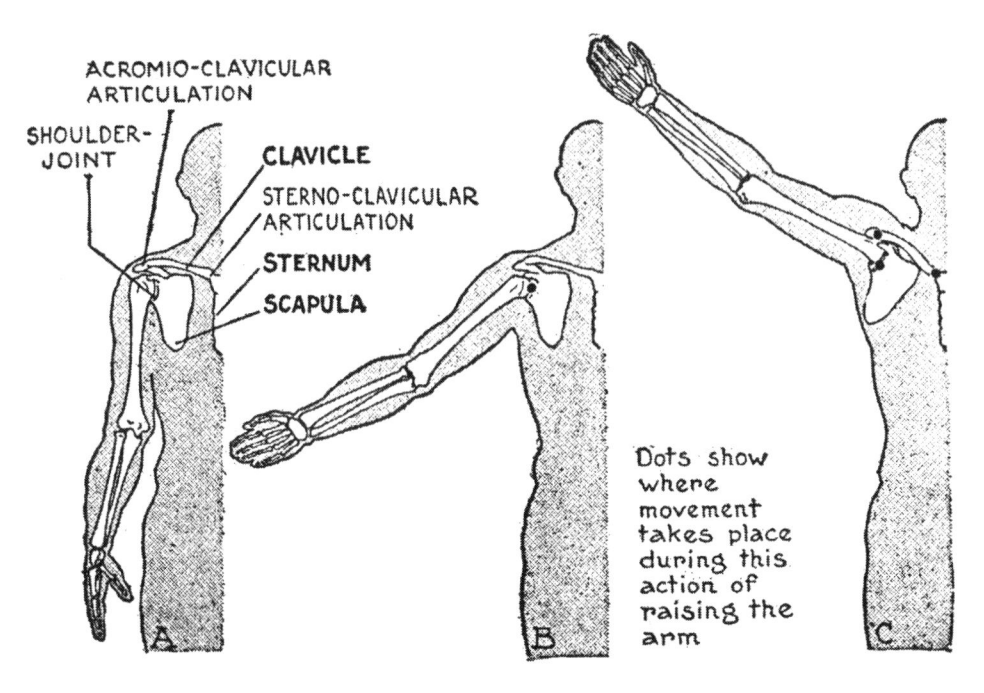

WHERE ARTICULAR MOVEMENTS TAKE PLACE IN THE SHOULDER GIRDLE WHEN THE ARM IS RAISED.

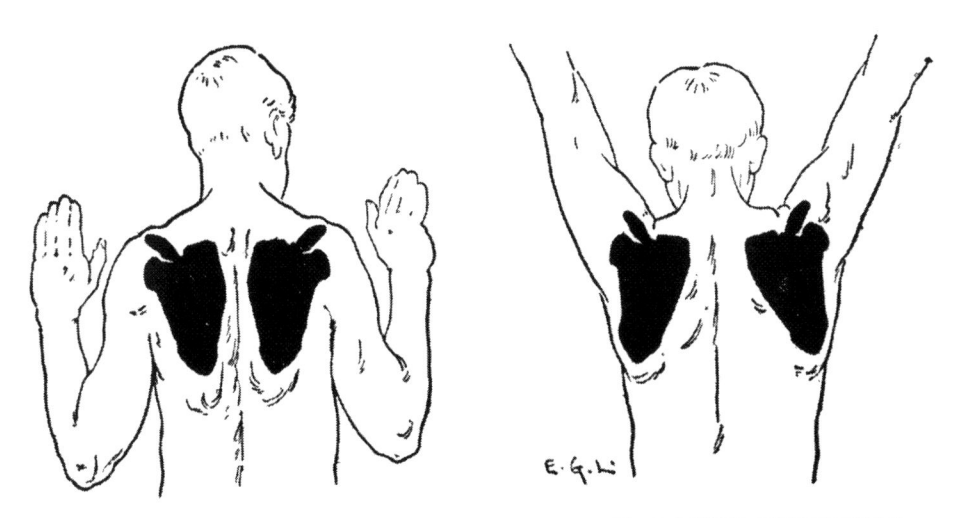

THE SCAPULÆ DURING CERTAIN MOVEMENTS OF THE SHOULDERS AND ARMS

ANATOMY CHARTS 337

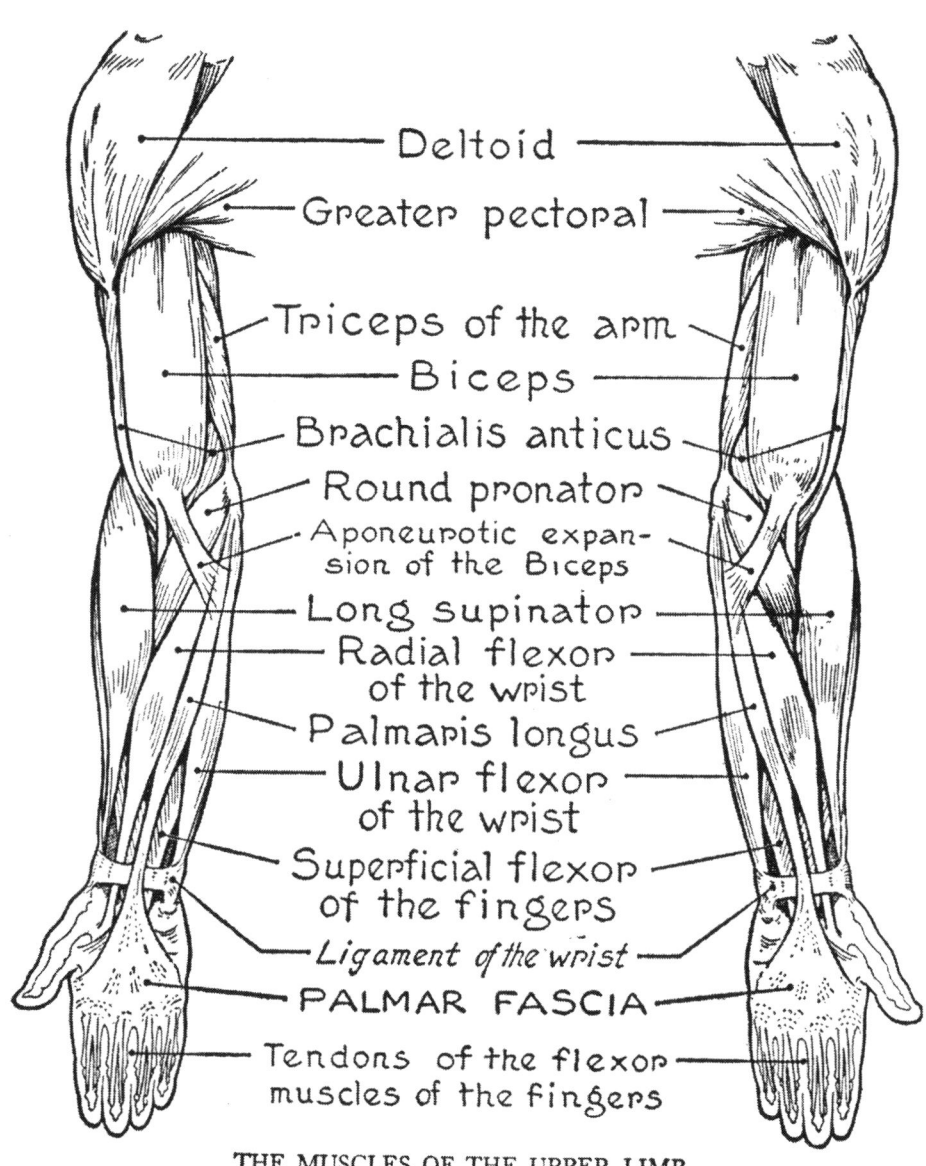

- Deltoid
- Greater pectoral
- Triceps of the arm
- Biceps
- Brachialis anticus
- Round pronator
- Aponeurotic expansion of the Biceps
- Long supinator
- Radial flexor of the wrist
- Palmaris longus
- Ulnar flexor of the wrist
- Superficial flexor of the fingers
- Ligament of the wrist
- PALMAR FASCIA
- Tendons of the flexor muscles of the fingers

THE MUSCLES OF THE UPPER LIMB.
Anterior view.

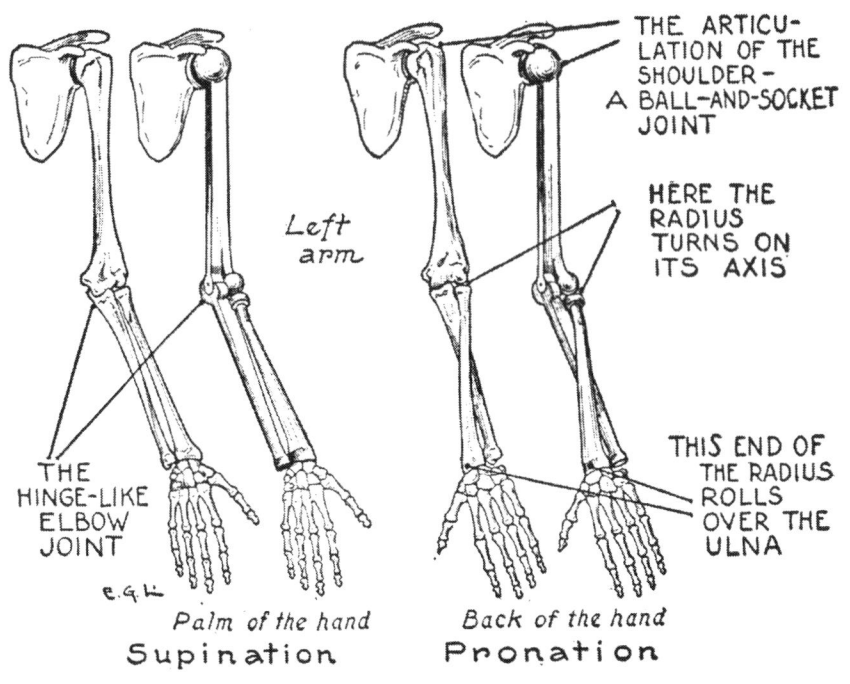

THE SKELETAL COMPONENTS OF THE ARM ARRANGED AS A MECHANISM.

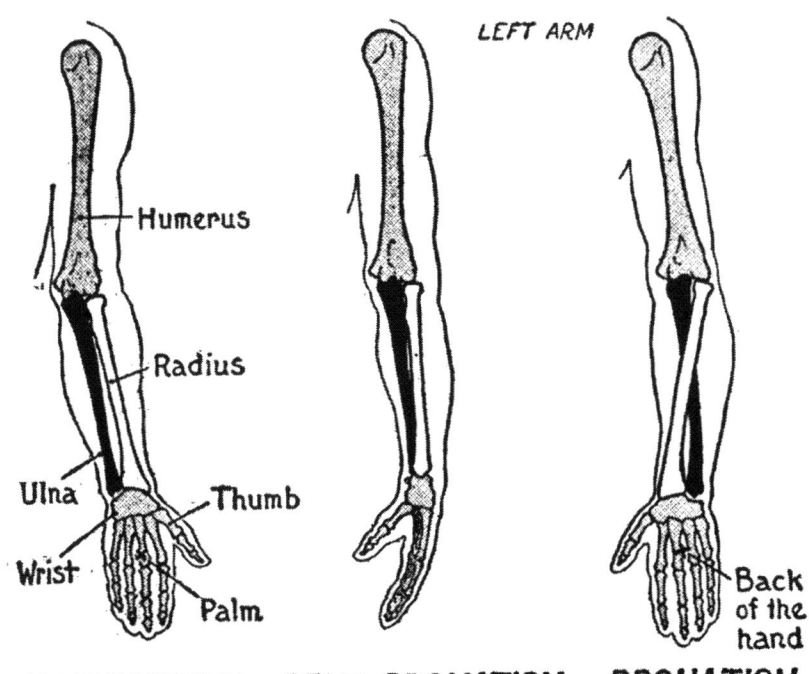

THE ACTION OF THE RADIUS IN THESE MOVEMENTS.

ANATOMY CHARTS 339

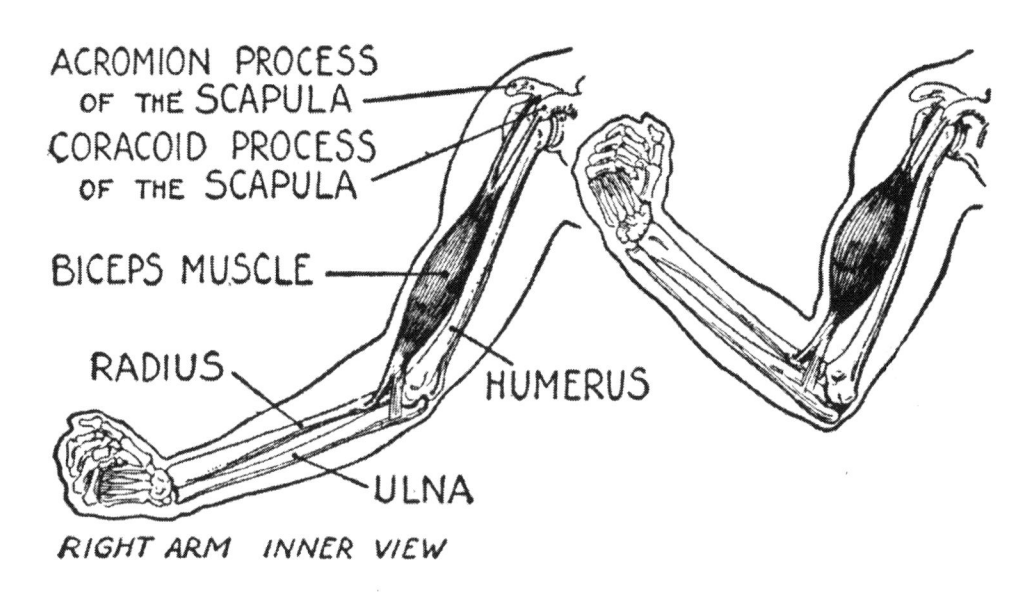

ACROMION PROCESS OF THE SCAPULA
CORACOID PROCESS OF THE SCAPULA
BICEPS MUSCLE
RADIUS
HUMERUS
ULNA
RIGHT ARM INNER VIEW

A MUSCLE IN ACTION.

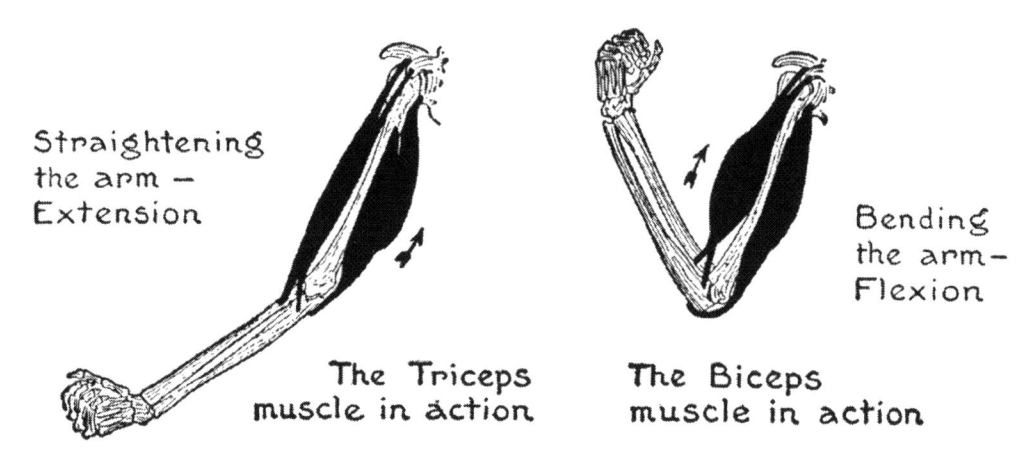

Straightening the arm — Extension

The Triceps muscle in action

Bending the arm — Flexion

The Biceps muscle in action

A PAIR OF ANTAGONISTIC MUSCLES IN ACTION.

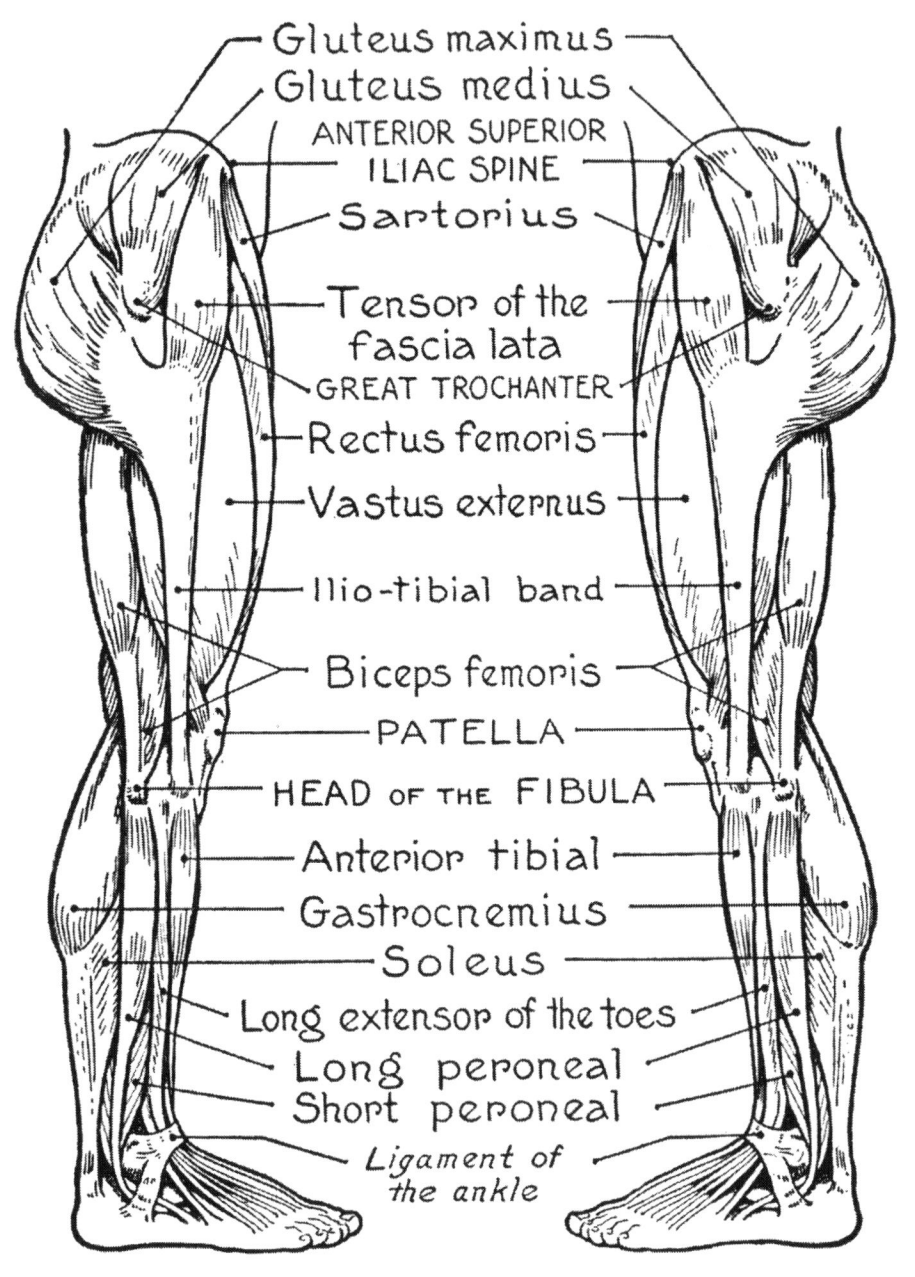

THE MUSCLES OF THE LOWER LIMB.
Outer view.

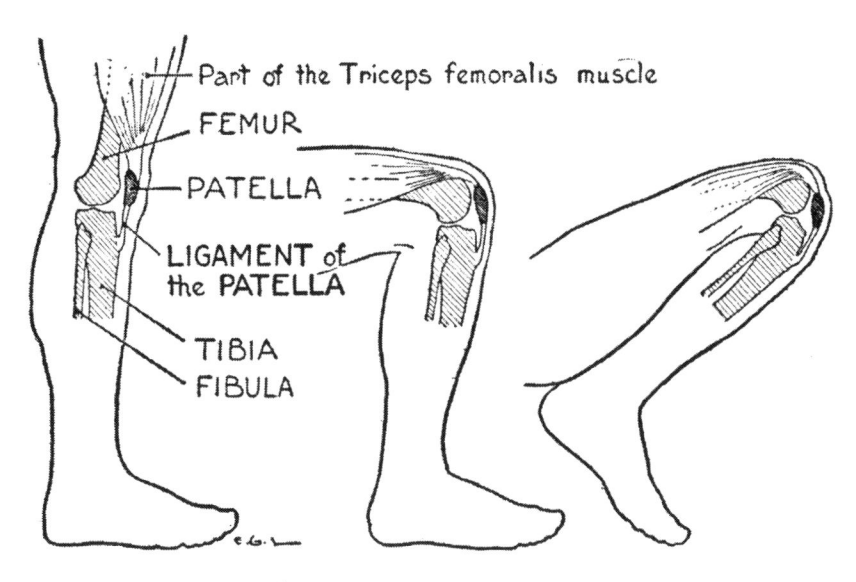

ANATOMY CHARTS 341

- Part of the Triceps femoralis muscle
- FEMUR
- PATELLA
- LIGAMENT of the PATELLA
- TIBIA
- FIBULA

DIAGRAMMATIC REPRESENTATION OF THE MOVEMENT IN THE KNEE-JOINT.

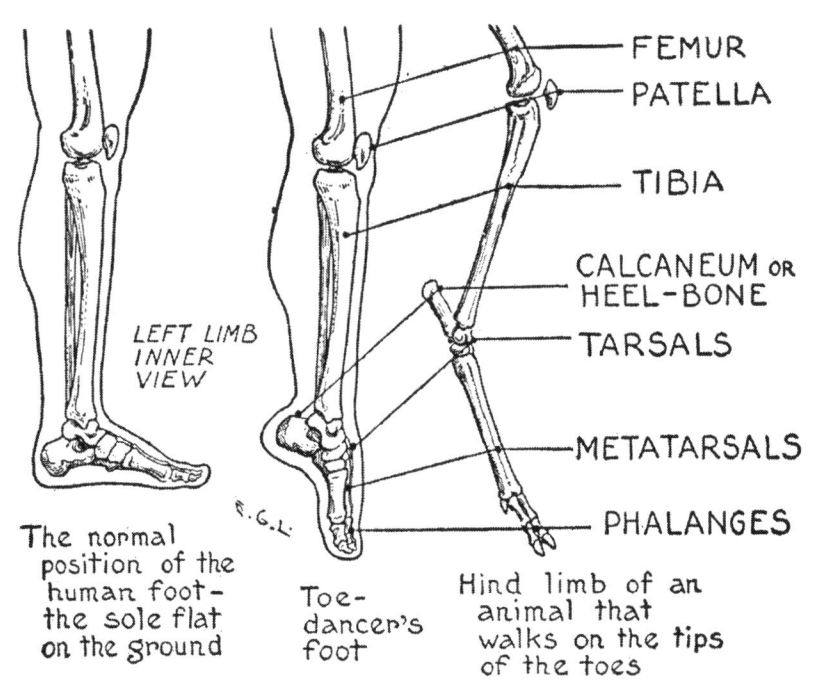

- FEMUR
- PATELLA
- TIBIA
- CALCANEUM OR HEEL-BONE
- TARSALS
- METATARSALS
- PHALANGES

LEFT LIMB INNER VIEW

The normal position of the human foot — the sole flat on the ground

Toe-dancer's foot

Hind limb of an animal that walks on the tips of the toes

THE POINTS IN COMMON IN THE SKELETAL STRUCTURE OF THE LEG AND FOOT OF A BALLET-DANCER, AND IN THAT OF THE HIND LIMB OF AN ANIMAL THAT PROGRESSES ON THE TIPS OF THE TOES.

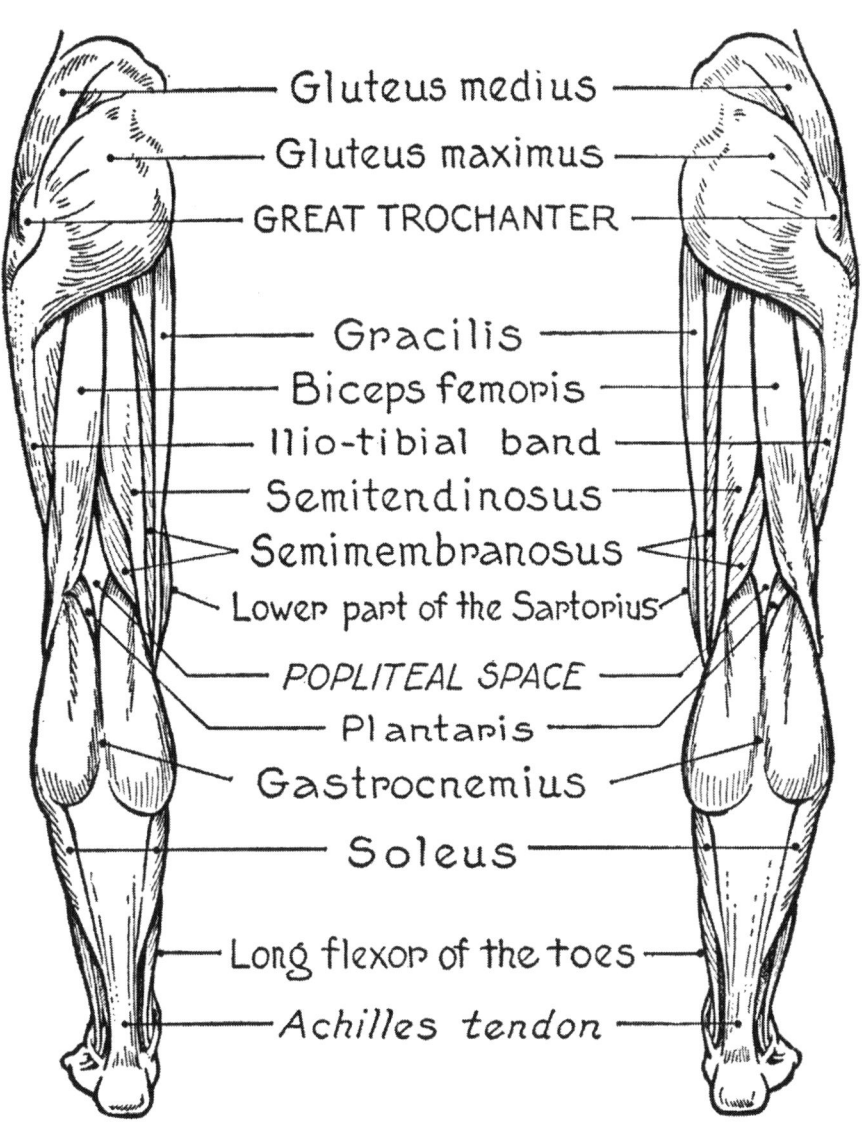

THE MUSCLES OF THE LOWER LIMB.
Posterior view.

CHAPTER TWENTY TWO

Glossary

Aerobic Exercise: Aerobic Exercise involves moderate activity that utilises oxygen-using, or oxidative, pathways to supply energy or muscular contractions. A persons capacity for aerobic exercise is limited by his or her cardiovascular conditioning.

Anaerobic Exercise: This term relates to muscular exercise or fitness activities in which speed, power, etc, are not limited by cardiovascular conditioning as the energy derives largely from non oxygen-utilising pathways to achieve muscular contractions.

Barbell: A sort of long dumbbell which is grasped in both hands and used for bodily exercises.

Crucifix: Old-time exercise in which the athlete holds two weights first overhead before slowly lowering them to an outstretched position at the side of the body (held for a time) - this can also be done with a set of rings.

Definition: Vernacular bodybuilding term used to describe and indicate how clearly visible or defined a persons muscles are.

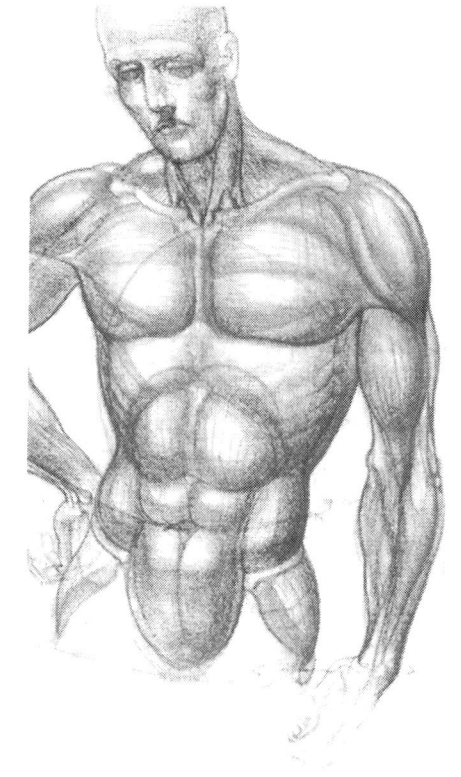

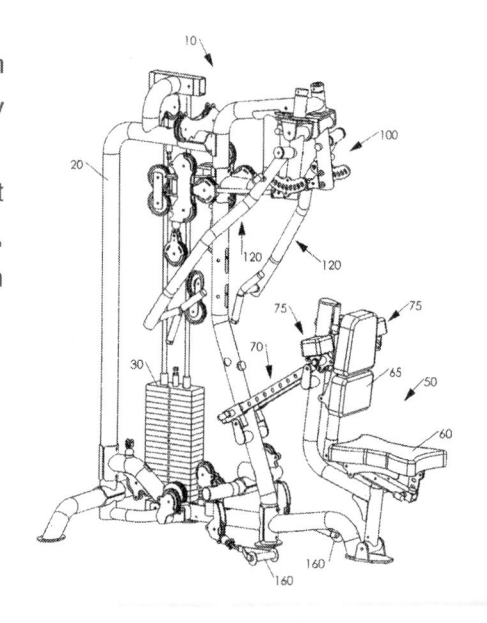

Dumbbell: Weight that is short and compact enough to be held with one arm at a time, usually of 2 different kinds, solid ones with globular or other shaped weights on either end; and disc or plate loading ones that can be adjusted in weight.

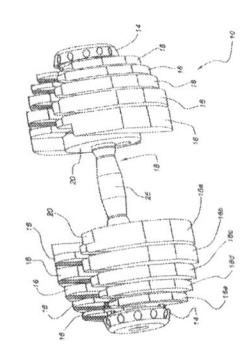

Extensor: Muscle used to extend a limb or part of the body into its fully extended position, for example the knee extensor muscles which move the lower leg up to the straight position.

Flex and Flexor: Contraction of a muscle, for example, flexing your biceps, Muscle used to move a limb or part of the body back towards its fully bent position, for example, the leg biceps muscles are used to move the lower leg into the fully contracted position.

Gymnasium: From the Greek meaning educational centre for mind and body.

Kettle-Bell: Like a dumbbell except the handle is located somewhat above the weights centre of gravity position; used for shoulder and back exercises.

Muscle: Fibrous tissue covering the skeleton and employed to effect movement of the various levers of the body. Comes in two kinds, those under voluntary control and those that move in response to survival responses like the heart etc.

Olympic Bar: Type of revolving sleeve barbell used in the Olympic Games, which is 7 feet long and takes plates with a 2 inch hole.

Repetitions: The number of times a lift is performed.

Sets: Term used to indicate the number of cycles of an individual exercise; for example 3 sets of 10 repetitions.

Steroids: Tissue-building drugs first used in the 1950s to build the muscles of the body to an unnatural size. Most definitely associated with health risks including cancer, heart attacks and early death.

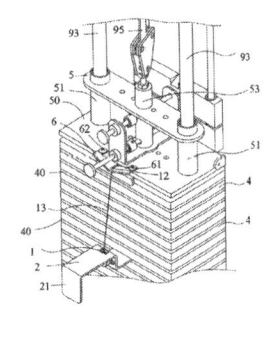

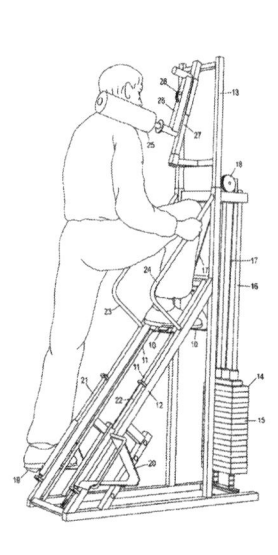

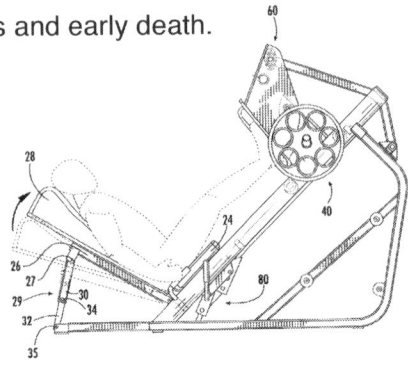

CHAPTER TWENTY THREE

Dangers of Machines

TODAY MOST resistance training performed world-wide is on machines. My own views on machine training should be clear at this point. In fact I feel so strongly about the dangers of training with machines that I have decided to include this section on safety with respect to their use.

It is commonly believed that gymnasium machines are intrinsically safer than free weights, and require less skill in using them. These are false beliefs however. The ability to use a machine properly depends on an adequate knowledge of the merits, deficiencies and principles underlying the design and proper use of the same. One also needs to know the similarities and differences between a machine exercise and the equivalent free-weights exercise.

In particular, when using a machine, we need to pay close attention to which muscles act as prime movers and which work as stabilisers at all stages of the movement. Good machines are: cable, rowing (concept) and seated cycles (some).

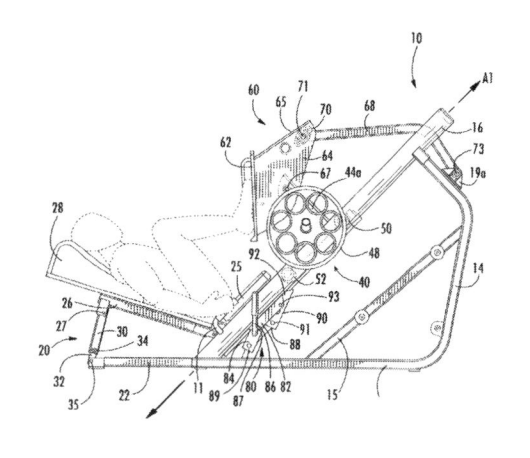

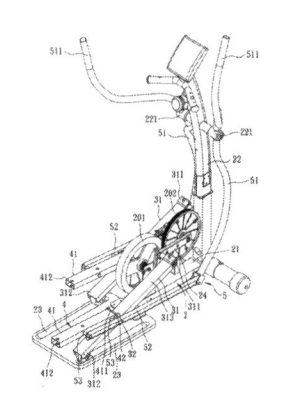

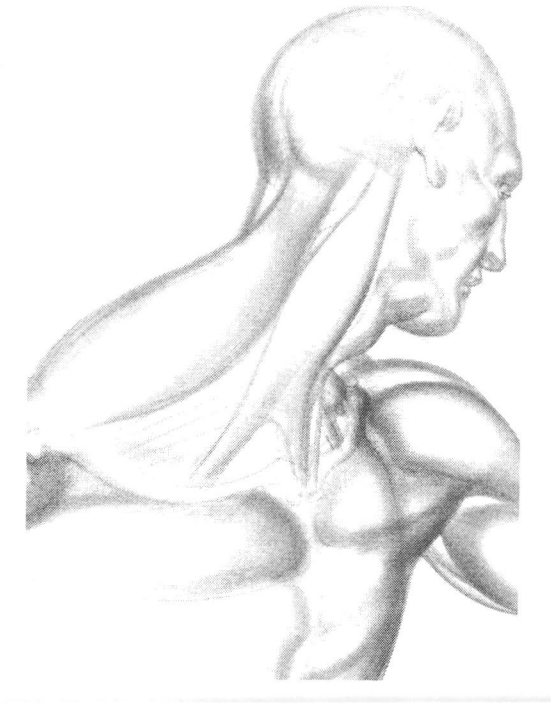

Bad and unsafe machine exercises:

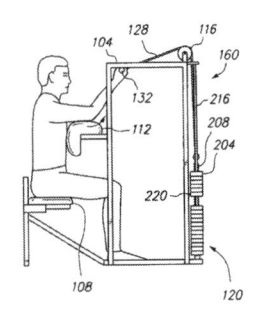

- Seated vertical pressing machines often force you to round the back, lean forward and hyperextend the lumber region. More stress is placed on the lumber region overall than with the free weight alternatives according to scientific studies!

- Seated pressing machines often have foot-rests situated in unnatural positions; making it difficult to use your hips and/or to stabilise/arch the back (lower).

- Seated leg-press machines provide backrests which do not match the natural curvature of the back, hence promoting lumber flexion which is dangerous with maximum loads.

- Lying / incline leg press machines allow you to bend your knees until they hit the abdomen thus forcing lumber flexion. Prone leg curl machines force the lumber into hyper-flexion due to the shape of the flat/angled surface.

- Hack squat machines can impose excessive shearing on the knee. Plus they tend to flatten the lower spine.

- All bench press machines force you to start the movement from the weakest bio-mechanical position.

- Calf-machines often force you to flex the spine, particularly with heavy loads.

- Seated back extension machines force you to start with a flexed lumber spine and end with loaded hyperextension.

- Seated lumber twist machines often allow you to flex the lumber spine whilst rotating and can cause ballistic type injuries. VERY DANGEROUS. NEVER USE!

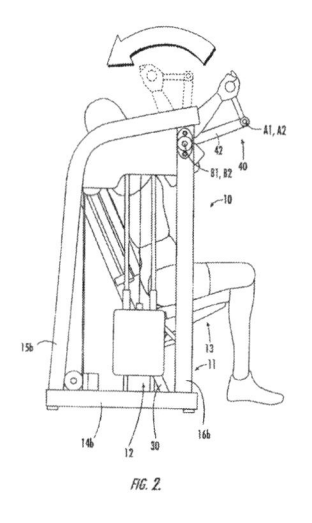

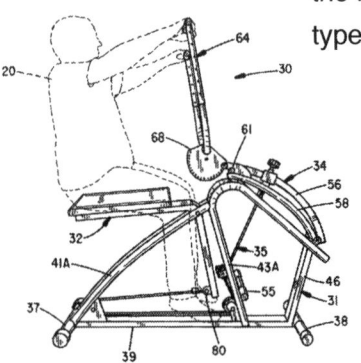

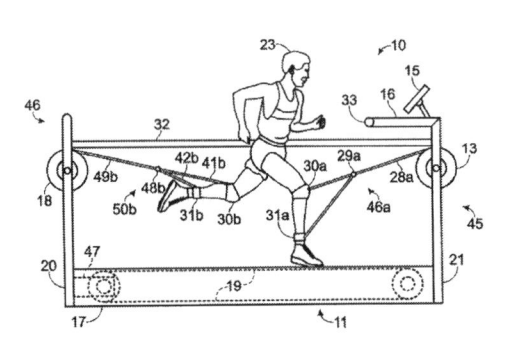

- Many abdominal machines force the abdominal and hip flexors to work in an unnatural "separated" manner.

- Standing hip adduction/abduction machines require you to push and pull the straightened leg against a loaded lever arm and can permit excessive simultaneous spinal rotation and/or flexion/extension of spine to occur.

- Many pullover machines force the lumber spine into hyperextension if used in the wrong fashion.

- "Smith" vertical press machines impose a larger load on the spine, shoulders and wrists than pressing with weights.

- Most hyperextension machines increase the stress on the hamstrings and soft tissues of the knee.

- Any machine that requires you to sit prevents you from using your hip, knee and ankle joints to absorb shock and/or redistribute loading. The posture of neutral pelvic tilt becomes far more difficult to maintain throughout the exercise and spinal hyperextension or hyper-flexion occurs more easily and spinal stress becomes far more likely. Poorly designed (and even well-designed) machines often impose large loads and/or unpredictable patterns of resistance on the body.

- Numerous machines force you to start and/or to perform the exercise with limbs in a bio-mechanically weak or vulnerable position, increasing likelihood of injury.

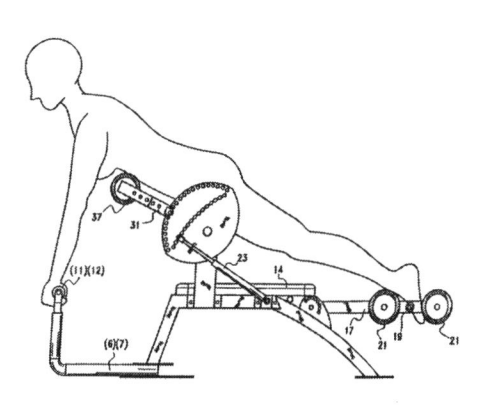

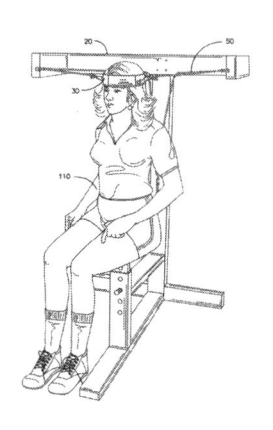

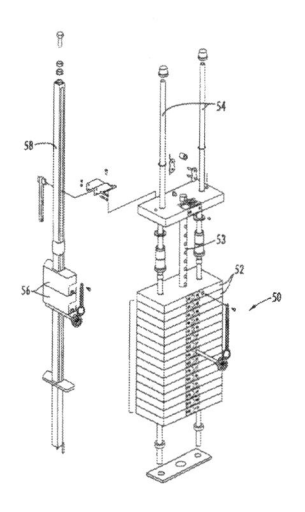

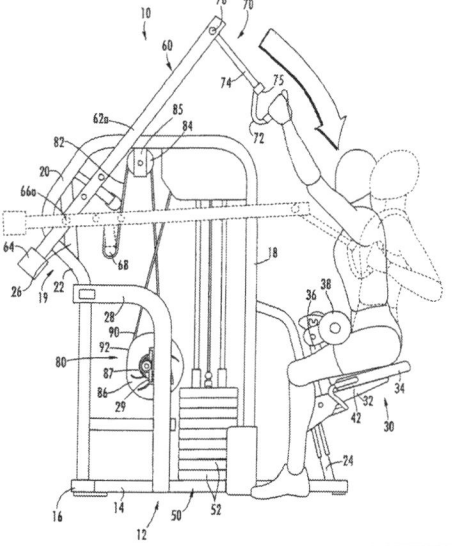

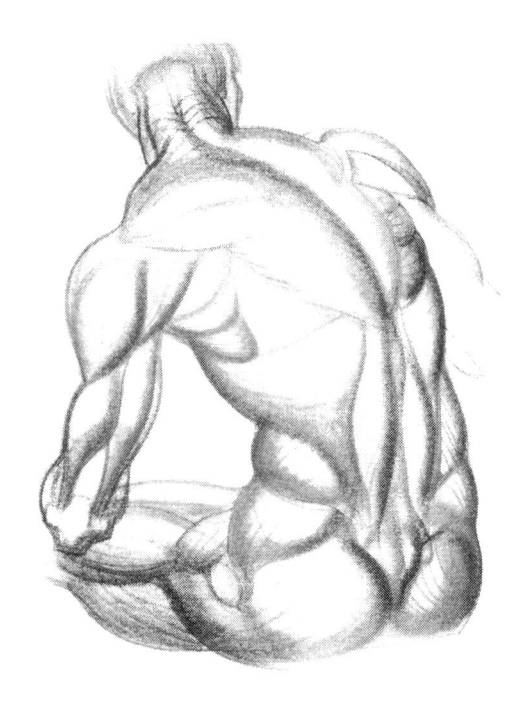

CHAPTER TWENTY FOUR

Exercises to Avoid

IN ALL fields there is disagreement, and we observe that fundamental theories sometimes contradict one another. Even so-called scientific "experts" fall-out over indisputable matters of "fact". The field of weight-training is no different in this respect, and opinions are many and varied. I can offer no solutions in this respect.

I am afraid that all I can do is to present my own views as expressed in the words and images of this book. Perhaps (in terms of fitness training) all any of us can offer is to present our beliefs, and in terms of what we have discovered to be true, and what has worked for us. Having said that, I have spent much of my life learning about the field of strength/fitness training, and I have attempted to present here a balanced and educated perspective.

Especially controversial is the question of which exercises to employ, and which (if any) to avoid due to danger (safety), poor effectiveness and/or lack of "fit" to the individual. It is my belief that certain exercises are to be avoided (generally) and I list the same here, complete with my reasons for such categorisation.

- **Barbell/Dumbbell Lunges:** (in place or "walking forward): this is a very dangerous exercise for several reasons. Firstly it places excessive (and unnecessary)

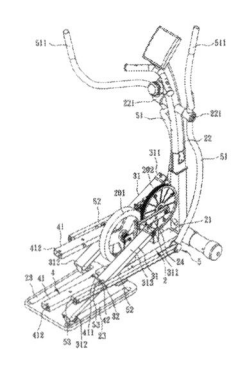

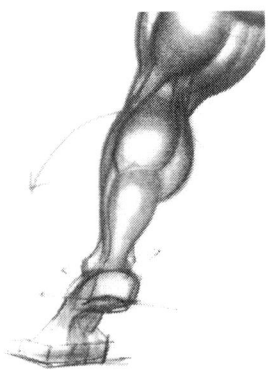

Avoid all exercises where the body is held in a "fixed" or braced position; and which then requires you to lift heavy weights without being able to maintain a natural lumbar arch, and/or where you are unable to adjust the position of the hips, legs, torso and back (during the lift) relative to the direction of gravity (or direction of the resistance) and in order to position/balance the resistance correctly with respect to the body. Stick mostly to standing exercises.

stress (pressure) on the knee joint and related structures. Secondly it is quite difficult to maintain form, and if you do loose balance and fall, slip or twist at the foot or knee then you could very well have a nasty accident. AVOID!

• **Press Behind the Neck**: During the behind the neck barbell press, the tendon of one of these muscles, the supraspinatus, can be rubbed and compressed between the head of the humerus and the surrounding articular features. This leads to inflammation and pain and, if not treated, can lead to permanent damage of the tendon resulting in the inability to lift your arm overhead. The general motion of the shoulder during this exercise, extreme external rotation and abduction, can also increase the shoulder's already unstable nature and result in damage to the joint capsule as well as torn muscles, ligaments or tendons. The neck is also at risk during the behind the neck barbell press. With each repetition you have to flex your neck forward in order to avoid hitting the back of your head with the barbell. This movement can lead to strained muscles in the neck, and especially if you're working with heavy weights. AVOID!

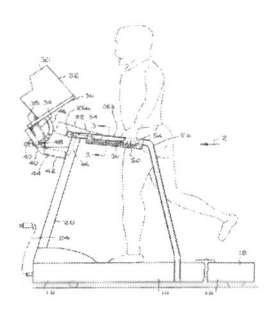

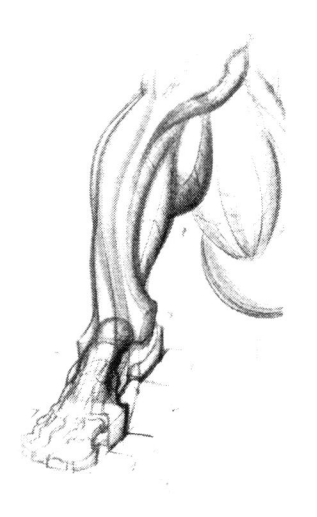

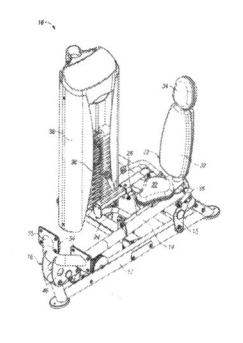

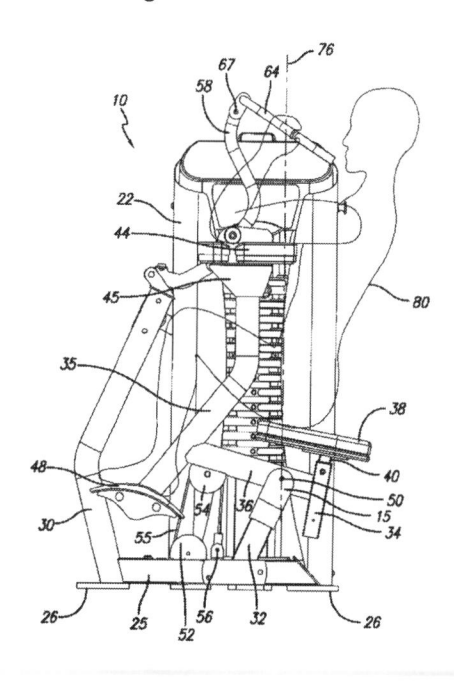

• **StairMaster / Elliptical Machines**: Many people on the StairMaster are slumped over the machine, with bodies that hang sluggishly over handlebars, programming boards and any other part of the cardio machine that will hold their weight. If you can't fully support yourself during the workout, then you're not doing the work or getting the benefit of the "program" you've selected. There may be safe way to use a StairMaster - but you will probably be better off (and safer) going for a walk outside and up a hill! And ellipticals, although apparently scientific, do force the body into entirely unnatural positions, and provide an even more unnatural movement pattern. Surely people do not really think that such machines are a good substitute for running or walking. It is my belief that the unnatural movement actions of all these kinds of "walking-substitute" machines can and will cause injury with continued use over time. AVOID!

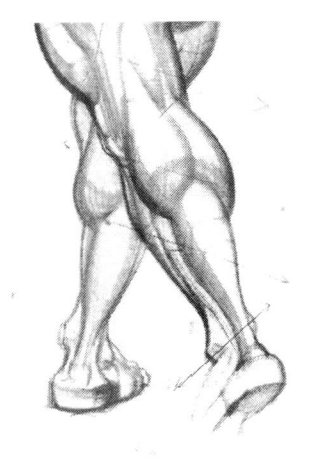

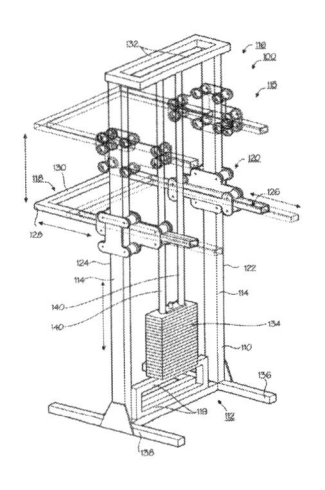

- **Early Morning Stretches**: Back injury/performance experts now state that we should never perform stretches for the spine early in the morning and immediately after getting out of bed. This is because the back is vulnerable until you have been awake and walking about for at least half an hour. The reason is that overnight the vertebral discs loose water (height and cushioning) and become susceptible to injury until we have stood up and allowed them to "puff-up" once-more due to a natural response to the stress of gravity. AVOID UPON RISING!

- **Broom Twists & Fast Twisting Motions:** Ever see those people doing fast and crazy whipping side-to-side motions with a broom handle across the back of their necks? Ouch. When done properly (slowly), twists may have good benefits for flexibility, but don't do them at great speed whereby you get a "ballistic" bounce at the far end of the movement. AVOID!

- **Unnatural Joint Movement(s):** Whilst I do believe that Yoga is a very good form of exercise, I also think that some of the extreme body positions can be dangerous for certain people to perform. Especially dangerous is the Plough (or similar neck pressure moves) posture whereby extreme stress is placed on the neck region. Such a movement may be extremely dangerous for heavier individuals, and I myself injured my neck with this move. You should use common sense when it comes to demanding Yoga postures and only perform postures that seem natural for yourself.

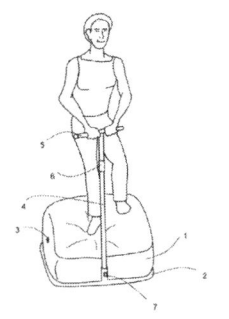

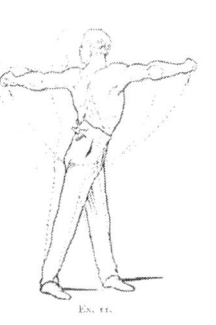

- **Behind Neck Presses / Lat Pulldowns / Pull-up:** Only people with extremely flexible shoulder joints can do any behind-the-head movement safely, and even they have to be very careful about not hitting the back of their necks with the bar. Never perform. AVOID!

• **Seated Leg Extension(machine):** This is a very popular exercise for targeting the muscles on the front of your thighs (quadriceps). **The Problem?** This exercise poses major risks to the knees. Lifting heavy weights in this position (with all of the resistance focused at your ankles), is not what the knee was designed to do. AVOID!

• **Inner and Outer Thigh Machine Exercises:** Both involve sitting with your knees bent in front of you. The adduction machine is designed to target the muscles of the inner thighs, and the abduction machine helps target the outer thigh muscles. **The Problem?** Using your inner and outer thighs to lift weight while in a seated position puts you at risk of straining these relatively small muscles and aggravating lower back and hip problems. In addition, your inner and outer thigh muscles are designed to support movement, not to be prime movers like they are in these types of exercises.

• **Easy-Bar Curls**: Places your hands in a semi-supinated position which is not so good either for stretching the biceps at the bottom or fully contracting the biceps at the top. However easy bar curls with the hands reversed (over-hand grip) are a good exercise for the brachialis and brachioradialis muscles of the forearm (preacher or standing).

• **Seated Shoulder Presses / Curls**: In general it is better to avoid all seated presses and curls because they place the back in a potentially weak and unnatural position. Exceptions are incline dumbbell presses and incline dumbbell curs which are both excellent.

• **Smith Machine:** Almost any exercise on a smith machine is performed in a very unnatural manner; largely because your back may be in an unnatural (loaded) position, and also your joints are forced to follow an unnatural movement arc. AVOID!

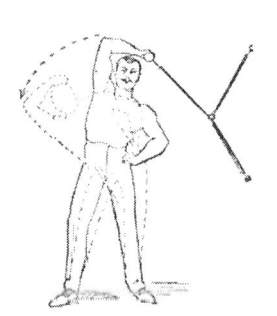

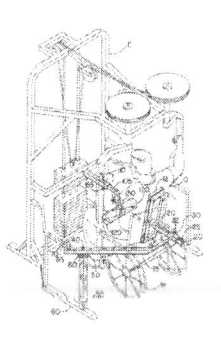

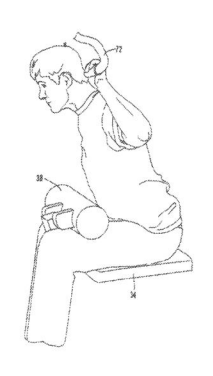

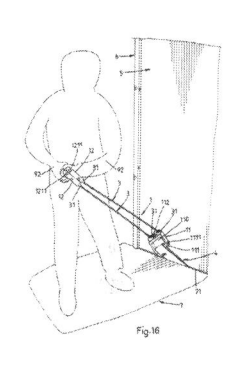

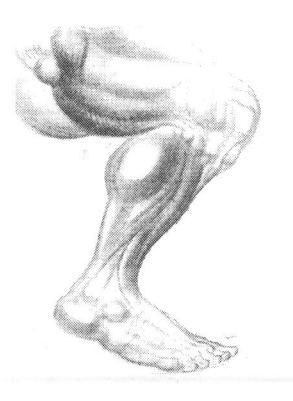

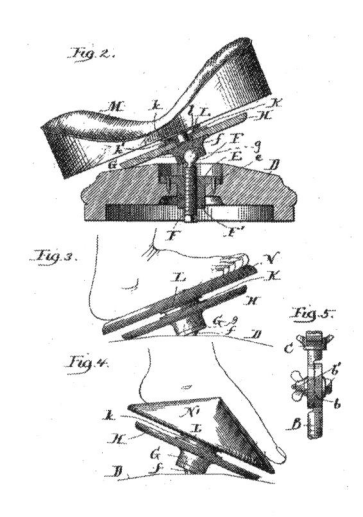

- **Upright Row:** There is much controversy currently in relation to this movement. Some say it is a good, effective exercise, whilst others claim it to be very unsafe. When people pull their hands (carrying weight) up to their chin, they may compress the nerves in the shoulder area, impinging the shoulder (dumbbells preferred). Make up your own mind. I think high pulls make a good substitute.
- **Balance Boards / Wobble Boards:** It is difficult to adequately describe the lunacy of such methods - and especially when wobble-boards are used in combination with weights. You force the spine to work in a wholly unnatural way, without a solid base, often ballistically and over fast/time-varying and gross/unpredictable ROMs. Trendy fitness gurus may tell you that lifting weights on a "wobble-board" is somehow good for the "core muscles", but in fact you could damage your spine permanently by such a practice. These crazy methods are in fact not new, and W.Masden in 1892 obtained a Patent on a wobble board (left). However this idea never took off - and for good reasons - it is dangerous and effectively useless.

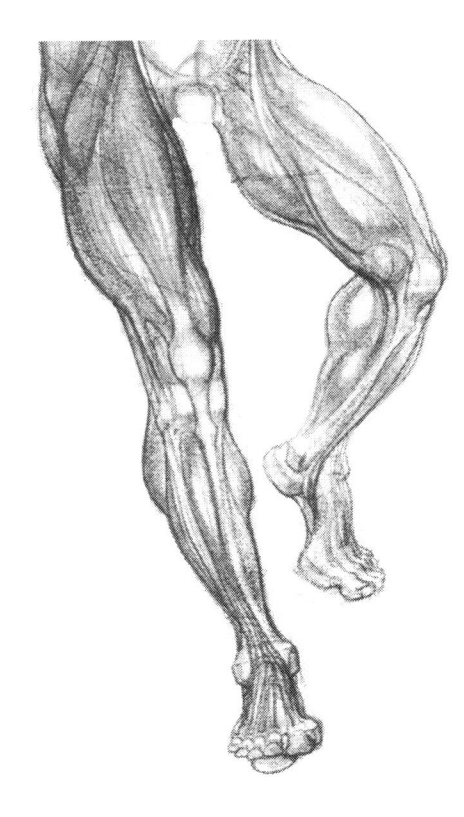

In conclusion, whilst some exercises may be bad for human beings in general, you will have to decide for yourself (or else discover) which exercises are safe and effective to perform in your own case. Do the research yourself. Also my advice is to use common sense, and if a movement looks dangerous or else unnatural, then avoid it. Avoid overly complex moves whilst holding weights. When evaluating any exercise - ask yourself - would our ancestors have moved in such a way during their normal day-to-day activities?

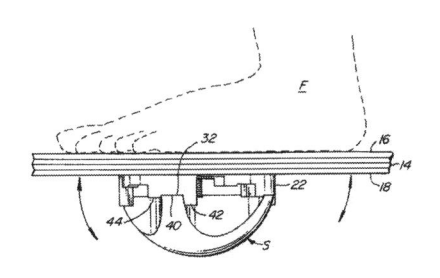

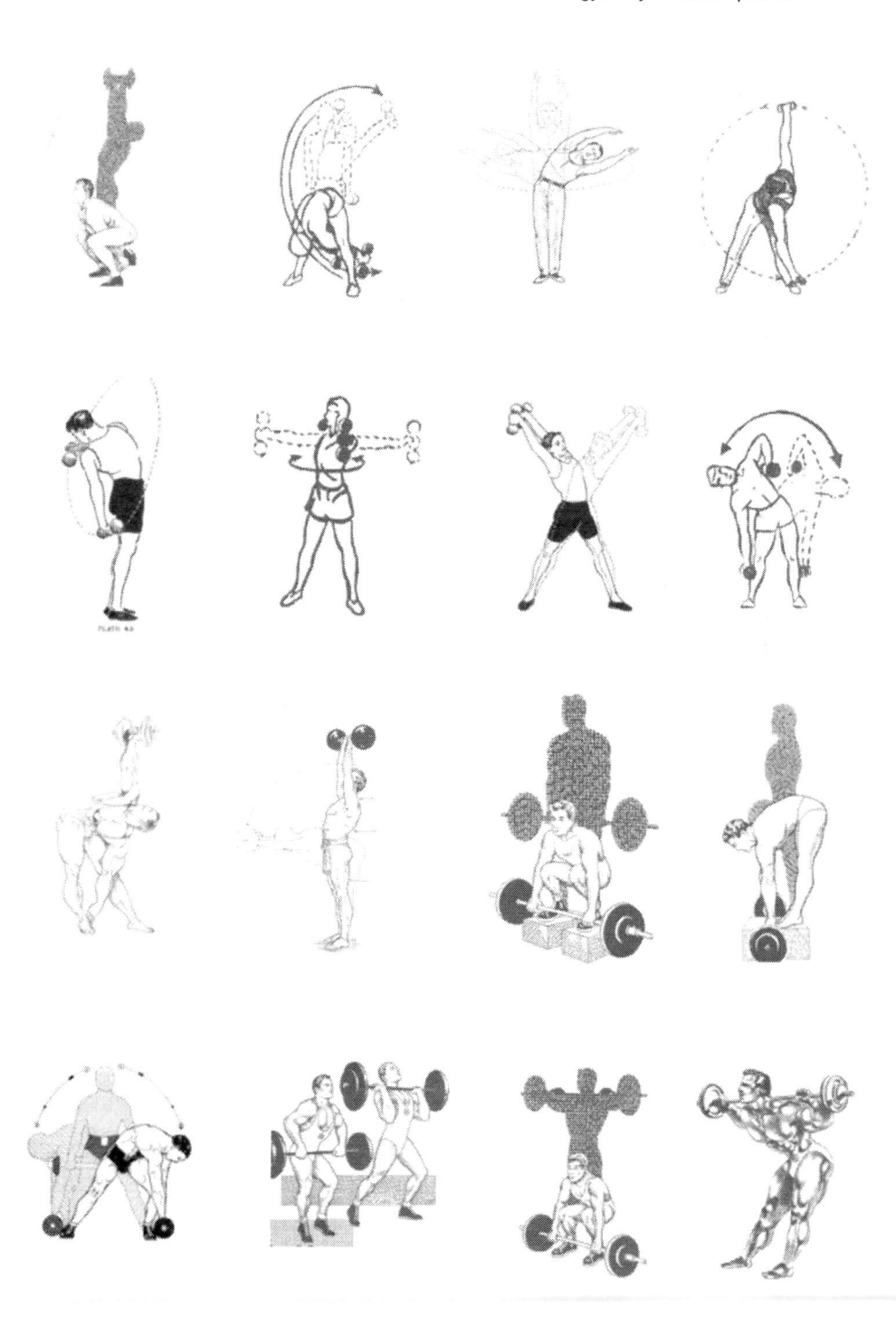

CHAPTER TWENTY FIVE

Exercise Charts

These charts depict 55 exercises from the fitness programs in this book. I suggest that you photograph the charts and carry them to the gym in your mobile phone.

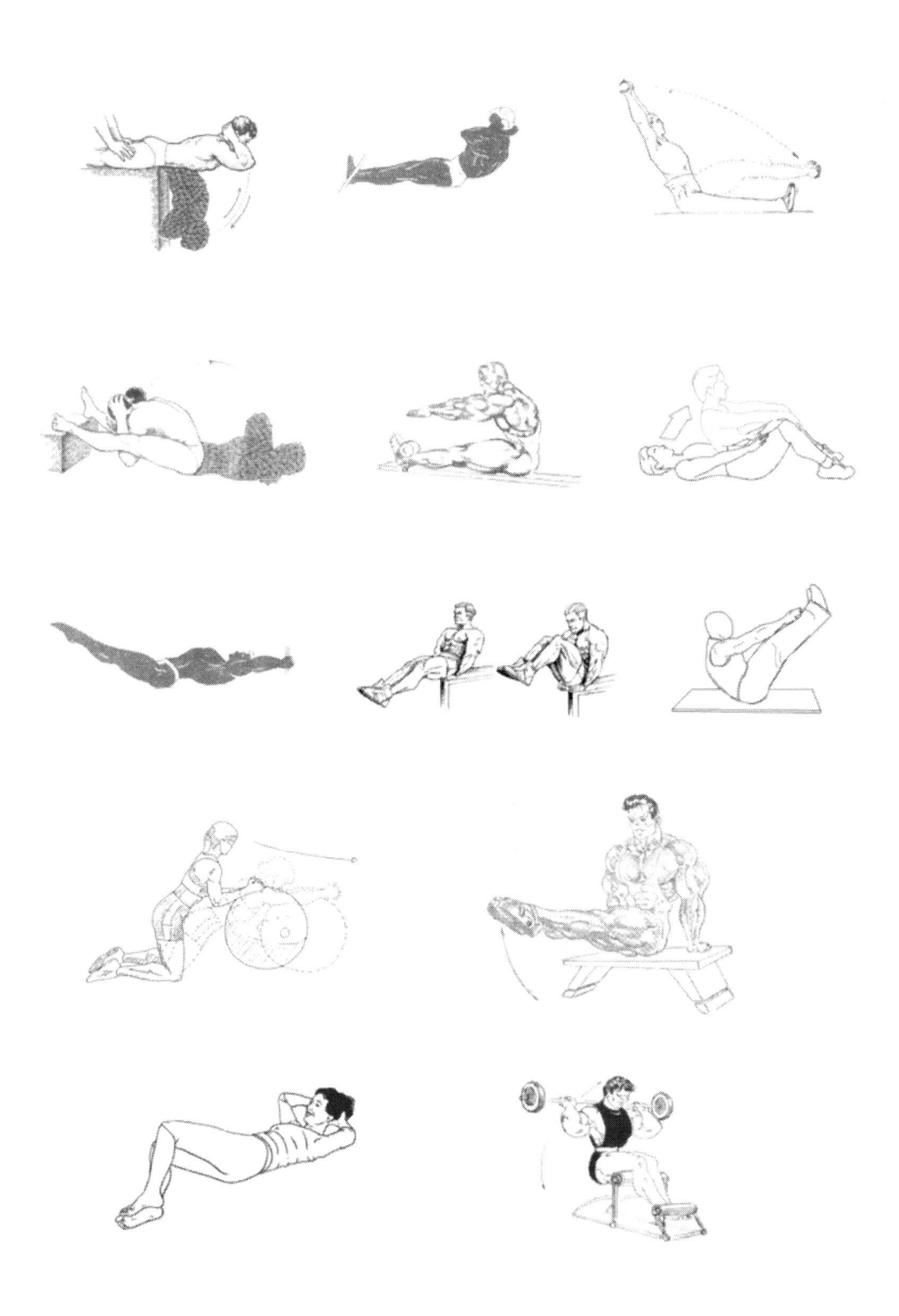

EXERCISE CHARTS 355

**6.
TRICEPS
CIRCLES**

SHOULDER CIRCLES

The Crucifix (left Turn) (arms lowered to shoulder level, palms upwards), is the second movement for followers of this body-building exercise.

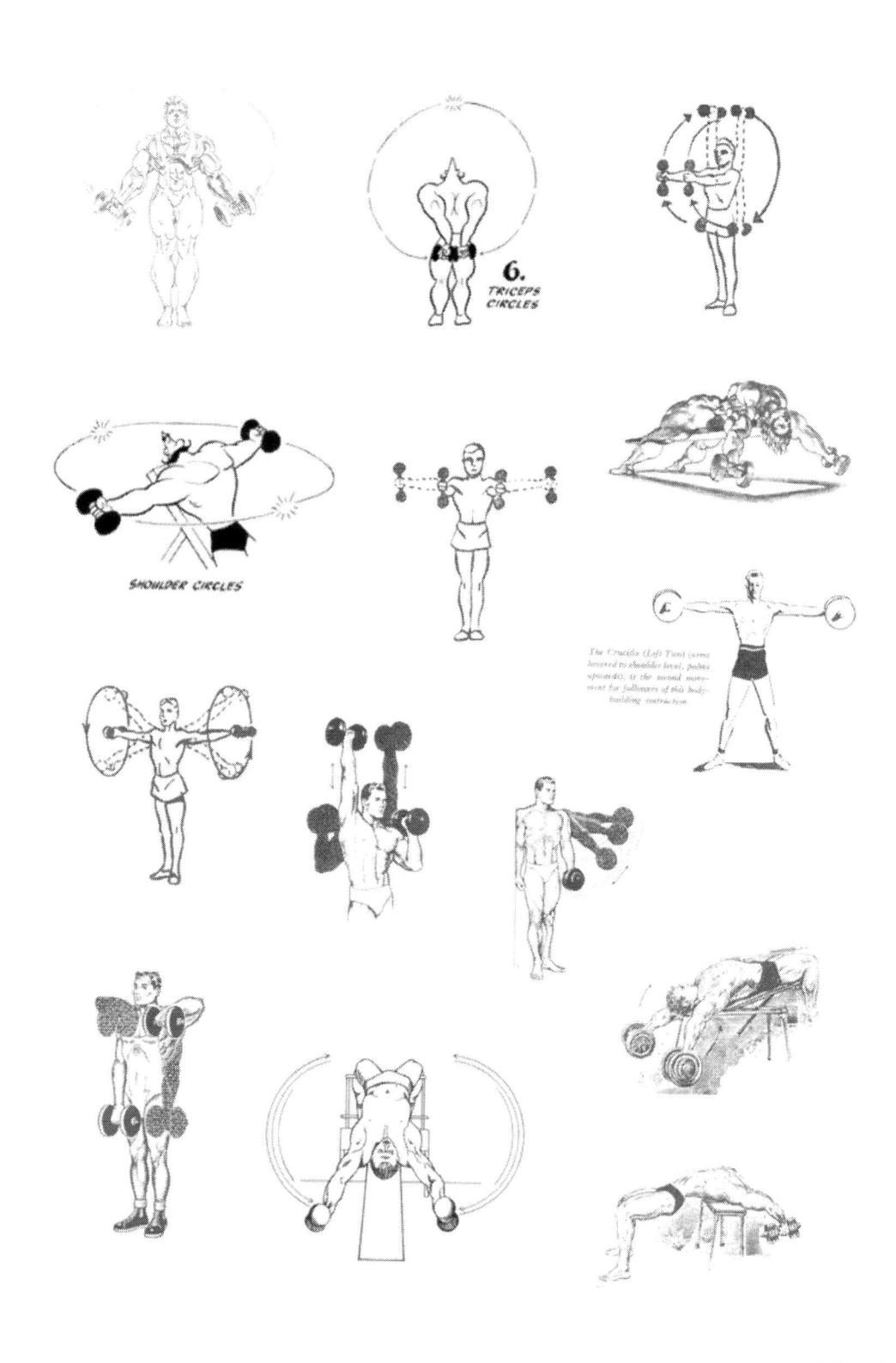

356 ZEN OF DUMBBELL TRAINING

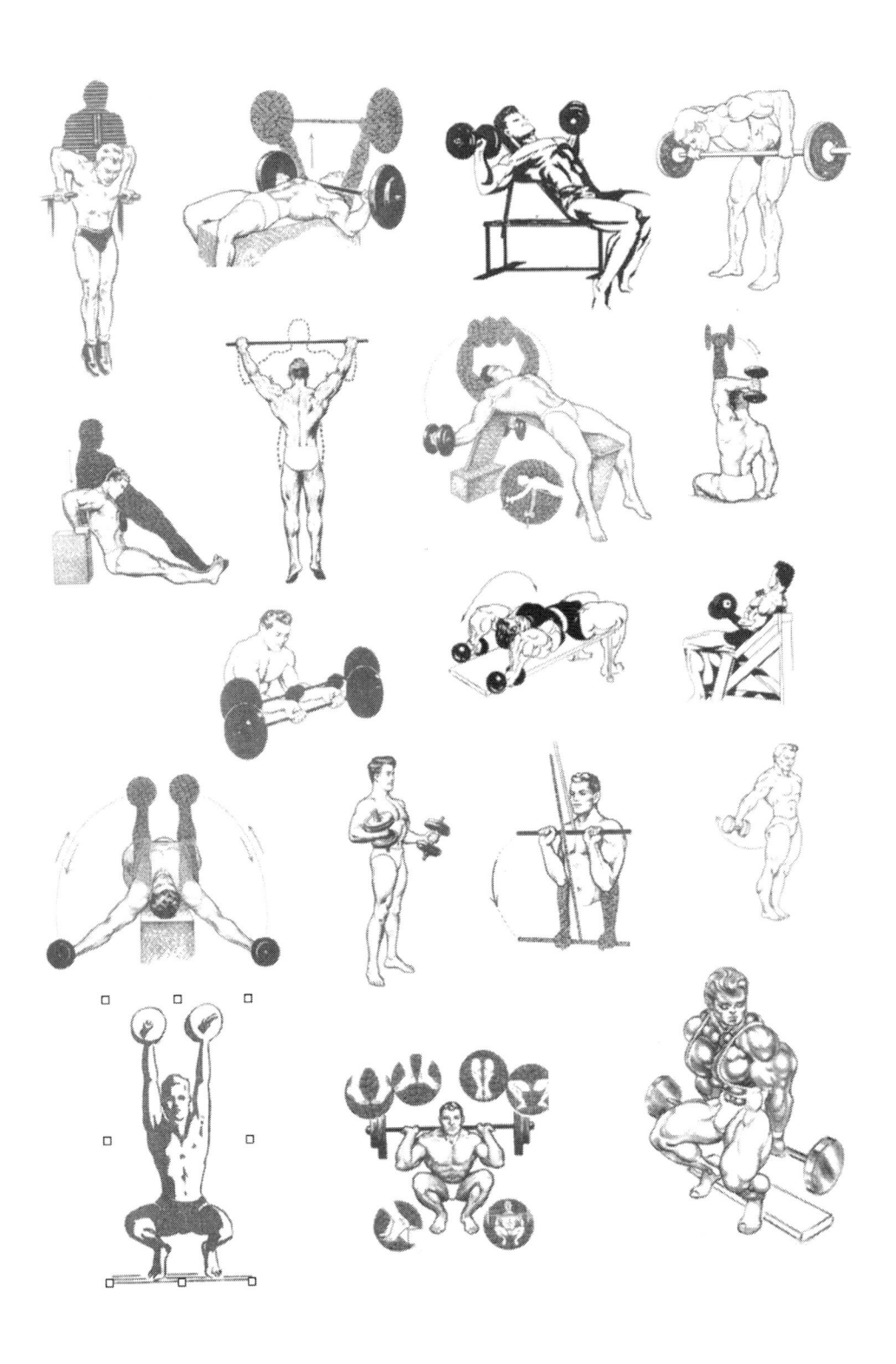

CHAPTER TWENTY SIX

Natural Movement Patterns

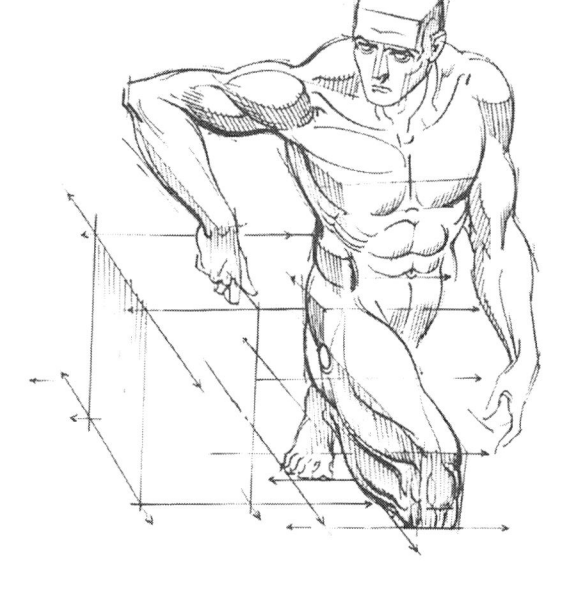

A MAJOR goal of the present book is to put forward the view that the trainee should perform only the most natural movements. That said, the problem becomes identification of useful ways to attain the same. Unfortunately, quite a few modern coaches complicate the issue by using excessive terminology. So much so, in fact, that it seems as if you need a sports science degree to even begin to understand recommended exercise techniques.

In this book we have given "scientific" details largely for reference alone. Our philosophy is that knowledge of human movement anatomy can help the trainee, but that it is not necessary to become an expert on all of the different ways in which the human body can, and does, move. We want you to get the maximum benefits, but with the minimum knowledge. The focus is on obtaining the right (useful) knowledge; as opposed to the pointless remembering of facts.

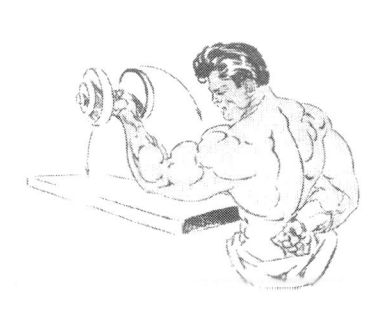

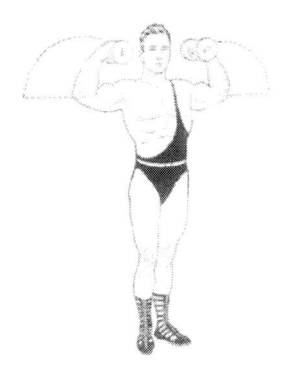

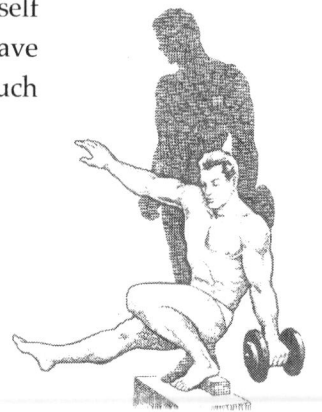

Our discussion has centred on the joints of the human body; and we recommend that you familiarise yourself with the basic ROMs of certain key joints. Largely we have ignored knowledge of musculature, because such knowledge is next to useless in practical terms, and also because whenever we move many muscles are involved. It would be difficult to remember all of these muscles, complex, and entirely unhelpful and/or pointless.

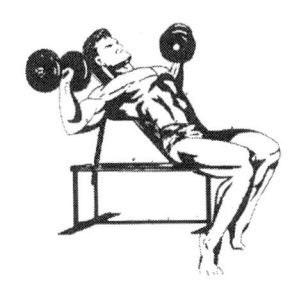

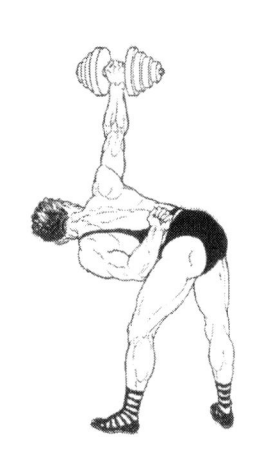

Our approach has placed emphasis on the position and movement of the underlying joints. And in the following paragraphs we shall overview how to employ certain key joints whilst exercising. But do not fall into the trap of believing that the mind always knows best, and that you should completely override your natural instincts whilst exercising. Our philosophy of Zen Training is that we must listen to the body whilst moving (in real-time); and follow it's instruction above all else. In particular we must ignore "scientific" advice when it conflicts with our personal experience. Listening to both mind and body is key.

And the listening relates to all aspects of dumbbell practice. Start with ambiance/mood of the place where you practice, and do not go to gyms where they play loud music, or have annoying types of people walking about. I would rather get myself some dumbbells and lift at home. Think of exercise as a type of yoga practice; and so it should be performed silently (you can use loud rock music if you like, once you become an expert). Also take great care over what you wear whilst exercising, the space you move in and also give yourself plenty of time. Move slowly and with complete concentration.

Choose the right weights for each movement, because this is the second most important choice you make - after the choice of which specific exercises to perform.

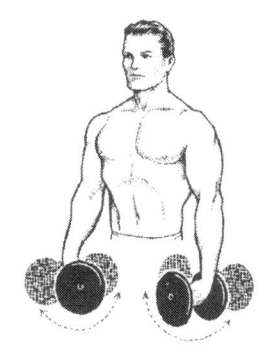

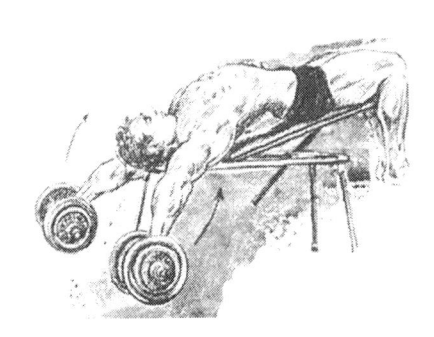

I recommend having a complete set of lighter dumbbells at home for ROM movements; say 1,2,3,4,5,6,7,8,9,10 kg pairs. Plus have a set of heavier dumbbells (with bigger increments between each), or get yourself a high-quality set of adjustable dumbbells (see IronMind in the USA).

I think that it is best to exercise at home and alone. Partners always bring another (unnecessary) opinion; and/or they provide an annoying distraction (they cannot help it). Use a coach if you must, but find one who really knows what he/she is talking about, and choose one who understands that you must find your own path, and so they must not be too "bossy".

Finally, I do believe that if you exercise according to the general recommendations given here, including choosing the right exercises and not going too heavy etc; that your own body will (over time) teach you everything that you need to know about how to train with dumbbells.

But you must listen carefully to your inner voice. It is not that you don't need (some) conscious control over exercise movement patterns, or that you do not need to study correct form; but rather that you must not over intellectualise performance with lots of fancy terms and complex thoughts. I recommend picturing (in your head) how each body-part moves whilst you lift. Use of cues can help, including instructions on: body-part position(s) at the movement start/end points, and 3D movement patterns etc.

Listen carefully to what your body tells you, and slightly adjust hand positions, joint engagements etc and pay attention to simple things like head/neck position, eye gaze, foot position, and dumbbell / hand positions etc.

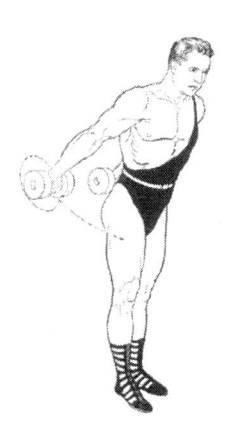

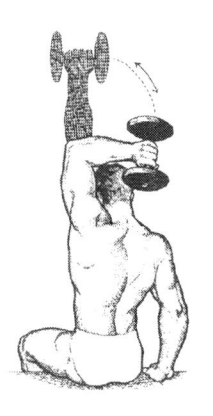

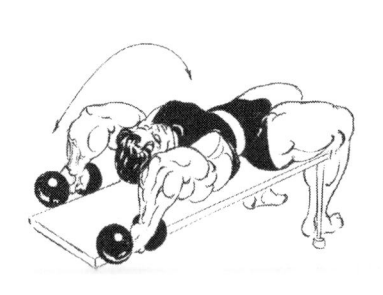

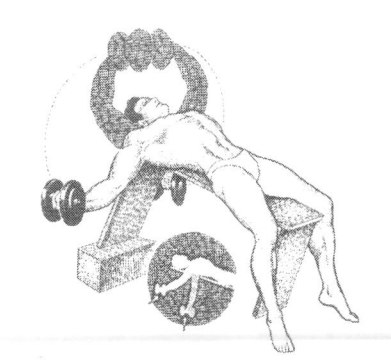

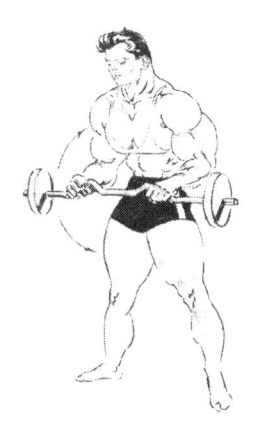

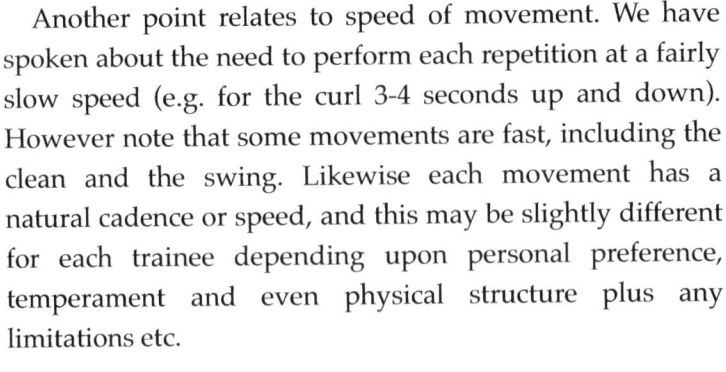

Another point relates to speed of movement. We have spoken about the need to perform each repetition at a fairly slow speed (e.g. for the curl 3-4 seconds up and down). However note that some movements are fast, including the clean and the swing. Likewise each movement has a natural cadence or speed, and this may be slightly different for each trainee depending upon personal preference, temperament and even physical structure plus any limitations etc.

Coaches: do not be mini-Hitlers in relation to your clients, but allow them to develop as they see fit. Correct gross mistakes; but be aware that each person's practice will be to some extent unique. Allow room for creativity and personal preference - always.

In the followings sections we provide *cues* to help you to find the most natural movement patterns on each exercise. (The word cue is defined as anything said or done, on or off stage, that is followed by a specific line or action.)

We do not believe that it is always best (for everyone) to consider these cues whilst exercising, we only say that it may help some people. It is nice to have this information for reference, in any case. Remember coaches, that some people are more visual and they may not like to hear lots of words during/prior to a workout, and in such a case demonstration of exercise form(s) is essential.

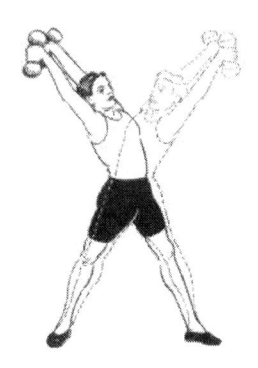

Spine / Hip Position

We spoke at length about the importance of using the correct spine and hip positions in Chapter seven. We shall not repeat that information here.

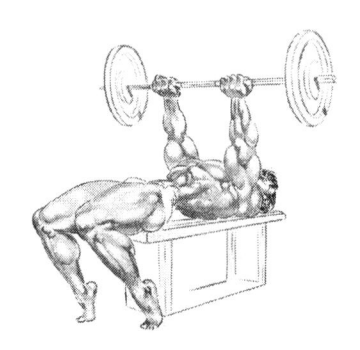

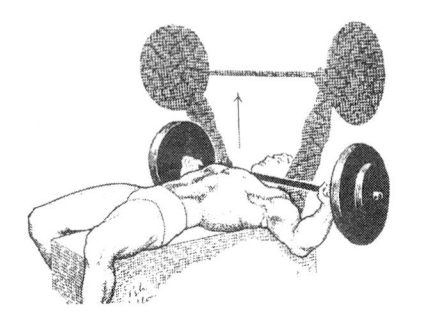

Suffice it to say that all trainees should know (when they bend at the waist); which type of bending they are engaged in: hip or spine, or both. Plus they must know how to set the spine (lower back) into a concave (extended) position prior to lifting heavy weights and in movements such as the squat, dead-lift and overhead press etc.

Trainees do not have to know much theory here - apart from the difference between bending with the hips and bending with the spine and which to use on each exercise. Plus they should be aware of the need to avoid a loaded spine. For example, remember that you do not want to "collapse" the spine when lifting weights at any time. The only exception is when lying down; and on exercises such as the crunch and possibly some abdominal exercises.

Overall, I do not think that anyone has any business lifting weights without such basic knowledge. Coaches: discuss/explain spinal and hip anatomy at length - but only if the trainee is especially interested.

I recommend that all trainees use a neutral spine normally. Neutral spine is good for many exercises, but not all. Obviously squats and dead-lifts (where the trainee fights to maintain lower spine concavity) are an exception. All trainees need to be aware of spine position, and to emphasise lumbar arch, on heavy standing moves such as squats, dead-lifts, cleans, rows and overhead presses etc.

Remember that nobody gets a movement pattern right first/every time, and constant practice is required to "evolve" and also to maintain correct form on any exercise. Remember also that everyone has a different physical structure, thus each of us will move differently from others when performing any specific lift.

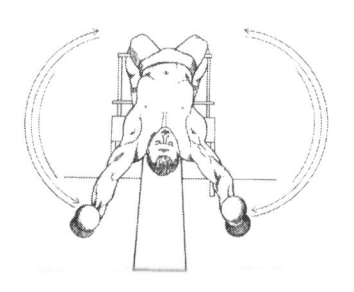

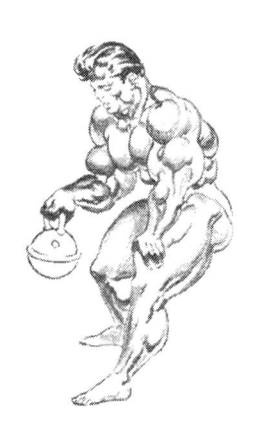

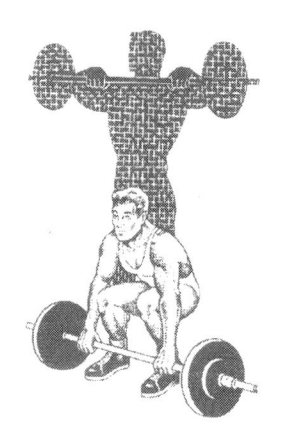

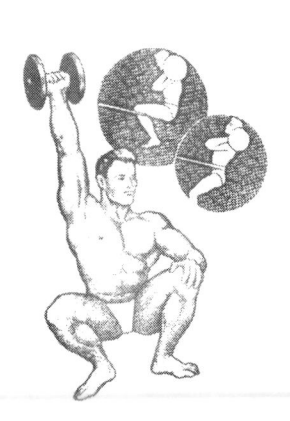

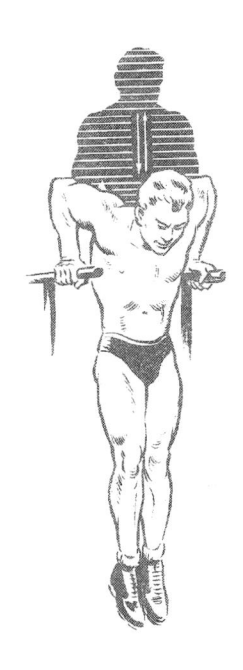

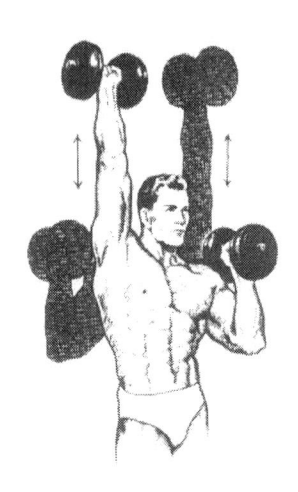

Scapula Position

Many personal trainers give clients cues on how to move the shoulder blades during back and chest strengthening exercises. Here in our exercise descriptions we have given scapula position for each and every exercise. We have done so because we think that setting the shoulder position is just as important as spinal position on many exercises. When both areas are correctly set, it becomes difficult to do any exercise incorrectly.

I know that consideration of scapula position sounds complex, and it is - to some extent. But here I have not crowded the reader's mind with useless descriptions of muscular actions, for example. Rather we have left "space in your head" for specific "cues", being spine/hip and scapula position, and because these are the key to effective movements of almost any kind.

Generally speaking, your shoulder blades should be allowed to move "naturally" during pushing and pulling exercises. Natural movement means the scapulae are moving in a smooth and controlled manner into retraction (on specific exercises). It is my belief that efficient scapula movements will naturally happen, given sufficient practice on any given movement.

However people with movement disfunction's or else unusual moving patterns may need coaching on how to optimise scapula movements. Plus it is nice to set beginners on the right path in this respect.

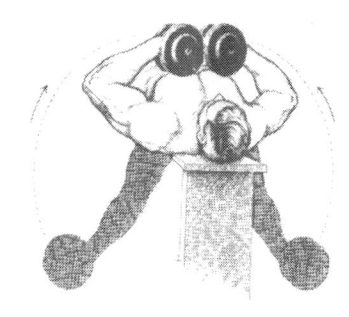

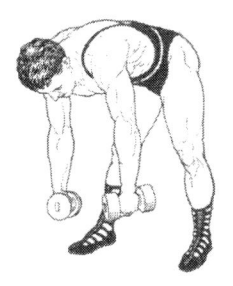

On the whole for normal people simply being aware of correct form when starting out with an exercise pattern will set them on the path to natural movements. Thus we focus on scapula starting position. It is important also, on any exercise, to manage the weight appropriately, that is to use a resistance that you can perform in good form. Sacrificing form for load teaches faulty movement patterns. As the weight exceeds a person's functional range of loading, there will be secondary (compensatory) movements induced, such as bobbing of the head, hiking of shoulders or overuse of the back etc.

Always check the neck position on any exercise. During each exercise the head should (normally) be in neutral. If the head is dropped, the scapulae will elevate as the upper trapezius becomes more involved in movement.

Also consider the rib cage. The rib cage is the forgotten workhorse of the upper body. Frequently, the rib cage relies on outside sources for movement, such as the spine, lungs, low back, and even the neck. Although the rib cage may seem like a passive guardian, in reality it is actively involved in most shoulder and back exercises by helping to stabilise the arms for any type of movement.

Place emphasis on first aligning the ribcage to create a good platform for the scapula to glide upon in rowing and pressing movements. First make sure the torso (and hence rib-cage) is facing the front and is not tilted or angled in a any way. Next try filling the lungs fully with air and then completely emptying them, and this will give you a feel for the two extremes of position.

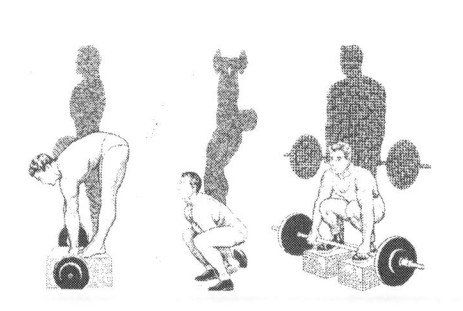

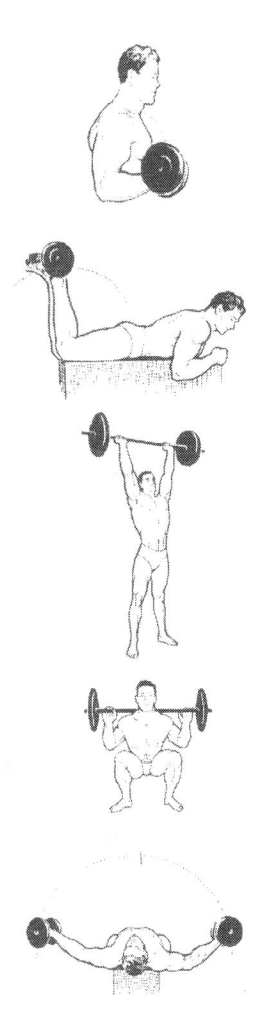

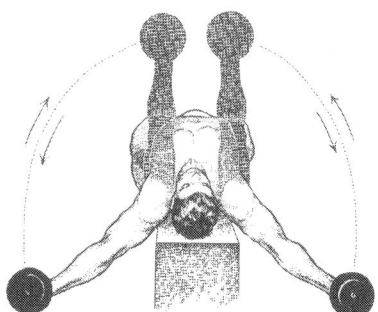

To obtain a strong position for the torso, we need to create a "centred" ribcage, and without bringing the head forward into a weak position and/or flexing the lower back into a crunched position. We also need to maintain a natural curve to the entire spine whilst getting the rib-cage into a neutral position, being neither too expanded nor too contacted.

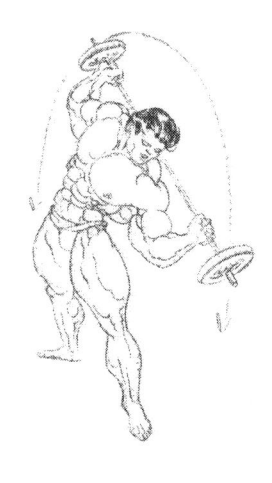

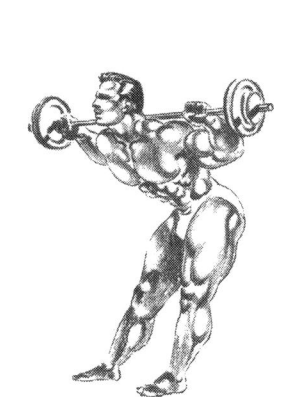

So how do we achieve a centred rib cage, neutral head, and neutral spinal posture simultaneously? First, we need to set the rib cage in neutral. You can set the rib cage just with flexion and no breath assistance, but it is better to breath maximally and then just let the rib cage settle into its most natural and comfortable position and hold it there. Get used to the feeling of placing your rib-cage into neutral prior to lifting. It will come naturally once you are an experienced lifter (on some lifts rib-cage expansion is required).

Back to scapula position. Do we retract it throughout an exercise? Or protract throughout? Or just move it freely? It all seems a bit complex. We shall take you through some common movements in order to explain scapula movements in detail. On the whole, however, and when in doubt, I would say that the scapula position should be left to take care of itself (e.g. experienced lifters).

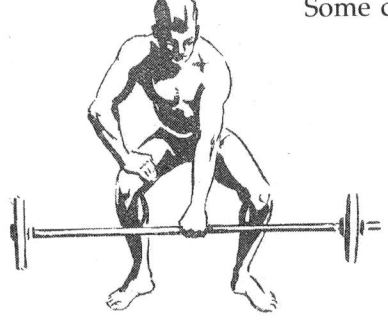

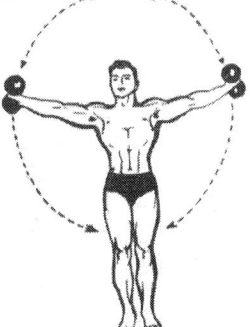

Rows: Firstly let us consider low pulley rows and dumbbell/barbell rows. On such moves, the scapula should protract and outwardly rotate as the arm reaches forward. As the arms pull the weight back the scapulae should retract and inwardly rotate back to the starting position. Scapula movement will change slightly as the arm raises or lowers, or if the width of the grip is altered. In order to manage or cue the movement correctly; watch out for over-activation of the upper trapezius (seen as a raising or shrugging of the shoulders during the exercise). Some coaches verbally cue trainees to move the shoulder blades "back and down," and to raise the sternum up during the concentric (pulling in) phase of the row.

BenchPress: When considering the bench-press things get a little more technical. We do not have sufficient space to go into all of the details, but rather we shall try to hit the main points of good form. There are several different styles of bench pressing; including ones performed for bodybuilding and/or powerlifting etc. Note that the bench press is a very technical, full body lift that requires a lot of practice.

A stable, and properly positioned, scapula will create a solid platform that your humerus can move around. The most common issue, and cause of injury, with the bench press is the lack of internal rotation in the shoulder. This is pretty easily traced back to your scapula.

Setting the scapula close to the correct position for benching can be easily performed simply by taking a deep breath. The key thing about your lungs is that when you fill them up completely and properly, they push everything back where it goes. This is essential. You've got to create the "shelf" when you press. Tighten your shoulder blades, and maintain tight shoulder blades for the duration of the set. It helps to arch your lower a bit, which is why you see the experts arching during the bench. On the bench the scapulas are retracted as completely as possible to get the chest up as high as possible (powerlifting style).

Push-Ups: Now let us consider push-ups. The scapulae should retract and slightly inwardly rotate (depending on how wide the hands are placed apart) on the down phase of the push-up. As the arms push away from the body, the scapulae should protract and slightly outwardly rotate.

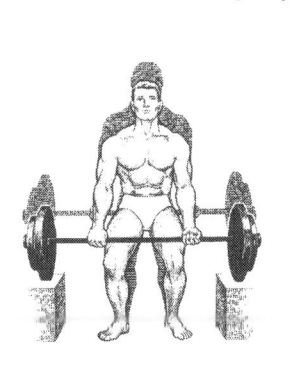

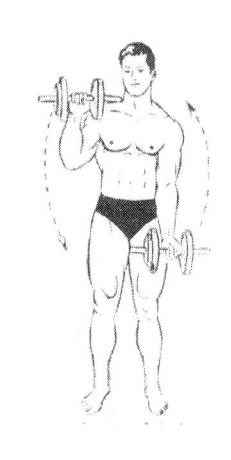

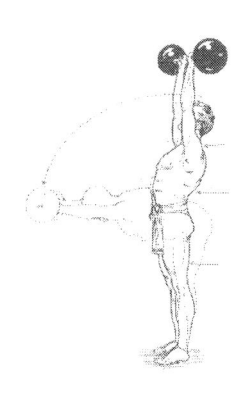

The scapula movement will change if the arm or hand positions are altered.

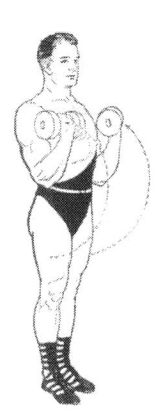

Chin-Ups: Now to chin-ups. The scapulae should outwardly rotate and elevate as the arms reach upward. As the arms pull the body back down, the scapulae should inwardly rotate and depress back to the starting position. As with low rows, move the shoulder blades "back and down".

Squats: With squats (barbell on back type) you need to likewise breath in deeply and retract the scapula fully (prior to start) and in order to create a shelf for the bar to rest on.

Standing Press: Let us now consider the standing press (with barbell or dumbbells). Here we do not attempt to retract the scapula fully at the start as we do in the bench press. Rather we stand upright with chest held high and with a slightly arched lumber, with lats flared and shoulders fully "down" in their sockets. As the bar is pressed up and back to position over the rear of the head, the scapulae should move together as the lifter reaches upwards. The scapulae rotate and push together as the press proceeds to form that stable base. Also, at the set position for any type of standing shoulder press, the scapula are not retracted - but rather are somewhat neutral. Note also that overhead work is always a lot more stable when flaring the lats.

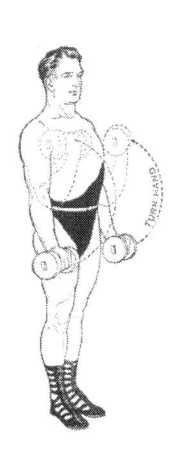

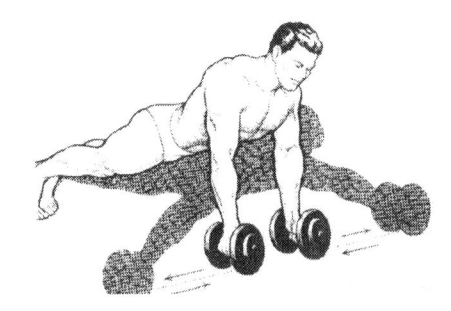

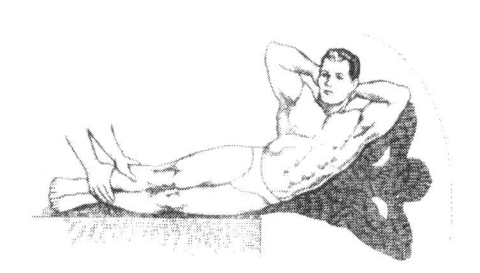

On the standing press, the chest is up, the elbows are slightly in front of the bar, and the upper back is tight. Part of this upper back tightness is traps, part is rhomboids, and part is lats being used isometrically to reinforce the chest position. This produces a firm platform from which to press, but it is not complete scapula retraction. You should stand tall during the press, dig your heels into the ground, squeeze the glutes and brace the abs. Don't put your heels together but shoulder-width apart. This will increase stability and thus strength. Hands about shoulder-width apart (barbell version). Hands should never touch your shoulders. Bar close to your wrist, in the base of your palm, not close to your fingers. Make a big chest & lift it up. Looking up is bad for your neck. Look forward, fix a point on the wall before you. Squeeze shoulders, traps & back. Lock your elbows. "Pull *through* the scaps" on the way down or back, and "push *through* the scaps" on the way up or forwards.

Flying motions (lying lateral raise): In flys, round the world, hang etc; I would prefer to keep the scapula in a neutral position, and without "forcing" any protraction or retraction as the movement progresses. The scapula may naturally retract as the arms come back in any case. Concentrate instead on the position of the elbow and dumbbell in space, and move according to the exercise being performed. Leave the scapula to take care of itself.

Lateral motions (standing): Let the scapula move naturally. Each "scap" tilts upwards once the dumbbell gets beyond horizontal or shoulder level. On regular dumbbell lateral raises, another option is to go to full range of motion (ROM) as recommended by Dr. Michael Yessis. As the arm passes 90 degrees, you may want to externally rotate the humerus to continue the motion so that the palms are facing each other at the bottom and top of the movement.

According to Yessis, "*The deltoid is most active from the shoulder level position to the above-the-head position. Stopping at shoulder level as typically done in the lateral arm raise exercise limits flexibility in the shoulder joints and full muscular development.*"

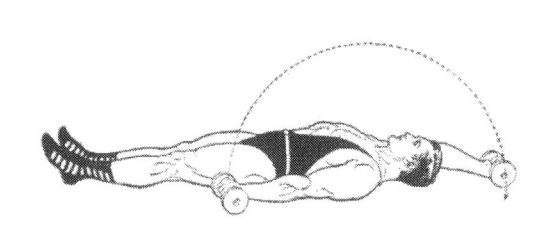

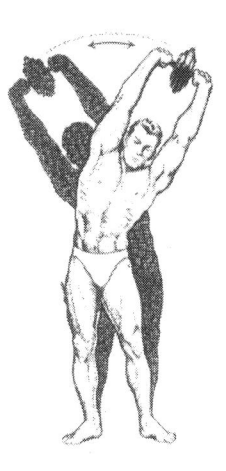

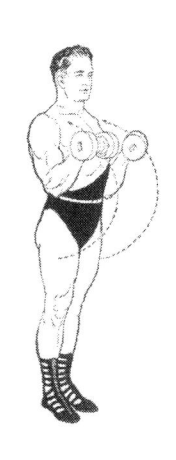

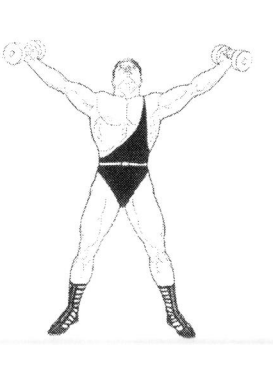

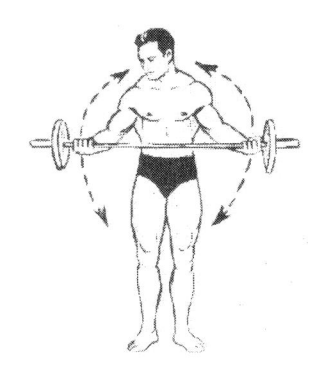

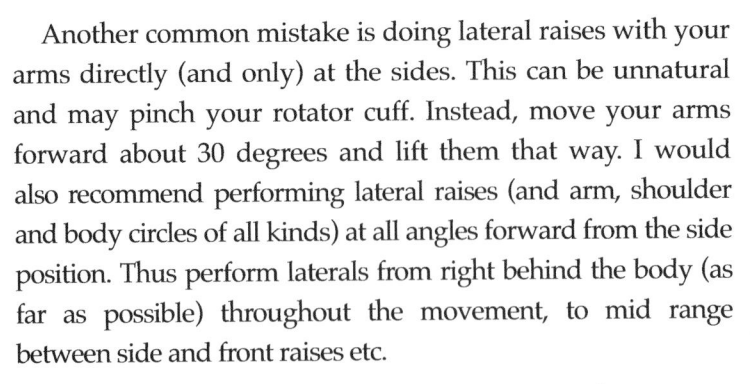

Another common mistake is doing lateral raises with your arms directly (and only) at the sides. This can be unnatural and may pinch your rotator cuff. Instead, move your arms forward about 30 degrees and lift them that way. I would also recommend performing lateral raises (and arm, shoulder and body circles of all kinds) at all angles forward from the side position. Thus perform laterals from right behind the body (as far as possible) throughout the movement, to mid range between side and front raises etc.

Thats about it in terms of our discussion of the scapula. Note that we have not the space to discuss scapula position for all of the recommended exercises in this book. Perhaps a neutral scapula should be considered the standard fall-back for most exercises; or simply let the body find its own way of holding the shoulder in place.

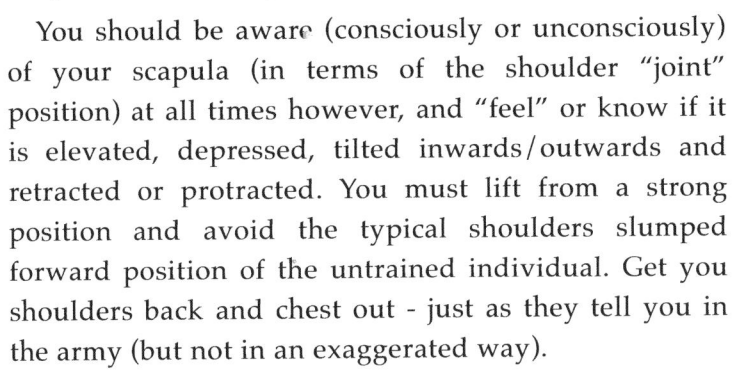

You should be aware (consciously or unconsciously) of your scapula (in terms of the shoulder "joint" position) at all times however, and "feel" or know if it is elevated, depressed, tilted inwards/outwards and retracted or protracted. You must lift from a strong position and avoid the typical shoulders slumped forward position of the untrained individual. Get you shoulders back and chest out - just as they tell you in the army (but not in an exaggerated way).

Stand up straight when exercising, get your head back, but do not over-correct the shoulder position, just get into a fully upright anatomical position prior to picking weights off the floor (for example).

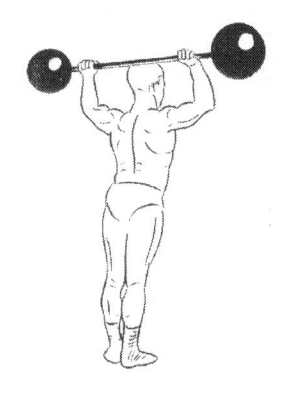

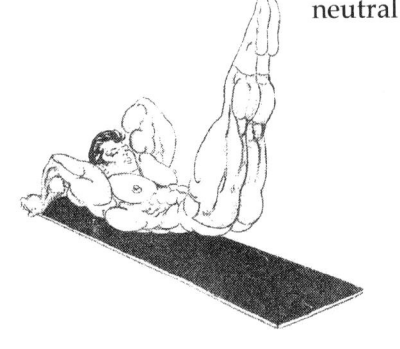

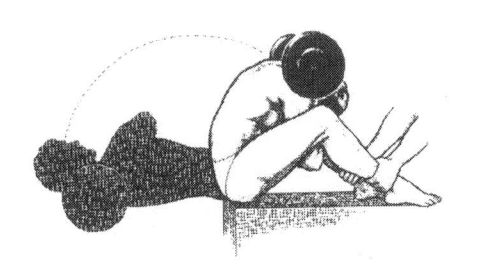

Be aware also of the degree (if any) of rotation of the humorous in its socket and learn how to set this into a neutral position. You need to concentrate on all parts of the body together at once when lifting; and especially the spine, scapula, legs, knees, ankles etc. Learn how to get your body into anatomical position prior to setting yourself up for a lift of any type.

I could probably go on giving recommendations, tips and advice forever in relation to weight-training. And when I reached the limits of my own experience and/or understanding, I could easily find other teachers who would be happy to continue your instruction. Such "learning" overload is unnecessary however, and may in fact be detrimental. Remember the Zen notion that the truth that can be told is not the real truth. In other words dumbbell training is not really something that can be told from one person to another - rather it must be experienced by the trainee himself. Dumbbell practice will be very different in each case, due to personal capabilities and limitations, plus as a result of the natural tendency of the individual to uniquely express himself (as Bruce Lee used to say). Therefore one should not compare oneself to others (difficult I know), but rather see "mindful" dumbbell training as a route to becoming better attuned to your true self; in terms of mind, body and spirit.

Rather than look for external gurus and teachers who instruct you in how to be, reach deep inside yourself and realise that it is you, and you alone, who manages your affairs in life. Do not let others - anyone in fact - tell you how you should train. Take advice - and collect knowledge - to be sure. But enlighten yourself to the truth; that you are, in fact, the master of your own destiny in life and that it is you who must be the ultimate guide. Have faith in yourself, and in your own opinions. Listen to friends, but rely on yourself.

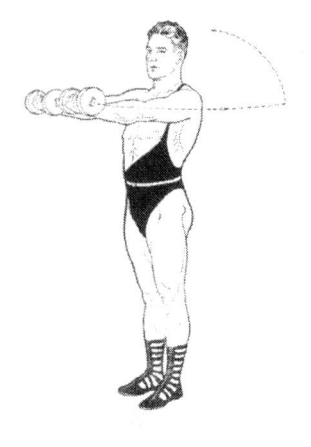

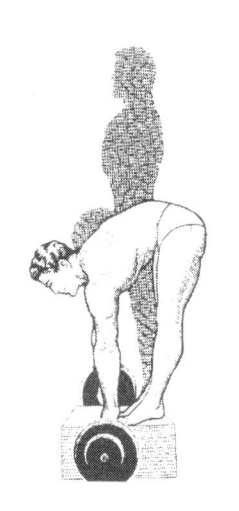

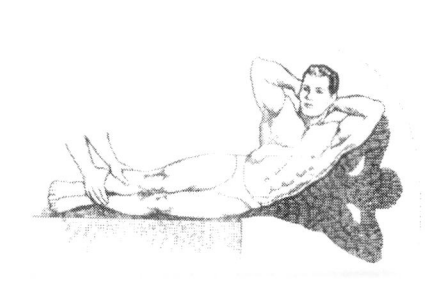

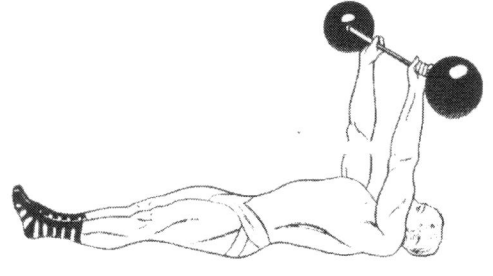

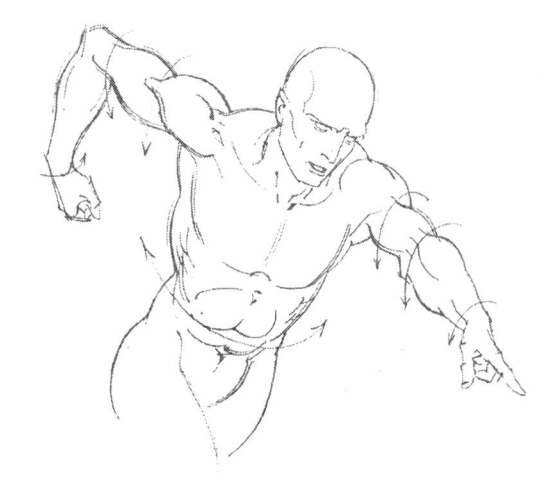

Conclusions

It is interesting to note how many and varied are the opinions on weight-training. For example, over the last 20 years or so certain exercises have been demonised; including stiff legged dead-lifts and side-lateral raises above the horizontal position. However 100 years ago physical culture adherents performed all kinds of lateral raises up and overhead, and the stiff-legged dead-lift was considered to be an essential part of anyone's program.

Today experts like Dr. Michael Yessis are once again recommending performing lateral raises right overhead. And recently a physiotherapist said of the stiff-legged dead-lift:

"The stiff leg dead-lift is highly therapeutic for someone with a "flat" lower back, a lower back that has lost its natural lordosis (e.g. as a result of a seated lifestyle). The stiff leg dead-lift, by strengthening the muscles behind the lumbar vertebrae, can gradually ease your lower spine back into its natural position over weeks and months of performing this exercise. As such, the stiff leg dead-lift will improve your posture, lower the likelihood of you suffering a back injury during your daily tasks (e.g. gardening, moving groceries); and make sitting more comfortable, flatten the profile of your stomach, and stabilise your pelvis."

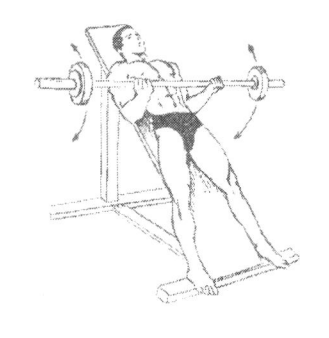

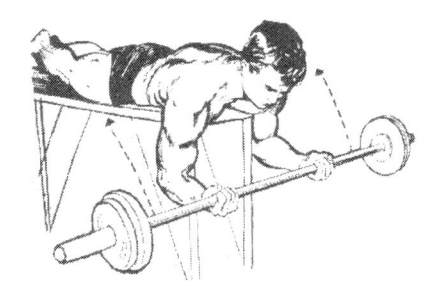

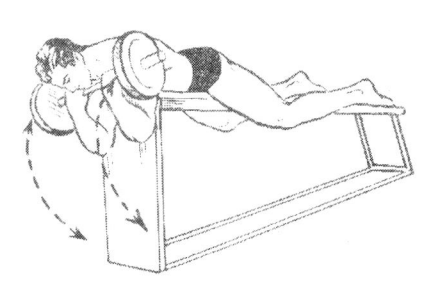

Overall, you will have to decide for yourself what is, in fact, a safe and beneficial exercise for yourself to perform. Pay close attention to style, weight used and speed of performance etc. Remember that any exercise is dangerous when using too much weight. Some exercises are best performed with lighter weights (ROM moves), and especially the stiff legged dead-lift and other bending and twisting moves.

In this book I have presented my own findings after a lifetime of study and also practical experience lifting weights. Hopefully you can find something useful from what I have had to say. But in one book we do not have the space to make a comprehensive examination of all of the different factors that relate to the field of dumbbell training. Therefore, you must gather training knowledge wherever you can find it. Seek out scientific information constantly, but test the findings against your own ideas. Remember to ask yourself if our ancestors would have moved in that way when evaluating any new exercise. And feel free to ignore everything that I have said (mostly), and allow your body to move in the specific way(s) that it tells you are the most natural (for you).

It is my position that scientific descriptions of exercise performance should be used only as a guide. I believe that your own body will teach you how to perform each exercise, through constant feedback obtained whilst performing natural movement patterns (3D paths in space). The most efficient form on each exercise will evolve with practice. The body has to be left to teach itself how to move. You can coach the body, but it is in charge! To some extent your aim is to create an efficient muscle-memory; whereby each movement must be learned - and memorised - by the body itself. Therefore give yourself plenty of time to learn each movement, and use dumbbells in order to obtain free movement paths.

The body is wise and if you listen closely it will be your ultimate instructor. Finally good luck. I feel certain that dumbbell training is the fastest, safest and most efficient route to exceptional fitness, super strength and first-class movement ROMs.

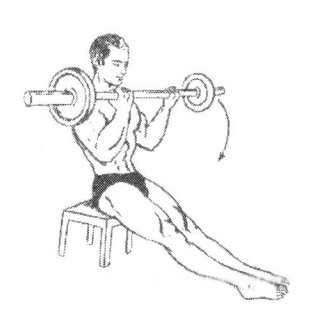

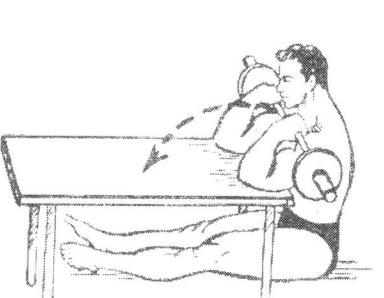

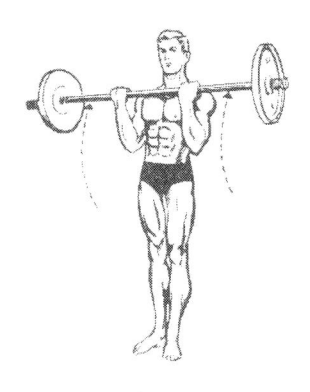

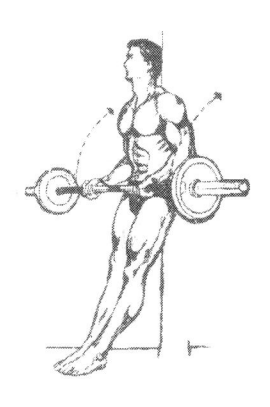

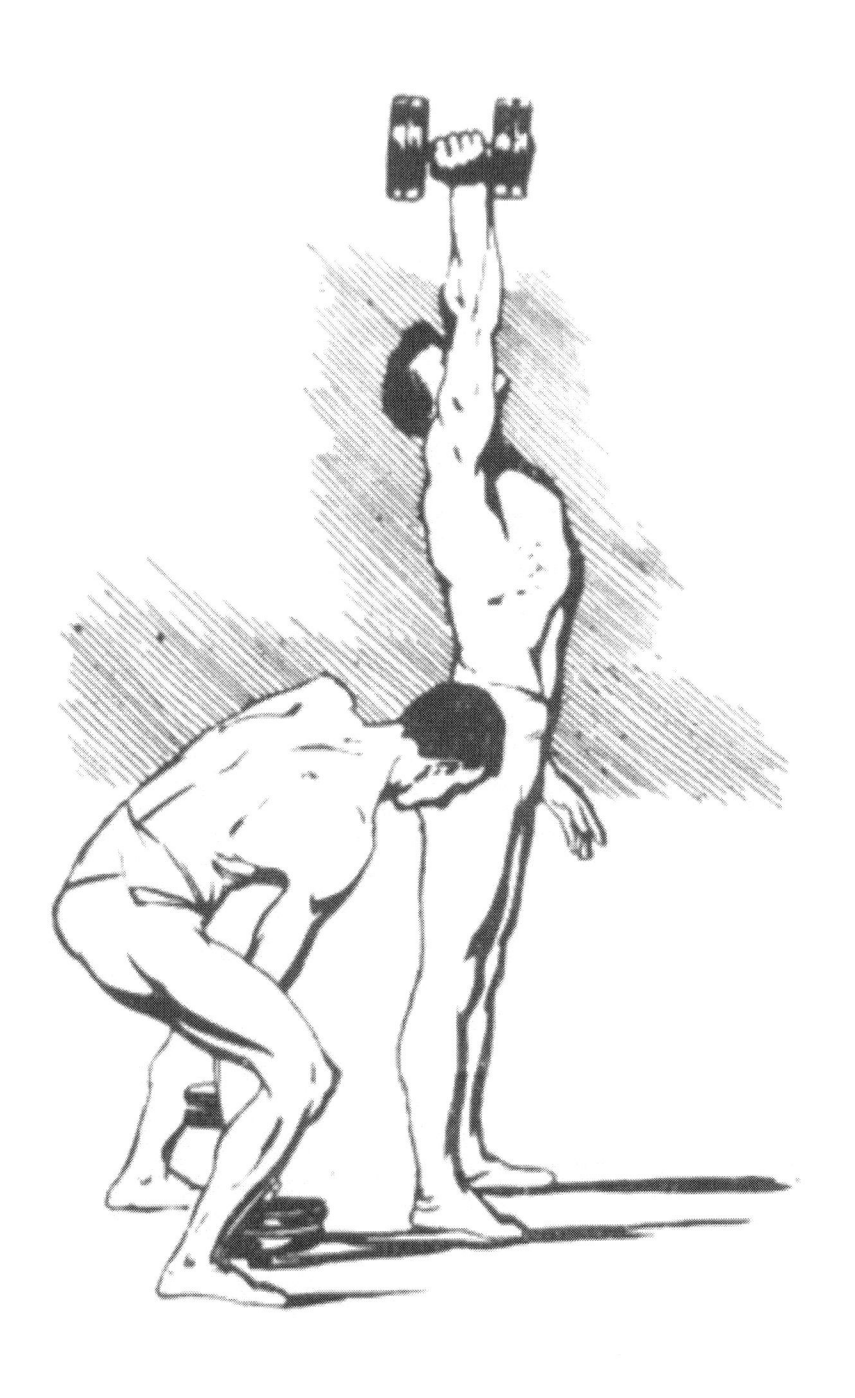

CHAPTER TWENTY SEVEN

MECHANICS OF DUMBBELL TRAINING

IN THIS last chapter I would like to address some important topics related to the mechanics of dumbbell training. In particular, I shall examine the lifting process itself, in practical terms, and in order to develop a *how to* guide for perfect lifting technique.

This book is aimed at the beginner or intermediate lifter; being someone who has either; no lifting experience whatsoever, or who has been lifting for less than one year. I want people who have not yet learned any bad-habits - or alternatively who are willing to unlearn the same!

I recommend that it is best to get the advice/coaching of a real expert on lifting technique; perhaps a weight-lifting coach would be best, or someone involved in the sport of powerlifting or strength athletics. You want to find someone who knows about the biomechanics of lifting; that is, how to use the spine, hips and legs etc. I also suggest that you first learn how to lift whilst standing up; and before doing any lying down movements whatsoever (ideally).

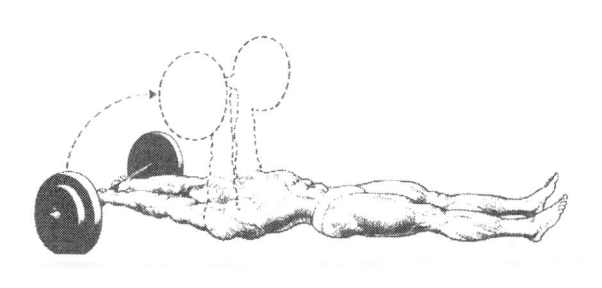

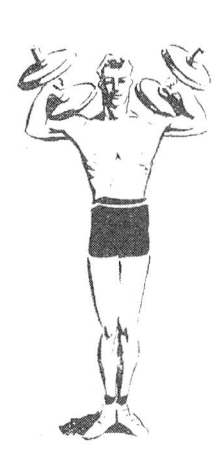

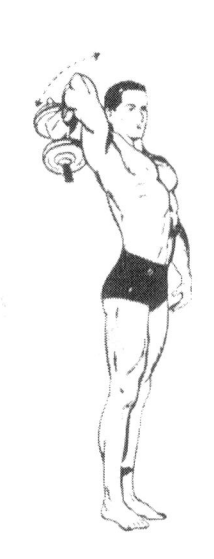

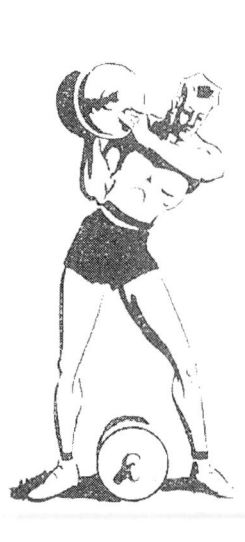

I do realise that unfortunately not everyone will be able to find such a coach. Hence this book. You can learn how to lift alone, but it is more difficult, and progress will be slower than if you had the help of an expert. If you do decide to go-it-alone in this respect, then I suggest that you read everything you can about weight-lifting technique - and especially information on exercises like the squat, dead-lift and the clean and press. Learn how to perform these movements correctly first-of-all. Once you have done so, then you will have learned the core principles of how to use the body in order to lift heavy objects. Such knowledge can then easily *cross-over* into the other movements, and you will find that you can make faster progress in this respect.

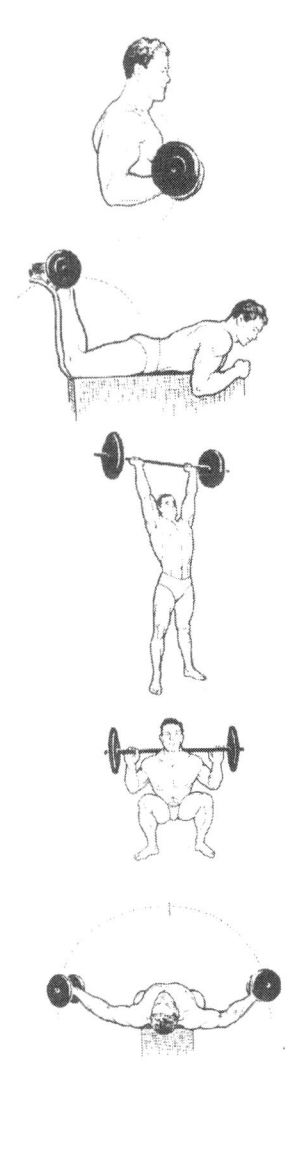

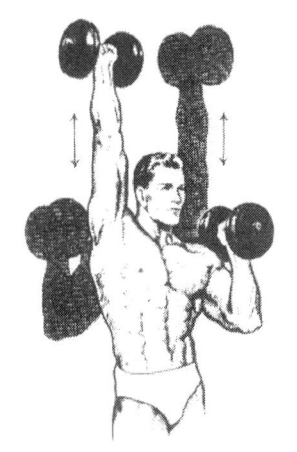

You will be aware at this stage that I do not like machines very much. I prefer free-weights. Plus I do like kettle-bells for some movements - for example they are excellent for the swing, windmill, standing press and for certain rowing moves etc. But on the whole the dumbbell is superior to a kettle-bell because the hand position allows a far greater variety of exercises to be performed. You will know by now that I also prefer dumbbells over barbells. However I do believe in the use of barbells for lifts such as squats, dead-lifts, rowing, and (sometimes) the clean and press.

I have split resistance training into two specific types, being strength and ROM training. In this book I have given detailed explanations of my reasons for so doing, and I have also explained how to train according to the resulting principles.

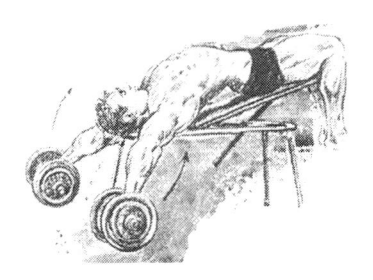

For ROM training I explained that the shoulder and hip joint are the main ones that require such an approach, and also that certain bending and twisting moves should be performed in a ROM style for the spine as well. I would like to re-iterate the fact that in ROM training one would normally explore all of the different joint angles (positions) - or at least as many as possible - and within a single workout. This is in order to be certain that you are working the joint from as many angles as possible - hence developing the *total flexibility of the joint* (i.e. shoulder and spine). Note that people have varying joint ROMs; and so ROM training will be specific to the individual. In other words, the movement patterns will be unique in terms of the 3D path(s) of the limbs/body-parts/dumbbell in space. It is important that nobody else try to force you to attempt (or else to follow) a movement path that is beyond your capacity; or rather that your body "tells-you" is wrong. Remember that zen training is all about feelings, and has your own body as the ultimate guide/teacher.

Be careful with ROM training for the spine, and do not use heavy weights and/or fast moves. Do use a variety of feet-widths for squats; and also a variety of grip-widths when using barbells, and so to work the ROM of the hip/shoulder joints from as many angles as possible. On standing and lying laterals etc; one would also want to explore as many positions of the shoulder joint as possible. Overall, use a great variety of different movement paths/arcs on ROM lifts. This type of training is all about exploring as many movement paths as possible; and in fact trying to get them all (those possible for you).

The way I see dumbbell *strength* training is more in terms of weightlifting practice. I have a background in this particular sport myself, but this is not the reason that I have placed such an emphasis in my teaching. Rather it is because of the poor techniques that I see in most gyms around the world. Trainees commonly have no idea how to *get-set, ready and go*; in relation to lifting; and thus how to place/align the feet, knees, hips, lower back and shoulders etc. Most have no clue how to get into the correct set position before even starting to lift (essential).

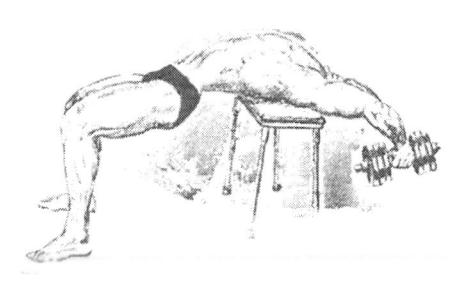

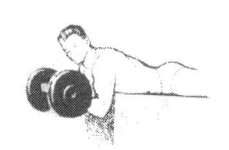

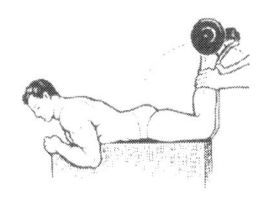

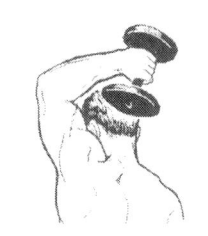

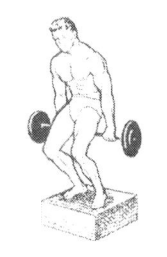

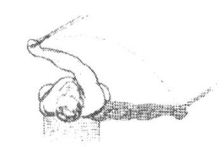

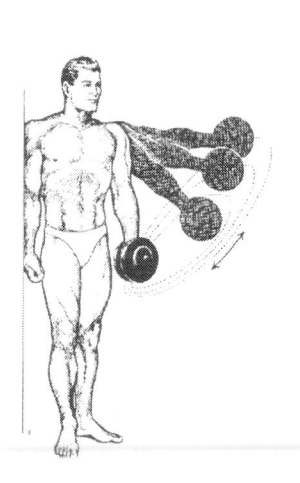

Many trainees have sloping shoulders, uneven feet, flat back, hips entirely un-involved - and all whilst lifting! But correct lifting technique (or body set-position) is the same no-matter if you are performing curls, standing presses, lateral raises or dead-lifts etc. The basic posture is the same, and should be known and learnt by all. You will never progress in dumbbell training unless you have learned the basics of how to first correctly set and then move your body; and in order to lift a heavy object.

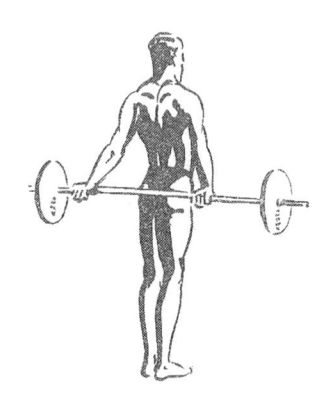

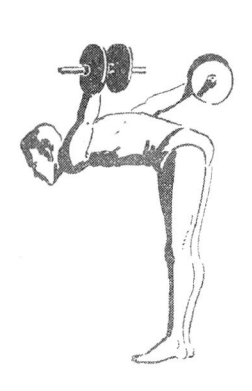

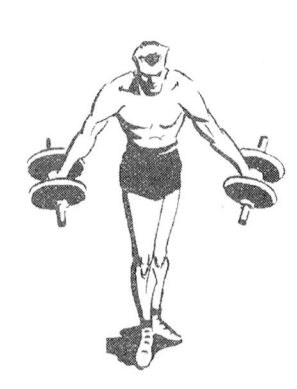

Dumbbell training is basically weight-lifting - no matter if you are training for bodybuilding, athletics, or running. The core principles are the same - and must be learned first; and because these principles are the foundation of all resistance training. One must learn how to move the entire body in an integrated fashion - as a unit. You must first learn the clean and press, dead-lift and squat - the basic standing-up exercises. For a beginner, I would not even attempt to do any other exercises for the first month of training. I recommend spending 1 hour 2-3 times weekly simply learning how to perform these specific lifts.

It is best for beginners to learn how to lift weights with a barbell - at first that is. This is so for several reasons, and notably because you want to learn a relatively simple movement pattern as offered by the barbell. Here the number of variables (movement paths/arcs) is reduced (relative to dumbbells) and you can concentrate on how the body itself should move whilst performing the lift. And so the beginner's job is to learn the basic movement biomechanics in terms of lifting weights whilst standing upright.

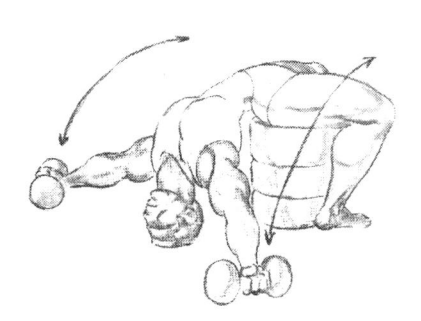

The fundamental exercise in weightlifting is the clean and press with a barbell. Once you learn how to perform this move, then you will be ready to transfer what you have learned to other exercises. When performing the clean and press you will learn all of the basic (underlying) theory of weightlifting and weight-training in one go. You will learn how to arch the lumbar, move, flex and extend the hips, bend at the knee and ankle, plus how to use and set the positions of the shoulder, head and arms. It is a mini-master's degree in lifting technique.

Lets get to it - and learn the clean and press.

The clean and press is a movement that involves both strength and speed. Although this exercise targets primarily the front deltoids, it also works the trapezius, erector spinae, the quadriceps, the hamstrings, the buttocks, and the triceps.

Place an Olympic barbell on the floor. Load the bar with an appropriate poundage, place your feet approximately shoulder width apart, and make sure that the bar is over the tops of your feet. Check that your feet are aligned correctly (one or the other is not askew) - and do the same for the shoulders. From this position, bend down and grasp the bar with an overhand grip. Look forward (before you lift), and set the rib-cage by breathing in. Make sure that your knees do not shoot out over your toes, lower your buttocks to the floor until your thighs are parallel to the floor. Now arch your lower back - that is flex your erector spinae muscles to maintain a strong (extended) lower back. After you have followed the above instructions, you are ready to start the movement. The first part of the move is the barbell clean.

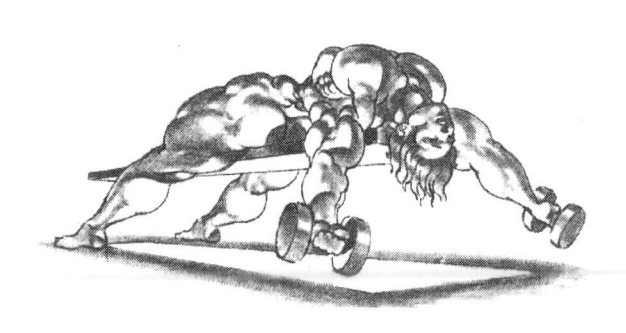

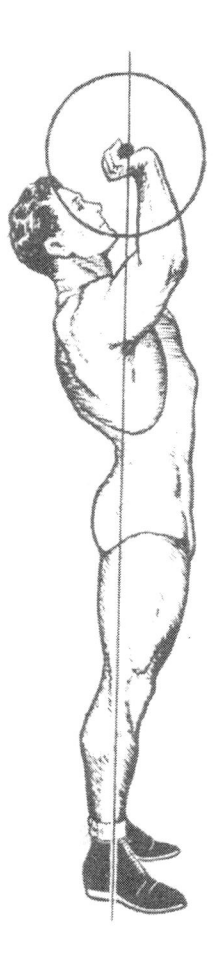

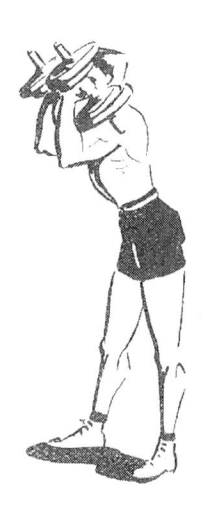

The clean is a quick movement. Position the shoulders over the bar, with back arched tightly. Arms are straight with elbows pointed along bar. Pull the bar up off the floor by extending hips and knees. As the bar reaches the knees vigorously raise the shoulders while keeping the barbell close to thighs. When the barbell passes mid-thigh, allow it to (slightly) contact the thighs. Jump upward extending the body. Shrug the shoulders and pull the barbell upward with the arms allowing the elbows to flex out to the sides, keeping the bar close to the body. Aggressively pull the body under the bar, rotating the elbows around bar. Catch the bar on the shoulders while moving into a squat position. Hitting bottom of a (partial) squat, stand up immediately.

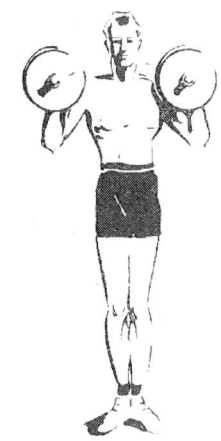

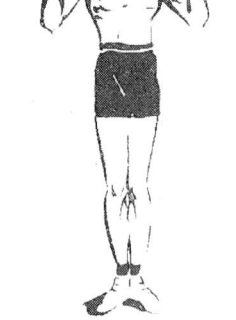

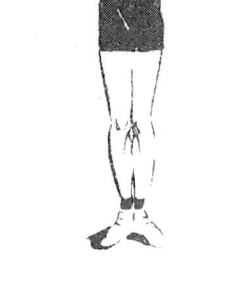

The whole "cleaning" movement is indeed complex - but the main learning point is that most of the strength of the body in weightlifting comes from the hips. Note that I am explaining the power clean here. The power clean is a fluid and non-stopping movement in which the barbell is lifted from the floor up and onto your shoulders, and all done in less than a second. You will be transferring all of your power to the barbell; so as to be able to accelerate the barbell and move it upwards against gravity.

There are 4 stages to the power clean: pull from the floor, second pull, triple extension (ankle, knees and hips) and catching. I do not have the space here to explain these stages in detail, but I suggest that you read-up and practice the clean by using such knowledge.

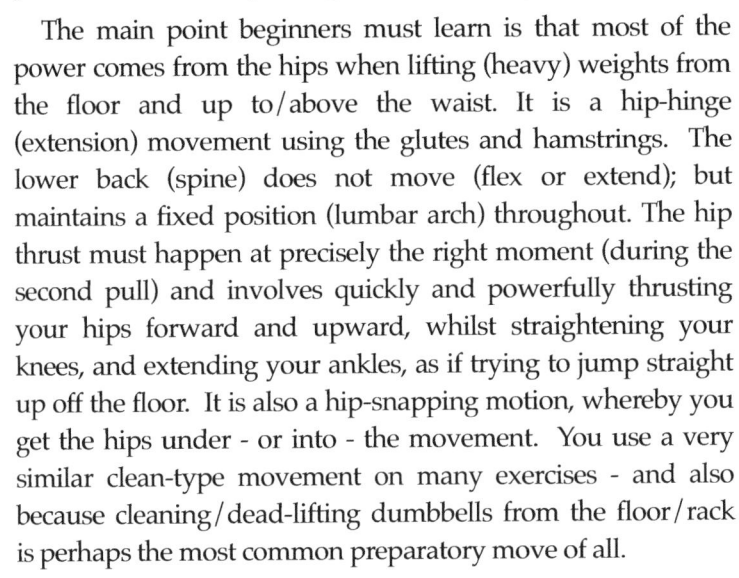

The main point beginners must learn is that most of the power comes from the hips when lifting (heavy) weights from the floor and up to/above the waist. It is a hip-hinge (extension) movement using the glutes and hamstrings. The lower back (spine) does not move (flex or extend); but maintains a fixed position (lumbar arch) throughout. The hip thrust must happen at precisely the right moment (during the second pull) and involves quickly and powerfully thrusting your hips forward and upward, whilst straightening your knees, and extending your ankles, as if trying to jump straight up off the floor. It is also a hip-snapping motion, whereby you get the hips under - or into - the movement. You use a very similar clean-type movement on many exercises - and also because cleaning/dead-lifting dumbbells from the floor/rack is perhaps the most common preparatory move of all.

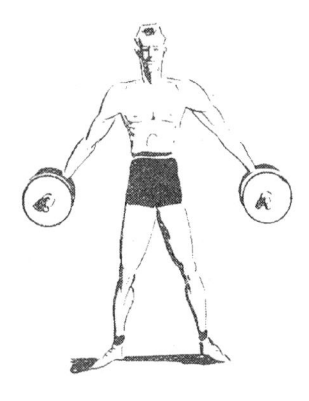

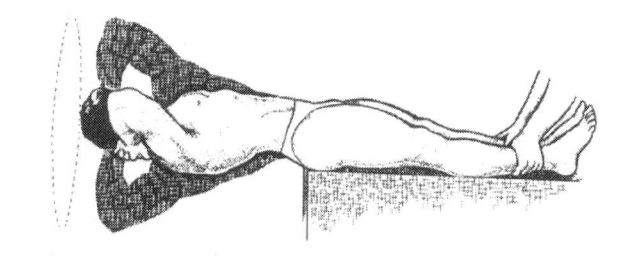

I do not want to spend any more time explaining hip movements here - because to some extent this is a skill that you must practice to learn - and being one that will come naturally if you simply perform lots of standing cleans. What you must understand is that the correct placement of one's hips is the essential weightlifting technique for lifting weights off the floor. Furthermore that you must learn how to hold the hips in the correct position relative to heavy weights; at all-times and on all-types of lifts.

Likewise you must not flex the lower-spine (and so try to lift with a loaded spine or rounded/flat lower-back) or else hyperextend the spine when lifting weights from the floor. Yet I often see people using their hips and lower back (lumbar) incorrectly during exercises such as curls, squats, presses, laterals etc. When this happens, I tell myself that if the same person had first learnt how to clean a barbell correctly then they would not now be having so much trouble.

Most do not even know that they are lifting incorrectly, because they fail to realise that lifting is all about using the hips and lower-back appropriately. The hips and lower back, must both be used in the correct manner before any other considerations are taken into account (position/movement of other joints and muscle actions); and thus before any other movements can happen efficiently.

And when using dumbbells - correct movement of the hips becomes even more important; because (when using one dumbbell alone) you need to obtain the full benefit of twisting and leaning motions. Here if you do not know how to position the hips, then injury could be the result. My advice is to study weight-lifting technique, and became adept in how to set - and move - the hips and lower back whilst lifting - and before attempting to learn any other "bodybuilding" exercises and/or any lying or seated movements etc.

I shall not go on to explain the pressing part of the clean-and-press in this Chapter, because it is adequately dealt with in the text.

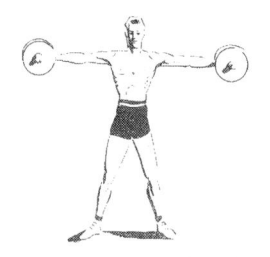

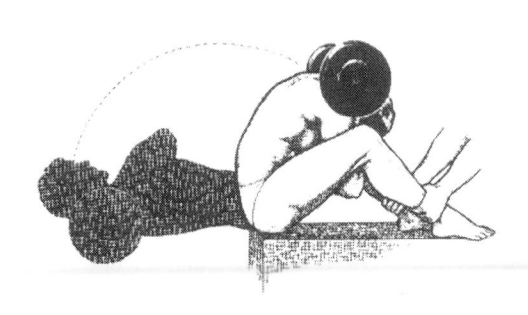

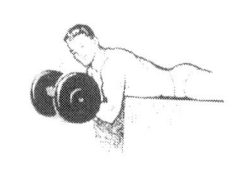

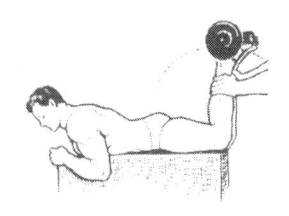

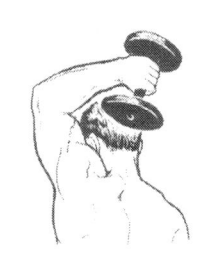

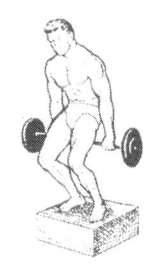

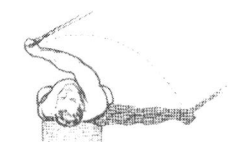

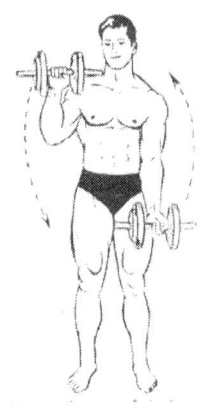

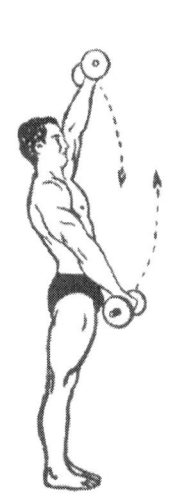

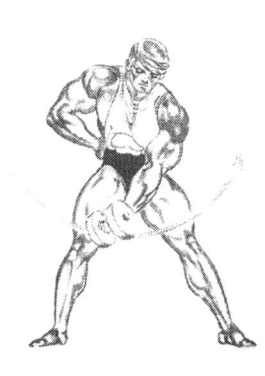

I would like to finish by introducing a set of 5 "mottos" that encapsulate the principles of zen dumbbell training, and that can be used as a handy shorthand by trainees when applying the zen method:

- Free the joints
- Light weights are heavy
- Set the joints
- Work the angles
- Explore the paths

Motto number one, *free the joints*; refers to the first principle of zen training; being the need to allow the joints and levers of the human body to move independently and along unrestricted and "free" movement paths. This motto indicates that dumbbells offer the most natural movement patterns, and promote healthy joint range of motions (ROMs). Dumbbell methods also involve full ROM, exercise the most muscles at once, and involve many stabilising muscles also; thus the potential for strength gains is often greater than when training with barbells and/or machines.

Motto number two, *light weights are heavy*, has been discussed previously and brings attention to the fact that even seemingly light weights are in actuality heavy (from the bodies perspective). Lighter weights do sometimes (in a real sense) provide greater resistance to specific muscles due to the avoidance of the structural re-arrangements that often occur when using very heavy weights. Everyone should use very light weights (regularly) as a result - and not only for ROM moves.

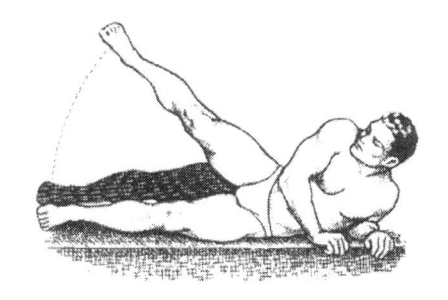

Motto number three, *set the joints*, refers to the fact that when performing any exercise; it is vital to hold certain body-parts - and hence joints in specific location(s) and also in fixed (motionless) position(s); and in order to give other joints the freedom to move with strength and confidence. We spoke about the fact that even simple movements involve many joints (body-part movements being combinations of circular motions).

Dumbbell-training is complex and involves the learning of multiple skills - and in order to perform each lift correctly. As a solution to this complexity; we have recommended using both theory and also listening to - and learning from - your own body. We think that such a dual approach is the best method to attain optimal movement related skills and knowledge.

Motto number four, *work the angles*, refers to ROM training (on the whole), and brings attention to the requirement (ideally) to work each joint (primarily the shoulder, hip and spine) from as many different angles as possible. In fact it would be best to work each joint from all possible (natural) angles - and as frequently as possible. Here one turns the movement itself into an exploration of multiple movement paths - and in order to explore the different ROMs that are possible with that joint. For example on shoulder round-the-worlds, and on hangs; I attempt to hit every possible shoulder joint angle (limb position); in terms of the arms being located behind the back. Thus I move the limb(s) through all-kinds of different positions. Do likewise on laterals and circles when the arms are in-front of the body; and when standing upright. Such training will dramatically improve joint ROMs, and increase the length of movement paths/arcs plus develop muscular flexibility.

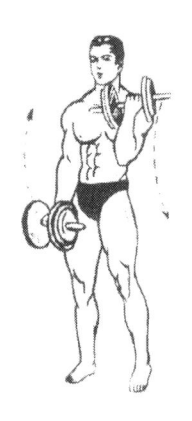

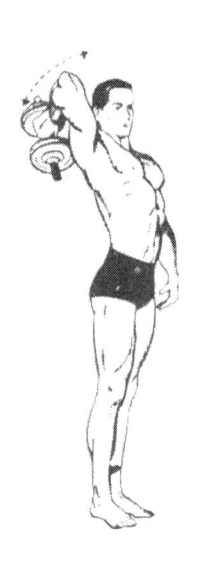

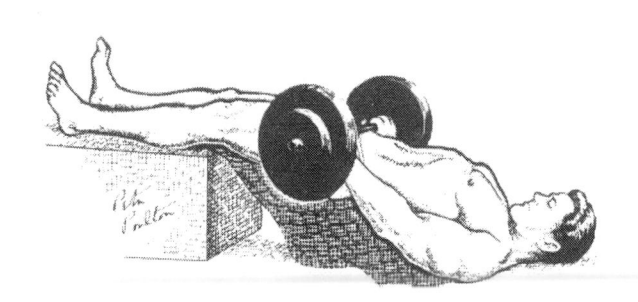

Motto number five, *explore the paths*, refers to a method of training whereby one uses multiple and different movement paths/arcs for the same body-part - but using slightly *different* exercises and/or exercise variations. One example would be on the barbell squat. Here the trainee performs many different versions of the squat; and so to work multiple and slightly different movement paths. We recommend performing overhead squats, plus one legged and jumping squats, and deep-knee-bends, plus hack squats etc; and with barbell, kettle-bell and dumbbell versions etc (probably in different workouts). Such an approach has the key advantage that one is exploring many different movement paths/arcs for the same basic movement pattern, thus strength and ROM improvements are magnified.

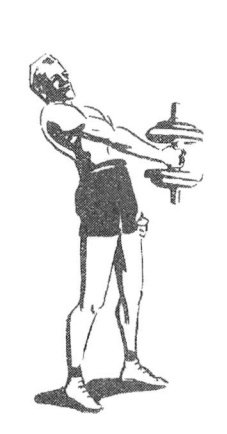

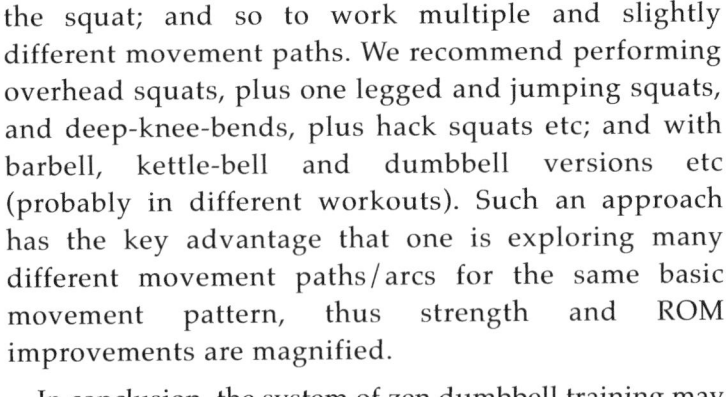

In conclusion, the system of zen dumbbell training may not actually contain any *truly* novel concepts - and especially in terms of the basic principles of resistance training. However the zen approach eliminates much that is useless, dangerous and/or less than optimal for any trainee. Thus it will help you to avoid wasted effort - and time - which would otherwise have been the case when following less-than-ideal training methods.

The Zen method is based on a single new training principle; and also on five mottos which guide your choice of exercises, performance techniques and overall training strategy. Once armed with such knowledge, it is hoped that you will then be able to formulate an ideal training program and so to maximise your physical potential.

Remember also that all knowledge is ultimately self-knowledge; and you will need to adapt all that you are told, read, see - and learn - to your own requirements and individual circumstances. In fact this is why dumbbells are the ultimate fitness training tools; because you can tailor them to your own specific needs.

Dumbbell training is the most natural, advanced and versatile system for improving the human body.

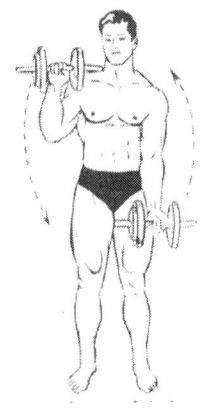

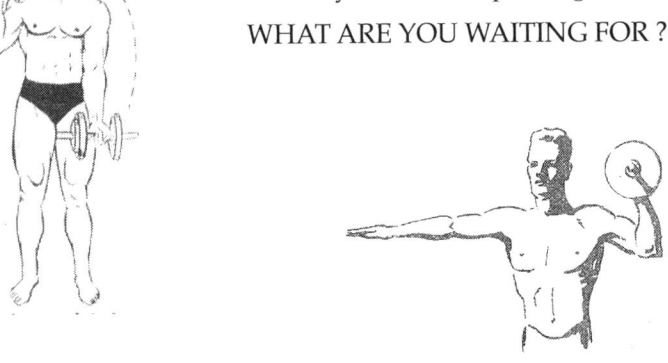

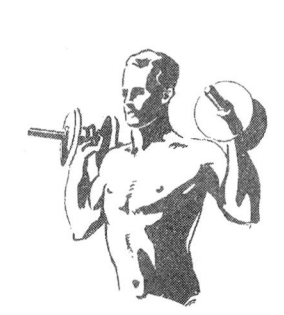

WHAT ARE YOU WAITING FOR ?

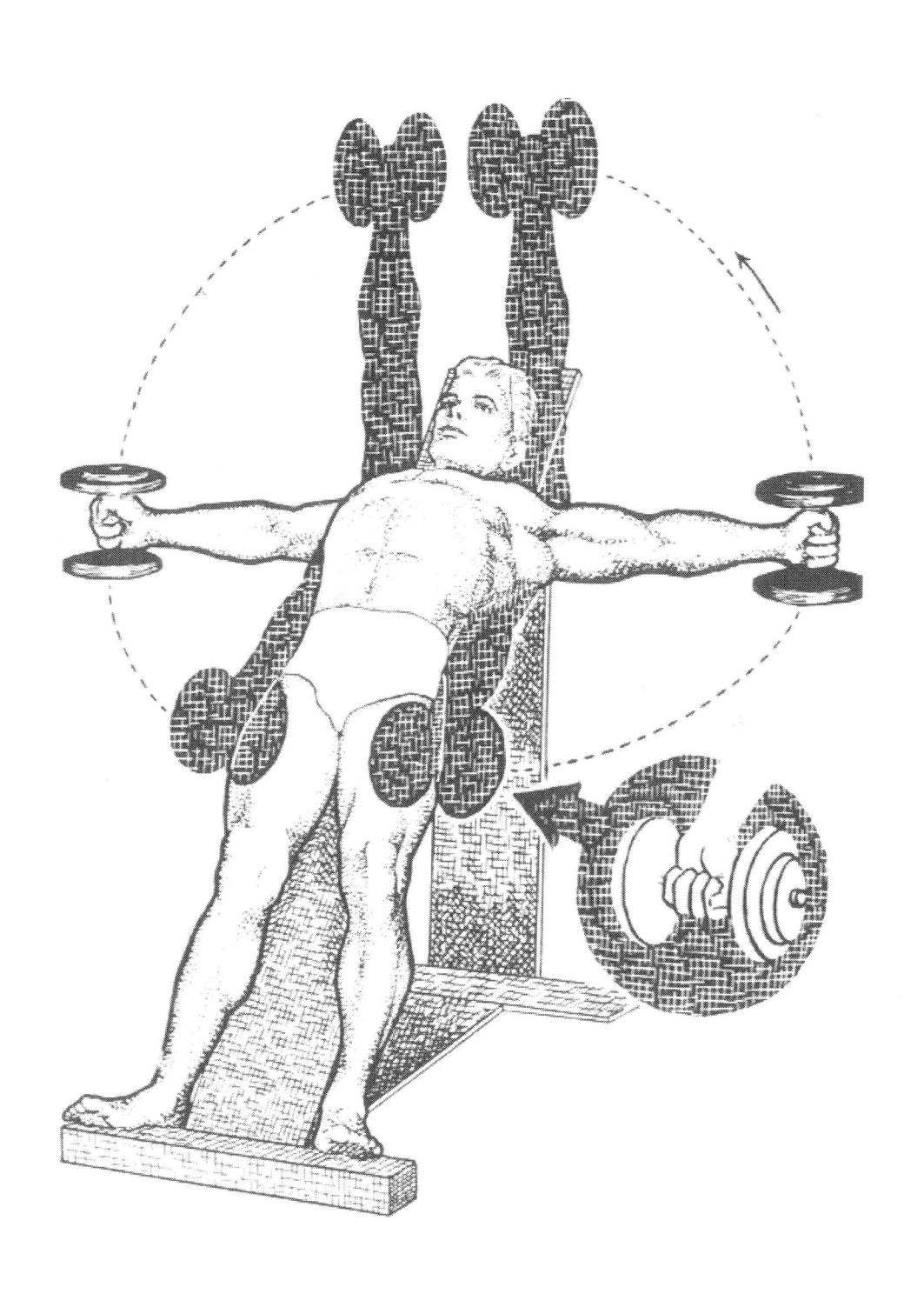

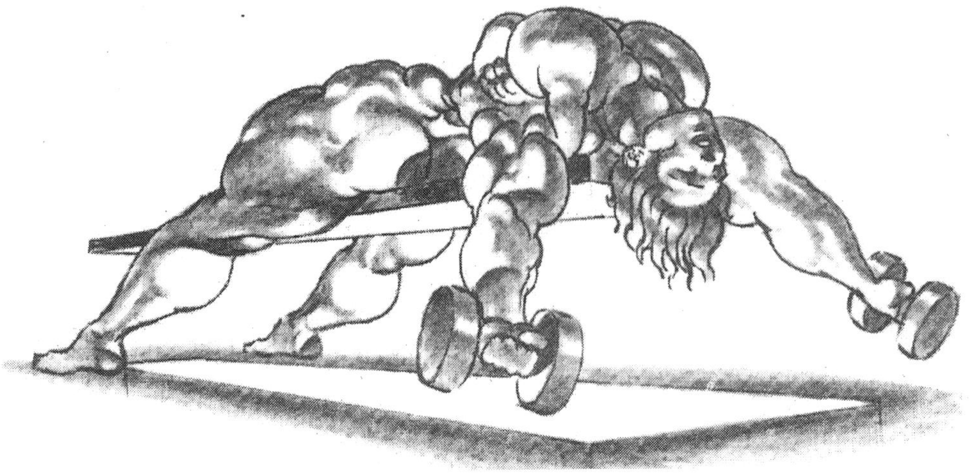

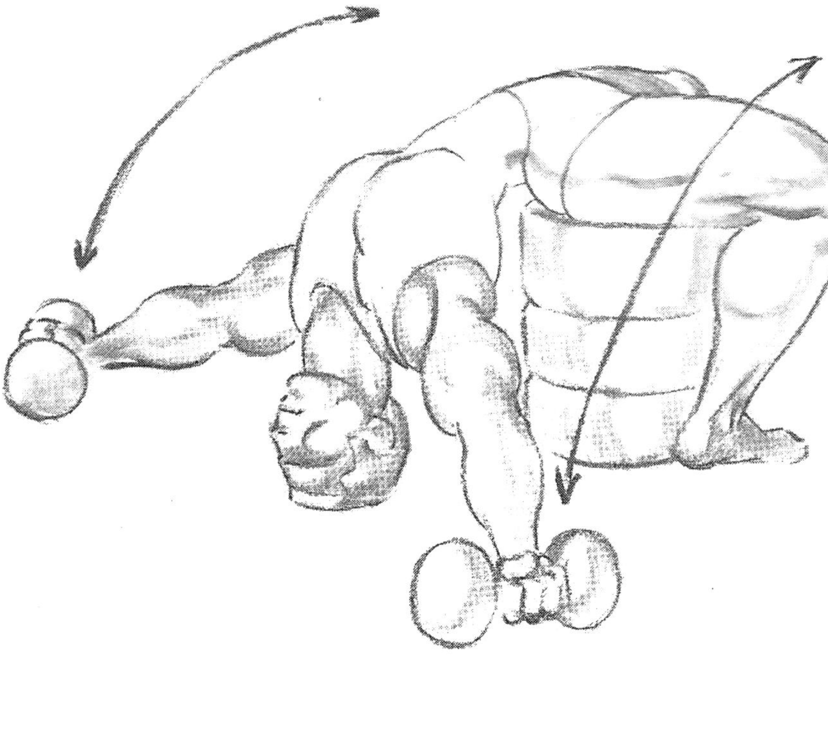

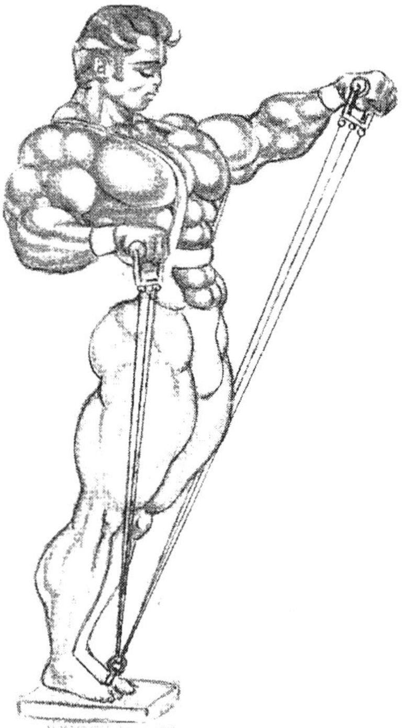

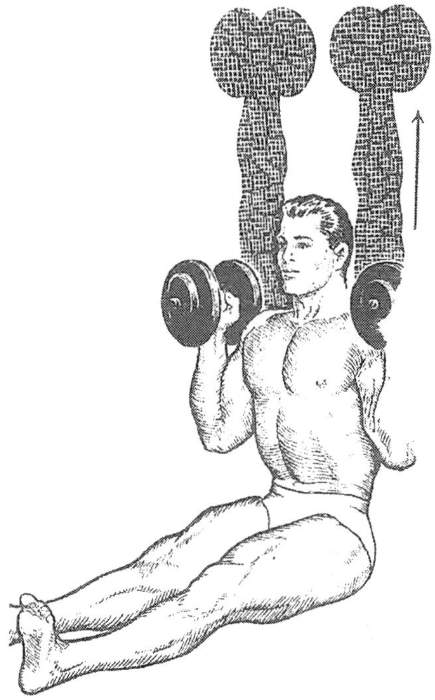

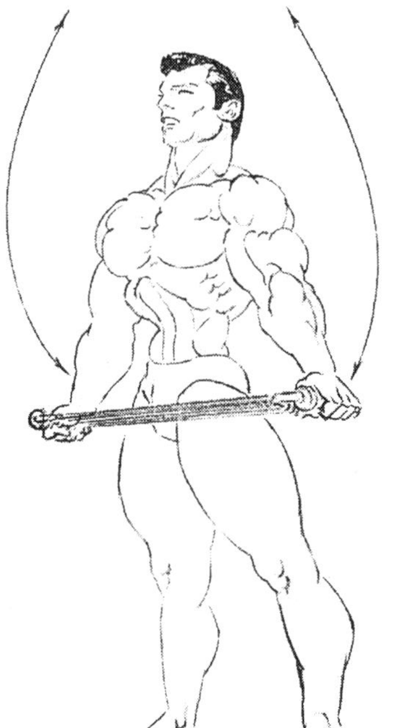

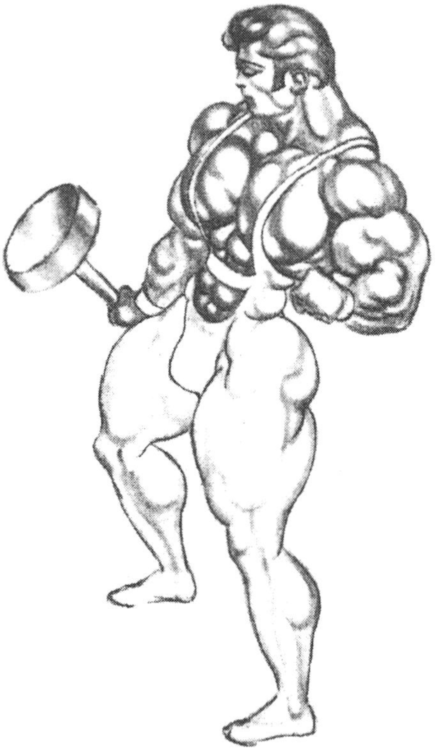

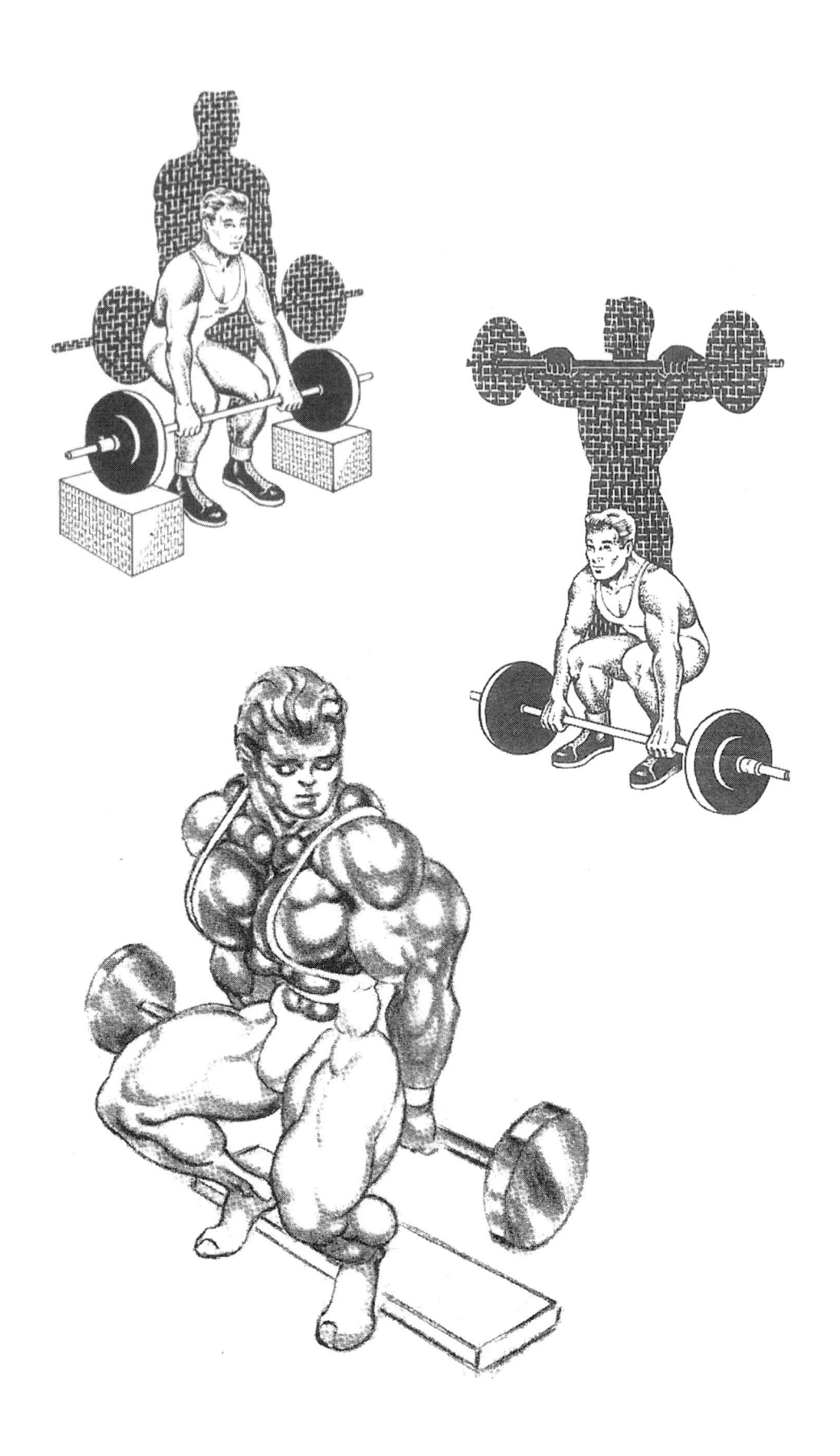

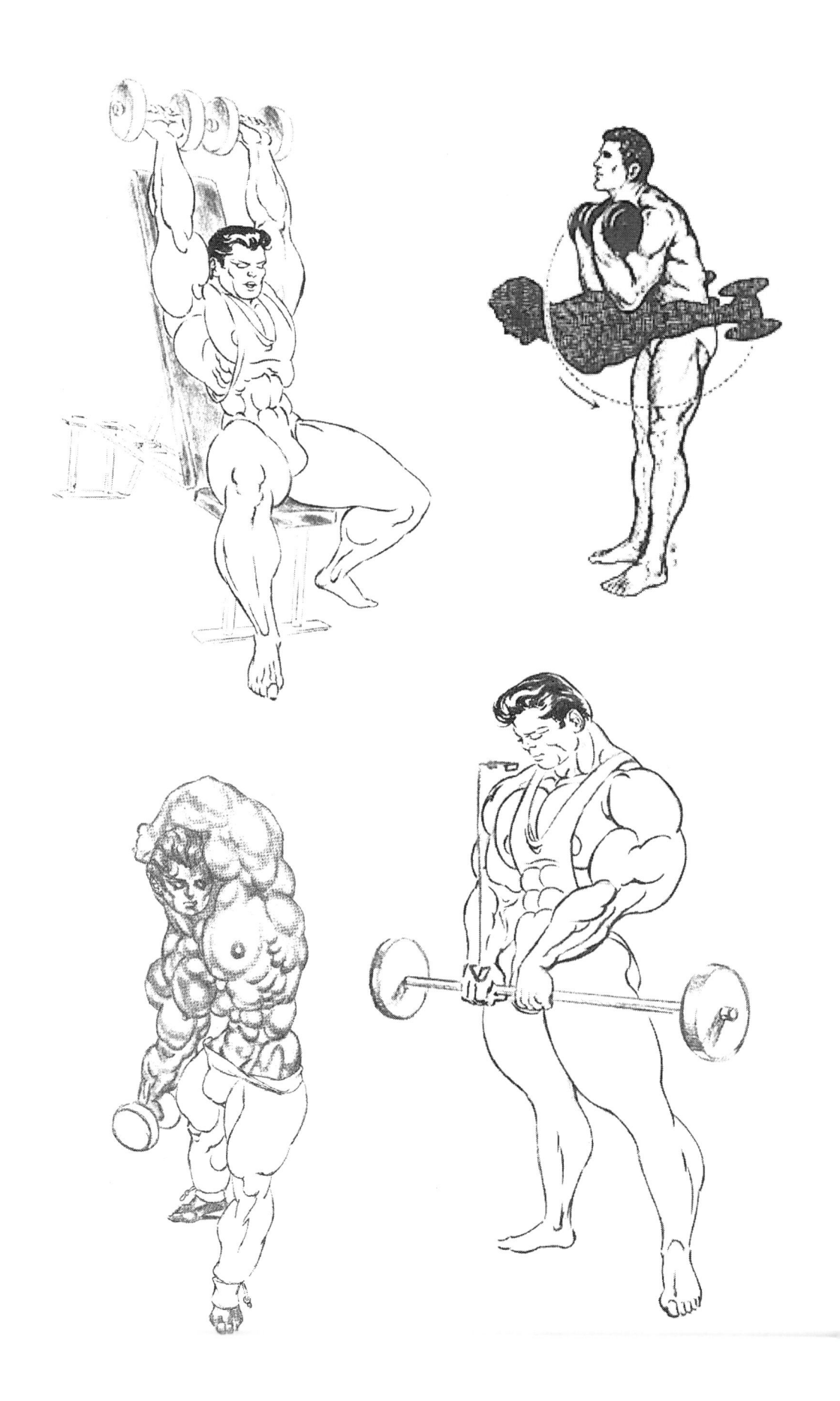

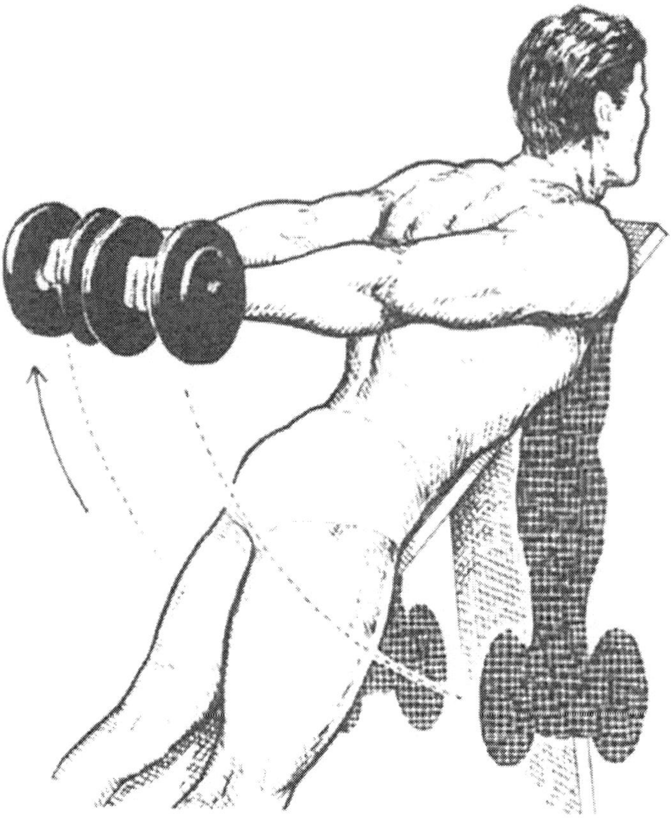

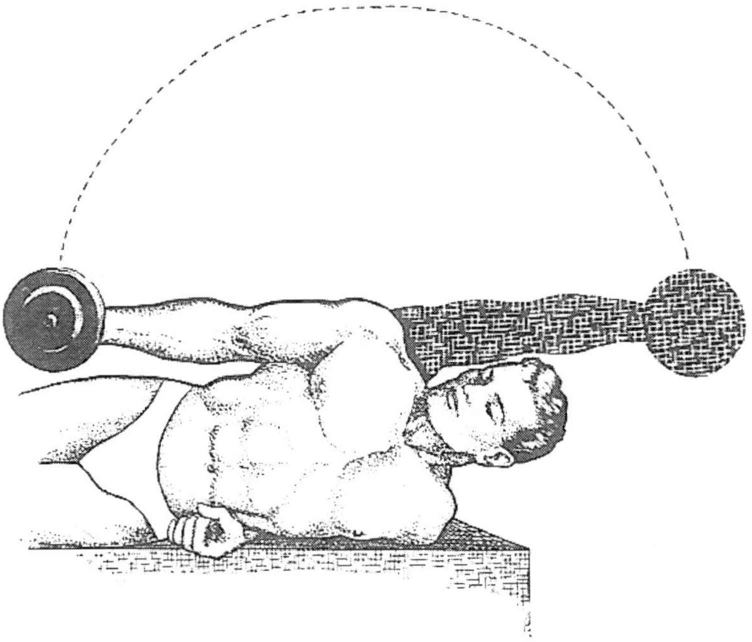

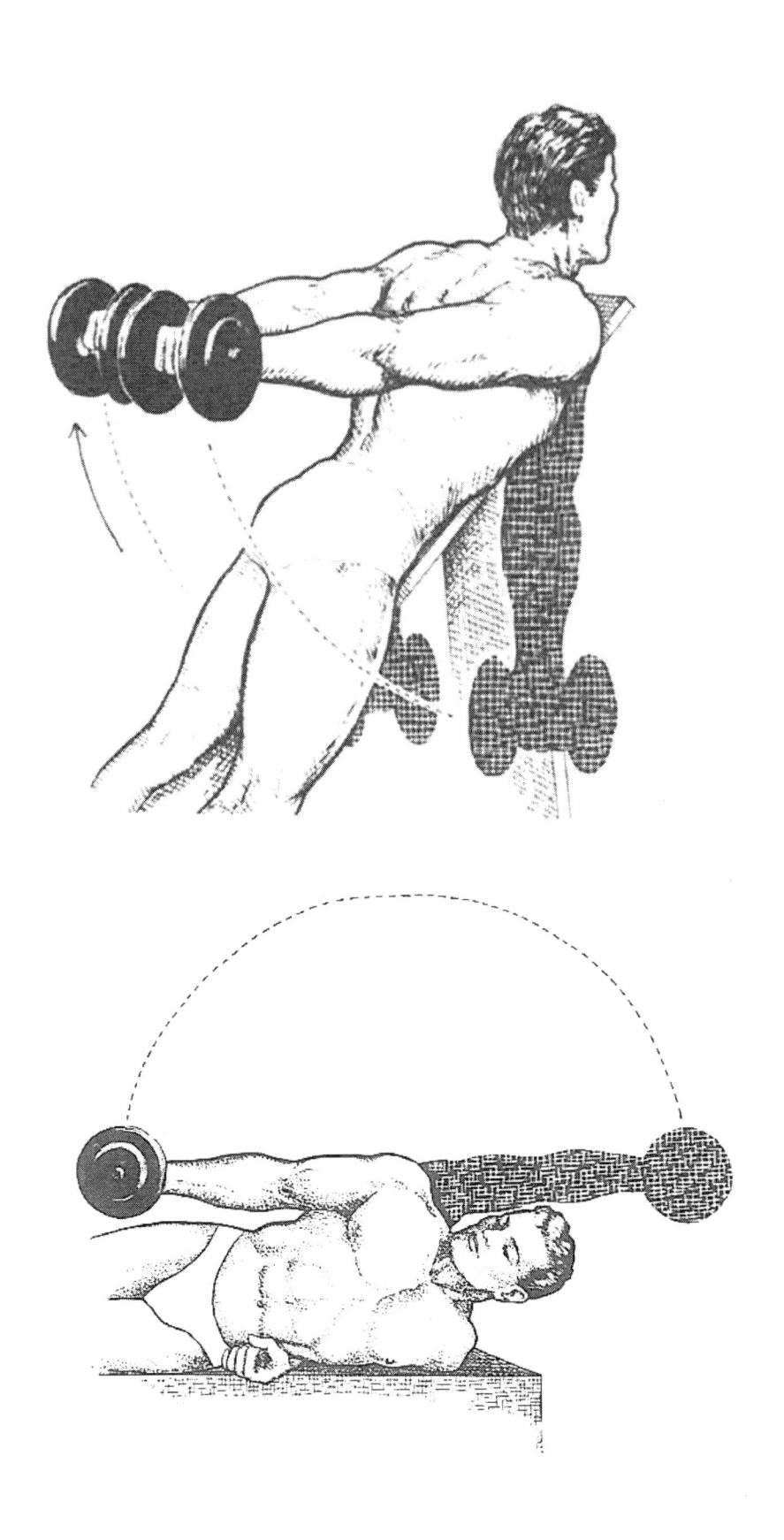

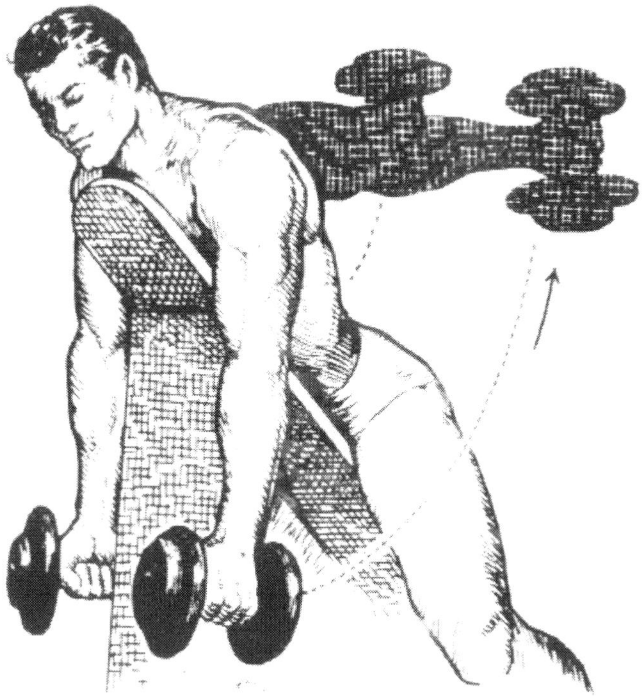

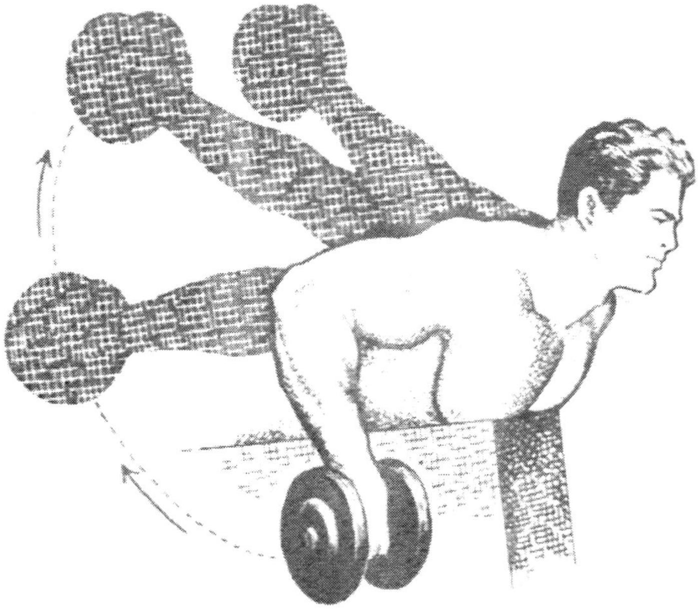

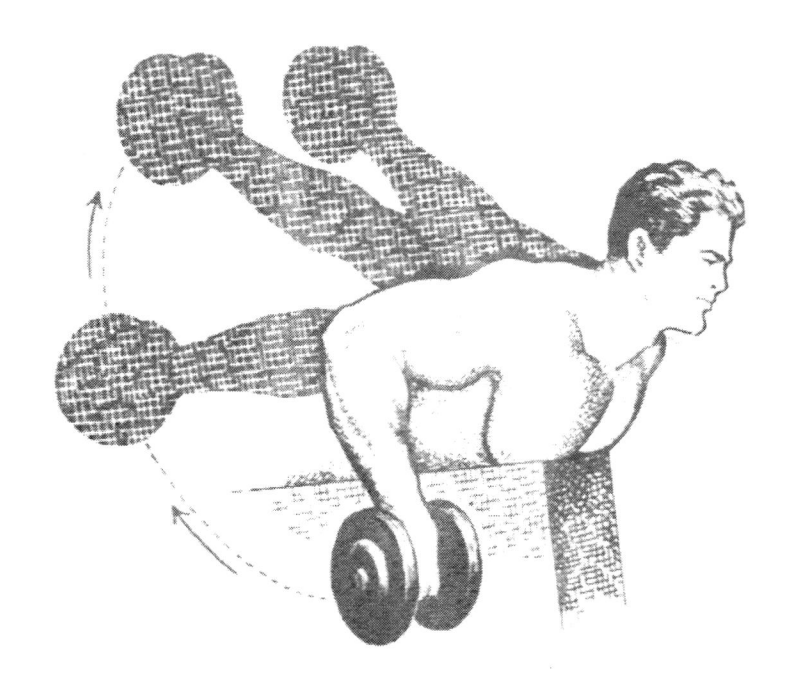

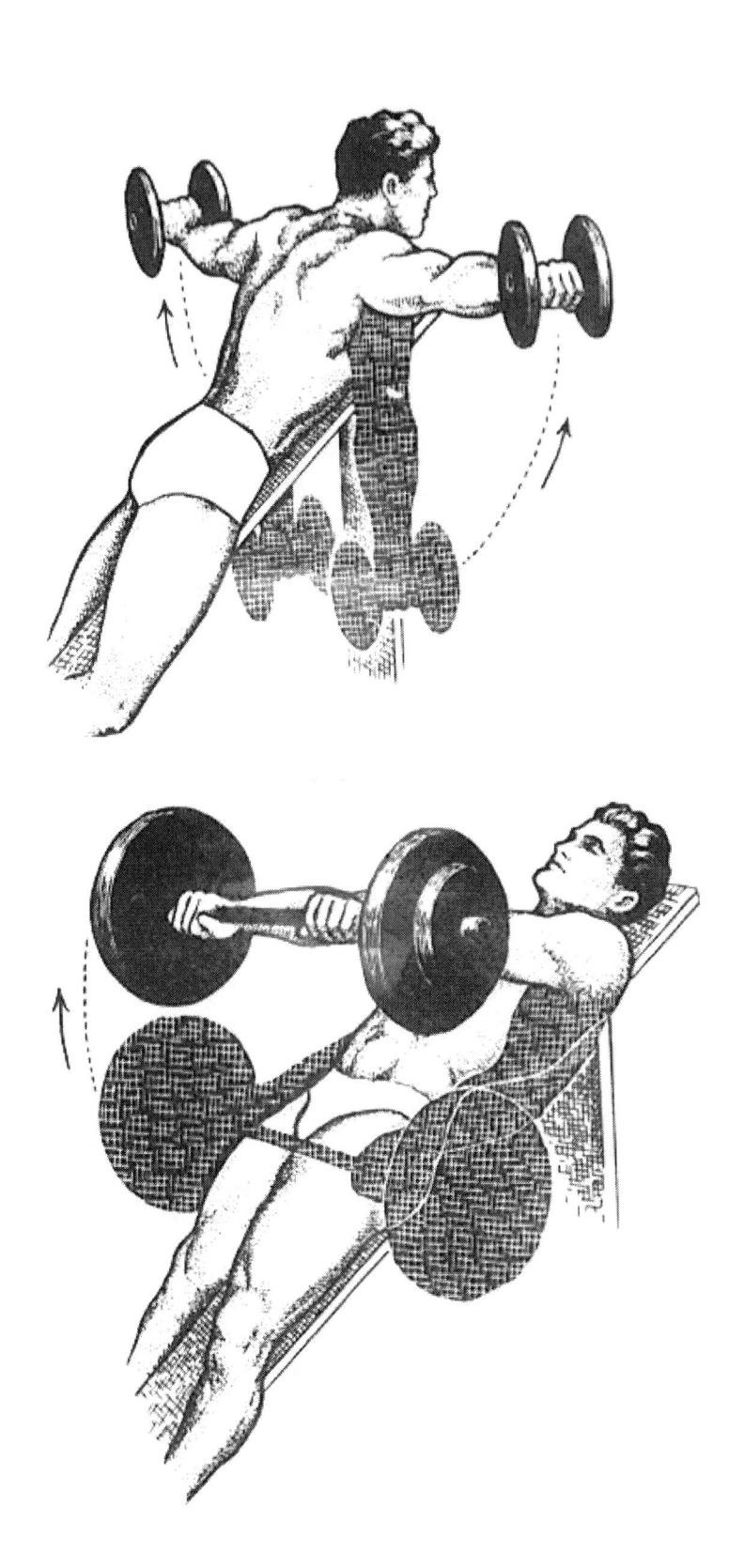

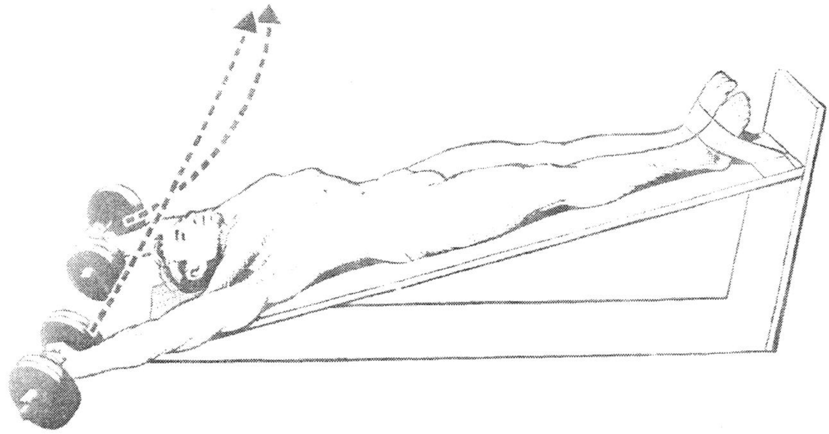

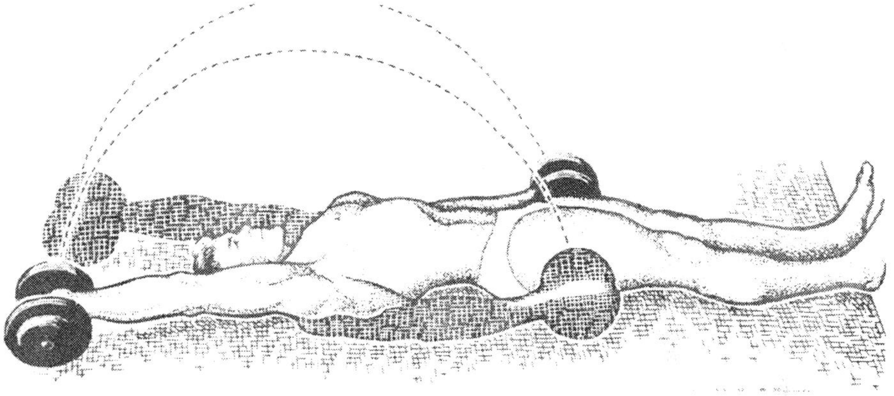

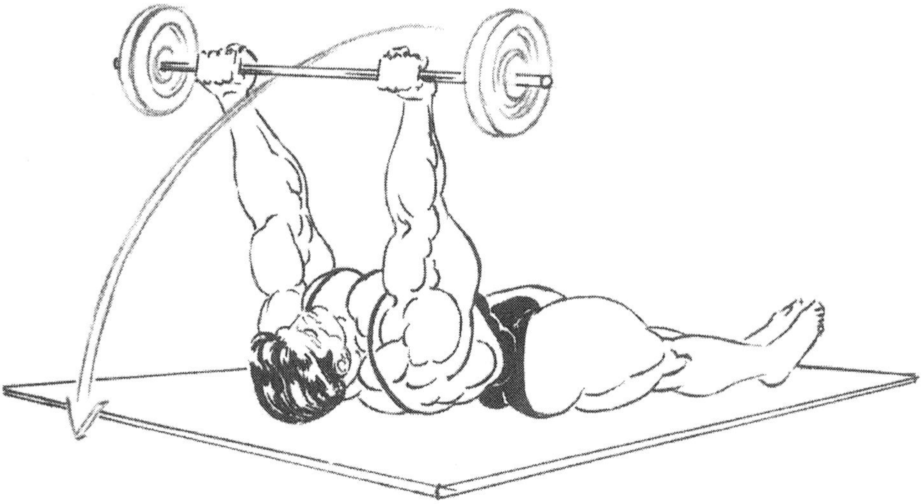

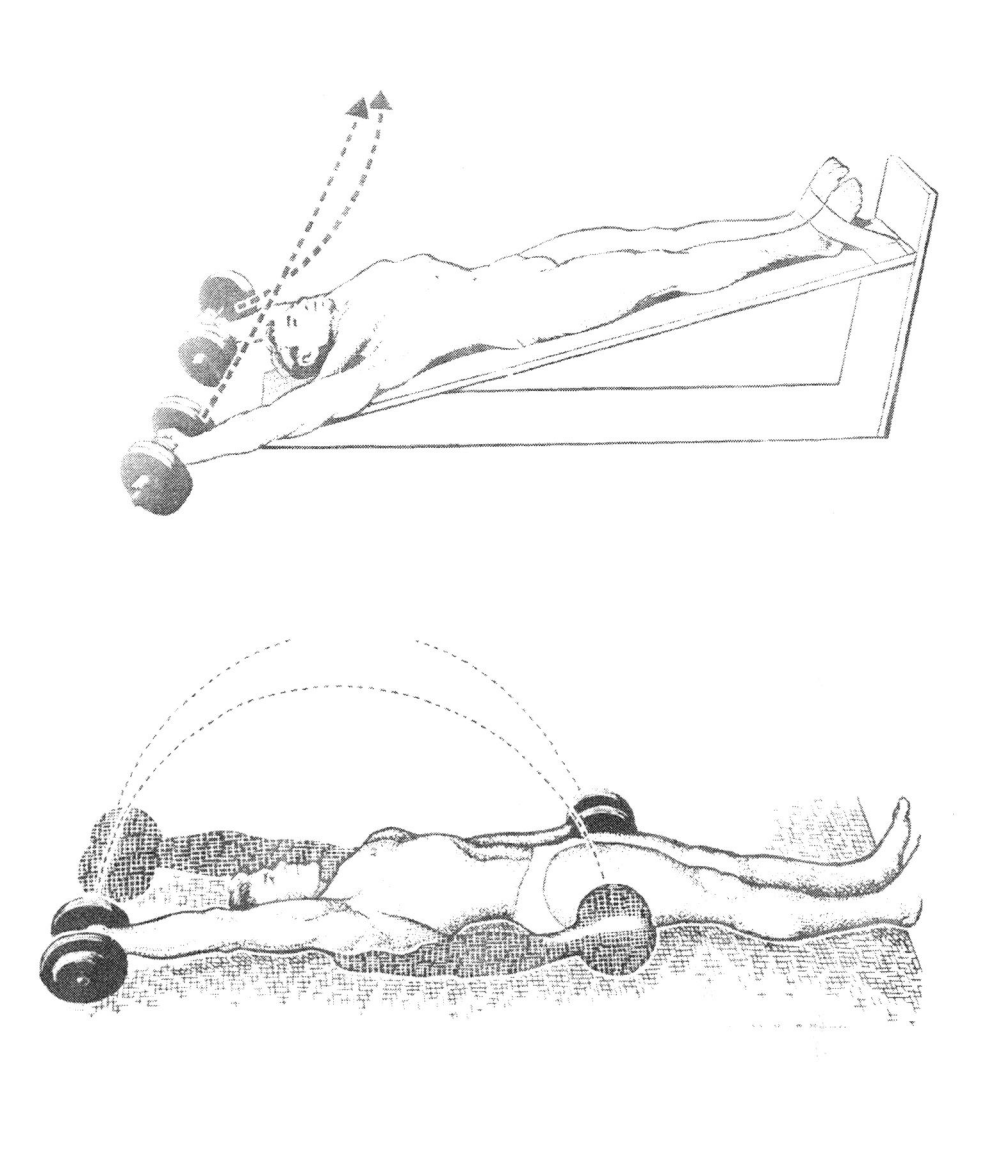

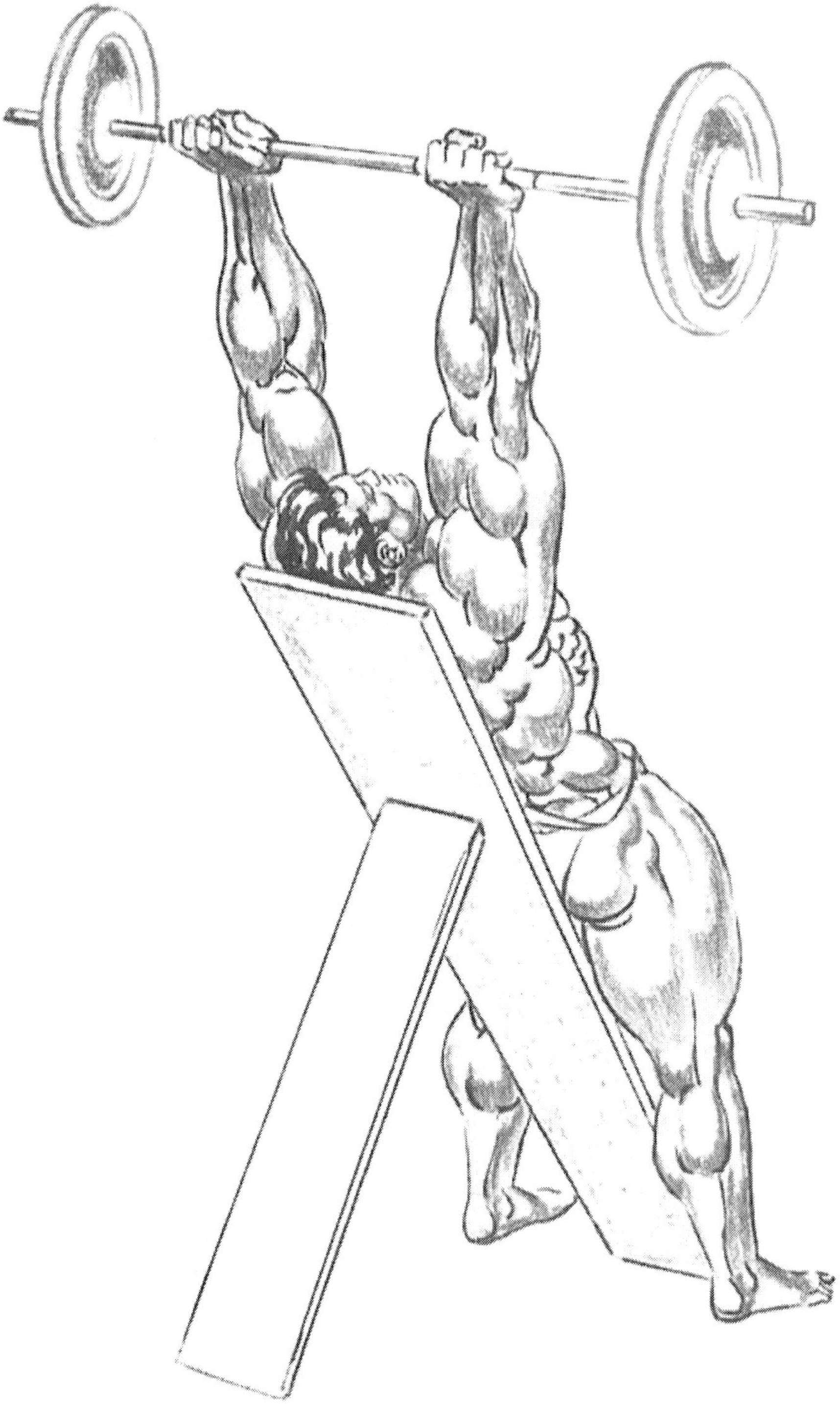

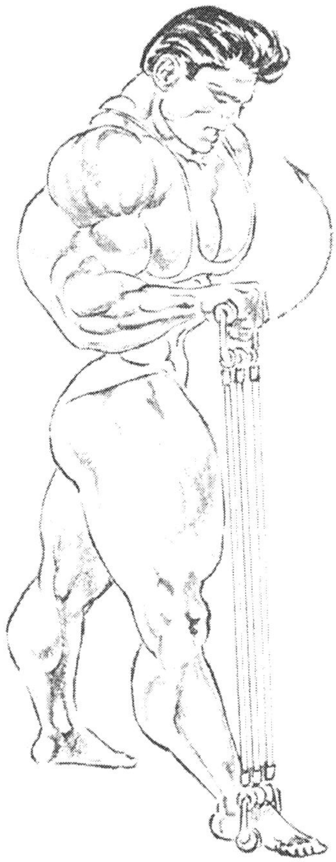

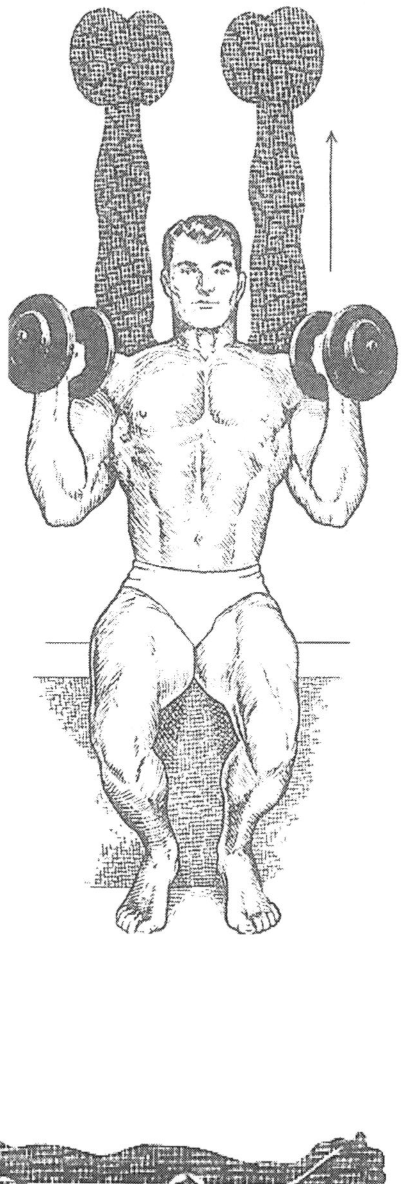

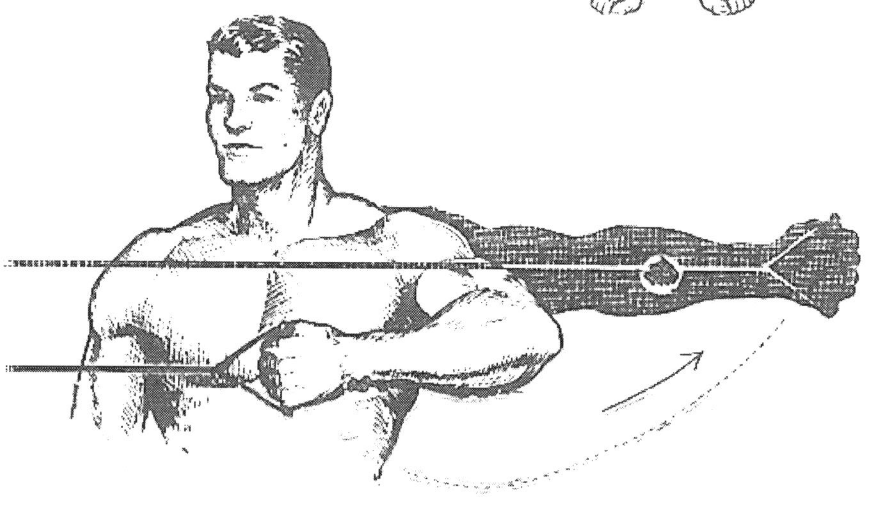

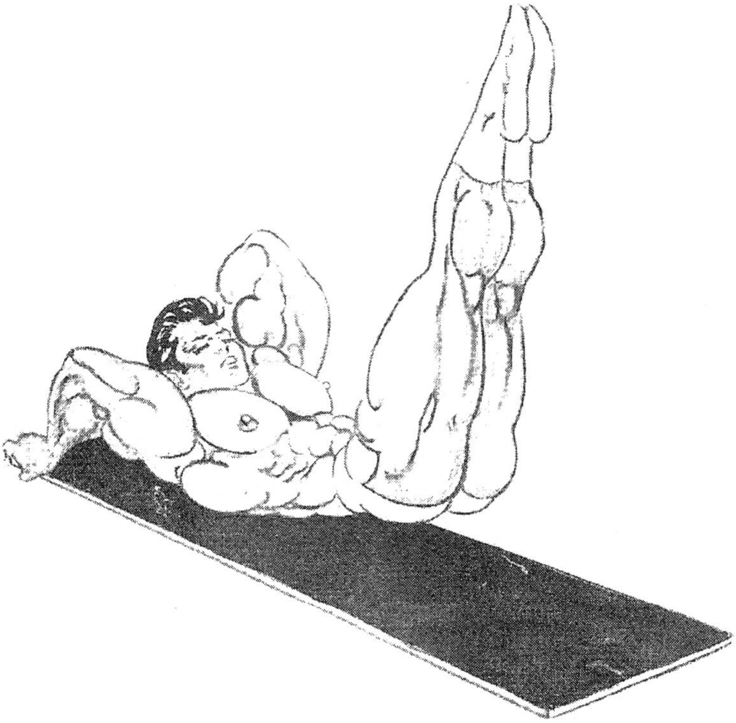

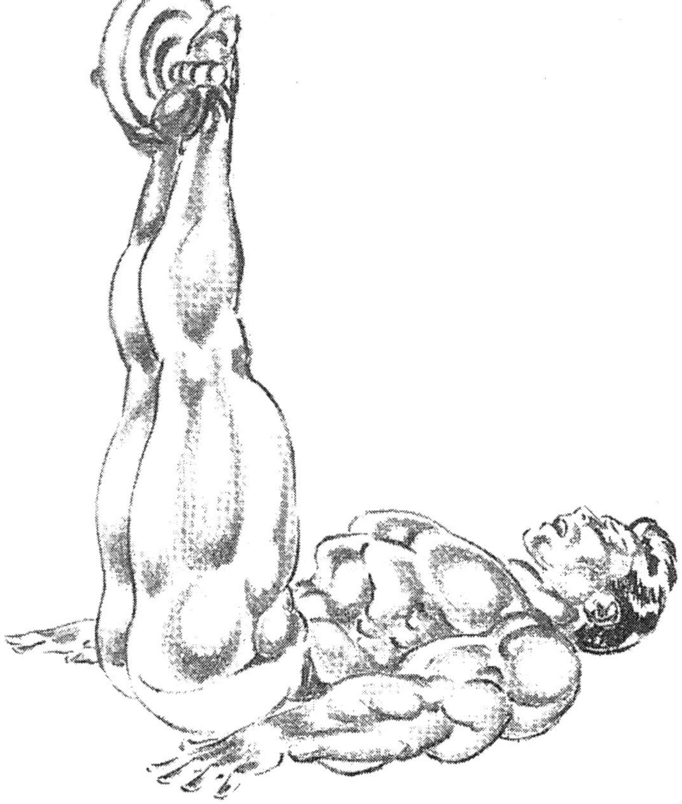

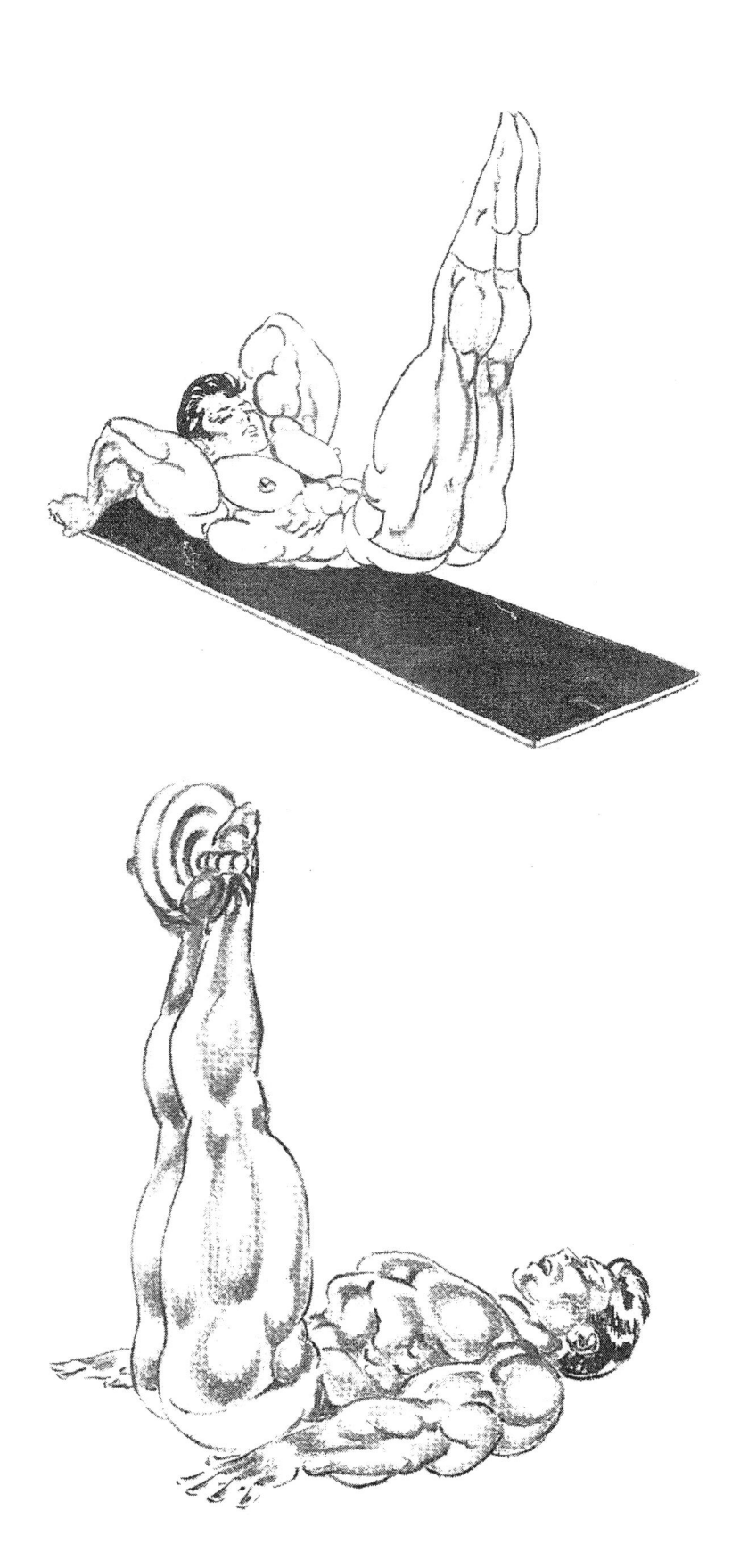

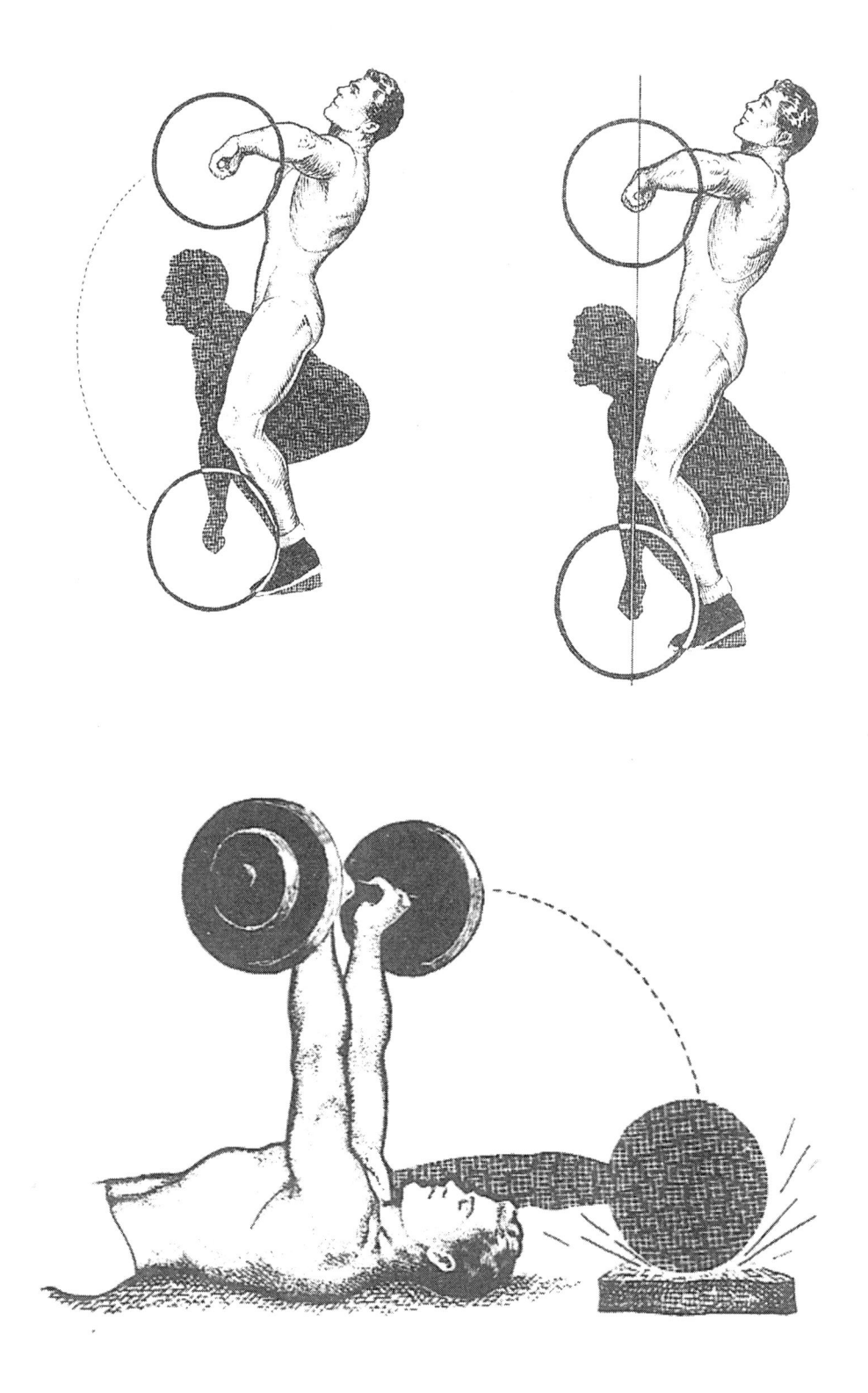

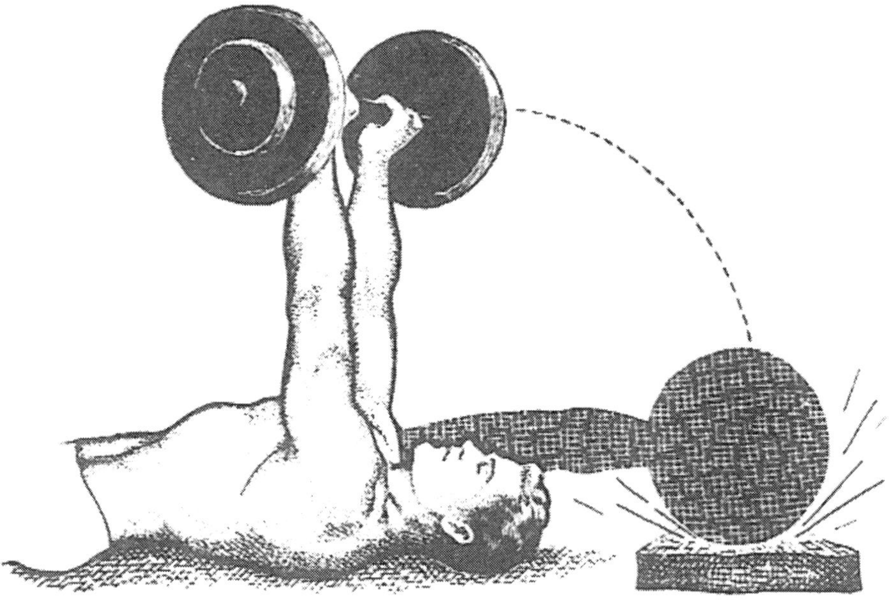

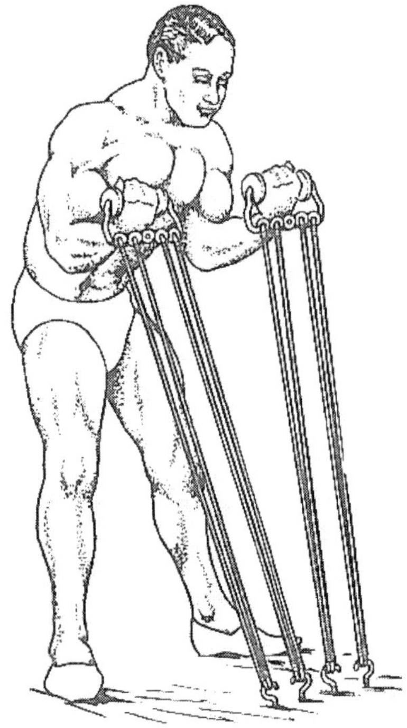

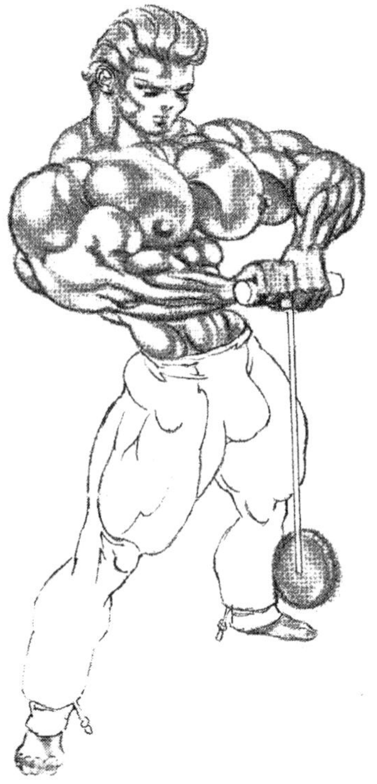

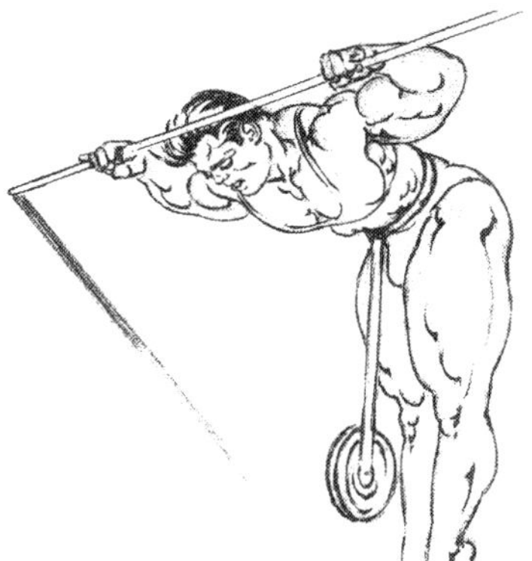

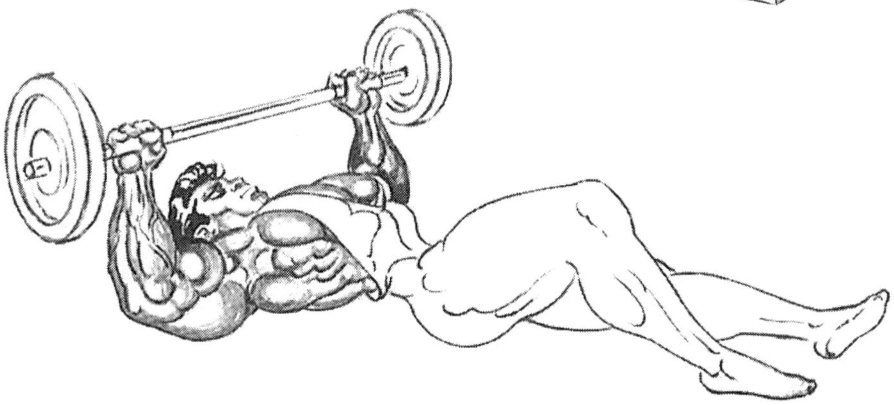

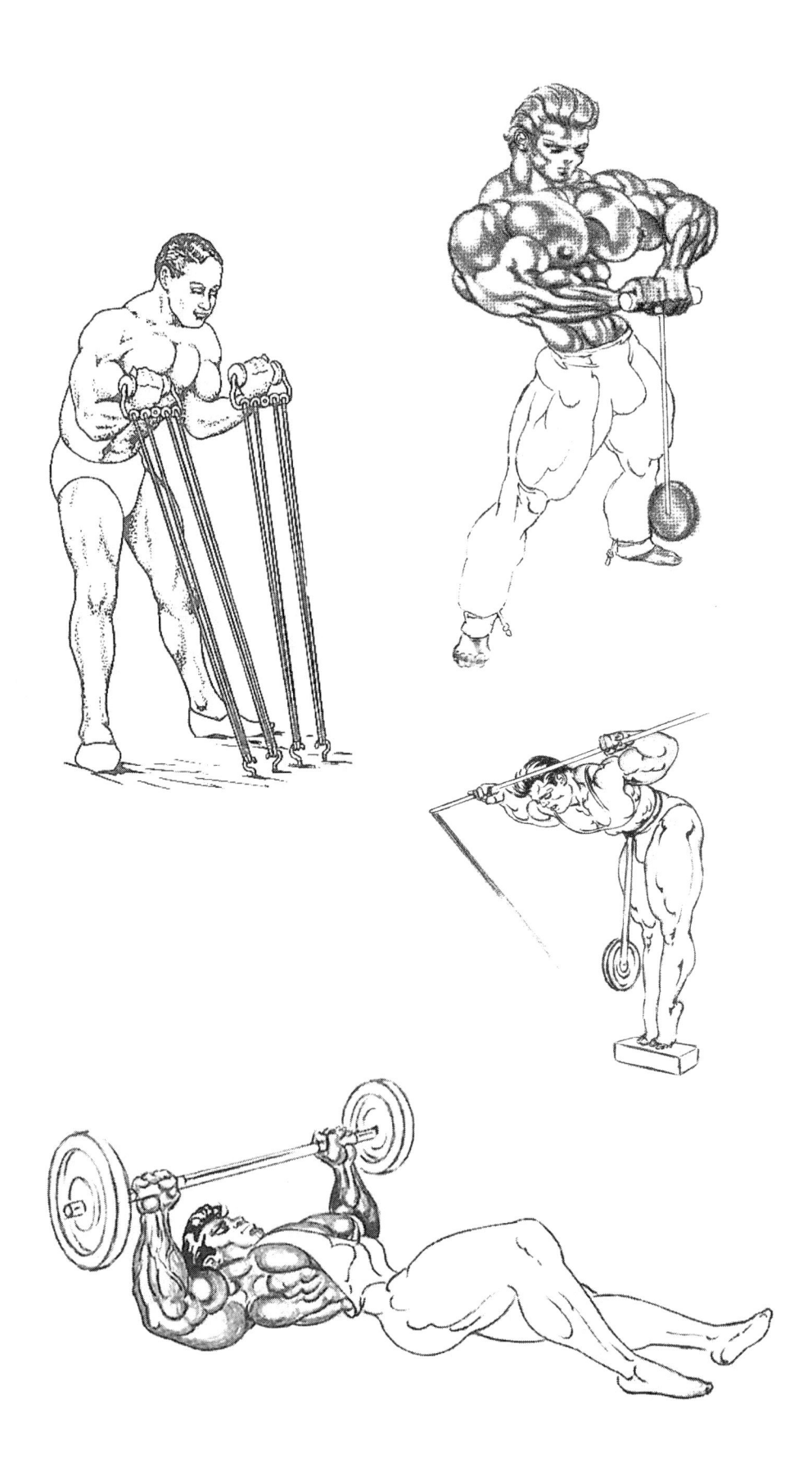

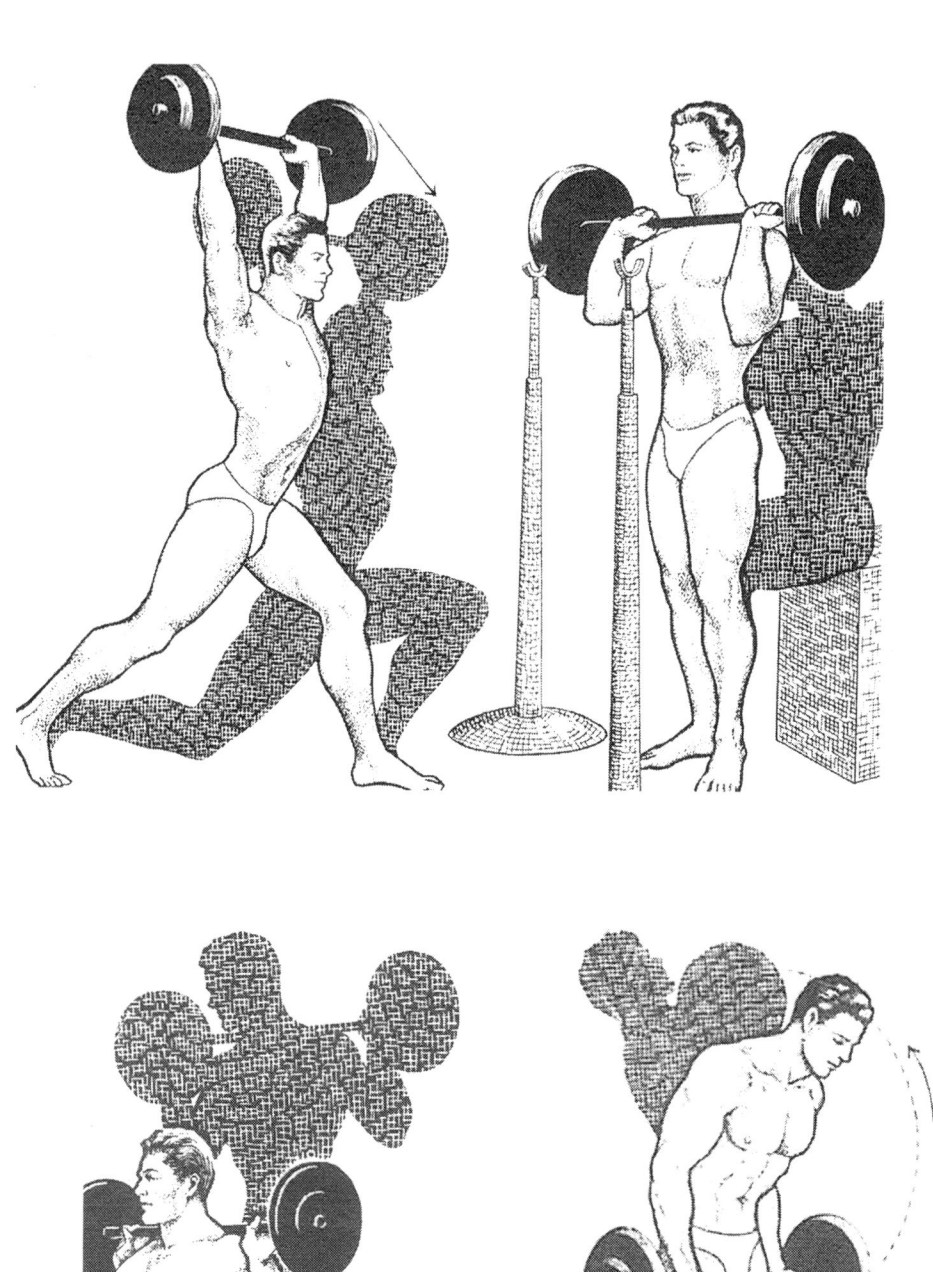

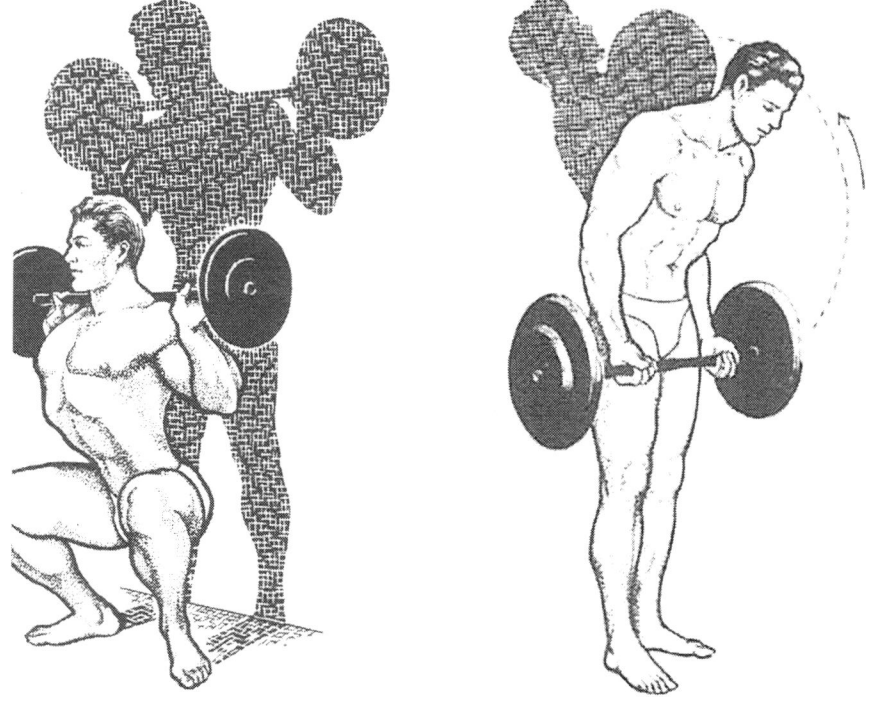

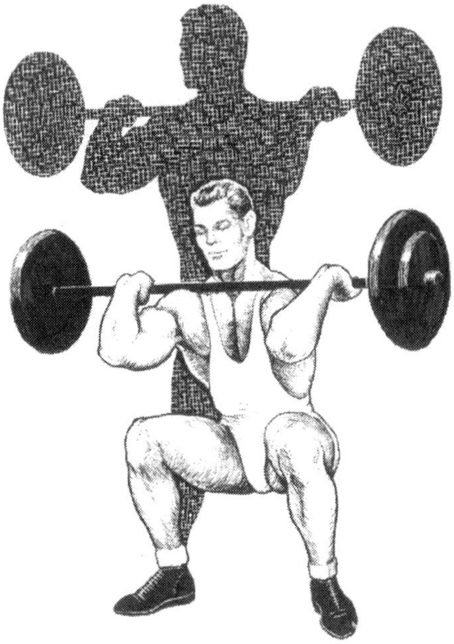

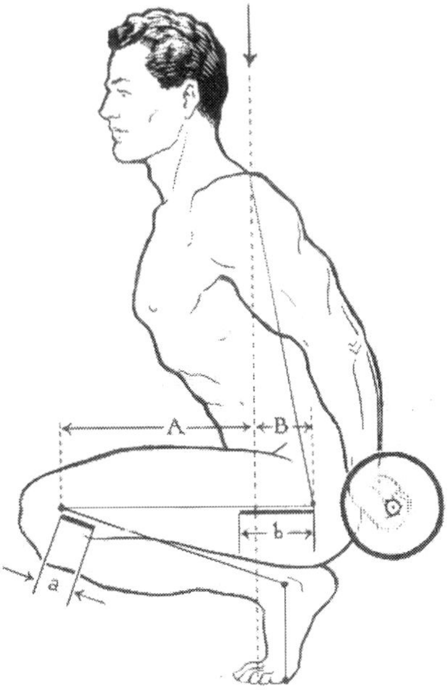
A
B
b
a

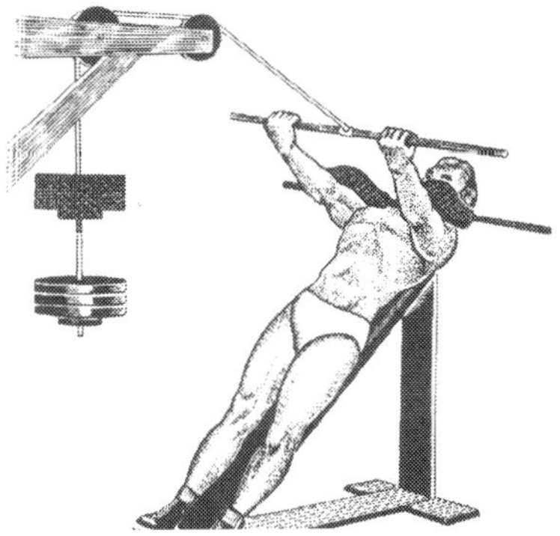

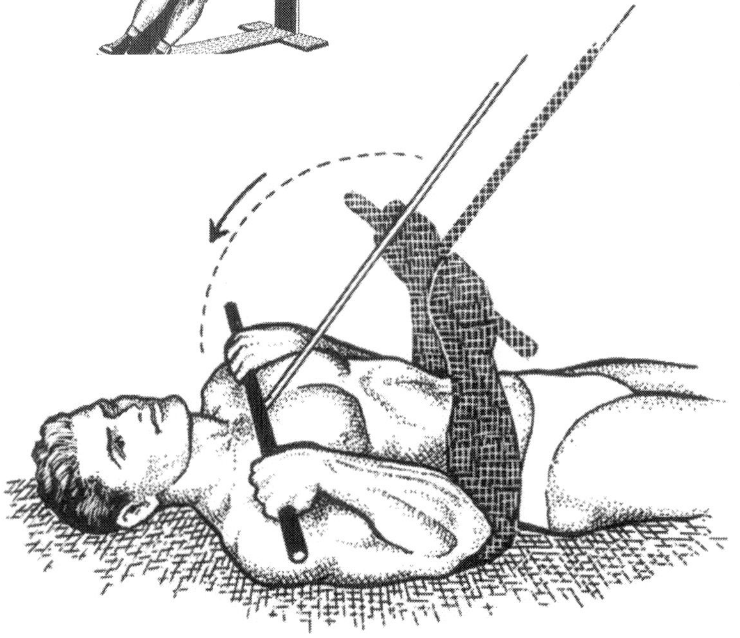

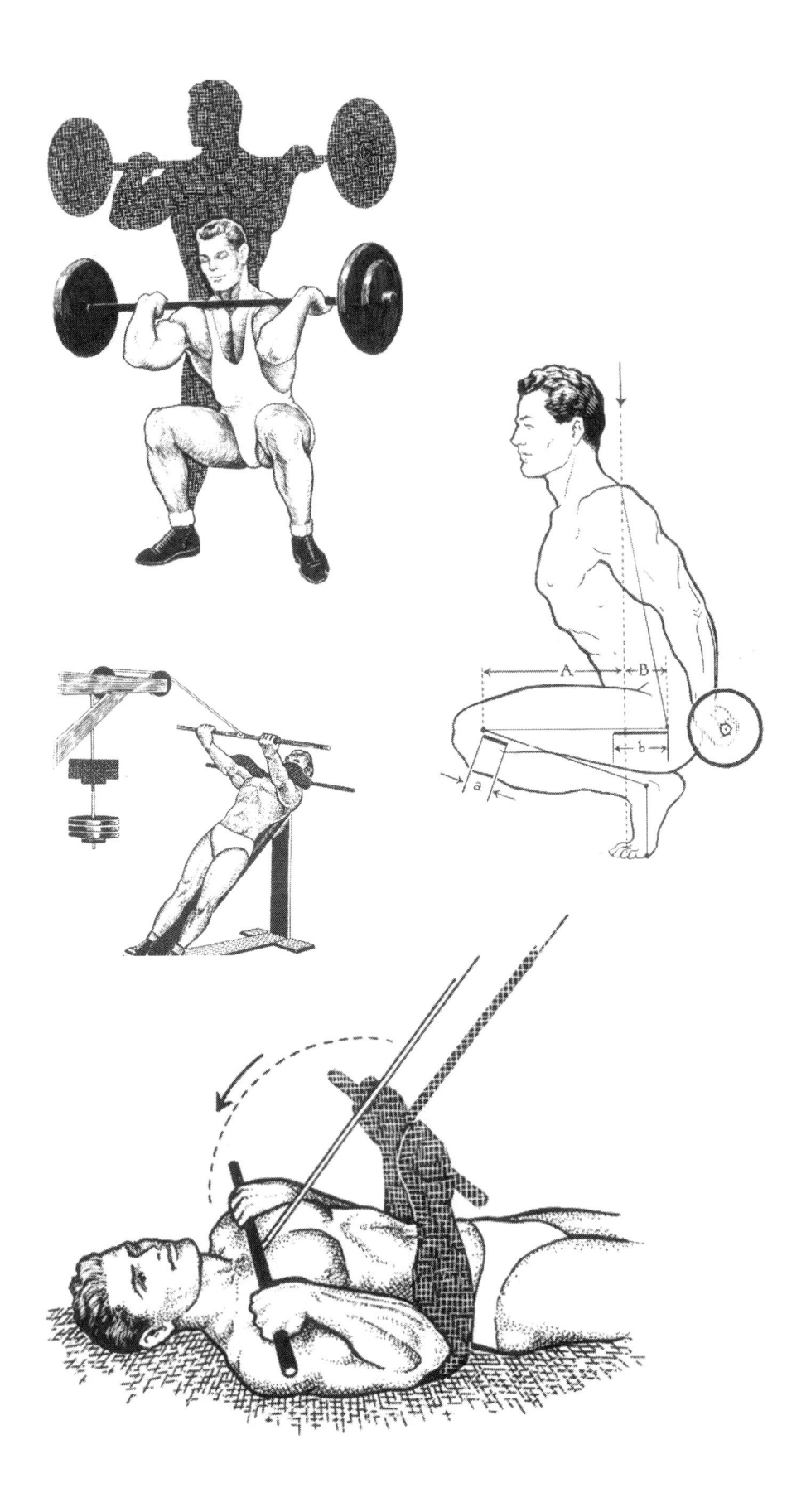

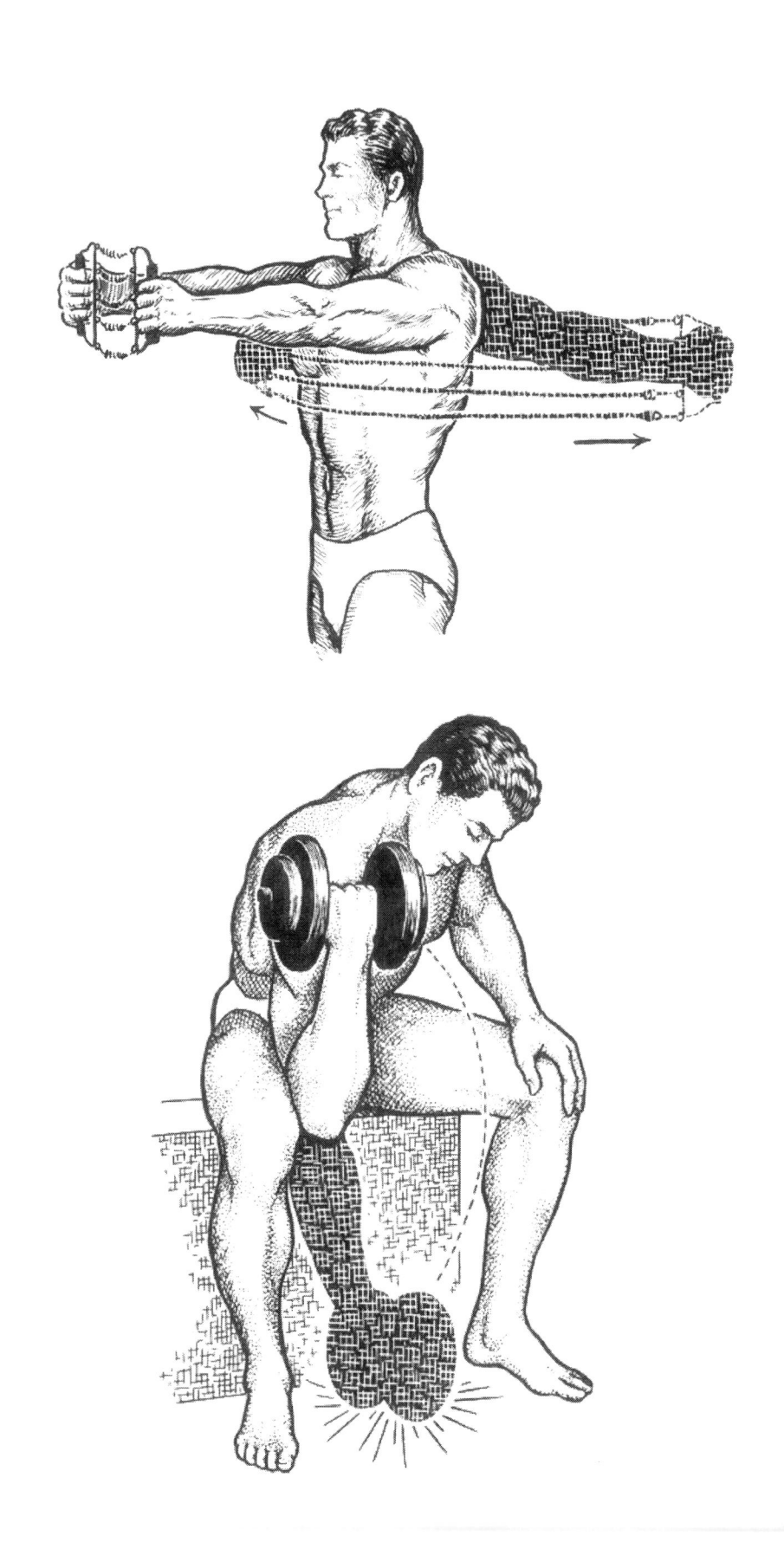

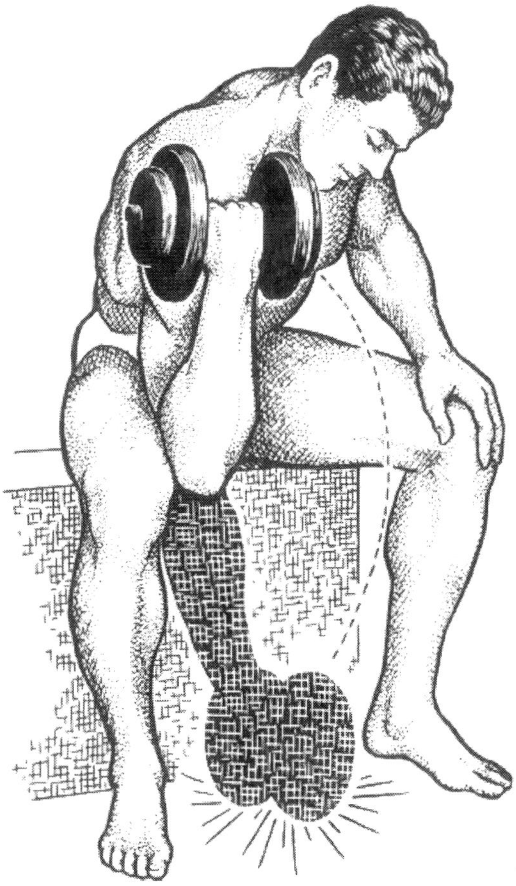

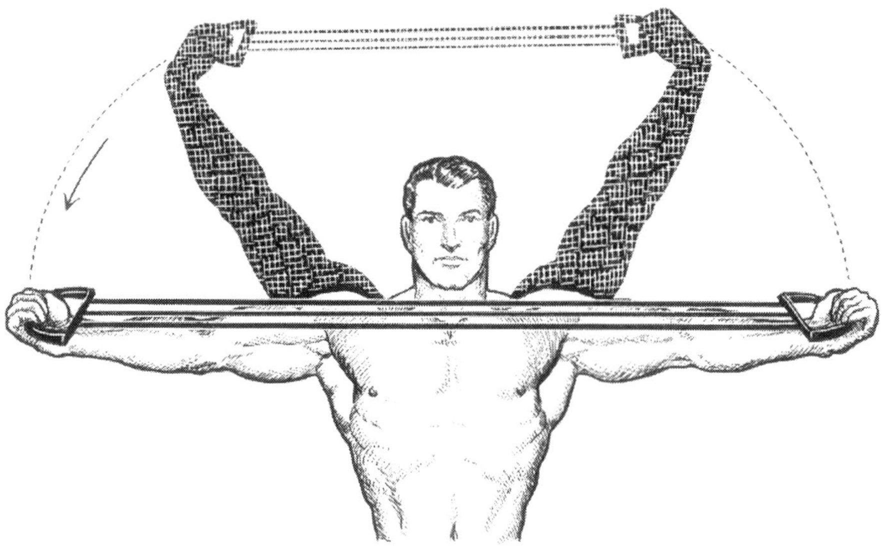

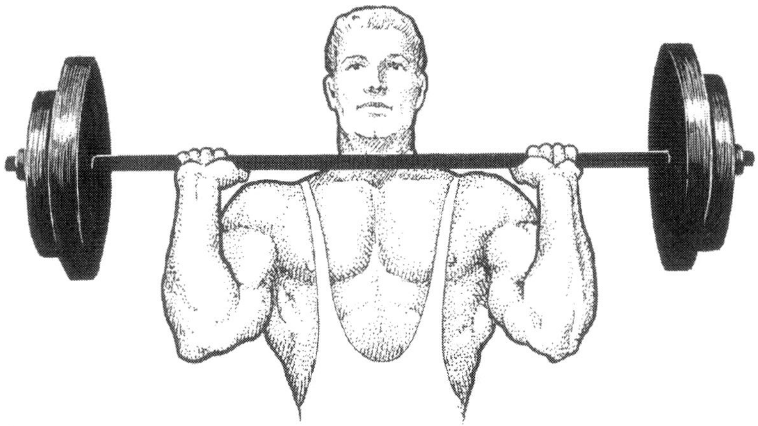

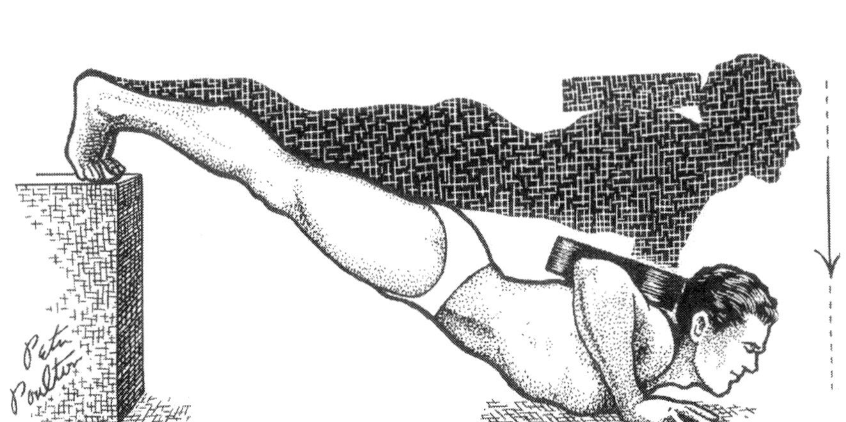
Peter Poulton

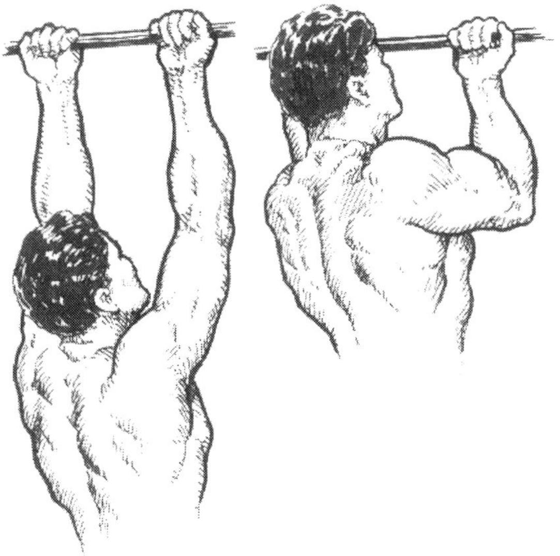

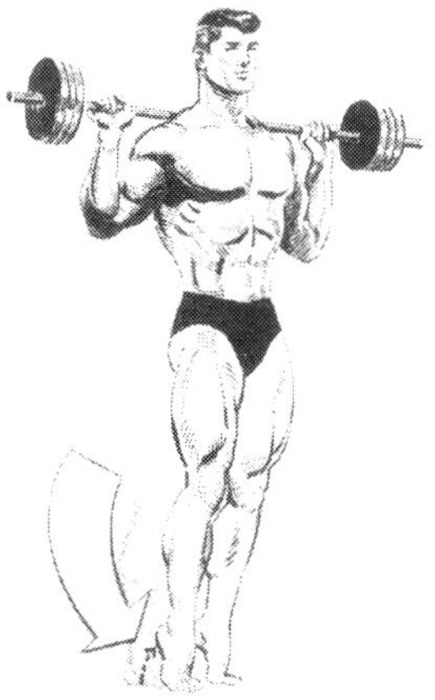

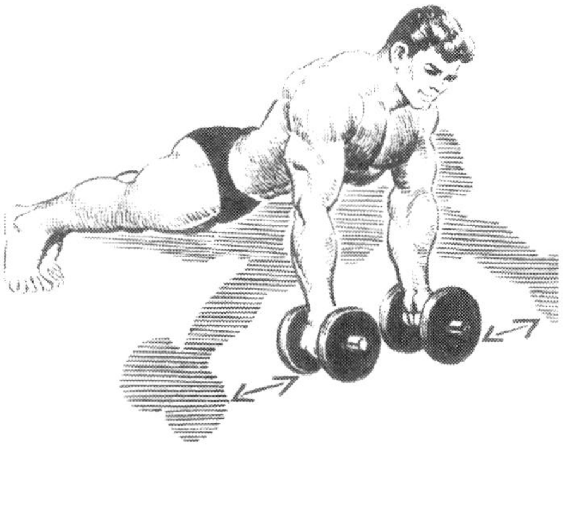

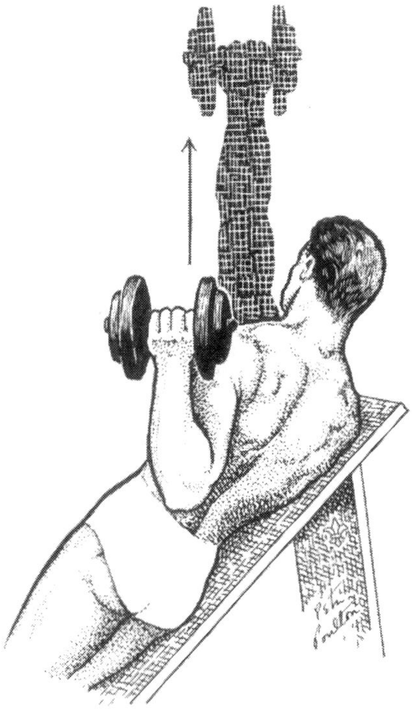

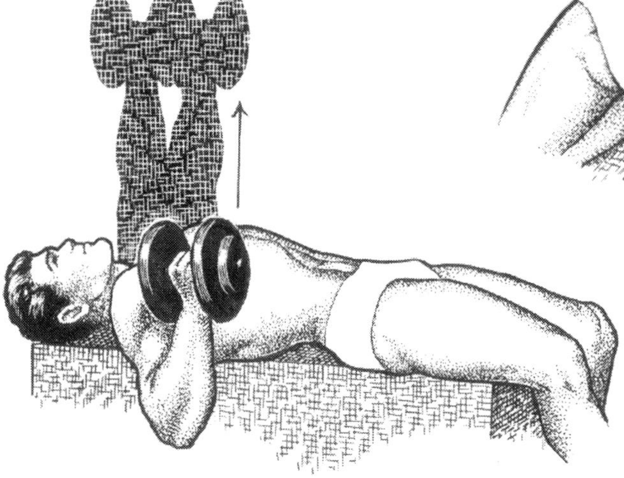

Printed in Great Britain
by Amazon